Molecular Toxicology

Molecular Toxicology

P. DAVID JOSEPHY
University of Guelph

with

BENGT MANNERVIK, University of Uppsala

and

PAUL ORTIZ DE MONTELLANO, University of California,
San Francisco

New York   Oxford
OXFORD UNIVERSITY PRESS
1997

Oxford University Press

Oxford   New York
Athens   Auckland   Bangkok
Bogota   Bombay   Buenos Aires   Calcutta
Cape Town   Dar es Salaam   Delhi
Florence   Hong Kong   Istanbul   Karachi
Kuala Lumpur   Madras   Madrid   Melbourne
Mexico City   Nairobi   Paris   Singapore
Taipei   Tokyo   Toronto
and associated companies in
Berlin   Ibadan

Library of Congress Cataloging-in-Publication Data
Josephy, P. David.
Molecular toxicology / P. David Josephy.
      p.   cm.   Includes bibliographical references and index.
ISBN 0-19-509340-2
1. Molecular toxicology.   I. Title.
RA1220.3.J67   1996   615.9—dc20   95-24812

9 8 7 6 5 4 3 2 1

Printed in the United States of America
on acid-free paper

To my mother and father

Contents

Preface

The modern science of toxicology brings together scientists from a wide range of disciplines, including chemistry, biochemistry, biology, and medicine. An introductory course in toxicology typically adopts a broad, interdisciplinary, and descriptive approach. The characterization of the responses of organisms to toxicants forms an essential component of the science of toxicology: We must characterize and measure toxic responses before we can begin to ask mechanistic questions. On the other hand, the measurement and quantitation of toxic effects are sometimes carried on with little attention to the biochemical processes underlying these effects.

In recent years, our understanding of toxicology at the molecular level has developed rapidly (1). Several advances in basic sciences have facilitated this maturation of molecular toxicology. The development of sophisticated techniques for chemical trace analysis allows toxicologists to detect and characterize metabolites present in tiny concentrations— in some cases, as little as one molecule per cell. Before the evolution of methods for the purification, sequencing, and structural characterization of proteins (especially membrane-bound proteins), biotransformation was a mysterious process leading from an administered drug or toxicant to a bewildering spectrum of metabolites; now, these reactions can be studied with mechanistic precision, and we can sometimes predict accurately the metabolic fate of a newly prepared compound. Once the mechanism of toxicity of a compound is understood, we may be able to "redesign" it—that is, propose a structure which will retain the desirable properties of the original compound while reducing or eliminating its toxicity (2). As we will see, many important biotransformation processes are catalyzed by families of closely related enzymes; often, many isozymes are present in a given cell or tissue. Therefore, mechanistic analysis has benefited greatly from the improvement of protein separation technology.

Even more dramatically, the flowering of molecular biology has opened new vistas in toxicology. Cloning of the genes coding for the enzymes of biotransformation has led to a deeper understanding of their evolutionary histories and biological roles. Expression of these genes in appropriate vectors allows precise analysis of their activities in metabolic activation or detoxication; site-directed mutagenesis provides a powerful tool for elucidation of chemical mechanisms of catalysis.

Since the mid-1980s I have offered a course in biochemical toxicology to a small class of senior students at the University of Guelph. This book is an outgrowth of that course, which has attracted students in toxicology, chemistry, biochemistry, and other disciplines, and is most suitable for students who have a similar academic background. These students have already taken an introductory course in general toxicology. Therefore, this text focuses on the biochemical fundamentals of toxicology. Throughout, I try to emphasize the close relationship of biochemical toxicology to the more familiar biochemistry and cell biology of intermediary metabolism and the mutually supportive interaction of biochemical and molecular biological approaches.

The principal focus of our attention is mammalian and, especially, human biochemistry. For obvious reasons the characterization of the enzymes of biotransformation emphasizes studies of humans and common laboratory animals (rat, mouse, rabbit, hamster). In a few cases which we discuss (e.g., arylamine N-acetyltransferase, cytochrome P-450_{cam}), bacterial systems have been important for the analysis of the structure and function of enzymes of toxicological importance. Plants also produce such enzymes as cytochrome P-450 and glutathione transferase (3). However, the study of the comparative distribution and function of xenobiotic metabolizing enzymes throughout the biological kingdom is still in its infancy.

A theme throughout this text is the connection between the biochemistry of metabolism of environmental toxicants and drugs (traditionally viewed as the province of toxicologists and pharmacologists) and the metabolism of endogenous compounds (the domain of biochemists). The major enzymes of drug biotransformation all act on endogenous as well as exogenous compounds: Cytochrome P-450 is the catalyst of steroid transformations as well as polycyclic aromatic hydrocarbon activation; glucuronidation eliminates both bilirubin and chloramphenicol; sulfotransferases act on bile acids as well as minoxidil; and so on. The distinction between endogenous compounds and xenobiotics, although heuristically valuable, is biochemically arbitrary: To an enzyme, molecules are just molecules, regardless of their origins. If this were not the case, humans could never have evolved the capacity to oxidize, conjugate, and detoxify compounds never before encountered, such as synthetic drugs, solvents, and pesticides.

Guelph, Ontario   P. D. J.
January 1996

NOTES

1. Marshall, E., Toxicology goes molecular, *Science* 259:1394–1398, 1993.
2. Flam, F., EPA campaigns for safer chemicals, *Science* 265:1519, 1994.
3. Sandermann, H., Jr., Plant metabolism of xenobiotics, *Trends Biochem. Sci.* 17:82–84, 1992.

Acknowledgments

Six chapters of this book were written by contributors, and then revised and edited by P.D.J.: Manfred Brauer and Philippe Couture, Department of Chemistry and Biochemistry, University of Guelph (lipid peroxidation); Denis M. Grant, Department of Clinical Pharmacology and Toxicology, Hospital for Sick Children, Toronto (N-acetyltransferase); Patricia Harper, Department of Clinical Pharmacology and Toxicology, Hospital for Sick Children, Toronto (Ah receptor); Jean Jordan, Department of Biochemistry, University of Ottawa (oncogenes and tumor suppressor genes); Bengt Mannervik, Department of Biochemistry, Uppsala University, Sweden (glutathione and detoxication); Paul Ortiz de Montellano, University of California, San Francisco (cytochrome P-450).

The following people contributed material for sections of chapters: John Barta, Department of Pathology, University of Guelph (malaria and antimalarial drugs); John Lowe, Department of Chemistry, Pennsylvania State University (molecular orbital theory of polycyclic aromatic hydrocarbons); John Phillips and Arthur Hilliker, Department of Molecular Biology and Genetics, University of Guelph (*sod* mutants in *Drosophila*); Greg Reed, Department of Pharmacology, Toxicology, and Therapeutics, University of Kansas, and Monique Cosman, Lawrence Livermore National Laboratory (PAH-DNA adducts); and Herb Schellhorn, Department of Biology, McMaster University (bacterial catalases).

I also wish to thank Robert Keates, Department of Chemistry and Biochemistry, University of Guelph, for many helpful suggestions; Steven Kruth, Ontario Veterinary College, for discussion of glucuronidation in felines; my former students Ruth Wallace and Panadda Kosakarn, for permission to use excerpts from their theses; and my mother, for reminding me of the passage from *Oliver Twist* quoted in Chapter 19.

Several people reviewed sections of the draft manuscript: Bruce Demple, School of Public Health, Harvard University; David Evans, Department of Molecular Biology and Genetics, University of Guelph; Richard Weinshilboum, Department of Pharmacology, Mayo Graduate School of Medicine; Robert Hanzlik, Department of Medicinal Chemistry, University of Kansas; Kirsten Skov, B.C. Cancer Research Centre; Paul Howard, National Center for Toxicological Research. I thank the members of my research group, who have tolerated my obsession with the manuscript and who carried on working very independently during my repeated "absences in spirit."

I did the final proofreading of the text in April 1996, while I was guest in the laboratory of Dr. Takehiko Nohmi, National Institute of Health Sciences, Tokyo, Japan. I wish to thank Dr. Nohmi and the Japan Research and Development Corporation for making this visit possible.

Responsibility for any errors and omissions lies with me, and I would appreciate receiving comments, suggestions, and corrections from readers. My Internet address is JOSEPHY@CHEMBIO.UOGUELPH.CA.

Finally, I wish to thank Ingrid Krohn for her advice and encouragement during the initial planning of this book, and I also wish to thank my editors, Kirk Jensen and Bob Rogers.

1

BIOCHEMICAL BACKGROUND

PREPARATION OF SUBCELLULAR FRACTIONS

As early as the mid-nineteenth century, biotransformation products had been isolated from the urine of animals or persons treated with foreign compounds. For example, as we will discuss later, urinary excretion of aryl sulfate esters was observed in the 1870s. One of the most important early experiments on the biotransformation of foreign compounds was the work of Knoop on the metabolism of fatty acids. His observation (1904) that ω-phenyl fatty acids were excreted as conjugates (glycine amides) of either benzoic acid (odd-chain) or phenylacetic acid (even-chain) provided the first evidence for the β-oxidation pathway of fatty acid metabolism.

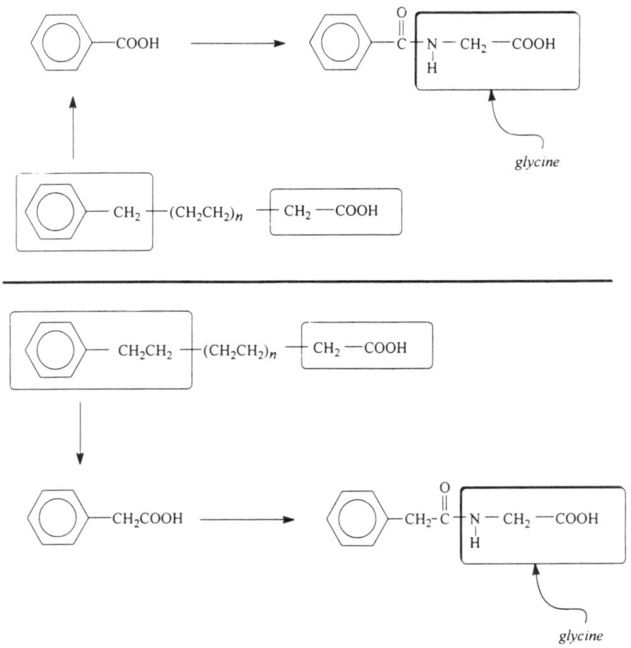

This chemical-labeling strategy foreshadowed the development of radioactive labeling in the post–World War II era, which would prove to be decisive for the sorting out of the pathways of intermediary metabolism. Knoop's experiments also demonstrated that lipophilic foreign compounds—in this case, benzoic acid and phenylacetic acid—are excreted by conjugation to polar endogenous compounds such as glycine. This approach to

1

studying the metabolism of foreign compounds is *pharmacological*: A compound is administered to an animal (dogs, in Knoop's experiments) and metabolites are isolated from the urine or feces. We can make only limited inferences about the mechanisms of biotransformation from a whole-animal study.

The hallmark of the *biochemical* approach to investigating metabolism is an emphasis on the purification of the enzymes which catalyze the individual reactions of biotransformation. A great deal of effort in the development of molecular toxicology has been devoted to the identification and characterization of these enzymes. As we will see, this approach has led, in recent years, to the successful cloning of the genes encoding most of the important enzymes. Before individual proteins can be purified, the researcher will first prepare the appropriate subcellular fraction in which the desired enzyme is found. This step eliminates or reduces contamination by enzymes localized in other compartments. The most important fractions we will consider are nuclei, mitochondria, "microsomes," and cytosol. For a complete introduction to the structure and function of subcellular components, the student should consult a text such as *Molecular Cell Biology* (Darnell, Lodish, and Baltimore, Chapter 4). The monograph *Biochemical Toxicology: A Practical Approach* (K. Snell and B. Mullock, eds., IRL Press, 1987) is a useful reference for detailed protocols.

Homogenization

The first step is homogenization of the tissue. The technique applied depends on the physical characteristics of the tissue sample; mechanical disruption with a motor-driven Teflon pestle is commonly used for organ preparations (such as liver or kidney, which are rich sources of biotransformation enzymes). The tissue homogenate may be prepared in an appropriate isotonic buffer, such as 50 mM Tris buffer, pH 7.4, plus either 0.15 M KCl or 0.25 M sucrose. Protease inhibitors and chelators, such as EDTA (ethylenediaminetetraacetic acid), may be added to maintain enzyme integrity; all steps are carried out at low temperature (typically, 4°C).

Centrifugation

The force on a molecule or particle in a centrifugal field is proportional to the centripetal acceleration applied by the spinning rotor ($a = r\omega^2$); this acceleration is commonly measured relative to g, the acceleration due to gravity at the earth's surface (9.8 m sec^{-2}), so we quote centrifugation conditions as, for example, $20,000 \times g$. The force is also proportional to the difference in densities of the particle and the solution; that is, the effective mass of the particle is reduced by the buoyant force exerted by the solution. (The *buoyant density* of a solute or particle may vary, depending on the nature of the solution, and is equal to the reciprocal of the *partial molar volume*, the change in solution volume per unit mass of dissolved solute.) The marked differences in densities of proteins, DNA, and RNA, as measured by sedimentation on CsCl density gradients, reflect mainly the relative amounts of Cs$^+$ bound to the molecules; the negatively charged phosphodiester linkages of DNA and RNA bind Cs$^+$ stoichiometrically.

Centrifugation techniques can be used to separate cellular components either on the basis of *sedimentation rate* (velocity), measured in Svedberg units, or (by equilibrium sedimentation in density gradients) on the basis of *buoyant density*. By placing each component on a two-dimensional plot of density versus sedimentation rate, we can see what separations can be achieved by centrifugation. The further apart two components occur on the plot, the better our ability to separate them. If two components overlap, they can-

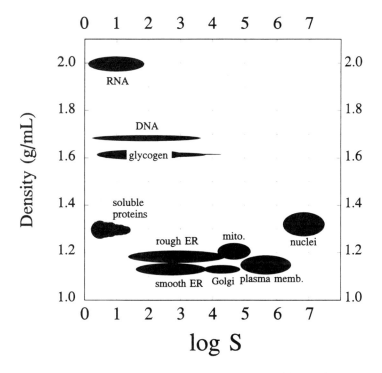

Sedimentation properties of cellular components: S-ρ diagram.   Densities are those measured on CsCl gradients (for macromolecules) and sucrose gradients (organelles). Buoyant densities vary substantially, depending on the nature of the medium.

not, in principle, be separated centrifugally. However, it may be possible to find special conditions under which, for example, one fraction will be selectively destroyed; this is the basis of a method for separating lysosomes from mitochondria (1).

In *zonal density gradient* centrifugation, particles are spun on a preformed concentration gradient. The gradient may be continuous (formed by mixing two solutions of different densities in continuously varying proportions) or consist of discrete layers. Sample is layered onto the top of the gradient, and centrifugation results in separation into bands, according to s values (velocity sedimentation), density, or both. In *velocity* (or rate) separations, the gradient serves only to minimize convective mixing (for example, analysis of DNA strand breaks on alkaline sucrose density gradients). In *equilibrium* separations, the gradient is chosen to provide a layer of appropriate density. For the separation of cells or intact organelles, polymeric materials such as Ficoll or Percoll are usually required, since dense solutions of low-molecular-weight solutes such as sucrose would be hypertonic and cause the organelles to shrink osmotically (2).

Microsomes

A very important procedure in toxicology is the preparation of postmitochondrial fraction (S9) and microsomal fraction. Microsomal fraction (loosely called "microsomes") consists of vesicles produced by homogenization of membranous structures, especially smooth and rough *endoplasmic reticulum*. Microsomes prepared by differential centrifugation, as described below, will also contain some plasma membrane, nuclear membrane, and ribosomes. Endoplasmic reticulum is a membranous organelle composed of approximately equal amounts of protein and lipid (by weight). Since the microsomal fraction is composed of membranes, we should expect that microsomal enzymes are membrane-bound, hydrophobic proteins. Rough endoplasmic reticulum membranes are studded with ribosomes and are the chief site of synthesis of membrane-bound proteins; smooth endoplasmic reticulum does not contain ribosomes, but is the locus of enzymes responsible for lipid (e.g., cholesterol, phospholipid) biosynthesis. The smooth endoplasmic reticulum, and hence the microsomal fraction of mammalian tissues, is a rich source of the enzymes which catalyze "phase 1" reactions of drug metabolism, such as the cytochrome P-450 system, prostaglandin H synthase, and epoxide hydrase; all these enzymes are discussed in later chapters. In addition, some enzymes of "phase 2" metabolism, such as UDP-glucuronosyltransferase, are also microsomal. The liver is the major organ carrying out drug metabolism, and hepatocytes have particularly large amounts of smooth endoplasmic reticulum. Microsomes contain about 20% of the total protein in an hepatocyte cell.

   The protocol described here

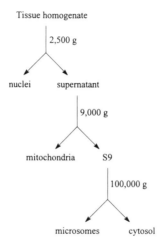

allows the preparation of S9, microsomes, and cytosol fractions. All steps are carried out at 4°C. Tissue homogenate is centrifuged at low speed in a bench-top centrifuge (15 min at 2500 × g). The pellet consists mainly of unbroken cells and intact nuclei and is discarded. Next the supernatant from the first step is spun for 15 min at 9000 × g. The pellet consists mainly of mitochondria and is discarded. The supernatant, known as PMS (postmitochondrial supernatant) or S9 (9000 × g supernatant), consists of both cytosol (soluble proteins and other molecules) and microsomes. This preparation may be used, for example, as an activation system in mutagenicity assays, to be discussed later. If desired, S9 can be further separated by a high-speed spin in an ultracentrifuge, typically 60 min at 100,000 × g. The supernatant from this spin appears clear and is referred to as *cytosol*. The pellet (microsomes) can be used directly, or washed with buffer and repelleted, to remove traces of cytosol.

   The success of a protocol for preparation of subcellular fractions may be evaluated by the electron microscopic evaluation of the product and by the assay of marker enzymes known to be associated with a particular fraction. For example, respiratory proteins (such as cytochrome c) are uniquely mitochondrial, cytochrome P-450 isozymes are microsomal or nuclear, acid hydrolases are lysosomal, and so on.

PROTEIN PURIFICATION

Biochemistry is largely the study of enzymes, and so the purification of proteins—and the maintenance of biological activity during purification—is the touchstone of progress toward an understanding of biochemical processes at the molecular level. Only following the purification of an enzyme protein can we make decisive progress in understanding its structure and catalytic mechanism. Purification of a protein is a necessary prerequisite to determination of its primary sequence and greatly facilitates the molecular cloning of the gene coding for the protein. As Arthur Kornberg stated recently: "I cannot recall a single instance in which I begrudged the time spent on the purification of an enzyme. . . . So, purify, purify, purify." The scientific maturity of the science of biochemical toxicology is evidenced by the great progress made, in recent years, toward the purification and characterization of most of the enzymes of xenobiotic metabolism, which we discuss later in this book.

Why does the purification of proteins continue to be such a challenge to biochemists? Proteins are molecular machines, which have evolved to perform specialized tasks as catalysts, receptors, structural components, and so on. Each protein interacts with its environment: the complex aqueous milieu of the cytosol or a particular subcellular compartment, or the hydrophobic milieu of a membrane. Enzyme proteins selectively bind their particular substrates. Proteins can also sense the concentrations of effector molecules, and they can undergo subtle conformational changes in response to these concentrations. Many proteins aggregate into multimers (quaternary structure) or form complexes with other proteins. All of these phenomena depend on the ability of proteins to exploit noncovalent chemical interactions, both for the generation of secondary and higher-order structure within the protein molecule and for interaction with other molecules. These chemical interactions are mediated by electrostatic forces, van der Waals forces, hydrogen bonding, and other noncovalent forces. Only by exploiting such weak intermolecular interactions can a protein respond to subtle changes in environmental conditions, as is required for biological homeostasis and regulation. Consequently, proteins are typically very delicate molecules, whose conformation and biological activity are easily destroyed by exposure to nonphysiological conditions. Unfortunately, most of the methods of protein purification, such as chromatography, require conditions under which the interaction of the target protein with its normal physiological milieu is severely disrupted. Maintaining activity and achieving purification are, therefore, frequently at odds.

The fragility of proteins contrasts with the remarkable stability of DNA. The biological activity of a protein depends on its conformation, whereas the information content of a nucleic acid is dictated by its covalent structure (sequence). The stability of the covalent bonds of DNA is so great that, in recent years, genetic information has been recovered from samples with ages of tens of thousands of years, such as insects preserved in amber. For the same reasons, experimental methods for the preparation of DNA from different organism are usually very similar, whereas the preparation of each protein is, typically, task-specific.

Methods of Protein Purification: An Overview

The goal of an enzyme purification procedure (3) is to reach chemical homogeneity while maintaining high yield and activity. Before we can begin such a procedure, we must have an assay for the enzyme activity. We will discuss many examples of enzyme assays in later chapters. For the moment, let us assume that a convenient assay is available—say, a colorimetric assay for the formation of a given product—and can be applied to a crude sample. We can now restate our goal: to reach maximum *specific activity* (units of enzyme activity per milligram of total protein) while maintaining acceptably high recovery (total units of enzyme activity in the purified preparation).

The first question to be addressed is the choice of a source or starting material (4). Since the major organs of drug metabolism include the liver, kidney, and lungs, these organs are often used. Before beginning a purification procedure, it is usually worthwhile to screen potential sources of the enzyme, with the goal of selecting a system with particularly high activity. This may involve the comparison of different experimental animals and different organs. Many of the enzymes of drug metabolism are *inducible*; that is, the level of enzyme activity increases following exposure of the animal to unusual conditions, especially treatment with certain chemicals. *In the case of cytochrome P-450 (see Chapter 14) the discovery of induction of the enzyme, by exposure of animals to xenobiotic chemicals, was a critical advance in understanding the enzyme family, since the levels of many forms of the enzyme are virtually undetectable in uninduced animals.*

The development of systems for the expression of proteins from recombinant genes introduced into bacterial, insect (baculovirus system), or mammalian cells provides an increasingly important alternative source for the purification of mammalian proteins. Additionally, such systems can be exploited for the production of engineered proteins—for example, site-specific mutants in which particular amino acid substitutions have been made. Such modified proteins may have altered catalytic activities (not only quantitatively different, but even qualitatively—that is, formation of different products) and are of great value in testing structure–function relationships.

Once a source has been chosen, the tissue must be homogenized and, in most cases, a specific subcellular fraction will be prepared, as discussed earlier. Most purification techniques are only applicable to soluble proteins. Since many proteins are not soluble under physiological conditions (for example, structural proteins and integral membrane proteins), it may first be necessary to achieve solubilization. Many of the enzymes of drug metabolism act principally upon hydrophobic (often, water-insoluble) substrates. Not surprisingly, many of these enzymes are themselves poorly soluble in aqueous solution; physiologically, they are sequestered in membranes. The purification and analysis of membrane proteins has lagged behind the study of soluble proteins because of the great technical obstacle presented by the requirement for solubilization. Procedures for solubilization without loss of enzyme function, usually by the addition of appropriate detergents, have been obtained for many membrane proteins, but achieving success remains a great challenge.

In this chapter we briefly review the most important methods of protein purification. A successful purification procedure almost always involves the successive application of several of these techniques. After each step, the protein fractions yielded by the purification procedure are assayed for total protein content and enzyme activity, and the active fractions are combined and carried forward to the next step. The most successful procedure is one which greatly increases specific activity—that is, which separates the desired protein as much as possible from all other proteins. The overall protein composition of the partially purified preparation can be examined, using an analytical method which can separate and characterize most protein components of a complex sample. Most commonly, this is effected by SDS-PAGE (sodium dodecyl sulfate–polyacrylamide gel electrophoresis; see below); more recently, time-of-flight mass spectrometry has become a useful alternative.

Precipitation

Any soluble protein remains in solution only over a limited range of ionic strength. Typically, solubility decreases rapidly at high ionic strength, since the activity of water decreases; but the exact relationship varies from protein to protein. Thus, by gradually raising the ionic strength of a protein solution in steps [typically, by the addition of aliquots of ammonium sulfate, $(NH_4)_2SO_4$], successive fractions of protein can be precipitated, and recovered as solids by filtration (5). In favorable cases, the desired enzyme will precipitate at a particular percentage of ammonium sulfate saturation (e.g., 10–20%) and can then be redissolved in a buffer of lower ionic strength. However, in some cases, precipitation may be irreversible or destroy activity. Precipitation is typically used as an early step in a purification procedure.

Ion-Exchange Chromatography

Virtually all proteins contain some charged amino acid residues: positively charged bases (arginine, lysine, histidine) or negatively charged acids (aspartate, glutamate), and usually both. In addition, proteins are often charged due to the presence of modifications introduced posttranslationally, such as phosphate groups attached to threonine, serine, or tyrosine residues. Therefore, every protein has a characteristic titration curve, reflecting the net charge on the protein as a function of pH. [Such a titration curve can be measured directly, either by conventional titration or by a two-dimensional isoelectric focusing technique (7).] Conversely, at a given pH value, each protein will have a characteristic net charge. Typically, acidic residues are more common than basic residues in proteins, and thus the majority of proteins are negatively charged near neutral pH, although there are numerous exceptions to this generalization.

Ion-exchange chromatography (6) separates molecules on the basis of charge: The protein solute binds reversibly via electrostatic interactions with the (charged) column matrix. The column matrix is a chemically modified support based on cellulose or dextran, incorporating covalently bound charged groups. For example, DEAE (diethylaminoethyl) Sephadex bears a positively charged tertiary amine functionality. Net charge neutrality is maintained by the presence of a solute counterion—in this case, an anion. Since the exchanger separates solute anions on the basis of their affinities for the column matrix, this is an *anion exchanger*. Conversely, a negatively charged support such as CM (carboxymethyl) cellulose functions as a *cation exchanger*. Initially, an anion exchanger is equilibrated with positive counterions, by washing with an appropriate buffer; for example, we can prepare DEAE Sephadex in the chloride form by washing with a buffer containing sodium chloride. Next, a protein sample is applied, and proteins with net charge opposite to the matrix may bind to the exchanger, displacing buffer ions. Proteins with near-zero net charge, or the same charge as the matrix, are not bound. The bound proteins may then be eluted by washing the matrix with competing ions—for example, by increasing the concentration of salt in the wash buffer. Alternatively, one may alter the pH so as to reduce the charge on the protein. As the wash buffer is changed, protein fractions are successively eluted. Ion exchange chromatography is typically carried out with the chromatographic matrix packed into a column, either an open column operating under the low pressure of a gravity head or peristaltic pump, or a sealed column connected to a high-pressure pump in the FPLC (fast protein liquid chromatography) approach. Alternatively, if high efficiency is not essential, the technique may be used in a "batch" mode: The exchanger is stirred in a slurry, and eluted fractions are collected by filtration of the solid exchanger matrix.

While net protein charge is the most important criterion of binding to an ion exchanger, other effects also contribute to the protein–matrix interaction, including the local distribution of charges, especially on the protein surface, and non–ion-exchange effects, such as hydrogen bonding interaction with the matrix.

Gel Filtration Chromatography

Gel filtration (or gel permeation) chromatography (8) separates molecules on the basis of molecular size, which is roughly correlated with molecular weight. The physical basis of gel filtration is very different from that of other familiar forms of chromatography, such as reversed-phase or ion-exchange chromatography. There is *no attractive interaction between the column matrix and the proteins*; separation is achieved because the volume accessible to large molecules is less than that accessible to smaller molecules. The column is formed from beads of a porous gel. The pore size can be controlled during the preparation of the gel material. The total volume occupied by the column bed consists of three distinct regions: the solid volume occupied by the matrix material itself, the *excluded volume* (or *void volume*), and the solvent volume within the interior of the beads. Sufficiently small molecules can penetrate the beads, and hence they must pass through the total solvent-accessible volume of the column. Larger molecules are unable to penetrate the beads; they pass through the excluded volume only, and they elute earlier. Because proteins are not actually bound to the column matrix, gel filtration can only be performed in column chromatography mode, not as a batch process. The separation power of the technique is limited, for the same reason. No solute can elute in less than the excluded volume or more than the total volume of the column (*compare with ion exchange*).

Gels are manufactured from relatively inert, uncharged, cross-linked polymers, such as dextran, a branched polysaccharide produced by fermentation (*Leuconostoc mesenteroides*); dextran is chemically cross-linked to form "Sephadex" (Pharmacia). Other commonly used gel filtration materials are polyacrylamide (Bio-Gel P, Bio-Rad) and agarose, a neutral polysaccharide prepared from agar. Agarose is used for very-high-molecular-weight-range fractionation ($>10^7$).

An illustrative application of gel filtration is desalting. When a protein has been subjected to a high concentration of buffer or salt (as would occur during ammonium sulfate fractionation, for example), it may be desirable to remove the salt prior to the next step. This can be done with a gel having a low exclusion limit (e.g., Sephadex G-10); the protein sample will elute in the (low-ionic-strength) solvent used to run the column; the original solvent (and salt) remains trapped on the column in the internal volume of the beads.

For protein purification, gel filtration columns are typically "long and thin," since the molecular weight selectivity is limited. Gel filtration is also used for estimation of native molecular weight; elution volume can be calibrated by running a series of standard proteins of known molecular weight. Nevertheless, such measurements are only approximate, since the shape of the protein, as well as its molecular weight, influences molecular volume; elongated or rod-shaped proteins behave anomalously.

At best, about 10 proteins can be resolved in a gel filtration run. Therefore, the method is generally applied late in a purification procedure when the number of contaminating proteins is small.

Affinity Chromatography

Affinity chromatography (9) refers to separations based on a specific binding interaction between a protein and a ligand which the protein recognizes; thus, unlike the separations described previously, affinity chromatography exploits the specificity of biochemical binding processes. For this reason, very high purification may be achievable with this technique. For example, we may take advantage of the specificity of binding of an enzyme with a substrate, substrate analogue, cofactor, inhibitor, or allosteric effector. The ligand is covalently attached to the column matrix; various chemical coupling methods have been developed (10). Usually, a chemical "spacer arm" is inserted between the matrix and the ligand; otherwise, steric interactions between the matrix and ligand might interfere with binding. Following addition of the sample, the column is washed to remove unbound material. The bound protein is then eluted by disruption of the interaction between ligand and protein. Of course, we wish to achieve elution without denaturing the protein. *Specific* elution refers to elution by addition of a high concentration of the free ligand, which will compete with the covalently linked ligand on the column matrix. *Nonspecific* elution relies on modification of the eluting buffer such that the favorable interaction between ligand and protein is disrupted—for example, altered pH or ionic strength or addition of chaotropic agents (urea, guanidine).

A particularly powerful technique combines affinity chromatography with molecular engineering of protein structure. For example, a recombinant gene for a protein of interest (see Chapter 2) can be modified by fusion (see sidebar "Gene Fusions" in Chapter 4) with a sequence coding for a domain of the enzyme glutathione transferase. The resulting fusion protein can be purified on an affinity matrix bearing immobilized glutathione moieties (see Chapter 11). Provided that the modification does not modify the protein's structure and activity unacceptably, this approach allows the efficiency and simplicity of the affinity method to be extended to almost any protein for which a cloned gene is in hand. In a further refinement of this approach, specific protease-sensitive sites are engineered into the fusion gene, so that the glutathione transferase domain can be cleaved from the fusion protein after purification. The vectors, columns, and reagents required for this approach have been assembled into a commercially available kit (Pharmacia GST Gene Fusion System).

PROTEIN CHARACTERIZATION

Electrophoresis

Since proteins are charged molecules (at least at appropriate pH values), they may be separated under the influence of an electric field: electrophoresis. Electrophoretic methods (11) are ubiquitous in modern biochemistry for the characterization of proteins and, in some cases, as a preparative method. All nucleic acids are negatively charged, and thus electrophoresis is also of enormous importance for analysis of these biomolecules.

In an electrophoretic system, an electric potential is applied across a solution; in modern gel electrophoresis, the solution is trapped in a semisolid gel, which minimizes convection and diffusion processes. A charged particle in an electric field experiences a coulombic force:

$$F = Eq$$

where E is the strength of the electric field and q is the charge. In a solution, a charge carrier will very quickly accelerate to a constant velocity v such that the frictional drag on the moving molecule is equal and opposite to the electrical force:

$$Eq = fv$$

where f is the frictional coefficient. Neither q nor f is readily predictable, even if we know the sequence of the protein. Any charged solute attracts a shielding cloud of electrolyte ions, which reduce the effective charge. The frictional coefficient is determined by the shape and size of the molecule. Empirically, we define the mobility (velocity per unit field):

$$\mu \equiv \frac{v}{E} = \frac{q}{f}$$

In an electrophoresis experiment, current flows in a closed circuit from an electrical power supply, through electrodes immersed in solution, and through the gel. In the electrical wires, current is carried, of course, by electrons. In the solution, current is carried by a variety of charged species, both positive and negative. The multiplicity of current carriers makes the analysis of the physics of electrophoresis more subtle than conventional electrical circuitry. The flow of charge between the electrodes and the solution is mediated by electrolysis reactions. At the anode, oxidation generates positive charge in solution:

$$H_2O \rightarrow \frac{1}{2} O_2 \ (g) + 2H^+$$

while, at the cathode, reduction generates negative charge:

$$2H_2O + 2e^- \rightarrow H_2 \ (g) + 2OH^-$$

These electrolysis reactions balance the electrophoretic flow of anions to the anode and cations to the cathode; it must be borne in mind that the net charge in any volume element remains neutral throughout the electrophoresis process, even though anions and cations are moving in opposite directions.

Electrophoresis was first developed as an analytical tool for the study of proteins by the Swedish chemist Tiselius in the 1920s. However, the resolution of electrophoresis experiments carried out in free solution was greatly hindered by diffusion. Routine high-resolution analytical use of protein electrophoresis was made practical by two developments: (i) the use of gels as supporting media and (ii) the invention of the discontinuous ("disc") electrophoresis technique by Ornstein, Davis, and others in the 1960s. These developments are discussed in greater detail elsewhere (12); the exploitation of these ideas allowed the development of routine methods capable of achieving very-high-resolution separation of proteins on electrophoretic gels.

Protein electrophoresis is usually carried out in a supporting polyacrylamide or agarose gel. As a result, the process of electrophoresis is combined with gel permeation effects (as in gel filtration chromatography), which separate on basis of molecular weight. The pore size and, hence, molecular weight sieving range of a polyacrylamide gel is fixed by the concentration of acrylamide monomer used in forming the gel (typically, 2.5–30%). Such gels are useful for separating proteins up to about 250 kD; above this, proteins cannot penetrate the gel pores. Agarose has a larger pore size and is used to separate very large protein complexes and nucleic acids.

The net charge on a protein cannot be predicted without sequence analysis, and even that may not be sufficient because of posttranslational modifications, strong interactions with charged ligands or counterions, and so on. As a result, the position of a protein on an electrophoresis gel, although characteristic, tells us little about its structure or composition. A variation on the method, however, allows us to use protein electrophoresis to determine protein molecular weight with reasonable accuracy. In the SDS-PAGE technique, proteins are denatured by boiling in SDS, an anionic detergent. SDS binds to almost all proteins, mainly by interaction with the peptide backbone, with a stoichiometry of about 1.4 parts SDS to one part protein by weight. Since SDS is negatively charged, this binding masks the protein's intrinsic charge: All SDS–protein complexes have a similar ratio of charge to mass. When separated by electrophoresis, the mobility of SDS–protein complexes is a function only of their molecular weight. By comparison to standards, the molecular weights of unknown proteins can be estimated. (This approach is not generally applicable to protein purification, however, since the procedure virtually always causes irreversible denaturation.)

Protein bands on electrophoresis gels can be detected by staining with Coomassie Brilliant Blue or other dyes, or by the highly sensitive silver-staining technique. If newly synthesized proteins have been labeled, for example, by growth of cultures in ^{35}S-methionine-containing medium, then autoradiography can also be used.

SIDEBAR: PROTEIN CHARACTERIZATION BY MASS SPECTROMETRY

The supremacy of SDS-PAGE for characterization of protein molecular weights has recently been challenged by the surprising extension of mass spectrometry —previously a technique limited to small molecules—to the analysis of proteins (13). Mass spectrometry relies on the separation of electrically accelerated ions in a magnetic field in vacuo. Ion beams are produced by thermal volatilization of the sample, followed by, for example, electron ionization (EI). Electrons, emitted by a heated tungsten wire cathode (much as in a television tube), are accelerated to an energy of about 70 eV and bombard the neutral molecules, stripping off electrons and generating analyte cations.

It seems improbable that a huge, nonvolatile molecule, such as a protein, could be successfully converted into a gas phase ion suitable for analysis by mass spectrometry. Nevertheless, this can now be achieved by the application of several special techniques for sample volatilization ionization and mass analysis. In the *matrix-assisted laser desorption ionization* (MALDI) approach, the protein sample is dissolved in aqueous solution, dried onto the sample probe, inserted into the vacuum system, and bombarded with ultraviolet laser. Determination of the masses of the huge ions produced can be achieved by *time-of-flight analysis*: Each laser pulse sets off a pulse of ions moving down a drift tube toward the detector; the time of arrival of the ions following each pulse is measured. The mass can be determined from the velocity by simple kinematics. In *electrospray ionization*, an aqueous solution of the protein is sprayed into the vacuum system through a fine needle held in a strong electric field; tiny droplets of solution evaporate into the vacuum. These techniques have been used successfully to measure, with unprecedented accuracy, the masses of proteins with molecular weights of up to hundreds of kilodaltons. This opens up new vistas in protein analysis. For example, the sickle-cell mutant form of β-hemoglobin (glu → val) can be resolved from the normal protein, on the basis of its lower mass (30 mass units out of nearly 16 kD). Posttranslational modifications, such as phosphorylation and glycosylation, can be detected. Complex protein mixtures can be profiled, as by SDS-PAGE. Several commercial systems for protein mass spectrometry have been introduced, and, with continuing development, the technique is likely to become the method of choice for protein mass characterization.

Antibodies

Antibodies (also called *immunoglobulins*) are proteins produced in specialized white blood cells (plasma cells, derived from B lymphocytes) and secreted into the blood plasma. (Some classes of antibodies are also found in the interstitial fluid and in secretions such as sweat, tears, saliva, and milk.) Antibodies (Ab) are produced in response to exposure of an animal to foreign substances, especially macromolecules, and constitute a key component of the immune defense system. The foreign substance which elicits an immune response is called an *antigen*. An antigen may be a macromolecule: protein, nucleic acid, polysaccharide, lipopolysaccharide, and so on. *Even an antibody can itself be an antigen*; for example, rabbit antibodies injected into a goat are recognized by the goat's immune system as foreign and will elicit an immune response. Antigens have varying effectiveness as elicitors of antibody production: We speak of some substances as being more "antigenic" or "immunogenic" than others.

Small molecules (e.g., DNA adducts; see Chapter 16) are usually poorly antigenic.* However, antigenicity can often be greatly enhanced by covalently linking the small molecule to a large molecule (such as serum albumin). This is useful if we wish to produce antibodies to a particular small molecule. In this situation, we refer to the small molecule as a *hapten* and to the large molecule as a *carrier*.

In vivo, antibodies instruct other elements of the immune system to attack and destroy foreign materials, such as invading microorganisms. The antibodies recognize and bind to foreign molecules displayed on the surface of, say, an invading bacterium. The bound antibodies are recognized by the *complement system*, a family of soluble plasma proteins which attack the membranes of microorganisms and thereby kill them. Also, the bound antibodies mark the cell for attack by the *phagocytic* cells of the immune system (e.g., neutrophils, macrophages), which engulf and kill foreign cells. Note that antibodies do not destroy antigens directly: Antibodies recognize and bind to antigens, marking the antigens for destruction by other elements of the immune system.

Antibodies bind to antigens with very high affinity: The dissociation constant for the antibody–antigen complex is typically 10^{-7} to 10^{-10} M. *The high binding affinity of antibodies for specific antigens is the basis of all biochemical and analytical applications of antibodies.* We can exploit this specificity to detect the presence of a tiny amount of antigen, even in the presence of a large excess of other molecules. A given antibody protein (immunoglobulin) specifically recognizes a single antigen, much as a given enzyme specifically recognizes a single substrate. (The intermolecular forces involved in antibody–antigen binding are very similar to the forces involved in enzyme–substrate binding.) In fact, an antibody recognizes a particular site on the surface of the antigen; we call this site an *epitope* or *antigenic determinant*. A single macromolecule will have many different surface features, just as a person has a nose, toes, fingers, and so on, each with distinctive shape and surface characteristics. (In the case of a protein, for example, epitopes may be determined by the primary/secondary structure of a stretch of primary sequence, or they may be formed by the tertiary structure of the protein.) Thus, *different antibodies can recognize different epitopes on a single antigen molecule.* However, a given antibody may also recognize molecules other than the antigen, if they happen to share very similar epitopes with the antigen. We call this phenomenon "cross-reactivity."

The standard approach to producing antibodies is *immunization*. An antigen (e.g., a protein or a hapten-carrier conjugate) is injected into an experimental animal (often, a rabbit). If the antigen is sufficiently immunogenic, antibodies to it will appear in the serum. Soon after immunization, IgM-class antibodies appear. After a few weeks, IgG-class antibodies appear. At the appropriate time, the rabbit is bled, and the serum is prepared (by

---

*Stimulation of the immune response requires that an antigen be processed within a B lymphocyte (e.g., degraded by proteolysis) and that a fragment of the antigen bind to a protein of the MHC (major histocompatibility complex) family. Small molecules generally fail to do so.

allowing the blood to clot, centrifuging, and removing the clear fluid supernatant). This preparation is called *immune serum*. If desired, the immunoglobulins can be purified from the serum, but often the serum is used directly.

Any animal is exposed to a multitude of foreign antigens. Therefore, the immune serum will contain antibodies to countless substances other than the injected antigen. These other antibodies might interfere with our later uses of the serum. Therefore, as a control, it is routine to obtain serum from the animal before immunization with the antigen of interest: *preimmune* serum.

A single antibody-producing plasma cell synthesizes only a single species of antibody. Studies of a form of leukemia known as *multiple myeloma* first made this fact clear. In these patients, an antibody-producing white cell has proliferated uncontrollably. The patients excrete large amounts of a single species of antibody (to an unknown antigen), called "Bence-Jones protein" after the physician who first observed this phenomenon. (Of course, one has no idea what antigen reacts with a particular patient's Bence-Jones protein antibody.)

If the cell encounters antigen to its antibody, it is stimulated to proliferate into a clone of daughter cells, all making the same antibody. *An individual animal can produce millions of different antibodies.* [The genetic mechanisms for generation of antibody diversity are discussed in Voet and Voet (14).]

Normally, antibody-producing lymphocytes cannot be grown in tissue culture. In 1975, Kohler and Milstein developed a technique for accomplishing this. Antibody-producing cells, isolated from the spleen of a mouse, are induced to "fuse" with "immortal" myeloma cells, by treatment with polyethylene glycol. The resulting cells, called *hybridomas*, combine the antibody-producing characteristics of the lymphocytes with the immortality (capacity for continuous growth in culture) of the myeloma cells. A hybridoma clone produces only a single form of antibody, just as in the case of Bence-Jones proteins. If we first immunize a mouse with the antigen of interest, then there is a good chance that some of the lymphocytes subsequently isolated from the animal's spleen will produce antibody to this antigen, as desired. If we can identify the hybridoma cell producing the desired antibody, that cell can be cloned and propagated in culture, and it acts as a tiny "factory." The cell's immunoglobulin product is called a *monoclonal antibody*. The great advantage of this approach is that it provides a single, pure, homogeneous antibody recognizing a specific epitope. (Different monoclonal antibodies will probably recognize different epitopes on the antigen.) In contrast, immune serum (*polyclonal antibody*) is a complex mix of desired antibodies (antibodies to epitopes on the immunizing antigen) and countless other unwanted antibodies produced by the animal.

IgG class immunoglobulins are proteins with a molecular weight of ~150. Each molecule consists of two "heavy chains" (50 kD) and two light chains (25 kD), linked by disulfide bridges (15). Both heavy and light chains contain *variable regions*, which have different primary sequences for each type of antibody, and *constant regions* (primary sequence shared by all the antibodies of a given class). This conclusion was also deduced from studies of Bence-Jones protein sequences, in the 1960s (16). Different species have different constant regions, with the degree of homology reflecting evolutionary relatedness. *The variable regions determine antigen specificity.*

Western Blotting (Immunoblotting)

The so-called Western blotting technique (the name is a pun on the earlier, unrelated technique of Southern blotting) is a modification of the SDS-PAGE technique. Western blotting combines the separation power of electrophoresis with the specificity of the antigen–antibody reaction. The technique is applicable once an antibody to the protein of interest has been prepared. Proteins are separated as in SDS-PAGE, and then they are detected by their reaction with an antibody (Ab). After electrophoresis is complete, proteins are transferred from the SDS-PAGE gel onto a thin sheet of *nitrocellulose*. The blot is first incubated with BSA (bovine serum albumin) or gelatin to block subsequent nonspecific binding of antibody to the membrane, then incubated with the antibody (17).

To detect the bound antibody, various methods can be used. Protein A from *Staphylococcus aureus* binds antibodies of many mammalian species with high affinity, so ^{125}I-labeled protein A (prepared by iodination) can be used to indicate the presence of the bound antibody. Alternatively, a second Ab can be used to detect the first. For example, "goat-antirabbit" is an antibody preparation from the serum of a goat immunized with rabbit antibodies. The goat's immune system recognizes the rabbit antibodies as foreign protein, and it generates antibodies which recognize the constant regions of the rabbit antibodies. These regions are common to all rabbit antibodies, so the goat-antirabbit will recognize any rabbit antibodies. The second Ab can be obtained commercially as a conjugate linked covalently to an enzyme, such as alkaline phosphatase or horseradish peroxidase, which oxidizes a substrate to an insoluble colored product. Thus the gel can be treated with the first antibody, then the second antibody, and finally with the substrate; the gel will stain at bands where the original antibody bound.

(Since the SDS-PAGE-separated proteins are denatured, it is sometimes desirable to use a similarly denatured protein preparation for immunization: structural epitopes on the native protein are unlikely to be present in the denatured form.)

Isoelectric Focusing

The isoelectric point (pI) of any polyelectrolyte is defined as the pH at which the protein does not move in an electric field. This is a characteristic property of a protein, determined by its content of acidic and basic functional groups (termini, side chains, and posttranslational modifications) and their interactions with one another and with the solution. Most proteins have acidic pI values, between about pH 4 and pH 7. Isoelectric focusing is a high-resolution technique for protein separation based on this property.

Isoelectric focusing (18) is performed in an agarose or polyacrylamide gel with large pores, so that diffusion is restricted, but negligible molecular sieving effects occur. The key to the technique is the use of *polyampholytes* (amphoteric electrolytes): low-molecular-weight synthetic polyaminocarboxylic acids which act as buffers covering a wide range of pI values (e.g., 4–10). The ampholytes are required to stabilize the pH gradient which forms during electrophoresis.

The pH gradient is established by applying acid (e.g., phosphoric acid) to the anode reservoir and base (triethanolamine) to the cathode reservoir. When voltage is applied, the small polyampholytes migrate quickly to their individual pI points and maintain a stable, linear gradient of pH along the gel. A protein anion moves toward the anode, encountering decreasing pH as it travels; eventually, it reaches the point in the gradient corresponding to its pI, where it stops. Different proteins are *stopped* at different points, as opposed to conventional electrophoresis, in which *rates* of migration are compared. This accounts for the excellent resolving power of isoelectric focusing. The technique can be applied both as an analytical method and on preparative scale. Under favorable conditions, one can separate proteins with pI differences as small as 0.01 pH units.

Two-Dimensional SDS-PAGE

This combined technique, introduced by O'Farrell in 1975, is the most powerful analytical tool for separating proteins (19). The method combines isoelectric focusing in one dimension and SDS-PAGE in a perpendicular dimension. Thus, each dimension separates proteins using a different property: pI (isoelectric focusing) and molecular weight (SDS-PAGE). Proteins of similar weight are unlikely also to have similar pI values, and vice versa. The two-dimensional approach permits resolution of over 1000 different proteins in a single analysis. This technique is invaluable for detecting regulatory responses to growth conditions or other environmental factors: Proteins whose expression is markedly altered can be pinpointed as spots whose intensity differs substantially between analyses of cells grown under different conditions. In recent years, computer-assisted image analysis of the complex two-dimensional patterns has improved the accuracy and power of the approach. For example, in a recent publication, a tabulation of more than 1200 protein species present in the liver of the Fischer 344 rat has been compiled as a computer database (20).

NOTES

1. Dobrota, M., in: *Biochemical Toxicology: A Practical Approach*, K. Snell and B. Mullock, Eds., IRL Press, Oxford, UK, 1987, Chapter 10.
2. Detailed methods for the preparation of mitochondria, plasma membranes, lysosomes, and peroxisomes are given in Snell and Mullock; also see Fowler et al., *Principles and Methods of Toxicology*, 2nd ed., A. W. Hayes, Ed., Raven Press, New York, 1989, Chapter 29.
3. Deutscher, M. P., Ed., *Guide to Protein Purification* (*Methods in Enzymology*, Vol. 182), Academic Press, New York, 1990.
4. See Section III, Optimization of starting materials, in: Deutscher, M. P., Ed., *Guide to Protein Purification*.
5. See Section VI, Bulk Methods, in: Deutscher, M. P., Ed., *Guide to Protein Purification*.
6. Rossomando, E. F., Ion exchange chromatography, in: Deutscher, M. P., Ed., *Guide to Protein Purification*, pp. 309–317.
7. For an example of this technique, see Beyer, W. F., Jr., and Fridovich, I., In vivo competition between iron and manganese for occupancy of the active site region of the manganese-superoxide dismutase of *Escherichia coli*, *J. Biol. Chem.* 266:303–308, 1991.
8. Stellwagen, E., Gel Filtration, in: Deutscher, M. P., Ed., *Guide to Protein Purification*, pp. 317–328.
9. Ostrove, S., Affinity Chromatography, in: Deutscher, M. P., Ed., *Guide to Protein Purification*, pp. 357–371.
10. *Biochemical Techniques, Theory and Practice*, J. F. Robyt and B. J. White, Waveland Press, 1987, pp. 96–98.
11. Section VIII, in: Deutscher, M. P., Ed., *Guide to Protein Purification*, pp. 357–371.
12. Freifelder, D., *Physical Biochemistry*, 2nd ed., W. H. Freeman, New York, 1982.
13. Chait, B.T., and Kent, S.B., Weighing naked proteins: practical, high-accuracy mass measurements of peptides and proteins, *Science* 257:1885–1894, 1992.
14. Voet, D., and Voet, J. G., *Biochemistry*, 2nd ed., Wiley, New York, 1995, pp. 1218–1223.
15. Stryer, L., *Biochemistry*, 4th ed., W. H. Freeman, New York, 1995, pp. 367–369.
16. Stryer, L., *Biochemistry*, 4th ed., W. H. Freeman, New York, 1995, p. 368.
17. Timmons, T. M., and Dunbar, B. S., Protein blotting and immunodetection, in: Deutscher, M. P., Ed., *Guide to Protein Purification*, pp. 679–688.

18. Garfin, D. E., Isoelectric focusing, in: Deutscher, M. P., Ed., *Guide to Protein Purification*, pp. 459–477.
19. Dunbar, B. S., Kimura, H., and Timmons, T. M., Protein analysis using high resolution two-dimensional polyacrylamide gel electrophoresis, in: Deutscher, M. P., Ed., *Guide to Protein Purification*, pp. 441–459.
20. Leigh Anderson, N., Esquer-Blasco, R., Hofmann, J.-P., and Anderson, N. G., A two-dimensional gel database of rat liver proteins useful in gene regulation and drug effects studies, *Electrophoresis* 12:907–930, 1991.

2

MOLECULAR BIOLOGY AND ITS APPLICATIONS IN TOXICOLOGY

The extraordinary growth of the science of molecular biology, following the development of methods for the sequencing of nucleic acids in the mid-1970s, constitutes a revolution in the understanding of biological science, comparable only to the transformation of physical science by quantum mechanics in the 1930s. The combination of molecular biological (i.e., nucleic acid-oriented) and biochemical (i.e., enzyme-oriented) approaches to the study of biological problems is synergistic. In most bioscience laboratories, the integration of molecular biological/genetic and biochemical approaches has become routine.

The significance of these developments for the science of toxicology is profound. Proteins which metabolize or interact with toxic chemicals were first identified on the basis of their biochemical activities; of their structures, we knew next to nothing. Now, most of these proteins, such as the Ah receptor or the many isoforms of cytochrome P-450 and glutathione-S-transferase, have been cloned and sequenced (see later chapters). The proteins can then be expressed in organisms ranging from bacteria to yeast to rodents, produced in large quantities, engineered into new forms by site-directed mutagenesis, and often, crystallized and studied by high-resolution X-ray diffraction analysis. Their evolutionary history can be traced, and the regulation of their transcription and translation can be studied in cells and tissues. All these vistas hardly seemed possible a generation ago.

In this chapter we present a brief introduction to the tools of modern molecular biology. For a more thorough treatment, the student is referred to other texts (1).

NUCLEIC ACIDS ARE THE GENETIC MATERIAL

DNA is the genetic material of all cellular organisms. This fundamental unifying fact of biology was appreciated rather late in the game; only the discovery of the double helix structure of DNA, by Watson and Crick (1953), brought widespread appreciation of the biological roles of nucleic acids. Nucleic acids were first isolated by Miescher in the 1860s. Why were they almost ignored for so many decades? After all, their presence in the cell nucleus hinted at a connection with the chromosome, and by the early twentieth century the central role of chromosomes in heredity was already apparent. But protein, a much more abundant biomolecule, became the focus of attention, especially once the identification of enzymes as proteins became clear in the 1930s. The macromolecular nature of nucleic acids was not appreciated until much later. Finally, nucleic acids from all sources seemed to have very similar chemical properties, apparently at odds with the concept that nucleic acids carry genetic information.

Evidence for the genetic role of DNA was actually available early on. In 1930,

F. L. Gates (2) examined the killing of bacterial cells by ultraviolet (UV) radiation. *Escherichia coli* or *Staphylococcus aureus* cells were prepared as a monolayer and irradiated with UV light. The survival of the irradiated cells, as measured by their ability to grow into colonies on Petri dishes, was measured as a function of wavelength. The resulting *action spectrum* indicates the killing efficiency, per photon, of UV light. Gates noted that the effectiveness peaked at about 265 nm and was much reduced at 280 nm or above. In subsequent years, the same wavelength peak was reported for induction of mutations in bacteria. These action spectra correlated closely with the known absorption spectrum of DNA ($\lambda_{max} \sim 260$ nm), but not with that of protein ($\lambda_{max} \sim 280$ nm), and were interpreted as evidence that DNA, not protein, was the genetic material. However, these results were largely ignored.

Another lead came from the study of *bacterial transformation*. In the 1920s, Frederick Griffith was studying the pathogenicity of the gram-positive bacterium *Diplococcus pneumoniae* in mice. He knew that some strains of the bacterium, called "smooth" because of the shiny appearance of the colonies on culture dishes, were *virulent* and would infect and kill mice into which they were injected. Other strains, called "rough" because of the mottled appearance of the colonies, were nonvirulent. Griffith wanted to understand the basis of this difference. Today, our very first guess would probably be that the difference was genetic, but bear in mind that in Griffith's day, it was still not clear that bacteria possessed genes at all! Griffith hypothesized that the smooth strains produced some chemical factor, absent in the rough strains, which conferred pathogenicity. *Today, we know that this factor is the production of a lipopolysaccharide coat. The complement protein system in animal serum attacks the bacterial membrane and kills the cells. The lipopolysaccharide coat shields the bacterium from this attack. The rough strains lack this protective coat and are readily killed by serum. The presence of capsule also interferes with the ability of phagocytic white blood cells to engulf and kill the bacterium.*

To test his hypothesis, Griffith sterilized a culture of the virulent smooth strain, by boiling it, and mixed the resulting cell debris with a live culture of the nonvirulent rough strain. The mixture proved to be pathogenic! Griffith discovered that *both smooth and rough colonies could be cultured from the blood of the infected mice*. He hypothesized that an unknown factor, released from the smooth cells during boiling, *transformed* some of the rough strains to the smooth phenotype. This factor is now understood to be a gene required for synthesis of capsule. *Griffiths was lucky, as well as imaginative, because it is usually more difficult to move genes between bacteria, or other organisms. The strains he was studying become highly "competent" for transformation following growth in culture.* Griffith's nomenclature has stuck, and we still refer to the passage of DNA directly from one organism to another as *transformation*.

What was the chemical nature of Griffith's *transforming principle*? Oswald Avery and his group at Rockefeller University, New York, embarked on a project aimed at purifying and characterizing the principle. [The history of this research effort has been recounted by Avery's colleague, Maclyn McCarty (3).] Naturally, they guessed that the principle might be a capsular polysaccharide; their expertise was in the analysis of capsule, and they already knew that this was the critical biochemical difference between smooth and rough strains. But chemically the transforming principle was completely unlike any polysaccharide; it did not seem to be a protein, since it resisted digestion by any of the known proteases. After 10 years of careful biochemical analysis, they announced their extraordinary conclusion in 1944. *Griffith's "transforming principle" was nucleic acid.*

Much has been made of the failure of the scientific community to appreciate immediately the significance of "Avery's bombshell." But it is perhaps not so surprising to a biochemist. The "Holy Grail" of biochemists is purification, and we know how difficult it is to free a molecule from all contaminants. It was easy to dismiss Avery's result on the mistaken assumption that, for example, some protein was still present in the purified "principle." But this objection could not be sustained long. In 1952, Alfred Hershey and Martha Chase used ^{32}P-phosphate and ^{35}S-methionine as selective radioactive labels for the nucleic acid and protein, respectively, of a T2 bacteriophage preparation. Their biochemical analysis showed that, when the labeled bacteriophage infected *E. coli*, the ^{35}S-protein coat was left outside the infected cell, whereas the ^{32}P-DNA entered the cell and was passed on to progeny bacteriophage. DNA was conclusively established as the genetic material.

THE STRUCTURE OF DNA

The double-helical secondary structure of DNA was elucidated by Watson and Crick in 1953 and was announced in a one-page paper in *Nature* that ranks among the most important in the history of science (as well as being a model of brevity!). We will not repeat a detailed exposition of the double-helical structure here, but it is worth noting a few features which are sometimes overlooked.

The deduction of the double-helical structure was based on the X-ray crystallographic analysis (by Rosalind Franklin and Maurice Wilkins) of DNA preparations which are sometimes described as "crystals" but which were really quasi-crystals because the DNA was heterogeneous. Consequently, only limited structural information could be gleaned from the X-ray analysis, such as the spacing of the repeating unit (base pair), the pitch of the helix, and the number of strands (2). But these clues were enough foundation for model-building based on chemical judgment and inspired intuition. (Detailed high-resolution structures of DNA were not obtained until the 1970s, when advances in molecular biology and nucleic acid chemistry had made possible the preparation of large amounts of DNA oligonucleotides of defined sequence. These developments confirmed the fundamental ideas of Watson and Crick, but they also revealed unsuspected novel aspects of DNA structure, such as the Z form adopted by certain sequences.)

The concept of the base pair, and hence of sequence complementarity between the two strands, fit the earlier analytical work of Erwin Chargaff. Chargaff had developed methods for the quantitative analysis of the base composition of DNA, and he determined that the rules A = T and G = C applied to DNA samples of widely varying (A + T)/(G + C) ratios. The consideration of this pairing relationship led Watson and Crick to envisage specific chemical interactions stabilizing the A–T and G–C pairings, and Linus Pauling's recent work on the protein α-helix drew attention to the importance of hydrogen bonding as a chemical basis for intermolecular recognition. A major obstacle to elucidating the base-pairing scheme was that the predominant tautomeric forms of the bases (enol versus keto) were still unclear, and most of the literature representations of the time gave the enol (or lactim) forms, not the keto (lactam) forms which we now know to be favored. Once Watson and Crick realized that the literature structures of the bases were misleading, they soon discovered the correct base-pairing interactions.

The phosphodiester linkage between each pair of adjacent nucleotide units joins the 3′ carbon of one deoxyribose with the 5′ carbon of the next. Thus, just as with polypeptide chains, each strand of nucleic acid has an intrinsic direction, which, by convention, we always write as 5′ to 3′. Furthermore, this means that each strand has two distinct ends, 5′ and 3′. *The two strands of the DNA double helix run in opposite directions in space (antiparallel).* This was deduced by Watson and Crick as a consequence of the geometric relationship between the two deoxyribose units of the Watson–Crick base-pair unit, and it was consistent with the X-ray diffraction data. [The direct chemical demonstration of the antiparallel orientation of the two strands was first achieved a decade later in Arthur Kornberg's nearest-neighbor analysis experiments (see Chapter 16).] Note that, since 5′dNTPs are the raw material for DNA synthesis, all DNA polymerases add on to the 3′ end of the growing strand: *Nucleic acid synthesis always proceeds in the 5′ → 3′ direction.*

Nucleic acid bases are uncharged, hydrophobic, planar, heteroaromatic structures and are poorly soluble in water. The bases are incorporated into DNA via attachment to the sugar–phosphate backbone. Glycosidic linkage of the base to the deoxyribose sugar gives the more soluble nucleoside; the addition of the negatively charged phosphate group gives the highly water-soluble nucleotide.

The main driving force behind the assembly of the double helix (which forms spontaneously when complementary single strands of DNA are allowed to anneal) is the hydrophobic effect. The polar sugar–phosphate backbone wraps around the outside of the double helix and interacts with solvent water and solute cations (such as Mg^{2+}), while the bases are forced into the hydrophobic interior of the helix. As with the protein α-helix, the core of the double helix is tightly packed with the atoms of the bases, making van der Waals contacts; solvent water is excluded. This arrangement also serves to protect the bases, which carry the informational content of the genetic code, from chemical damage by solute molecules. The hydrogen-bonding of the base pairs stabilizes the pairing of complementary sequences in the two helices. Furthermore, the bases in the double helix are *stacked* (roughly in the geometry of a stack of dinner plates; see Fig. 2.1), separated by about 3.5 Å. This allows favorable van der Waals interactions between successive bases and provides an additional large thermodynamic driving force for double-helix formation (4).

The DNA double helix can be reversibly heat-denatured ("melted") into single strands. This conformational change can be monitored optically: The UV absorbance at about 260 nm increases by about 40% upon denaturation ("hyperchromic effect"), due to unstack-

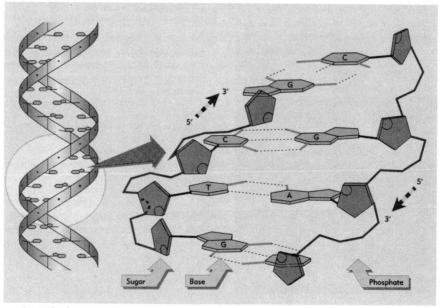

Figure 2.1.   Flat base pairs lie perpendicular to the sugar–phosphate backbone. From B. Lewin, *Genes V*, Oxford University Press, 1994, Fig. 4.12, p. 93, by permission.

ing of the bases (5). The denaturation process is a highly cooperative transition, occurring over a relatively narrow temperature range; the characteristic transition temperature (T_m) depends on the G + C content of the DNA and on the ionic strength. This cooperativity arises because the formation of a given hydrogen-bonded base pair greatly facilitates and strengthens the adjacent base pairs by bringing the partner bases into proximity and the correct orientation (6). As a result, the double helix "zips itself up" in a coordinated fashion, as a solution containing complementary strands is cooled through the transition temperature. This cooperativity is crucial to the biological role of DNA. In the absence of cooperativity (i.e., if the base pairs behaved completely independently), the double helix would not be stable at biological temperatures, because the Watson–Crick hydrogen bonds are individually weak. On the other hand, the cooperativity is not limited and is local rather than long-range. That is, the influence of a given base pair only extends over a few adjacent bases. If the cooperativity were much greater and longer-range, then the double helix would be held together too strongly to be melted at all. Melting is required for transcription and replication of DNA. DNA strands can also form mixed hybrid duplexes with complementary RNA. The reversible denaturation/renaturation of DNA strands forms the basis of many techniques in molecular biology, including Southern and Northern blotting, probe hybridization, and the polymerase chain reaction. Melting can begin at a free end of a double helix, where there is less opportunity for base stacking, or at an internal site, with the transient single strands stabilized by interactions with proteins, such as *single-strand binding protein*.

When the two bases of a Watson–Crick complementary pair are oriented in their favorable, hydrogen-bonded double-helical geometry, the angle between the two glycosidic bonds is only about 100°. As a consequence, the double helix has distinct "front" and "back" sides at any point along the helix. The helical twisting of these "front" and "back" sides creates the two distinct grooves of the double helix: the wide *major groove* and the narrow *minor groove* (see Fig. 2.2).

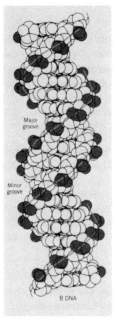

Figure 2.2. The double helix of B-form DNA. From B. Lewin, *Genes V*, Oxford University Press, 1994, Fig. 5.8 (middle panel, B-DNA), p. 121, by permission.

Although the bases are packed into the center of the helix, their edges are exposed in these grooves. The exocyclic substituents on one side of the base (e.g., the guanine O^6-keto group, adenine N^6-amino group, thymine C^5-methyl group) protrude into the major groove, while the substituents on the other side (e.g., the guanine N^2-amino group) protrude into the minor groove. The student should study the following figure:

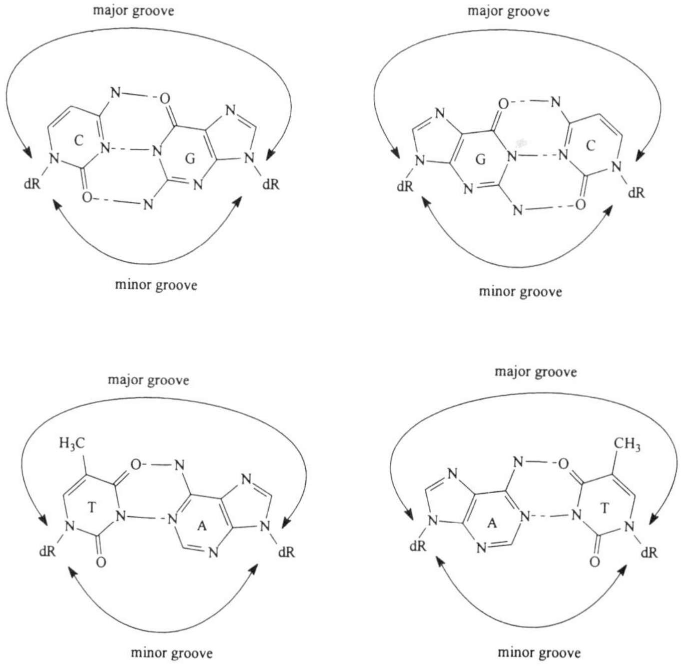

(and, if possible, a three-dimensional model of the double helix) carefully to appreciate this geometry. *The major groove is wider and much more accessible to interactions with other molecules than is the minor groove.* Consequently, the base sequence of DNA can be "read" by molecules which make chemical contacts with the protruding functional groups of the bases lining the major groove. This principle is the basis of the sequence-specific DNA interactions of restriction endonucleases, transcriptional repressors, and other DNA-binding proteins (7). (For the same reason, major groove substituents are more susceptible to chemical damage than are minor groove substituents.) Nevertheless, some proteins do make close chemical contacts with the minor groove. For example, the purine repressor PurR, in addition to making typical helix–turn–helix contacts with the major groove (8), also "pries apart" an adjacent minor groove by inserting the side chains of a pair of leucine residues (9).

RESTRICTION ENZYMES

The sequence analysis of both proteins and nucleic acids depends on the specific cleavage of long linear chains of monomer subunits into shorter chains. In the case of proteins, this is accomplished with proteolytic enzymes or reactive electrophilic chemical reagents (cyanogen bromide). These treatments make specific cuts in polypeptides, by recognizing the chemical functionalities of specific amino acid residues (basic side chains, in the case of trypsin: aromatic side chains, in the case of chymotrypsin; the nucleophilic sulfide of methionine, in the case of cyanogen bromide). Following cleavage, the fragments must be separated and sequenced. In the case of proteins, separation can be achieved by electrophoresis, and sequencing is carried out by the Edman degradation procedure. Finally, the order of the fragments is established by aligning the sequences of sets of fragments obtained by two different cleavage methods.

Until the 1970s, little progress was made in cracking the problem of DNA sequence analysis, because specific cleavage techniques were not available. Indeed, since DNA is comprised of only four different subunits (versus 21 in proteins) and chromosomal DNA molecules are far larger than any proteins, it seemed unlikely that much progress could ever be made. The situation changed dramatically with the discovery of Type II restriction endonucleases (restriction enzymes), bacterial enzymes which recognize and cleave DNA at specific sequences. The sequences recognized by restriction enzymes are 4, 6, or 8 base-pair palindromes (10), or inverted repeats.[*] That is, the sequences are the same on both strands, running in the $5' \rightarrow 3'$ sense, but in opposite directions—for example, *Xho*I, a restriction enzyme from *Xanthomonas holcicola*:

$5'$ ... C$^\downarrow$TCGAG ... $3'$

$3'$ ... GAGCT$_\uparrow$C ... $5'$

(the positions of the resulting strand breaks are indicated by the arrows).

The discovery of restriction enzymes opened the door to modern molecular biology, since it provided a tool for the cleavage (digestion) of high molecular weight DNA into specific small fragments. Hundreds of restriction enzymes, recognizing many different palindromic sequences, have been isolated from bacterial species.

GEL ELECTROPHORESIS OF NUCLEIC ACIDS

DNA fragments are easily separated by gel electrophoresis; since all DNA molecules have one negatively charged phosphate group per nucleotide, and the double-helix conformation of dsDNA varies but little, the mobility of dsDNA fragments on gels depends only on their molecular weights. In effect, DNA molecules behave just like sodium dodecyl sulfate (SDS)-denatured proteins. Using agarose as the supporting gel, DNA fragments ranging from a few hundred base pairs to a few thousand base pairs can be separated and their lengths (molecular weights) determined. (Fragments of millions of base pairs can be separated with pulsed-field electrophoresis techniques.) Polyacrylamide gel electrophoresis can be used to separate oligonucleotides (less than a few hundred base pairs) with very high resolution, for sequencing purposes.

The use of restriction enzymes and gel electrophoresis allows large DNA molecules to be cut into defined smaller pieces. Restriction enzymes recognize sequences of various lengths. For example, a restriction enzyme recognizing a 4-base sequence ("4-cutter") will encounter its target sequence approximately every 4^4 (~250) bases, along a random DNA sequence. Similarly, 8-cutters cut roughly every 4^8 (~64,000) bases, and 6-cutters cut every 4^6 (~4,000) bases. Thus by choosing the enzyme, or combination of enzymes, appropriately, even very long pieces of DNA can be cut reproducibly into smaller fragments, which are isolated by gel electrophoresis. For a very large piece of chromosomal DNA, this can be done in stages; using a 4-cutter directly would produce far more fragments than could be separated by electrophoresis. For example, first an 8-cutter is used; the fragments are separated, and each is cut with a 6-cutter, and so on. This process allows, in principle, the complete disassembly of the chromosome into characterized fragments.

---

[*] The sequence is not always continuous; for example, *Mst*II recognizes the sequence CCTNAGG, where N can be any base. Searchable databases of restriction enzymes and recognition sequences are available via the WorldWideWeb.

RECOMBINANT DNA

Many restriction enzymes make offset, or *staggered*, cuts in the phosphodiester bonds of the two strands, as shown above. Each of these offset strand breaks terminates with a 5'-phosphate and a 3'-OH residue. Such breaks[*] can be resealed by the action of the enzyme DNA ligase,

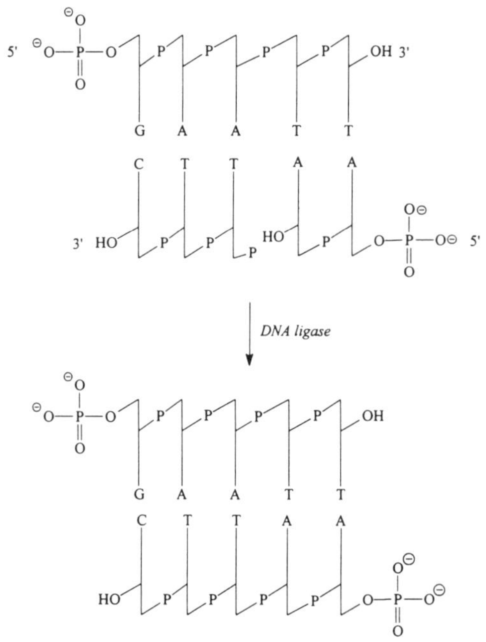

with the use of ATP free energy. Therefore, a restriction cut can be reversed, in the test tube, to regenerate the original DNA molecule. More importantly, fragments produced by the digestion of *different* DNA molecules with the same restriction enzyme can be ligated to create novel *recombinant* molecules. Since the chemical makeup of DNA from any biological source is fundamentally the same, differing only in sequence, this means that recombinant "chimeric" (11) molecules, created by the splicing together of DNA from different organisms, can be made without any fundamental limitations. This idea is the basis of all cloning techniques.

CLONING

Gene cloning refers to (a) the isolation of a desired gene in pure form and (b) its amplification, which can be carried out by the replication of a vector or by the polymerase chain reaction.

The first step in cloning a desired gene is usually the preparation of a *library*—a collection of vector DNA molecules, each bearing a piece of DNA from the organism being studied. Genomic DNA isolated from the organism is cleaved with restriction enzymes, and the fragments are ligated into a suitable vector. Bacterial plasmid vectors bear selectable marker genes (usually, antibiotic resistance genes). Plasmids can be introduced into bacteria by chemical treatment of the cells with $CaCl_2$ or by *electroporation*, the appli-

---

[*] Some restriction enzymes cut both DNA strands at the same point, producing *blunt-ended* fragments. Such fragments can also be rejoined by ligase, but much less efficiently.

cation of a brief (milliseconds) high-voltage electrical discharge to a suspension of cells (12). The presence of marker genes allows colonies bearing inserted foreign DNA to be identified or selected. The vector also incorporates an origin of replication; this allows the plasmid to be replicated along with the bacterial chromosome. Each colony, being of clonal origin, represents a specific fragment of DNA from the original digest: a "volume" from the complete gene "library." (Later, we will consider the problem of finding the *particular* volume for which we are looking.)

Bacteriophages (viruses) are also used as vectors. A central portion of the linear genome of the *E. coli* bacteriophage λ is not required for replication of the phage in the bacterial host. This section is excised from the linear phage genome by restriction enzyme digestion, and the "left" and "right" arms of the genome are isolated. Recombinant phage DNA, bearing inserted foreign DNA, is produced by restriction enzyme digestion of the foreign DNA, followed by ligation with the bacteriophage "arms." Only recombinant phage DNA bearing foreign inserts of suitable size can be packaged successfully into phage heads, in vitro. The resulting recombinant phage particles are then grown as plaques on a lawn of *E. coli*.

cDNA Cloning

Rather than cloning genomic DNA, messenger RNA isolated from the cytoplasm of any tissue can be used as a template for the synthesis of complementary DNA (cDNA), by the action of the enzyme *reverse transcriptase* (13). The cDNA can then be introduced into a vector and cloned. The use of cDNA libraries has important advantages over genomic cloning. First, the messenger RNA for a protein molecule produced in large abundance by a specific cell type or tissue will be present in very many copies per cell. The genomic DNA sequence, in contrast, is present only once (or twice, in a diploid cell). So, if we wish to isolate the gene encoding the subunits of hemoglobin, for example, the population of cDNAs prepared from reticulocytes (immature red blood cells) should be dominated by the desired gene. This enrichment facilitates isolation of the desired clone.

Second, the cloning of cDNA allows the coding sequence to be obtained without interruption by *introns*. The existence in eukaryotic genomic DNA of introns, a completely unexpected phenomenon, was revealed by the first experiments with eukaryotic genomic cloning (14). The coding DNA sequences for most eukaryotic proteins are not contiguous sequences on the chromosome. Rather, they are divided into several distinct pieces, known as *exons*, and separated by noncoding regions (*introns* or intervening sequences). In some cases, the exons correspond to particular domains of protein structure. The primary transcript, synthesized by the action of RNA polymerase in the cell nucleus, is *spliced* before it is used as a template for protein synthesis (translation). *Splicing* refers to the cleavage and ligation of the primary RNA transcript, removing the introns, and connecting the exons into the processed and mature RNA. Splicing is catalyzed by enzymatic machinery which recognizes specific consensus sequences at or near the intron–exon junctions. In some cases, more than one pattern of splicing may occur with a single molecular species of primary transcript (*alternative splicing*), allowing variant mature RNAs, and hence variant proteins, to be synthesized from a single gene (15).

Most processed eukaryotic mRNA molecules are also modified by the addition of a "poly-A tail": a series of consecutive A residues at the $3'$ end. The biological role of this tail is not clear, but it provides the basis for the convenient isolation of mRNAs on the basis of their binding to a polyT affinity column.

Bacterial genes do not contain introns. Perhaps, introns evolved after the appearance of the eukaryotic cell. More probably, all primitive genes were assembled from the "shuffling" of a primitive set of exons, separated by noncoding introns; bacteria later lost the intron sequences under the selective pressure of achieving the smallest possible genome and, hence, the most rapid possible replication and cell division (16).

Since the exons of a specific gene may be distributed over a long stretch of DNA, separated by long introns, a genomic clone often contains only a portion of the desired gene.

SOUTHERN AND NORTHERN BLOTTING

DNA strands can be separated by heating, and they will reanneal to form complementary dsDNA if allowed to cool gently. As Sol Spiegelman first demonstrated, RNA–DNA hybrid molecules can also be formed. The molecular recognition of one strand of nucleic acid by a complementary strand forms the basis of the techniques of Southern and Northern blotting.

In the Southern technique (named after its inventor, Edwin Southern), DNA molecules (usually, the fragments generated by restriction enzyme digestion of chromosomal DNA) are separated by gel electrophoresis, denatured (by soaking the gel in 0.5 M NaOH), and then transferred from the gel to a sheet of nitrocellulose (by "sandwiching" the gel against the sheet, followed by capillary or electrophoretic transfer). The nitrocellulose sheet is then incubated with a *probe*. A probe is a denatured (ss) DNA (or, in some applications, RNA) fragment which has been labeled (e.g., by radioactive labeling with ^{32}P). Probes can be made from homologous genes, already in hand, or can be synthesized chemically (see sidebar on page 28). The probe will anneal to bands on the gel where complementary fragments exist, and these bands can then be visualized by autoradiography. This process allows the presence of specific sequences to be detected, even in a digest containing fragments representing the entire genome. This specificity is analogous to the ability of an antibody to detect an antigen with high specificity and sensitivity, even in a very complex sample. In both cases the techniques's success derives from the specificity and high affinity of molecular recognition: by complementary nucleic acid strands, in one case, and by antibody-antigen binding, in the other.

Once a gene has been cloned from a given source (say, the rat genome), Southern blotting can be used to verify the presence in other samples (say, the genomic DNA of other mammals) of homologous genes.

Another important application of Southern blotting is *restriction fragment length polymorphism* (RFLP) analysis. Suppose we compare the Southern blots from two different organisms: One is wild-type for a particular gene, and the other bears a mutation. If the mutation is due to a large deletion or insertion in the gene of interest, then a comparison of the Southern blots may show a distinct shift in the position of the bands hybridizing with a probe for the gene. Alternatively, if the mutation is a base substitution at a site recognized by a particular restriction enzyme, in the wild-type sequence, then the mutant will lack this restriction site. A digest prepared with this restriction enzyme will show a band shift. (Heterozygotes would show two bands.) An illustration of this principle, as applied to the molecular diagnosis of the genetic disease sickle-cell anemia, is shown below:

β Hemoglobin	DNA Sequence	Protein Sequence
A (normal)	*CCT GAG G*AG MstII site	-pro-glu-glu-
S (sickle-cell mutant)	*CCT GTG G*AG No MstII site	-pro-val-glu-

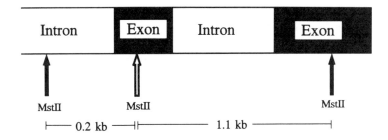

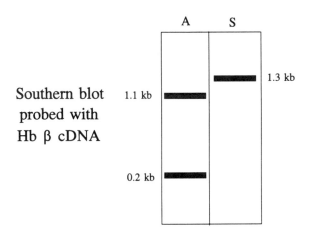

Southern blot
probed with
Hb β cDNA

The analysis of RFLPs is a key technique for mapping the human genome, positional cloning of disease genes (see below), and forensic applications (genetic fingerprinting) (17).

Northern blotting is an analogous technique, applied to RNA, and named as a pun on Southern blotting. mRNA is isolated from a tissue of interest and is separated by gel electrophoresis. The molecular weights of mRNA are typically a few kilobases. The RNA is transferred from the gel to nitrocellulose and is probed with DNA or RNA, as discussed before. The Northern blot reveals the presence, and approximate amount, of message derived from the gene of interest. Therefore, the Northern blot is a powerful tool for the analysis of gene expression.

STRATEGIES FOR CLONING SPECIFIC GENES OF INTEREST

We have explained how one can construct a library representing the genome or messenger RNA of a cell. But this library does not come with a card catalogue: How can one identify the particular clone (i.e., the gene) corresponding to a particular protein or enzyme activity? This is the key problem in applying molecular biological methods to the analysis of particular biochemical questions. Many strategies have been used.

If a purified protein is already in hand and has been (at least partially) sequenced, then a specific *DNA probe* for the corresponding gene can be designed. Hybridization is then used to pick out the desired clone. The genetic code is *degenerate*: a one-to-many mapping of protein sequences to DNA sequences. However, the degree of degeneracy varies among the amino acid residues. Some residues are specified by only a single codon, while others are specified by up to six different codons (see sidebar on pages 28–29). In designing a probe, one seeks stretches of protein sequence rich in less-degenerate amino acid residues. A corresponding oligonucleotide probe is then synthesized. Usually, a cocktail of degenerate probes is prepared, representing all of the possible coding sequences for the target protein sequence. The probe is labeled with ^{32}P and is used to screen the library by DNA–DNA hybridization. Positive clones are isolated by examining autoradiograms for hot spots. Note that in this approach the nucleic acid sequence itself is the target of the cloning: the corresponding protein need not be expressed. Because of the ambiguity resulting from degeneracy of the genetic code, along with the possibility of hybridization to only partially homologous genes, positive clones can only be regarded as putative or "candidate" clones of the desired gene, and further analysis of many such candidates (for example, by expression of the protein product) is usually required to verify that the desired gene has been cloned.

The physical principle underlying this technique is that the thermodynamic stability of a DNA duplex increases with its length, up to a limit, due to the cooperativity of base-pairing interactions (see above) and is weakened by the presence of any mismatches. At an appropriate temperature the target gene (complementary to the probe) will anneal, and mismatched, nontarget sequences will not. How long must a probe be, to identify a desired gene without ambiguity? The number of possible sequences of length L is 4^L. In a random piece of DNA of length C the number of possible target sites for annealing is $2C$, since annealing can occur to either strand. Thus, a sequence of length L, where $4^L = 2C$, should occur only about once in the genome. In practice, an oligonucleotide probe of about 20 bases length is usually sufficient to identify a given gene in a mammalian genome (18). Beyond this length, little additional duplex stabilization energy is gained, because the cooperativity of base-pairing is relatively short-range (see above).

SIDEBAR: DNA OLIGONUCLEOTIDES CAN BE SYNTHESIZED CHEMICALLY

Oligodeoxynucleotides can be synthesized conveniently by the phosphoramidite method. Nucleotide 3′-phosphoramidites are coupled to the 5′ end of the growing strand (the direction of strand growth is opposite to that of biochemical polymerization of nucleic acids), yielding phosphite triesters. These are converted to the natural phosphate triesters by iodine oxidation (19). Oligodeoxynucleotide synthesis is now a simple, automated procedure, and it is used routinely to prepare desired ssDNA fragments for use as probes or synthesis primers. Complementary ssDNA fragments prepared in this manner can be annealed to give dsDNA fragments.

SIDEBAR: CLONING FROM THE PROTEIN SEQUENCE: DESIGNING A PROBE BASED ON A KNOWN AMINO ACID SEQUENCE

The sequence is scanned for clusters of preferred residues. The preferred residues are (a) Met and Trp (1 codon each) and (b) Phe, Asp, Asn, Glu, Tyr, Gln, His, Lys, and Cys (2 codons each). The residues to be avoided are Leu, Arg, and Ser (6 codons each). For example, consider the hypothetical partial amino acid sequence . . . Phe Met Glu Trp His Lys Asn . . . :

Phe	Met	Glu	Trp	His	Lys	Asn
TTT	ATG	GAA	TGG	CAT	AAG	AAT
TTC	—	GAG	—	CAC	AAA	AAC

The corresponding degenerate mRNA sequences include

5′ TTTATGGAATGGCATAAGAAT 3′
5′ TTCATGGAATGGCATAAGAAT 3′
5′ TTTATGGAGTGGCATAAGAAT 3′
5′ TTCATGGAGTGGCATAAGAAT 3′

and so on, with a total of 32 possibilities. (For a detailed analysis of the design of oligonucleotide probes see reference 20.)

Antibody screening is an alternative strategy for identifying a clone of interest. For this strategy, the library to be screened must be composed of cells which *express the protein products of the recombinant genes*. The purified protein whose gene is sought is used as an antigen: An animal (e.g., rabbit) is immunized with the protein and antiserum is obtained. The genes in the foreign DNA library (e.g., mammalian cDNAs) are inserted into a plasmid or phage *expression vector*, such as λgt11. This phage construct carries most of the *lacZ* gene, encoding the enzyme β-galactosidase. λgt11-infected *E. coli* cells are rendered *lacZ*$^+$ and express this enzyme. When such phage plaques are grown on medium containing the synthetic β-galactosidase substrate X-gal (5-bromo-4-chloro-3-indolyl-β-D-galactopyranoside), the substrate is hydrolyzed by β-galactosidase, to produce a blue-colored product. An *Eco*RI site is present near the 3′ end of the *lacZ* gene in λgt11, so that foreign DNA can be inserted. The recombinant phage plaques can be identified easily, since insertion of the foreign DNA disrupts the *lacZ* gene; the infected cells are *lac*$^-$ and therefore produce colorless plaques.

If foreign DNA is inserted in the correct orientation and reading frame (one chance in six), a *fusion protein* of β-galactosidase and the foreign protein will be synthesized in the infected *E. coli* host. In most cases, this fusion protein will retain epitopes required for antibody binding to the foreign protein and therefore will be recognized by the antiserum. Identification of the desired clones can then be attempted, based on the specific binding of antibody. The methods are analogous to those used in Western blotting (discussed earlier).

The technique of *subtractive hybridization* is used to prepare libraries enriched with genes which are differentially expressed in two different cell types or tissues (A and B). mRNA is prepared from both tissues. Single-stranded cDNA copies are prepared from cell type A mRNA. This cDNA preparation is mixed with cell type B mRNA. Those mRNAs expressed in both cell types will form dsRNA–DNA hybrids; cDNAs expressed only in cell type A will remain single-stranded. Hydroxylapatite chromatography is used to separate the ds molecules (which bind to the column) from ss molecules, which are eluted. The eluted cDNAs represent a population enriched in genes expressed specifically in cell type A.

Complementation of function is a cloning strategy applicable even in the absence of a purified target protein, *if one can select for the biological function of the expressed pro-*

tein. For example, consider a mutant *E. coli* strain which is auxotrophic for a particular amino acid; that is, unlike the wild type, the mutant can only grow when supplied with this amino acid. The auxotrophy probably results from a mutation causing loss of function of an enzyme in the biosynthetic pathway for that amino acid. This mutant strain can be transformed with plasmids carrying genes from a library prepared from wild-type *E. coli* (or another organism). The transformants are plated onto minimal medium, in the absence of the amino acid required by the mutant. Only those cells in which the chromosomal gene (encoding the defective enzyme) is complemented by the corresponding wild-type gene (carried on the plasmid) will be able to grow and form colonies.

The same approach can be extended to selection of mammalian cells. We will discuss some successful applications of this strategy later in this book. For example, *oncogenes* (derived, for example, from tumorigenic viruses) confer the "transformed" phenotype (uncontrolled growth in tissue culture) on certain mammalian cell lines. The cloning of such genes can be performed by selecting, in culture, for the rapid-growth phenotype. Another example of this strategy is the cloning of genes encoding DNA repair enzymes. Cell lines defective in DNA repair (i.e., not expressing the functional repair enzyme) are often highly sensitive to killing by radiation or mutagenic chemicals. This sensitivity may be complemented by expression of a recombinant gene encoding the missing enzyme.

The genes responsible for many human genetic diseases, including cystic fibrosis and Huntington's disease, have been cloned by a purely molecular genetic strategy, without any knowledge of either the sequence or function of the target protein. The basis of this approach is genetic mapping: Analysis of the inheritance patterns of the gene in family pedigrees permits assignment of the location of the gene to a particular human chromosome. More precise mapping is accomplished by studying the linkage between the disease gene and other known polymorphisms (marker genes) on the chromosome, as well as by additional techniques such as chromosome walking; these specialized techniques will not be discussed further here.

In some cases the gene responsible for the disease, when finally captured, turns out to code for a known gene product, whose relationship with the disease was unsuspected. This is illustrated by the recent discovery that the gene for familial amyotrophic lateral sclerosis encodes Cu, Zn-superoxide dismutase (see Chapter 4).

DNA SEQUENCES CAN BE DETERMINED

The discovery and application of restriction enzymes and the development of cloning vectors (and, later, the PCR) allowed particular DNA fragments to be isolated and amplified. In the mid-1970s, several methods for the sequencing of DNA were developed, permitting the analysis of gene structure to be extended to the very finest level of resolution. The principles behind the two most commonly used sequencing methods will be presented here. Both of these methods generate four (one per base) collections of DNA fragments, whose lengths correspond to the positions of each of the four bases in the sequence. The fragment lengths are then analyzed by gel electrophoresis, taking advantage of the ability of this technique to (a) separate fragments according to their lengths and (b) resolve fragments which differ by only a single base pair in length.

In the Maxam–Gilbert (or chemical cleavage) method (21) the DNA to be sequenced is first labeled at one 5′ end by treatment with T4 polynucleotide kinase and $[\gamma\text{-}^{32}\text{P}]\text{ATP}$. (If dsDNA is used, *both* 5′ ends will be labeled; the product must then be restriction enzyme digested, so that a fragment labeled at one end only can be separated by agarose gel electrophoresis.) The labeled fragment is divided into four aliquots and subjected to each of four chemical treatments (see below). These treatments are designed to modify each of the bases (or pairs of bases, in some cases), remove the modified base by cleaving the glycosidic bond, and create a single-strand break at this site. The reactant is limited, so that only one site in 100 or so is attacked. Thus, for example, the "G" tube will contain a series of "nested" fragments, each beginning with the 5'-end label and extending to a "G" site on that labeled strand. Finally, the four reaction mixes are run in parallel lanes on a polyacrylamide gel; the 5'-end labeled fragments are detected by autoradiography, and the lengths of the fragments are assigned, by reading sequentially up the gel, from the smallest to the largest fragments. The sizes of the fragments for each lane indicate where the strand breaks occurred and, in turn, indicate the locations of that particular base.

CHEMICAL CLEAVAGES

The key to the success of this approach is the design of base-specific strand cleavage chemistry. These reactions are of particular interest to the student of toxicology, since each reaction represents a form of DNA damage. Indeed, one of the ingredients in the development of the chemical cleavage method was the work of Brookes and Lawley on DNA damage by alkylating agents. In the early 1960s, they observed that alkylated purine residues have labile glycosidic bonds. A decade previously, Erwin Chargaff and his colleagues had prepared "apurinic acid" by the acid-catalyzed hydrolysis of the glycosidic bonds of purine bases in DNA; they also showed that the phosphodiester bonds of apurinic acid, in contrast to those of DNA, are hydrolyzed by subsequent alkali treatment.

Walter Gilbert and his group (Harvard University) were studying the specific binding of *lac* repressor protein to the *lac* operator, a specific DNA sequence upstream from the structural genes of the *lac* operon of *E. coli* (see Chapter 17). Restriction enzyme digestion was used to prepare a fragment of DNA containing the operator site. Gilbert knew that the operator site bound repressor protein with high affinity, and he reasoned that *this section of the DNA fragment should be protected from attack by reactive chemicals.* (This idea is the basis of what is now called the "footprinting" technique: The protein leaves a "footprint" on the DNA sequencing ladder.) The approach was to label one end of the fragment with ^{32}P, alkylate the DNA fragment with dimethylsulfate (either with or without repressor present), release the labile purines by heating, create strand breaks by alkaline hydrolysis, and size the fragments on a polyacrylamide gel. The repressor-binding portion of the DNA fragment could be discerned by the absence of bands on the resulting gel, when compared to the control gel (the same DNA fragment alkylated in the absence of repressor). In fact, guanines could be roughly distinguished from adenines, since the former base reacts more quickly with dimethylsulfate than does the latter. Gilbert and his co-worker Alan Maxam recognized that they had the ingredients of a DNA sequencing technique (22). To realize the potential of this idea, they needed to improve the discrimination of G from A and to develop analogous reactions for the pyrimidines. (In principle, the pyrimidine sequence can also be deduced from the locations of the purines on the complementary strand.)

The pyrimidine-specific cleavages were developed from the existing work on the chemistry of hydrazine treatment of DNA, which had been studied by Chargaff and others. Hydrazine reacts with, and fragments, the pyrimidine ring. The refinement of this chemistry into a reliable pyrimidine-specific strand cleavage reaction is discussed by Maxam (22).

The four chemical cleavage reactions are listed below (23). Note that several variations on these conditions have been used; only one version is described here.

Guanine: The alkylating agent dimethyl sulfate [(CH$_3$)$_2$SO$_4$], in basic solution, methylates the purine bases to form ^{7}MeG and a smaller amount of ^{3}MeA

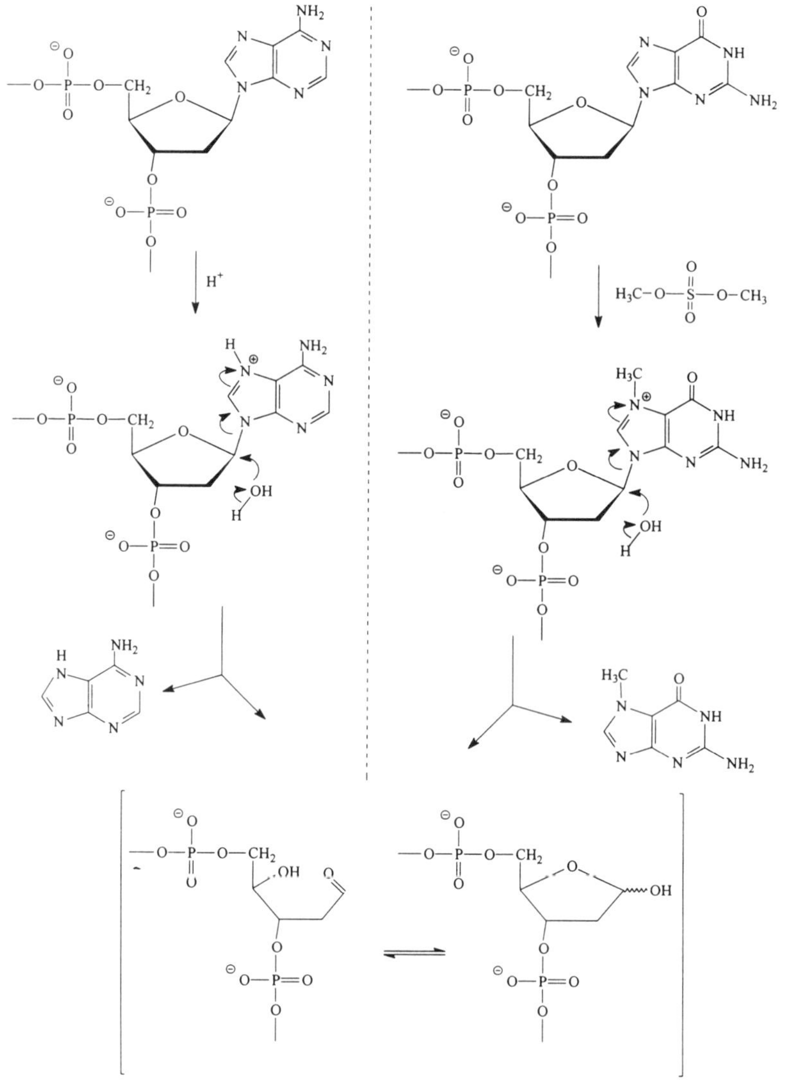

(DNA alkylation is discussed further in Chapter 16.) The positive charge on ^{7}MeG acts as an electron sink, facilitating hydrolysis of the glycosidic bond. The abasic site is converted to a strand break by subsequent treatment with piperidine (see below).

Adenine + Guanine: This cleavage is similar to the previous one, except that acid hydrolysis (pH 2) is used instead of alkylation. Adenine and guanine are both protonated and released, forming abasic sites. Adenine is determined by comparing the results of this reaction with the results of the previous one.

Cytosine + Thymine: Hydrazine attacks pyrimidines at the C-4 and C-6 positions, breaking the heterocyclic ring. The reaction scheme for cytosine is shown in

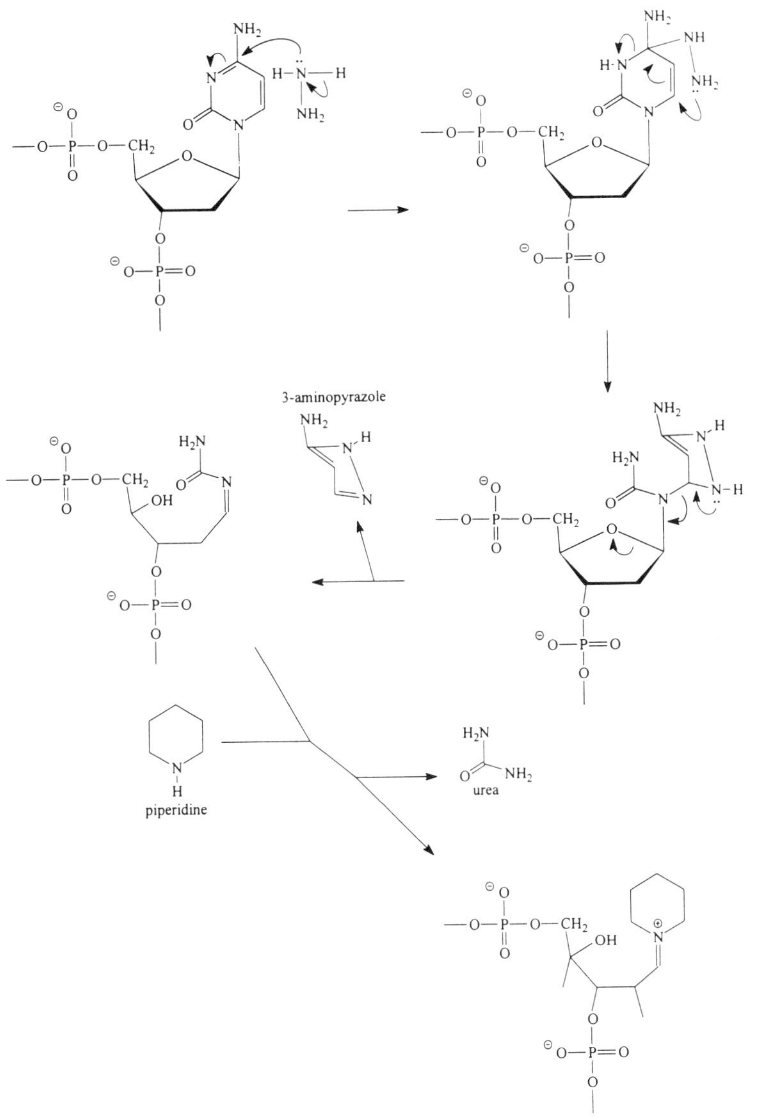

Cytosine carbons 4, 5, and 6, along with the exocyclic amino group, are released as 3-aminopyrazole. The other product is a hydrazone composed of deoxyribose (in its ring-opened form) and urea. Treatment with piperidine converts this into the piperidine hydrazone and releases urea; both phosphate ester bonds are then cleaved by β-elimination.

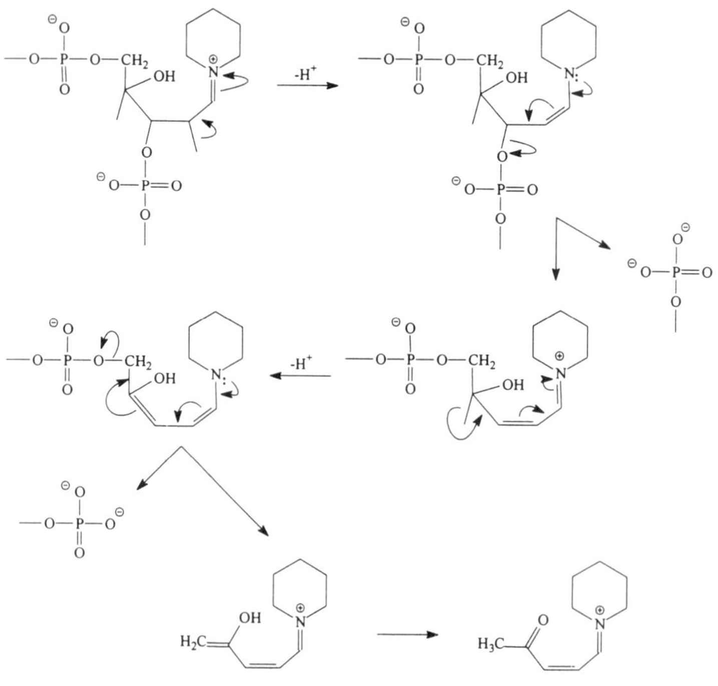

Cytosine: Maxam knew, from the chemical literature, that cytosine reacts with hydrazine slightly faster than does thymine. He observed differences in band intensities following hydrazinolysis, but he was frustrated by the irreproducibility of the intensities, which prevented him from making a clear assignment of C and T bands. Was this irreproducibility from experiment to experiment due to the salt carried over from the polynucleotide kinase labeling step? He tried adding excess salt. The thymine reaction, but not the cytosine reaction, was greatly inhibited! This was the key to distinguishing C from T. Cytosine bands are observed following high-salt hydrazinolysis; thymine is determined by comparison of the results of hydrazinolysis in the presence versus absence of salt.

While the Maxam–Gilbert approach has been replaced by the chain termination method (below) for many sequencing applications, it is still the method of choice for sequencing oligonucleotides. Also, the presence of the modified base 5-methylcytosine, which is found at specific sites in cellular DNA, can be deduced by a form of Maxam–Gilbert sequencing (24). (The biological significance of 5-methylcytosine will be discussed in Chapter 17.) The chain termination method, which analyzes a polymerase copy of the original strand, cannot be used for either of these analyses.

The chain termination approach to DNA sequencing (25) was devised by Fred Sanger of Cambridge University—20 years after his sequencing of the first peptide, insulin. These accomplishments won him two Nobel prizes: The first was for protein sequencing, and the second (shared with Gilbert) was for DNA sequencing.

The chain termination method is purely biochemical (enzymatic) in design. Rather than breaking an existing DNA strand, as in the chemical cleavage method, *a new strand is synthesized, ending at a given one of the four bases.* ssDNA is required for this method. Usually, DNA is prepared for sequencing by cloning into the ssDNA phage, M13, or by asymmetric PCR (see below).

DNA polymerase, in the presence of the four dNTPs, extends a primer strand in the

$5' \rightarrow 3'$ direction, copying a template strand. For the Sanger method, a primer strand is required. For example, if the DNA to be sequenced has been cloned into a restriction site of a *sequencing vector*, such as those derived from bacteriophage M13, then a primer complementary to the (known) vector sequence near that site can be used.

In each of the four reaction tubes (A, G, C, T), template ssDNA, primer, [α-^{32}P]dATP, all four dNTPs, and DNA polymerase are added. ([α-^{32}P]dATP will be incorporated into the newly synthesized strand, which can then be detected by autoradiography.) A small amount of a given 2',3'-dideoxynucleoside triphosphate (ddNTP) is also added. At a frequency dependent on the relative affinity of the polymerase for the ddNTP and corresponding dNTP, and their relative concentrations, the ddNTP will be incorporated into the growing strand. *The incorporated 2',3'-dideoxynucleotide blocks further chain elongation, since it lacks a 3'-OH group for addition of the next nucleotide.*

After strand synthesis, the samples are heated to separate the daughter strands, and the copied strands are run out on a gel. Each sample will have labeled strands that terminate at the location of the base *complementary* to the ddNTP used. The sequence of this strand can then be read from the four lanes of the gel.

[An entirely new approach to DNA sequencing has recently been developed. *Sequencing by hybridization* is based on the application of a solid-state "chip," onto which arrays of large numbers (e.g., 4^8) of oligonucleotides have been assembled, in a specific order. The DNA fragment to be sequenced is labeled with a fluorescent marker and hybridized to the chip. The complementary oligonucleotides on the chip are detected by fluorescence. In principle, long stretches of sequence can then be deduced, by aligning the known sequences of the hybridizing oligonucleotides (26). This approach has the great advantage of requiring no chemical or enzymatic reactions at all, but the potential of this method has yet to be explored.]

THE POLYMERASE CHAIN REACTION

"Cloning" means making many identical copies of an individual template. We have seen that gene cloning can be accomplished by inserting target DNA sequences into vectors, such as plasmids or phage. The amplification (copying) process is then carried out by the normal biological process of bacterial cell division (plasmid vectors) or virus replication (phage vectors). In the case of a plasmid, for example, we may have no interest at all in the host bacteria: They are simply a vehicle for the replication of many copies of the desired gene. Once the colony has reached sufficient size for preparation of the plasmid DNA to be practical, the cells are lysed and discarded and the plasmid is isolated.

The polymerase chain reaction (PCR) provides a purely biochemical in vitro method for the amplification of genes. The intellectual ingredients for the PCR had been present ever since the discovery of DNA polymerase in the late 1950s. Once DNA oligonucleotide synthesis became routine in the early 1980s, the PCR was an idea whose time had come. Yet, the creative insight of an imaginative individual was the spark needed to give birth to this revolutionary technique. That clear insight came to Kary Mullis of Cetus Corporation on a long automobile trip in 1983, as he "gripped the steering wheel . . . and snaked along a moonlit mountain road into northern California's redwood country" (27). In 1993, Mullis was rewarded with the Nobel Prize for Chemistry.

The polymerase chain reaction is a method for amplifying specific regions of dsDNA from a template, even in the presence of a vast number of other DNA molecules or genes. The specificity of the amplification process results from the use of two synthetic oligonucleotide primers.

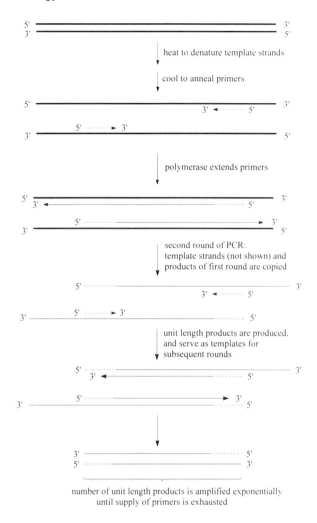

number of unit length products is amplified exponentially
until supply of primers is exhausted

The template DNA, two primer oligonucleotides, DNA polymerase, and all four dNTPs are mixed. In current protocols of the PCR, DNA polymerase from a heat-tolerant organism, such as the hot-spring bacterium *Thermus aquaticus* (*Taq* polymerase), is used; the enzyme is not denatured, even at the high temperatures required for the PCR process, and has maximum catalytic activity at ~72°C. The temperature of the incubation is raised to ~95°C to denature the template to ssDNA. Then the temperature is lowered to ~55°C, allowing the primers to anneal to the template by complementary base-pairing. The primers are located at either end of the segment to be amplified; they are designed to be complementary to opposite strands of the template and are "aimed" at each other. The temperature is increased to ~72°C; DNA polymerase now extends the primers through the target sequence. Both primers are extended in the 5' → 3' direction, of course, and thus the two primers are extended toward each other, copying the region of interest. *The key to the amplification power of the PCR is that the new copies of the target sequence, synthesized by the polymerase, serve as templates in subsequent cycles.* A large excess of both primers is added, so that replication of the templates is not limited by the availability of primers. Therefore, each successive cycle of denaturation, primer annealing, and polymerization doubles the number of copies of the target sequence present in the reaction mix. Nontarget sequences are not copied, since the required primers are not present.

With each cycle, the number of copies rises exponentially. Even if one starts with a small sample, such as a colony of bacterial cells, the amount of DNA present after, say, 30 cycles of the PCR is sufficient for direct analysis by gel electrophoresis and sequencing. PCR "machines" are commercially available; these are simply programmable heating/cooling blocks, which run through the cycles of temperature changes automatically. Each cycle lasts a few minutes.

A simple variation on the PCR technique is the *asymmetric* PCR: One primer is present in excess, but the amount of the other primer is reduced. Once the reaction has proceeded for about 20–25 cycles, the limiting primer is used up. Therefore, subsequent cycles of amplification only produce copies of one of the strands of the DNA template. From this point, amplification is only linear, not exponential, but the product is ssDNA, suitable for direct dideoxy sequencing analysis.

The PCR has many powerful applications. First, it eliminates the need for repetitive cloning in situations where the same gene is studied from many different sources. For example, as we will see when we discuss mutagenesis, we may wish to sequence a particular gene from a large number of mutant colonies (bacterial or eukaryotic), all derived from a single parental strain. Each mutant allele may be slightly different in sequence, due to the process of mutation, but the changes are unlikely to be so drastic as to interfere with primer binding. Thus the desired genes from all of the mutant colonies can be amplified simultaneously overnight, one sample per PCR tube. A similar case arises in screening clinical samples (such as blood samples) for particular genetic diseases.

The exponential growth inherent in the PCR means that exceedingly small DNA template samples can be amplified. In principle, a single molecule of dsDNA may suffice, and the practical limits of the technique are not far short of this ideal. This exquisite sensitivity has had extraordinary consequences in forensic science, since it allows genes to be amplified from vanishingly small traces of material. In combination with RFLP analysis of polymorphic human genes [such as the VNTR (variable-number tandem repeat) sequences], this may allow the identification of an individual, by comparison of the evidence sample with DNA from an authentic blood sample. Even DNA from hair, tears, or shed skin can be amplified. In 1993, one of the terrorist bombers of the World Trade Center, New York, was identified by PCR amplification of DNA in the traces of saliva remaining on the gummed envelope in which he mailed an "anonymous" letter claiming responsibility for the crime. The "genetic signature" is even more conclusive than a handwritten version.

PCR is also being used to amplify genes from the DNA of preserved museum specimens of extinct animals. Some researchers claim to have amplified DNA from ancient insects, preserved in amber (fossilized tree resin); this idea forms the basis of the far-fetched plot of the movie "Jurassic Park." If verified, this accomplishment would demonstrate that the covalent sequence of DNA can remain intact (at least over short stretches of sequence) for extraordinarily long periods of time: tens of millions of years, if the dating of the amber specimens is correct. [As of the time of writing, the case for preservation of multi-million-year-old DNA seems to be weakening (28).] The measurable rates of DNA-degrading reactions in aqueous solution (such as cytosine deamination and purine deglycosidation; see Chapter 16) would seem to rule out such ultra-long-term stability (29), but perhaps the desiccated amber environment has unexpected properties as a "DNA preservative."

Many other techniques in molecular biology have now been modified and extended by special applications of the PCR technology.

SEQUENCE DATABASES

Nucleic acid and protein sequence information is accumulating at an enormous rate, and its storage, verification, and dissemination is a major task. The development of the Inter-Net has greatly facilitated the job of obtaining sequence data, as well as other information of importance to biochemists and molecular biologists.

Several World Wide Web sites for access to biochemistry and molecular biology information now exist. An example is the ExPASy WWW server (30) at the University of Geneva. The URL for this site is http://expasy.hcuge.ch/. The ExPASy server allows users to search for sequence data on particular proteins or enzymes and is remarkably easy to use. One can also access graphic images of X-ray crystal structures of proteins, images of two-dimensional gels of proteins from various types of cells, and other valuable information.

Sequence data can also be retrieved by standard E-mail from the National Center for Biotechnology Information at the National Institutes of Health, USA. To learn how to search gene sequences by this method, send the one-line E-mail message HELP to: retrieve@ncbi.nlm.nih.gov; leave the "subject" line in the header blank. You will receive a reply containing a detailed set of instructions on use of the system.

PROTEIN EXPRESSION

Once a gene has been cloned and sequenced, the next goal is usually the construction of a recombinant system for expressing large amounts of the gene product ("overexpression") in a host cell. (*In the case of cloning via antibody screening, protein expression is necessary for the cloning of the desired gene, in the first place.*) If the host cell is different from the original source of the gene (which is the usual situation), we call this *heterologous* expression (31).

Why is protein expression a desirable alternative to purification of the protein from its original source? First, the original source may be scarce—or even extinct! Perhaps only trace amounts of the desired protein are present in the source. If we can arrange to have a bacterium or cultured cell line produce large amounts of the protein, then purification will be correspondingly easier. (In development of commercial products, such as peptide hormones or vaccines, this may be the difference between success and failure.) Second, protein expression systems based on the recombinant gene permit us to *modify the protein product.* It is relatively straightforward to introduce *site-directed mutations* into a cloned gene (32). For example, suppose we suspect that a particular *cysteine* residue is located at an enzyme's active site and that the cysteine −SH is essential for activity. We could replace the cysteine codon by a codon for *alanine*, by DNA engineering techniques. If we can express the mutant protein, we can then measure its activity and test our hypothesis. We can even splice pieces of different genes together. Many enzymes of biotransformation have two distinct binding sites: One site binds the xenobiotic substrate, and the other binds the conjugating agent (e.g., glutathione or UDP-glucuronic acid). If these binding sites are on two distinct domains of the protein, then we can experiment with *swapping* domains between two such enzymes and test the activities of these chimeric products. (We will look at experiments of this sort later on.) This can provide great insight into the relationship between protein structure and enzyme function. Third, expression allows us to study the physiological effects of the protein on the host cells, and this may give important clues to the biological role of the gene product.

Another aspect of gene transfer into eukaryotic cells is the construction of *transgenic* animals, expressing a foreign protein in some or all tissues. If foreign genes are introduced (by microinjection of DNA) into fertilized mouse egg cells, some of the offspring may have integrated the foreign DNA into their somatic cells and, possibly, their germ cells. The offspring derived from these transgenic germ cells may carry a stably integrated copy of the gene in some or all of their somatic and germ cells (33). Finally, the prospect of *gene therapy* (replacement of defective genes in patients with genetic diseases by the normal counterpart genes) depends on the introduction of the "foreign" (i.e., normal) gene into the patient's cells.

EXPRESSION IN *E. coli*

Expression strategies may be divided into two broad categories: expression in *E. coli* and expression in anything else (mainly eukaryotes). Expression in *E. coli* is usually easier. *E. coli* cells are simple (and inexpensive) to grow, even in industrial-scale quantities. Useful plasmid vectors for *E. coli* abound, and they are easily transformed into, and isolated from, the bacterial cell. *The key to protein overexpression is to ensure that large amounts of mRNA are transcribed from the sequence of interest.* This requires the use of a strong promoter (RNA polymerase binding site) sequence upstream of the desired gene. Many choices are available (34). *lac* is the promoter of the *lac* operon, and transcription is regulated under the control of the *lac* repressor in *E. coli*. A gene under the control of *lac* is expressed only when we add an inducer of the *lac* operon (usually the lactose analogue IPTG, isopropylthiogalactoside) to the cells (35). The ability to turn on protein expression, by adding IPTG, is very valuable. Many proteins are toxic to *E. coli* when expressed at high levels (they may catalyze undesirable reactions, disturb metabolic regulation, and so on). The *lac* promoter system allows one to keep synthesis of the foreign protein shut off while the *E. coli* culture grows up; once the cells have grown, we turn on production of the protein with IPTG. The cells may soon die, but we are now ready to harvest the protein.

Eukaryotic membrane-bound proteins (e.g., integral proteins of the endoplasmic reticulum membrane) can be expressed in *E. coli*. Since the bacterial cell does not contain organelles, the resulting proteins are likely to be found in the plasma membrane or to form insoluble precipitates (see below). In some cases, modification of the sequence, such as removal of the hydrophobic sequences responsible for membrane-binding, leads to synthesis of soluble, enzymatically active proteins. This strategy has recently been applied to the expression of cytochrome P-450 (36).

EXPRESSION IN EUKARYOTIC CELLS

Why should one wish to use any organism other than *E. coli* for protein expression? Some eukaryotic proteins are not translated well in *E. coli*; others are degraded rapidly. Many eukaryotic enzyme proteins are catalytically inactive when synthesized in *E. coli*, and electrophoretic or immunological analysis reveals that the expressed protein is very different from the native protein. The bacterium does not carry out many of the posttranslational modifications typical of eukaryotic cells. These may include specific disulfide bond formation, glycosidation, phosphorylation, or specific proteolysis reactions (37). Successful folding of the desired protein may depend on specific interactions with other eukaryotic proteins. Denatured or improperly folded proteins tend to accumulate as insoluble *inclusion bodies* within the bacterial cell. Many eukaryotic enzyme proteins are destined for incorporation into membranes, such as plasma membrane, inner mitochondrial membrane, or endoplasmic reticulum, and will not function properly in other environments. Finally, of course, the biological function of a eukaryotic protein is best studied in another eukaryotic cell.

Plant or animal cells are much slower-growing than bacterial cells (if they can be cultured at all) and may be finicky, requiring special media, growth factors, or serum. Yeast, on the other hand, are easily grown. *Saccharomyces cerevisiae* (bakers' yeast) has been used most often, but other yeasts, such as *Pichia pastoris*, have recently turned out to be very useful expression host cells (38). Introduction of foreign DNA into eukaryotic cells is often more difficult than in *E. coli*, especially if the cell is surrounded by a wall, as in plant and yeast cells. Unlike bacteria, eukaryotic cells do not normally harbor independent extrachromosomal genetic elements, such as plasmids. Nevertheless, many successful approaches for eukaryotic expression have been developed, in a wide range of host cells.

Viral replication depends on the introduction of viral genes into the infected cell: thus, viruses are "sensationally souped-up gene transfer vectors" (39). Following infection, viral promoters can support synthesis of very large amounts of viral transcript: They subvert the cell's protein synthesis machinery and use it to make viral, instead of cellular, proteins. This is pretty much what the experimenter wants to do, of course, so viruses are excellent tools for development of expression systems. One of the first successful approaches used the monkey (simian) tumor virus SV40 (originally isolated from Rhesus monkey cells), which replicates to a high copy number in monkey cells (40). The 5-kb SV40 genome encodes, among other proteins, the "large T" and "small t" antigens. T antigen must be present in the cell for viral replication to occur: T binds to the SV40 DNA replication origin.

Suppose we place the SV40 replication origin (but *not* the T antigen gene) on a plasmid, along with the gene of interest and a (eukaryotic) promoter (41). The plasmid is then introduced into the cultured monkey cell, by transfection or electroporation (42). Since the SV40 virus will not replicate in the absence of T antigen, a special host cell is required. *COS cells* are derived from the African green monkey kidney CV-1 cell line, transformed with an origin-defective SV40 virus (COS stands for **C**V-1 **o**rigin-defective **S**V40). That is, the cells carry an integrated SV40 genome on their chromosomes, but the replication origin is absent. The COS cells do not produce virus, but they *do* produce T antigen. When a plasmid bearing the SV40 origin is taken up, the "fuse" and the "bomb" are "connected," and the plasmid is replicated just as if it were a virulent SV40 genome. As many as 10^5 copies per cell of the vector may be synthesized, and transcription of the gene of interest may support synthesis of a large amount of the protein. Within a few days, the host cell dies, presumably due to the toxic effects of all this replication, so this system cannot be used to establish permanent cell lines expressing the heterologous gene: It is a *transient* expression system.

Another, increasingly popular, viral expression system is based on *baculovirus*, which grows on certain insect cell lines. The baculovirus coat protein is produced at extremely high levels after infection. Foreign genes can be inserted in place of the coat protein gene, under control of the coat protein promoter (43). This system is now being used to produce, for example, gp 160, the product of the *env* gene of HIV, for possible therapeutic use as an AIDS vaccine (38).

STABLE EXPRESSION SYSTEMS

For some purposes, we would prefer to achieve *stable*, rather than transient, expression of the desired gene. Foreign DNA introduced into mammalian cells is usually lost, but it occasionally integrates (more or less randomly) into a chromosome. Vectors based on retroviruses, which integrate into mammalian cell DNA as part of their life cycle, have been designed to facilitate integration (44). However, the random pattern of integration of foreign DNA means that, even if a strong promoter is used, the level of expression which will be obtained is hard to predict.

How can the successfully transformed cells be selected? One way is to link the gene of interest to a *selectable marker* gene, such as the bacterial gene for the enzyme *aminoglycoside 3'-phosphotransferase*, which confers resistance to the antibiotic *neomycin*. The parental cell line is neomycin-sensitive, so transformed cells can be selected for growth in the presence of the antibiotic.

In fact, the need to link the selectable marker and the desired gene can be avoided. Although foreign DNA is taken up at low frequency by cultured mammalian cells, the few cells that actually do so are good at it! Cells are transfected with the plasmid bearing the gene of interest and, *simultaneously*, with a much lower amount of a second plasmid, bearing the selectable marker gene. The odds are good that the antibiotic-resistant cells will also have taken up and integrated the vector bearing the desired gene. Suitable cells can be found by screening clones—for example, with an antibody to the protein of interest—and used to establish permanent cell lines.

Inducible promoters have also been developed to allow regulated expression. For example, genes under control of the promoter of the metallothionein gene are induced following exposure of the cells to Cd^{2+}, which normally induces metallothionein, a protein which chelates heavy metals (45).

NOTES

1. Stryer, L., Exploring genes, in *Biochemistry*, 4th ed., W. H. Freeman, New York, 1995, Chapter 6; Voet, D., and Voet, J. G., *Biochemistry*, 2nd ed., Wiley, New York, 1995, Chapter 28.
2. Gates, F. L., A study of the bactericidal action of ultraviolet light. III. The absorption of ultraviolet light by bacteria, *J. Gen. Physiol.* 14:31–42, 1930.
3. McCarty, M., *The Transforming Principle: Discovering that Genes Are Made of DNA*, Norton, New York, 1985.
4. Cantor, C. R., and Schimmel, P. R., *Biophysical Chemistry, Part I: The Conformations of Biological Macromolecules*, W. H. Freeman, San Francisco, 1980, pp. 182ff.
5. Freifelder, D., *Physical Biochemistry*, 2nd ed., W. H. Freeman, New York, 1982, pp. 508–510.
6. Freifelder, D., *Physical Biochemistry*, 2nd ed., W. H. Freeman, New York, 1982, pp. 21–22.
7. Lehninger, A. L., Nelson, D. L., and Cox, M. M., *Principles of Biochemistry*, 2nd ed., Worth Publishers, New York, 1993, pp. 948ff.
8. Branden, C., and Tooze, J., *Introduction to Protein Structure*, Garland Publishers, New York, 1991, Chapter 7.
9. Schumacher, M. A., Choi, K. Y., Zalkin, H., and Brennan, R. G., Crystal structure of LacI member, PurR, bound to DNA: Minor groove binding by α helices, *Science* 266:763–770, 1994.
10. In the "single-stranded" English language, a palindrome is a string of text that reads the same both forward and backwards ("A man, a plan, a canal: Panama"). DNA palindromes are analogous, but refer to the sequences on the two complementary strands.
11. Chimera: "The word has of course come to mean an unreal, monstrous creation of the imagination; but you will recall that the classical chimera was a monster of a rather special type. It

had the head of a lion, the body of a goat, and a serpent's tail. That is to say, it could exist only in dreams, being composed of elements which could not possibly be joined together in the real world." (Salman Rushdie, *Imaginary Homelands*, Granta Books, London, 1991, p. 63.)

12. Solioz, M., and Bienz, D., Bacterial genetics by electric shock, *Trends Biochem. Sci.* 15:175–177, 1990.

13. Lehninger, A. L., Nelson, D. L., and Cox, M. M., *Principles of Biochemistry*, 2nd. ed., Worth Publishers, New York, 1993, p. 994.

14. Witkowski, J. A., The discovery of split genes: a scientific revolution, *Trends Biochem. Sci.*, March 1988.

15. Smith, C. W., Patton, J. G., and Nadal-Ginard, B., Alternative splicing in the control of gene expression, *Annu. Rev. Genet.* 23:527–577, 1989.

16. Gilbert, W., Genes in pieces revisited, *Science* 228:823–824, 1985.

17. Nowak, R., Forensic DNA goes to court with O. J., *Science* 265:1352–1354, 1994; Nowak, R., How DNA fingerprinting is done, *Science* 265:1353–1353, 1994.

18. Sambrook, J., Fritsch, E. F., and Maniatis, T., *Molecular Cloning*, 2nd. ed., Cold Spring Harbor Laboratory Press, Cold Spring Harbor, NY, 1989, Sections 11.5–11.6.

19. Voet, D., and Voet, J. G., *Biochemistry*, 2nd ed., Wiley, New York, 1995, pp. 896–897.

20. Sambrook, J., Fritsch, E. F., and Maniatis, T., *Molecular Cloning*, 2nd ed., Cold Spring Harbor Laboratory Press, Cold Spring Harbor, NY, 1989, Chapter 11; Lathe, R., Synthetic oligonucleotide probes deduced from amino acid sequence data: theoretical and practical considerations, *J. Mol. Biol.* 183:1–12, 1985.

21. Maxam, A. M., and Gilbert, W., A new method for sequencing DNA, *Proc. Natl. Acad. Sci. USA* 74:560–564, 1977.

22. Maxam, A. M., Nucleotide sequence of DNA, in: *Methods of DNA and RNA Sequencing*, Weissman, S. M., Ed., Praeger Publishers, New York, 1983, pp. 113–164.

23. See also Voet, D., and Voet, J. G., *Biochemistry*, 2nd ed., Wiley, New York, 1995, pp. 888–892; Sambrook, J., Fritsch, E. F., and Maniatis, T., *Molecular Cloning*, 2nd ed., Cold Spring Harbor Laboratory Press, Cold Spring Harbor, NY, 1989, pp. 13–78ff.

24. Ohmori, H., Tomizawa, J., and Maxam, A. M., Detection of 5–methylcytosine in DNA sequences, *Nucl. Acids Res.* 5:1479–1485, 1978.

25. Sanger, F., Nicklen, S., and Coulson, A. R., DNA sequencing with chain-terminating inhibitors, *Proc. Natl. Acad. Sci. USA* 74:5463–5467, 1977.

26. Stryer, L., *Biochemistry*, 4th ed., W. H. Freeman, New York, 1995, p. 126.

27. Mullis, K. B., The unusual origin of the polymerase chain reaction, *Sci. Am.* 262(4): 56–65, April 1990.

28. Williams, N., Ancient DNA: The trials and tribulations of cracking the prehistoric code, *Science* 269:923–924, 1995.

29. Lindahl, T., Instability and decay of the primary structure of DNA, *Nature* 362:709–715, 1993.

30. Appel, R. D., Bairoch, A., and Hochstrasser, D. F., A new generation of information retrieval tools for biologists: The example of the ExPASy WWW server, *Trends Biochem. Sci.* 19:258–260, 1994.

31. Godowski, P. J., and Henner, D., Eds., Protein overproduction in heterologous systems, in *Methods, A Companion to Methods in Enzymology* Vol. 4, number 2, Academic Press, New York, 1992.

32. Stryer, L., *Biochemistry*, 4th ed., W. H. Freeman, New York, 1995, pp. 139–140.

33. Watson, J. D., et al., *Recombinant DNA*, 2nd ed., W.H. Freeman, New York, 1992, Chapter 14 and pp. 478ff.

34. Das, A., Overproduction of proteins in *E. coli*: vectors, hosts, and strategies, *Meth. Enzymol.* 182:93–112, 1990.

35. Stryer, L., *Biochemistry*, 4th ed., W. H. Freeman, New York, 1995, p. 950.

36. Waterman, M. R., Heterologous expression of cytochrome P-450 in *Escherichia coli*, *Biochem. Soc. Trans.* 21:1081–1085, 1993.

37. Sambrook, J., Fritsch, E. F., and Maniatis, T., *Molecular Cloning*, 2nd ed., Cold Spring Harbor Laboratory Press, Cold Spring Harbor, NY, 1989, p. 16.3.

38. Hodgson, J., Expression systems: a user's guide, *Bio/Technology* 11:889–893, 1993.
39. Watson, J. D., et al., *Recombinant DNA*, 2nd ed., W. H. Freeman, New York, 1992, p. 223.
40. Lewin, B., *Genes IV*, Oxford University Press, New York, 1990, p. 774.
41. Sambrook, J., Fritsch, E. F., and Maniatis, T., *Molecular Cloning*, 2nd ed., Cold Spring Harbor Laboratory Press, Cold Spring Harbor, NY, 1989, pp. 16.5ff.
42. Sambrook, J., Fritsch, E. F., and Maniatis, T., *Molecular Cloning*, 2nd ed., Cold Spring Harbor Laboratory Press, 1989, pp. 16.30ff.
43. Watson, J. D., et al., *Recombinant DNA*, 2nd ed., W. H. Freeman, New York, 1992, Fig. 12-12.
44. Lehninger, A. L., Nelson, D. L., and Cox, M. M., *Principles of Biochemistry*, 2nd ed., Worth Publishers, New York, 1993, p. 1006; Bradley, M. K., Overexpression of proteins in eukaryotes, *Meth. Enzymol.* 182:112–132.
45. Stryer, L., *Biochemistry*, 4th ed., W. H. Freeman, New York, 1995, p. 138.

3

BIOLOGICAL OXIDATIONS

Life first evolved by a process of chemical synthesis of complex organic molecules, probably driven by atmospheric electrical discharges or other geological sources of energy and possibly catalyzed by surface active materials, such as clays. The prebiotic assembly of relatively complex biochemical building blocks from simple precursors can be simulated experimentally, following the classic work of Stanley Miller, Melvin Calvin, and others in the early 1950s (1). The key to success in such experiments is the use of a highly reductive environment, dominated by gases such as ammonia and methane. Of course, the atmospheres of nonterrestrial planets have similar compositions. (In an oxidizing atmosphere, energetic discharges would cause combustion of organic materials to carbon dioxide, rather than synthetic processes.) Therefore, it is generally accepted that life began in an anaerobic environment. Oxygen arose at a later epoch, following the evolution of photosynthesis. The atmosphere of the earth today is, as far as we know, unique in being made up largely of molecular oxygen and nitrogen. This store of molecular oxygen represents a vast reservoir of free energy, which is consumed by oxidation processes and replenished by solar energy via photosynthesis.

The transformation of the atmosphere from reductive to oxidative conditions presented a new opportunity for life on earth, as well as a great threat. Oxidation of organic compounds could be exploited for the release of free energy far in excess of that yielded by anaerobic (fermentative) processes—if this energy could be harnessed and stored in a biologically usable form. But uncontrolled oxidation threatened the integrity of biomolecules. The peculiar chemical properties of the oxygen molecule permitted the development of biochemical processes which could realize the opportunity without succumbing to the threat: playing with fire without getting burned. Aerobic organisms thrived, while anaerobic organisms retreated to a few anoxic sanctuaries, such as the mammalian intestinal tract.

Although it may seem odd to treat oxygen as a toxic molecule, experimental evidence proves that it is. Obligate anaerobe bacteria are (by definition) only able to grow in the absence of oxygen, and most are killed by exposure to oxygen. (This group includes many pathogens, such as *Clostridium*.) Oxygen is also toxic to higher organisms. Exposure of a rodent to pure oxygen (1 atmosphere partial pressure) results in death within a few days, primarily due to lung damage. As we shall see, all aerobic organisms must deal with the toxic consequences of the formation of partially reduced oxygen species, and enzymatic defenses have evolved to control this hazard.

REDOX POTENTIALS

Any redox reaction

$$A_{red} + B_{ox} \rightarrow A_{ox} + B_{red}$$

is a chemical reaction of the general form

$$A + B \rightarrow C + D$$

The rate at which such a reaction will reach equilibrium depends on the rate of electron transfer in solution; in biochemical systems, such reactions are invariably enzyme-catalyzed (2). Where will the equilibrium for the reaction lie? That is, which species, B_{ox} or A_{ox}, will have a greater tendency to accept the available electrons? This is a special case of the general question of reaction equilibria. K_{eq} is determined by ΔG, the free energy change for the reaction. Free energy changes in redox reactions can be measured *electrically*.

We can write separate half-reactions:

$$A_{red} \rightarrow A_{ox} + ne^-$$
$$B_{ox} + ne \rightarrow B_{red}$$

Of course, isolated half-reactions cannot occur: a reduction must always be accompanied by an oxidation, since charge is conserved.

Here, n is the number of electrons transferred:

$$Fe^{3+} + e^- \rightarrow Fe^{2+} \qquad n = 1$$
$$NAD^+ + 2e^- + H^+ \rightarrow NADH \qquad n = 2$$
$$O_2 + 4e^- + 4H^+ \rightarrow H_2O \qquad n = 4$$

Any pair A_{ox}/A_{red} is called a *redox couple*. An *electrochemical cell* is an apparatus which allows us to separate physically the two half-reactions of a redox process. That is, the reduction and oxidation half-reactions are carried out in separate beakers or compartments; electrons flow between the compartments through a wire. This arrangement allows us to measure the "driving force" of the redox reaction (the potential difference, or "voltage"). As we will see, this potential difference is simply related to ΔG, the change in Gibbs free energy accompanying the reaction.

To rank the strengths of various oxidizing agents (i.e., their tendencies to accept electrons), we compare each one to a standard couple and measure the electrical potential difference. The generally accepted standard is the SHE (standard hydrogen electrode):

$$H_2 \rightarrow 2H^+ + 2e^-$$

We assign the potential $E_0 = 0$ to this half-cell. This is an arbitrary standard, like the 0°C point on the Celsius temperature scale. (In the earlier literature, pre-1960, other standard cells were often used.) Any other couple can be compared to this standard, at least in principle, by constructing the appropriate cell.

The concentrations of all reactants are set at 1.0 M (standard state). The potential developed by such a cell is referred to as the *standard reduction potential* of the half-reaction. (By convention, we always tabulate reduction potentials rather than oxidation potentials.) As usual in biochemistry, we set the standard state at pH = 7 rather than pH = 0; the modified potentials are indicated by E_0'. For the SHE, $E_0' = -0.42$ V.

Standard E_0' values for some important biochemical redox couples is shown in Table 3.1. The most powerful oxidants are at the top left (high E_0'), and the most powerful reductants are at the bottom right (low E_0'). Electrons "flow up" the list, toward the most positive couples—by convention, the electron charge is *negative*, and therefore electrons flow to *high* potential. Oxygen appears toward the top left of any such table, and NADH near the bottom right. A redox reaction can proceed spontaneously if $\Delta E_0'$ is > 0. (Some authors feel that it is more "natural" to have electrons "flow downhill." Therefore, some

Table 3.1. Standard Reduction Potentials of Some Important Redox Couples (25°C, pH 7.0)

Half-Reaction			E_0' (V)
$^1/_2O_2 + 2H^+ + 2e^-$	$\rightarrow$	H_2O	0.82
$NO_3^- + 2H^+ + 2e^-$	$\rightarrow$	NO_2^-	0.42
$O_2 + 2H^+ + 2e^-$	$\rightarrow$	H_2O_2	0.31
Cytochrome c $Fe^{3+} + e^-$	$\rightarrow$	Cytochrome c Fe^{2+}	0.25
$FAD + 2H^+ + 2e^-$	$\rightarrow$	$FADH_2$	-0.22
$GSH + 2H^+ + 2e^-$	$\rightarrow$	GSSG	-0.23
Cytochrome b_{558} $Fe^{3+} + e^-$	$\rightarrow$	Cytochrome b_{558} Fe^{2+}	-0.245
$NAD(P)^+ + H^+ + 2e^-$	$\rightarrow$	NAD(P)H	-0.32
$O_2 + e^-$	$\rightarrow$	$O_2^{\cdot-}$	-0.33
Ferredoxin $Fe^{3+} + e^-$	$\rightarrow$	Ferredoxin Fe^{2+}	-0.43

textbooks list redox potentials in the opposite order—that is, most negative couples at the top.)

We can use these tables to predict the electromotive force (potential difference) of any redox process. For example, can fumarate oxidize cysteine, under standard-state conditions?

Fumarate $+ 2H^+ + 2e^- \rightarrow$ Succinate	$+0.03$ V
(Cystine $+ 2H^+ + 2e^- \rightarrow$ 2 Cysteine	-0.34 V)
$\therefore$ 2 Cysteine $\rightarrow$ Cystine $+ 2H^+ + 2e^-$	$+0.34$ V
$\therefore$ **2 Cysteine + Fumarate $\rightarrow$ Cystine + Succinate**	**+0.37 V**

Thus, $\Delta E_0'$ is > 0 and the reaction can proceed spontaneously. However, the *rate* of the reaction will depend on kinetic, not thermodynamic, factors.

THE NERNST EQUATION

There is a fundamental connection between redox potential and Gibbs free energy. This is expressed by the relationship

$$\Delta G^{0'} = -n \, \mathscr{F} \, \Delta E_0'$$

Here $\mathscr{F}$ is the Faraday constant, the charge on one mole of electrons. $\mathscr{F} = 96{,}494$ coulomb mol^{-1} = 23.06 kcal V^{-1} mol^{-1}. The negative sign, again, arises from the negative charge of the electron. *Thus, redox potentials are simply Gibbs energies for redox reactions.* A knowledge of redox potentials allows us to predict whether a particular redox reaction will be thermodynamically spontaneous. Clearly, positive values of $\Delta E_0'$ correspond to negative (spontaneous) values of $\Delta G^{0'}$.

$$\textit{Since:} \quad \Delta G' = \Delta G^{0'} + \frac{RT}{nF} \ln \frac{[C][D]}{[A][B]}$$

$$\textit{Then:} \quad \Delta E' = \Delta E_0' - \frac{RT}{nF} \ln \frac{[A_{red}][B_{ox}]}{[A_{ox}][B_{red}]}$$

This relationship allows us to calculate redox potentials at nonstandard state conditions. The variation of cell potential with concentration allows us to determine concentrations of redox-active species electrochemically; this is the idea behind the pH meter, which is probably the most familiar electrochemical instrument.

SIDEBAR: HOW ARE REDOX POTENTIALS OF BIOCHEMICAL COUPLES MEASURED?

If the species involved are readily prepared, we can use electrochemistry; that is, we construct an appropriate half-cell and measure its electrical potential relative to a standard. However, preparation of an electrode capable of mediating electron transfer to the biochemical couple in solution may be difficult: Enzymes were not designed to transfer electrons to platinum wire! One approach is to add a redox-active compound such as methylene blue, which can act as a catalyst of electron transfer between the electrode and the couple. Alternatively, a chemical (nonelectrochemical) approach is possible: We measure the equilibrium constant for a redox reaction with a known couple, and we calculate $\Delta E_0'$ from $\Delta G^{0'}$. Again, a redox-active dye is useful, since the position of the equilibrium can be measured spectrophotometrically.

The reduction of oxygen to water is a process of particular interest. The overall four-step process requires four electrons: $O_2 + 4H^+ + 4e^- \rightarrow 2H_2O$. This process has a very large positive redox potential. *The reduction of oxygen to water by almost any biochemical reductant is thermodynamically favorable.* Molecular oxygen is one of a very few homonuclear diatomic molecules which exists as a *ground-state triplet*: The two highest-energy electrons occupy degenerate molecular orbitals (antibonding π^*) and have parallel spins. Therefore, the ground-state O_2 molecule has net electron spin of 1: Oxygen is paramagnetic. Consequently, the reaction of O_2 with most (diamagnetic) organic molecules and its reduction to water are hindered by spin restriction. *Molecular oxygen combines two characteristics which are often incompatible: thermodynamic potency and kinetic stability.* The energy available from the reduction of O_2 can only be released if the spin restriction on its reduction is overcome. This can be accomplished by very high temperatures (as in combustion processes), by interaction with enzymes, especially those bearing transition metal ions, or by the univalent reduction of oxygen to generate free radicals (3).

Consider the possible intermediates of the stepwise (univalent) reduction of molecular oxygen:

$$O_2 + e^- \rightarrow O_2{}^{\cdot -} \qquad \text{(superoxide anion)}$$
$$O_2{}^{\cdot -} + e^- \rightarrow H_2O_2 \qquad \text{(hydrogen peroxide)}$$
$$H_2O_2 + e^- \rightarrow OH^{\cdot} \qquad \text{(hydroxyl radical)}$$
$$OH^{\cdot} + e^- \rightarrow H_2O \qquad \text{(water)}$$

The values of these one-electron redox potentials are illustrated schematically below:

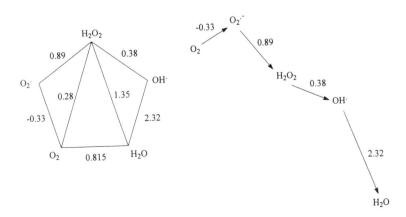

(4). This shows that the thermodynamic potential inherent in the reduction of oxygen is released mainly in the final step, reduction of the hydroxyl radical, which is an extremely potent oxidant and a highly reactive species kinetically. With respect to the reduction of oxygen to superoxide anion, oxygen is a poor oxidant; as we shall see below, superoxide is able to reduce many biochemical couples, such as cytochrome c.

SIDEBAR: HOW ARE THE REDOX POTENTIALS OF REDUCED OXYGEN SPECIES MEASURED EXPERIMENTALLY?

Hydrogen peroxide, of course, is a sufficiently stable compound to be kept in a bottle, so the redox potential for its reduction to water can be measured by conventional approaches, as discussed above. These measurements require the experimental analysis of redox processes involving the indicated species. But $O_2{}^{\cdot-}$ and $OH^{\cdot}$ are unstable free radicals, with short lifetimes in aqueous solution. Thermodynamic data on free radicals are generally scarce, compared to data on stable species, since special techniques are needed to generate and study these species (5). The redox potential of superoxide can be measured by the use of pulse radiolysis. In this method (6), a very brief (microsecond to picosecond) burst of radiation (e.g., from a linear accelerator) bombards a sample cell and generates radicals; the subsequent chemical processes (see Chapter 4, sidebar on radiolysis of water) are monitored, usually by absorption spectrophotometry. A less reliable approach is to use data for the gas-phase species, which are more stable and easier to study, and make educated guesses of the hydration energies. In the case of $OH^{\cdot}$, the values obtained by this approach proved to be misleading in the light of recent pulse radiolysis experiments, which employed the Tl^+/Tl^{2+} couple [see Stanbury (5)].

THE ROLES OF PYRIDINE AND FLAVIN COENZYMES IN BIOCHEMISTRY

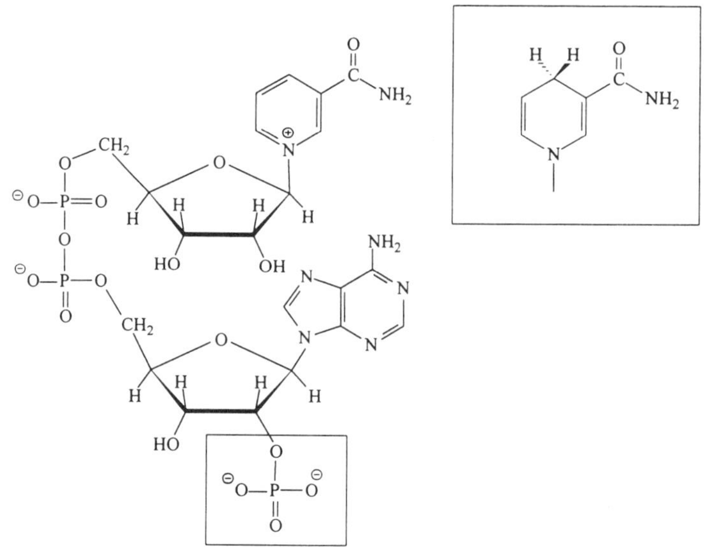

NAD(P)$^+$ and NAD(P)H

NADH/NAD$^+$ and NADPH/NADP$^+$ have almost identical redox potentials (-0.32 V); the reduced forms of these cofactors are therefore among the strongest reducing agents in the cell. Very few enzymes are able to use these two cofactors interchangeably. In most cases, NAD$^+$ is used in those reactions which conserve respiratory energy for ATP generation via the electron transport chain—for example, glyceraldehyde-3-phosphate dehydrogenase (glycolysis) and β-hydroxyacyl-CoA dehydrogenase (β-oxidation of fatty acids). In contrast, NADPH is used as a source of reducing power for biosynthetic reactions—for example, fatty acid synthase, cholesterol synthesis pathway, ribonucleotide reductase, and the cytochrome P-450 system.

Under typical cellular conditions, [NAD$^+$/NADH] is more abundant (about 1 mM) and mainly oxidized; [NADP$^+$/NADPH] is less abundant (about 0.1 mM) and mainly reduced. The maintenance of these two similar redox couples at very different redox poise, one mainly oxidized and the other mainly reduced, implies that the two couples are largely uncoupled from each other: Exchange of reducing equivalents between the two systems is slow. *This specialization of roles is essential, because cells must perform both oxidative (catabolic) and reductive (biosynthetic) tasks simultaneously.*

The nicotinamides, NAD$^+$/NADH and NADP$^+$/NADPH, are cofactors for many dehydrogenases. Generally, *these cofactors act as freely diffusible substrates*, which can associate with, and dissociate from, enzymes which use them. In contrast, the flavin cofactors, FAD/FADH$_2$ and FMN/FMNH$_2$, are usually *prosthetic groups* tightly bound to proteins to form *flavoenzymes*.

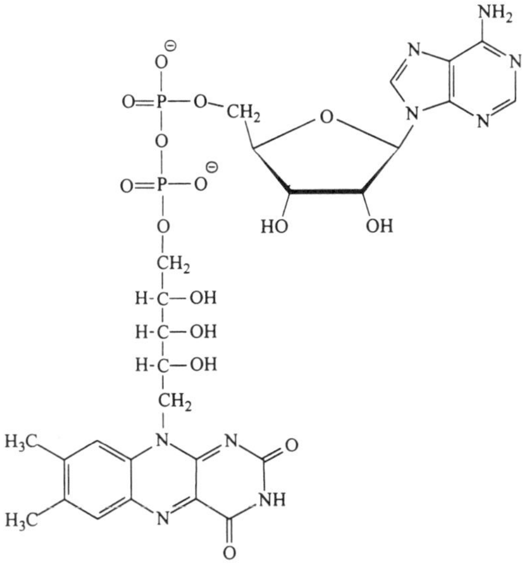

Since reduced nicotinamides are stronger reducing agents than are reduced flavins, the path of electron flow in electron-transfer systems often goes from a nicotinamide-linked dehydrogenase to a flavoenzyme.

Flavoenzymes are particularly versatile redox catalysts. If the apoprotein moiety of a flavoenzyme binds the reduced form of the flavin more tightly than the oxidized form, the protein stabilizes the *reduced* (bound) form, and the flavoenzyme will have a higher redox potential than the free flavin (the bound reduced form is a *weaker* reducing agent than the free reduced flavin). Conversely, if the protein stabilizes the *oxidized* (bound) form of the flavin more tightly, the flavoenzyme will have a lower redox potential than the free flavin (the bound reduced form is a *stronger* reducing agent than the free reduced flavin) (7). Nature exploits the strong chemical interactions between protein and cofactor to "tune" the chemical behavior of the small molecule. [*An even more striking example of this type of effect occurs in the visual transduction system: The same cofactor (11-*cis-*retinal) serves as the light-absorbing chromophore for all three protein pigments (blue, green, and red photoreceptor proteins) of color vision. The interactions with the proteins "tune" the absorbance band of the cofactor to the desired frequencies, over a range of nearly 200 nm (8).*]

Flavin coenzymes, unlike pyridine nucleotides, have relatively stable half-reduced (free radical) intermediates

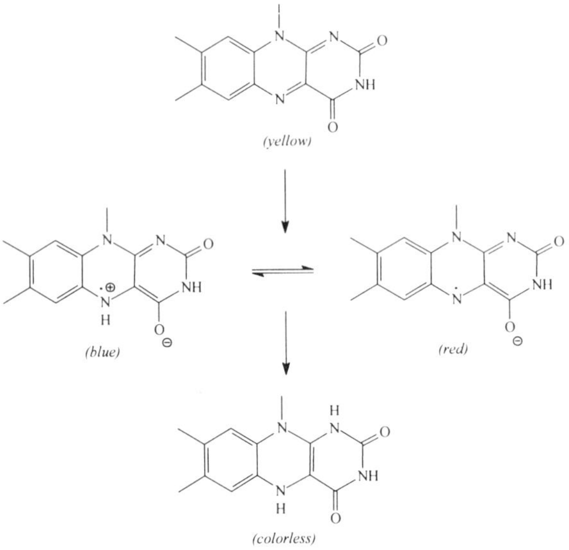

therefore, *flavoenzymes are characteristically involved in one-electron transfer processes,* such as the reduction of ferric iron in cytochromes. In many cases, the radical intermediate is sufficiently stable to be characterized spectroscopically, electrochemically (two distinct one-electron reduction potentials), or even crystallized, as in the case of flavodoxin (6).

From an inspection of the redox potentials listed in Table 3.1, we can understand the thermodynamic rationale for the commonly observed flow of reducing equivalents from nicotinamide cofactors to flavoenzymes, to cytochromes, and, finally, to the ultimate electron acceptor (e.g., oxygen). Although the *direct* transfer of reducing equivalents from strong reductants (such as NADH) to strong oxidants (such as oxygen) is thermodynamically highly favorable, *nature always chooses a stepwise path* via intermediate electron carriers: an *electron-transfer chain.* Why is this so? First, the direct route would release more free energy than can be stored in a chemical or chemiosmotic form. A weight lowered gradually on a pulley can be harnessed to do useful work (as in an old-fashioned clockworks), while the same weight, thrown from a tall building, will just make a big crater when it hits the ground. Second, as in this mechanical analogy, only the stepwise redox process can be controlled to meet changing metabolic requirements.

The most familiar electron-transport chain (although it is far from the simplest!) is that of the mitochondrion. In the mitochondrial electron transport chain, NADH is produced by dehydrogenases in the mitochondrial matrix (e.g., the citric acid cycle enzymes isocitrate dehydrogenase and malate dehydrogenase). These reducing equivalents are passed to the flavoenzyme *complex I*, then, via ubiquinone and cytochrome c, to oxygen. We will see many other electron-transport chains in the following chapters. For example, in the methemoglobin reductase system (see Chapter 8), reducing equivalents are passed from NADH to a flavoenzyme, cytochrome b_5 reductase, then to cytochrome b_5, and finally to (ferric) methemoglobin. A variation on this theme catalyzes the unsaturation of fatty acids in the fatty acyl-CoA desaturase system of the endoplasmic reticulum (10). In the microsomal cytochrome P-450 system (Chapter 14), electrons are passed from NADPH, via the flavoenzyme NADPH-cytochrome P-450 reductase, to cytochrome P-450.

OXIDATION MECHANISMS

From the time of Priestley, who discovered oxygen in the late eighteenth century, it was clear that oxidation was a fundamental life process: A mouse deprived of oxygen soon died. But the complete elucidation of the biochemical roles of oxygen has remained a challenge to the present day. With the beginnings of enzymology in the early twentieth century, it soon became clear that biochemical oxidations (such as the oxidation of ethanol to acetaldehyde to acetic acid) could occur (albeit to a limited extent) in anaerobic tissue extracts. Hence, the ultimate oxidant in such processes could not be oxygen itself. In the 1930s, Wieland proposed the now-accepted view that *enzymatic redox reactions involve transhydrogenations* (transfer of H^- equivalents) between organic donors and acceptors. We now know that the cofactors NAD^+, $NADP^+$, and FAD are the most important oxidizing agents in the reactions of intermediary metabolism. Subsequent reoxidation of the reduced forms of these cofactors by the respiratory chain is dependent on the presence of oxygen, and thus oxidative metabolism can only be maintained under aerobic conditions. (However, some bacteria can exploit alternative oxidants, such as nitrate, sulfate, and organic *N*-oxides, as terminal electron acceptors.) The Krebs (citric acid) cycle couples the complete oxidation of acetic acid (the product of carbohydrate and lipid catabolism) to carbon dioxide, with the stepwise generation of reduced cofactors, NADH and $FADH_2$. The β-oxidation of fatty acids proceeds by analogous biochemical steps. These oxidations are catalyzed by dehydrogenases:

$$MH_2 + Cofactor \rightarrow M + Cofactor \cdot H_2$$

The resulting reducing equivalents are then reoxidized in the mitochondrion, and this process provides the great majority of the energy yielded by catabolic processes.

The direct involvement of oxygen in intermediary metabolism is limited, then, to a single all-important enzymatic reaction: the reduction of oxygen to water at the final stage of the respiratory electron-transport chain. In the mitochondrion, this reaction is catalyzed by *cytochrome oxidase*. We reserve the term *oxidase* for an enzyme which catalyzes the reduction of molecular oxygen. The X-ray crystal structure of cytochrome oxidase, a huge multi-subunit protein complex, has recently been solved (9). This accomplishment should advance our understanding of the mechanism by which this enzyme carries out the reduction of oxygen to water. As discussed above, the respiratory chain must carry out the concerted four-electron reduction of oxygen. The thermodynamic value of combustion is mainly associated with the last one-electron step, and release of the intermediate products (superoxide, hydrogen peroxide, hydroxyl radical) must be avoided, as discussed later.

A few enzymes (e.g., amino acid oxidase, monoamine oxidase, glucose oxidase) reduce oxygen to hydrogen peroxide; these enzymes appear to be exclusively localized in peroxisomes, where the potential release of hydrogen peroxide into the cell is controlled by the presence of catalase.

The organization of the electron transport chain in the mitochondrial inner membrane allows the thermodynamically favorable flow of electrons (reducing equivalents) from reduced cofactors (through intermediary electron carriers) to oxygen, to be coupled to the vectorial transport of protons across the membrane. This transport establishes an electrochemical gradient and hence stores energy, in much the same manner as an electrical capacitor. According to the chemiosmotic theory, oxidative phosphorylation occurs as the return flow of protons down this electrochemical gradient is harnessed to drive the chemical conversion of inorganic phosphate and ADP into ATP.

In short, the thermodynamic value of oxygen as an electron acceptor is exploited by intermediary metabolic processes, but the chemical role of molecular oxygen is very limited: Its only interaction with metabolism is as a terminal electron acceptor.

The paradigm described in the previous paragraph remains valid for the energy-generating processes of intermediary metabolism. But a reevaluation of the role of oxygen in biochemistry was required following the discovery of the direct incorporation of oxygen atoms, from molecular oxygen, into organic substrates. This pivotal discovery was made twice in the same year, 1955. In the United States, H. S. Mason and his colleagues discovered the *monooxygenase* reaction (incorporation of one atom of oxygen from molecular oxygen into an organic substrate): the hydroxylation of a phenol derivative to give the corresponding catechol (*ortho*-dihydroxybenzene):

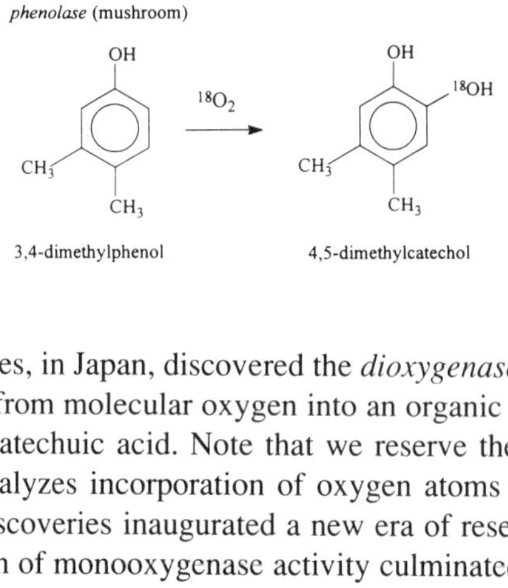

phenolase (mushroom)

3,4-dimethylphenol   4,5-dimethylcatechol

Hayaishi and his colleagues, in Japan, discovered the *dioxygenase* reaction (incorporation of both atoms of oxygen from molecular oxygen into an organic substrate): the oxidation of catechol to give pyrocatechuic acid. Note that we reserve the designation *oxygenase* for an enzyme which catalyzes incorporation of oxygen atoms from molecular oxygen into a substrate. These discoveries inaugurated a new era of research in biochemical oxidations. The investigation of monooxygenase activity culminated in the discovery of the enzyme cytochrome P-450, along with the elucidation of its central role in xenobiotic biotransformation. We will turn to a detailed consideration of cytochrome P-450 in Chapter 14.

NOTES

1. Calvin, M., *Chemical Evolution*, Oxford University Press, New York, 1969.
2. Testa, B., *Biochemistry of Redox Reactions*, Academic Press, New York, 1994.
3. Malmström, B. G., Enzymology of oxygen, *Annu. Rev. Biochem.* 51:21–59, 1982.
4. Wood, P. M., The potential diagram for oxygen at pH 7, *Biochem. J.* 253:287–289, 1988.
5. Stanbury, D. M., Reduction potentials involving inorganic free radicals in aqueous solution, *Adv. Inorg. Chem.* 33:69–138, 1989.
6. Simic, M. G., Pulse radiolysis in the study of oxgen radicals, *Meth. Enzymol.* 186:89–100, 1990; von Sonntag, C., *The Chemical Basis of Radiation Biology*, Taylor & Francis, London, 1987,

pp. 19–23; von Sonntag, C., and Schuchmann, H.-P., Pulse radiolysis, *Methods Enzymol.* 233:3–20, 1994.

7. Metzler, D. E., *Biochemistry: The Chemical Reactions of Living Cells*, Academic Press, New York, 1977, pp. 477ff.

8. Stryer, L., *Biochemistry*, 4th ed., W. H. Freeman, New York, 1995, p. 339.

9. Tsukihara, T., Aoyama, H., Yamashita, E., Tomizaki, T., Yamaguchi, H., Shinzawa-Itoh, K., Nakashima, R., Yaono, R., and Yoshikawa, S., Structures of metal sites of oxidized bovine heart cytochrome c oxidase at 2.8Å, *Science* 269:1069–1074, 1995.

10. Lehninger, A. L., Nelson, D. L., and Cox, M. M., *Principles of Biochemistry*, 2nd ed., Worth Publishers, New York, 1993, pp. 653–654.

4

SUPEROXIDE AND SUPEROXIDE DISMUTASE

THE DISCOVERY OF SUPEROXIDE DISMUTASE

The hypothesis that oxygen radicals are formed during aerobic metabolism, and that such radicals play a role in oxygen toxicity, is far from new. In the 1940s, Leonor Michaelis (best known as a founder of enzyme kinetics) proposed that respiration might proceed by one-electron steps. The connection between the action of radiation, which generates reactive oxygen radicals, and the mechanism of hyperbaric oxygen toxicity was appreciated by post–World War II radiation biologists (1). However, the breakthrough which marks the beginning of the modern era of oxygen toxicology was the discovery of the enzyme superoxide dismutase, by McCord and Fridovich, in 1968. This discovery has had profound consequences for biochemistry and toxicology, which could hardly have been envisaged at its beginnings: It is a fine illustration of the unexpected results of research driven by simple scientific curiosity. Several lines of investigation eventually converged on the discovery of superoxide dismutase and the concomitant realization of the biological significance of the superoxide radical. Let us follow one of these lines (2).

The story begins with the studies of Horecker and Heppel on the enzyme xanthine oxidase in the late 1940s. The purine nucleosides adenosine and guanosine are catabolized by convergent metabolic pathways. Adenosine is metabolized to hypoxanthine, and guanosine is metabolized to xanthine.

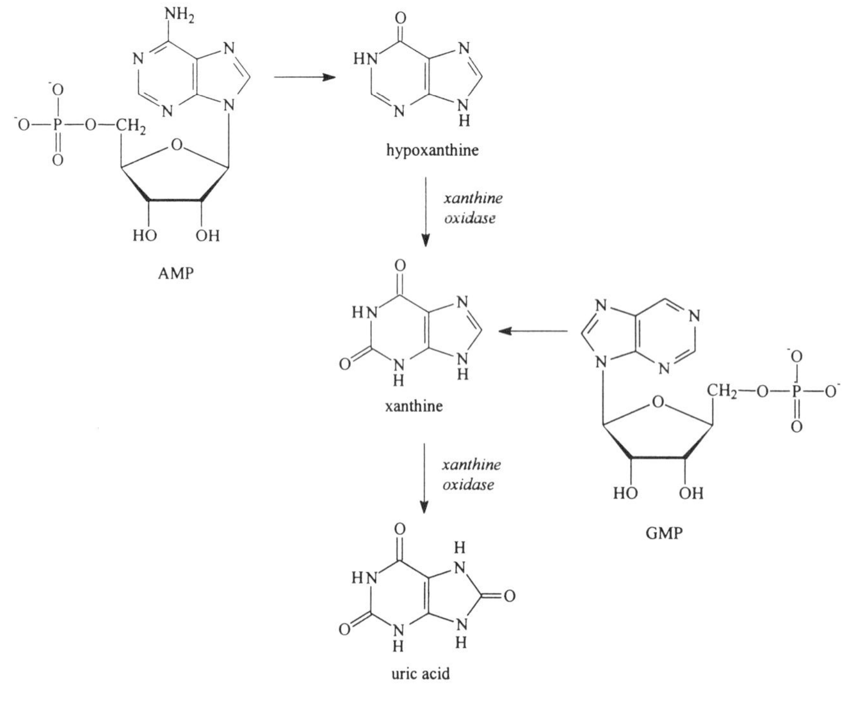

Both of these purines are converted to uric acid: hypoxanthine in two steps and xanthine in one. A single enzyme, xanthine oxidase, catalyzes the oxidation of hypoxanthine to xanthine and also catalyzes the oxidation of xanthine to uric acid.

[Uric acid is a substance of much toxicological importance. Primates, among other animals, excrete uric acid (derived from nucleic acid turnover or dietary purines) in the urine. As was first pointed out by Bruce Ames, the high levels of uric acid in human serum may serve an antioxidant role (3). However, excessive accumulation of uric acid (which is poorly soluble in water) results in *gout*, a painful condition resulting from the deposition of urate crystals in the joints and the kidney. Gout can be treated with the drug *allopurinol*, a xanthine oxidase inhibitor.]

Xanthine oxidase is a flavoenzyme which also contains molybdenum and four iron–sulfur centers. The enzyme can be isolated from milk, among other sources. The transformation of hypoxanthine to xanthine is, stoichiometrically, a hydroxylation, followed by tautomerization of the product from the enol to the keto form. Thus we can write a balanced equation:

$$\text{Hypoxanthine} + H_2O + O_2 \rightarrow \text{Hypoxanthine·OH} + H_2O_2$$

and, indeed, hydrogen peroxide is produced by the xanthine/xanthine oxidase/O_2 or hypoxanthine/xanthine oxidase/O_2 systems. Oxidants other than oxygen can drive the reaction, including $NADP^+$ (xanthine dehydrogenase activity) or organic nitro compounds. These alternative oxidants are, of course, reduced in the reaction. In 1949, Horecker and Heppel, investigating the ability of the xanthine/xanthine oxidase system to reduce such alternative substrates, discovered that oxidized cytochrome c was reduced from the ferric to the ferrous form (4). But ferric cytochrome c could not replace oxygen in the reaction, so the reduction could not be a simple redox reaction between cytochrome c and xanthine. Apparently, the xanthine/xanthine oxidase system was generating an unidentified reducing agent, which in turn could reduce cytochrome c. But what was it? One possibility was that the reductant was a reduction product of oxygen. N. O. Kaplan and colleagues studied the problem and suggested that "enzyme-bound H_2O_2 can act as the reductant" (5). Certainly, it seemed at odds with chemical common sense to invoke hydrogen peroxide as a reducing agent.

In the early 1960s, Irwin Fridovich, at Duke University in North Carolina, turned his attention to this unresolved problem. Noting conflicting published reports of the ability of cytochrome c to accept electrons from the xanthine/xanthine oxidase system, he surmised that the irreproducibility of the results might be due to varying purity of the cytochrome c preparations used by different research groups. Perhaps an inhibitor of the reaction had been present in some of the preparations. Indeed, first myoglobin and then carbonic anhydrase (erythrocyte proteins, which might well contaminate a preparation of horse heart cytochrome c) were found to be inhibitors of cytochrome c reduction (6). How could one account for the ability of these proteins to act as inhibitors? Perhaps they might block the interaction of cytochrome c with xanthine oxidase, say by binding to the latter enzyme, but there was no evidence that such a protein–protein interaction existed. And how could the ferric heme group of cytochrome c, buried deep within the protein, make contact with the active site of xanthine oxidase? All these observations amounted to a conundrum!

Fridovich and Handler speculated that the xanthine/xanthine oxidase/O_2 product which mediated cytochrome c reduction might be the one-electron reduction product of dioxygen, the superoxide radical, rather than hydrogen peroxide. Superoxide was known to be a product of radiolysis of aerated aqueous solutions. But the idea that an enzymatic reaction might produce superoxide, an unstable free radical associated with radiolysis processes, seemed extravagant; Fridovich and Handler confined themselves to postulating that an enzyme-bound form of superoxide might be involved.

SIDEBAR: RADIOLYSIS OF WATER

The damaging effects of ionizing radiation on biological systems can be divided into two chemical mechanisms: *Direct* damage results from the interaction of radiation with critical biological target molecules, such as DNA and protein; *indirect* damage is due to the effects of reactive species generated by radiolysis of water. Since water is by far the most common molecule in the cell, and since there are no radiation "chromophores," most of the absorbed radiation energy is absorbed by water, and indirect damage is probably a greater contributor to radiation effects than direct damage (7).

The interaction of high-energy irradiation with water (8) generates high-energy electrons by ionization: $e^- + H_2O \rightarrow e^- + H_2O^{+\cdot} + e^-$; the products react rapidly.

The electrons rapidly become hydrated:

$$e^- + nH_2O \rightarrow e^-_{aq}$$

$$H_2O^{+\cdot} + H_2O \rightarrow \,^{\cdot}OH + H_3O^+$$

$$e^-_{aq} + H_2O \rightarrow H^{\cdot} + OH^-$$

so that $H^{\cdot}$, $OH^{\cdot}$, and hydrated electrons, e^{-aq}, are the major transient products. These radicals can then recombine to give water, interact with one another to give H_2 and H_2O_2, or react with solutes. Therefore, the products of radiolysis will include both oxidizing (e.g., $OH^{\cdot}$) and reducing radicals.

In aerobic aqueous solutions, the reducing radicals (hydrated electron and hydrogen atom) can reduce molecular oxygen:

$$O_2 + e^-_{aq} \rightarrow O_2^{\cdot -}, \qquad O_2 + H^{\cdot} \rightarrow HO_2^{\cdot}$$

yielding superoxide and *perhydroxyl radical*, respectively.

For experimental studies, it is often desirable to limit the radiation products to only one major product, so that its chemistry can be studied without interference by competing reactions.

To produce a purely oxidizing system, nitrous oxide is useful:

$$e^-_{aq} + N_2O + H_2O \rightarrow N_2 + \,^{\cdot}OH + OH^-$$

To generate superoxide alone, formate is added. Formate scavenges $OH^{\cdot}$, a potent oxidant, and the resulting anion radical, in turn, reduces oxygen:

$$OH^{\cdot} + HCO_2^- \rightarrow CO_2^- + H_2O, \qquad CO_2^- + O_2 \rightarrow CO_2 + O_2^{\cdot -}$$

In 1968, Joe McCord, a graduate student with Fridovich, set out to measure the binding of carbonic anhydrase to xanthine oxidase, reasoning that such binding must be the cause of the inhibitory action of the former enzyme on the latter. When these attempts came to nothing, he suddenly realized that the *real* inhibitor might be neither myoglobin nor carbonic anhydrase, but rather some distinct erythrocyte protein which had contaminated all of the preparations, including the cytochrome c. An assay for this mysterious inhibitor was, of course, at hand: Inhibition of the xanthine/xanthine oxidase catalyzed reduction of cytochrome c, so go back to the original crude preparation (erythrocytes) and . . . purify! In short order, the inhibitory factor was found to be chromatographically separable from the other proteins. "The . . . activity was found not to belong to the proteins originally suspected of binding to xanthine oxidase, but to a trace impurity of amazing potency" (9). The desired protein was notably resistant to inactivation; it survived chloroform–ethanol denaturation, which removed much of the unwanted protein in the crude preparation. Precipitation with cold acetone, followed by ion-exchange chromatography, yielded a blue-green enzyme protein, which they named *superoxide dismutase* (9). ("Dismutation" refers to the redox reaction of a compound with itself, as is seen in the stoichiometry discussed in the next section.) They recognized the enzyme as "hemocuprein," a copper-containing protein of unknown function which had been isolated from erythrocytes 30 years earlier. Indeed, the protein had also been isolated, independently, from liver and brain tissue.

The identification of the enzymatic activity of "hemocuprein" as superoxide dismutase was, of course, not the end of the story, but the beginning. It was an unusual episode in biochemistry, because it marked not only the discovery of an important enzyme, but also the simultaneous recognition of the biological significance of its substrate, superoxide. Indeed, it was the first indication that free radical chemistry played a major role in biochemistry, fulfilling the much earlier prediction of Michaelis. Before we look at the biochemical implications of superoxide dismutase, we will consider the enzyme itself: how it is assayed, its catalytic mechanism, and the structure and distribution of the various forms of the enzyme.

CHEMICAL SOURCES OF SUPEROXIDE

The first requirement for an enzyme assay is a source of substrate. Potassium superoxide (KO_2) has long been known as a solid compound, formed by the high-temperature combustion of potassium. When this substance is dissolved in water, it yields hydrogen peroxide and oxygen, following the stoichiometry

$$2O_2^{\cdot -} + 2H^+ \rightarrow O_2 + H_2O_2$$

as determined by Harcourt in 1861 (10). The discovery, in 1934, that KO_2 is paramagnetic (i.e., possesses a magnetic moment) suggested that its structure should be represented simply as a salt of K^+ and $O_2^{\cdot -}$ (11).

The decomposition kinetics of the superoxide radical were studied by pulse radiolysis of aqueous solutions in the early 1960s and were found to be pH-dependent; this is a consequence of the properties of the conjugate acid, perhydroxyl radical, which has a strength comparable to that of acetic acid:

$$HO_2^{\cdot} \rightleftarrows O_2^{\cdot -} + H^+ \qquad pK_a = 4.8$$

The dismutation reaction of the basic form is very slow, due to the electrostatic repulsion of the anions. The reaction goes fastest at the pK_a.

$$2HO_2^{\cdot} \rightarrow O_2 + H_2O_2 \qquad\qquad k_2 \approx 8 \times 10^5 \text{ M}^{-1} \text{ sec}^{-1}$$
$$HO_2^{\cdot} + O_2^{\cdot -} + H^+ \rightarrow O_2 + H_2O_2 \qquad k_2 \approx 8 \times 10^7 \text{ M}^{-1} \text{ sec}^{-1}$$
$$2O_2^{\cdot -} + 2H^+ \rightarrow O_2 + H_2O_2 \qquad\qquad k_2 < 0.3 \text{ M}^{-1} \text{ sec}^{-1}$$

Stable solutions containing superoxide can be prepared under anhydrous conditions, since the dismutation reaction requires H^+. McCord and Fridovich used electrolytic reduction of O_2 in dimethylformamide; the dimethylformamide solution was then infused into the assay mixture. Alternatively, potassium superoxide can be dissolved in dry dimethylsulfoxide (DMSO) with the aid of a crown ether (12).

More commonly, superoxide is generated in the assay mixture by an enzymatic (xanthine/xanthine oxidase) or a photochemical process. The illumination of various dyes (riboflavin, methylene blue) in the presence of tetramethylethylenediamine (TEMED) generates superoxide. The mechanism of this process presumably involves photoexcitation of the dye, electron transfer from TEMED, and then reduction of oxygen by the reduced dye. (Riboflavin and TEMED can also be used as a radical generating system for forming polyacrylamide gels; in this case, oxygen interferes with the desired reaction, acrylamide polymerization, and thus the solutions are usually degassed.)

SUPEROXIDE DISMUTASES

Why is superoxide dismutase necessary at all, since the uncatalysed dismutation is fast, even at neutral pH? As Fridovich has pointed out, the spontaneous dismutation is second-order in the concentration of $O_2{}^{\cdot-}$. In contrast, the enzymatic dismutation, which is initiated by the interaction of a molecule of $O_2{}^{\cdot-}$ with a molecule of enzyme, is first-order with respect to superoxide concentration. Thus, at low concentrations of superoxide, the enzyme-catalyzed reaction dominates. The steady-state concentration of superoxide can be maintained at a much lower value in the presence of the enzyme. To put it another way, at low steady-state levels of superoxide, a superoxide radical is much more likely to encounter a molecule of superoxide dismutase than to encounter a second molecule of superoxide. The enzyme acts as the carrier of electrons from one superoxide radical to another.

All superoxide dismutases are metalloenzymes. Probably, the simplest interpretation of the mechanism of enzymatic catalysis is a "ping-pong" process

$$M^{n+} + O_2{}^{\cdot-} + H^+ \rightarrow [M^{(n-1)+}H^+] + O_2$$
$$[M^{(n-1)+}H^+] + O_2{}^{\cdot-} + H^+ \rightarrow H_2O_2 + M^{n+}$$

in which the metal center is first reduced, then oxidized, by superoxide, and the enzyme also facilitates proton transfer to the superoxide anion. Currently favored mechanisms are of this type; however, other possibilities cannot be excluded.

SIDEBAR: KINETICS OF THE SUPEROXIDE DISMUTASE-CATALYZED REACTION

The enzyme-catalyzed "ping-pong" reaction mechanism proposed for superoxide dismutase provides an interesting exercise in enzyme kinetics (13). We will assume that the reaction proceeds via two irreversible steps:

$$SOD^0 + O_2{}^{\cdot-} \xrightarrow{k_1} SOD^- + O_2 \tag{1}$$

$$SOD^- + O_2{}^{\cdot-} \xrightarrow[H^+]{k_2} SOD^0 + H_2O_2 \tag{2}$$

We make the steady-state approximation for the reduced-enzyme intermediate, SOD^-:

$$\frac{d[SOD^-]}{dt} = 0 = k_1[SOD^0][O_2{}^{\cdot-}] - k_2[SOD^-][O_2{}^{\cdot-}]$$

$$\therefore [SOD^-] = \frac{k_1[SOD^0]}{k_2}$$

But:

$$[SOD]_{total} = [SOD^-] + [SOD^0] = [SOD^-] \times (k_1 + k_2)/k_1$$

The fraction of the enzyme found in the reduced form, at steady state, is given by this equation, and it can be measured experimentally by observing the spectral bleaching of the cupric enzyme (14). The overall reaction rate is equal to the rate of disappearance of superoxide:

$$\frac{d}{dt}[O_2{}^{\cdot-}] = k_1[SOD^0][O_2{}^{\cdot-}] + k_2[SOD^-][O_2{}^{\cdot-}]$$

$$= [SOD]_{total}[O_2{}^{\cdot-}] \times 2\{k_1k_2/(k_1 + k_2)\}$$

Thus, we can express the turnover number for the enzyme, k_{cat}, in terms of the rate constants for the two steps of the reaction:

$$k_{CAT} = (k_1k_2)/(k_1 + k_2)$$

BIOLOGICAL SOURCES OF SUPEROXIDE

Is superoxide formed in biological systems? The presence of an enzyme capable of acting on this radical leads one to suspect that the substrate must be present as well. Direct evidence for the formation of superoxide has been harder to obtain, since the lifetime of superoxide is so short, especially in the presence of the enzyme (see discussion of SOD^- mutants below). But strong evidence exists for generation of superoxide in several biological systems.

1. When microsomes or mitochondrial membrane preparations are exposed to oxygen and electrons are supplied in the form of NAD(P)H, superoxide production can be observed by techniques such as electron paramagnetic resonance (EPR) spin-trapping (see below) and reduction of cytochrome c.
2. Plant chloroplasts harvest solar light energy for the generation of NADPH reducing equivalents, which are then used for the reductive synthesis of carbohydrates from carbon dioxide. Asada and colleagues have shown that chloroplasts generate superoxide on exposure to light (15), apparently from the autoxidation (oxidation by molecular oxygen) of components of photosystem I, including the powerful reductant ferredoxin (16).
3. The "respiratory burst" of neutrophils and macrophages is a specialized enzymatic system for the generation of superoxide and other reactive oxygen species, for the purpose of destroying foreign cells such as invading bacteria. This fascinating and important biological system is discussed later (Chapter 6).
4. Redox-cycling agents are chemicals which undergo enzymatic one-electron reduction, generating a transient radical. Subsequent reoxidation of this radical by oxygen generates $O_2{}^{\cdot-}$ (17–19). Reactive oxygen species are primarily responsible for the toxicity of redox-cycling agents. Well-known examples of such agents are *viologens*, such as paraquat (1,1'-dimethyl-4,4'-dipyridilium dichloride), and naphthoquinones, such as juglone, one of the allopathic chemicals secreted by the black walnut tree.

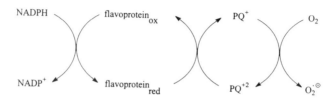

Viologens are so named because they can be reduced to long-lived radicals which are deep blue or violet in color. Paraquat is a herbicide; it was widely used to kill illicit marijuana crops in Mexico in the 1970s (20). Paraquat-mediated superoxide generation is driven by the photosynthetic generation of reducing equivalents, and paraquat's herbicidal effect requires the presence of light.

Redox-cycling activity can be measured in intact *Escherichia coli* cells as *cyanide-resistant respiration* (21). Dehydrogenases (e.g., NADH and succinate dehydrogenases) transfer two reducing equivalents to ubiquinone-8 in the cytoplasmic membrane of *E. coli*. The branched respiratory chain provides electrons from ubiquinone-8 to either of two terminal cytochrome oxidases, the cytochrome o and cytochrome d complexes, which reduce oxygen to water (22, 23). The rate-limiting step in *E. coli* respiration is the removal of electrons from metabolites, rather than the transfer of electrons to oxygen, so the net rate of respiration should not be affected by redox-cycling agents. However, cyanide, an inhibitor of both terminal oxidases, prevents the outflow of reducing equivalents from the respiratory chain. The flow of electrons to redox-cycling agents bypasses this metabolic block. Thus, a dose-dependent increase in the rate of cyanide-resistant respiration provides a measure of a compound's redox-cycling capabilities. A new variation on this method uses a mutant *E. coli* strain which is devoid of cytochrome oxidase activity. This strain has almost no baseline oxygen consumption activity, so the addition of cyanide is unnecessary (24).

SUPEROXIDE DISMUTASE: ASSAYS

Although superoxide absorbs ultraviolet (UV) light (below 300 nm), its concentration in enzymatic systems is usually much too small for direct detection. Consequently, any assay for superoxide dismutase is predicated on an assay for superoxide itself. The enzyme assays rely on the ability of superoxide dismutase to intercept $O_2^{\cdot-}$ and hence to inhibit alternative reactions of the form

$$O_2^{\cdot-} + D \rightarrow O_2 + D^-$$

where D is a detector molecule and D^- is a readily detected product.

Let's consider a few of the many assays which have been devised for superoxide dismutase, keeping the criteria of utility of an enzyme assay—sensitivity and specificity—in mind.

Reduction of Cytochrome c

As we have seen, superoxide dismutase inhibition of the reduction of cytochrome c by superoxide was the basis for the discovery of the enzyme, and this assay is still widely used. One unit of superoxide dismutase is defined as the quantity of enzyme which inhibits cytochrome c reduction by 50%; of course, the incubation conditions must be specified. Cytochrome c undergoes a large change in extinction coefficient upon reduction ($\Delta\epsilon_{418\,nm} = 7 \times 10^4\,M^{-1}\,cm^{-1}$; higher λ can also be used), which makes this assay potentially very sensitive. Even greater sensitivity is achieved by delaying addition of cytochrome c until the superoxide generating system has reached steady state, and then measuring the sudden burst of reduction upon addition of cytochrome c (25). The specificity of the assay relies on the inhibition by superoxide dismutase: Superoxide-independent pathways for cytochrome c reduction are also possible, but are not affected by superoxide dismutase. On the other hand, such alternative routes for cytochrome c reduction reduce the sensitivity of the assay, since they increase the baseline rate of change of ΔA against which the differential effect of superoxide dismutase is measured.

Another widely used assay is based on the reduction of the chromogenic reagent nitro blue tetrazolium (NBT):*

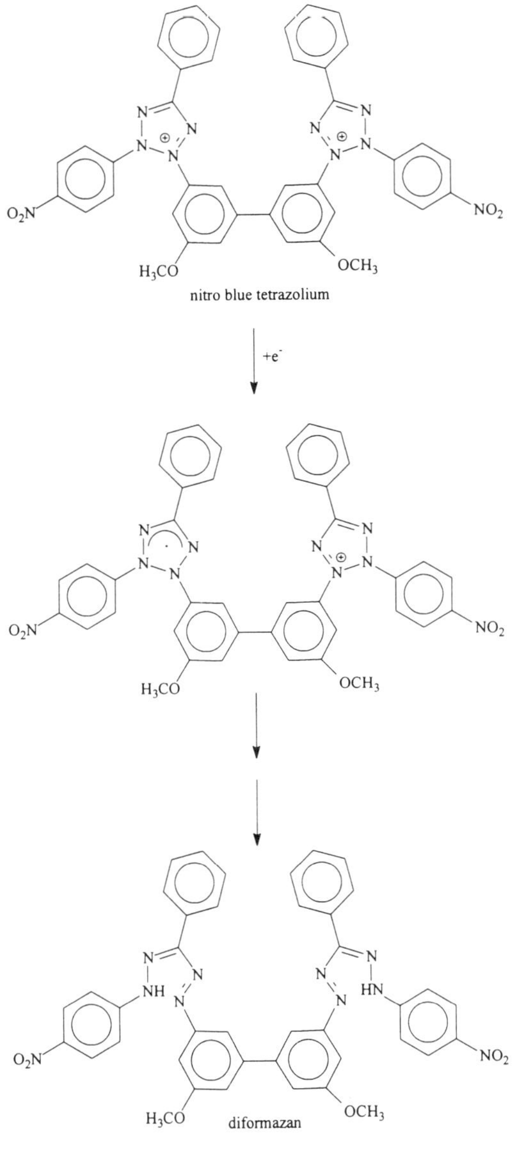

nitro blue tetrazolium

$+e^-$

diformazan

* Figure adapted from Bielski et al., *J. Phys. Chem.* 84:830, 1980.

NBT is yellow, but, upon reduction, it yields a pigment called *formazan*, which is purple-blue colored. The pigment is insoluble; as a consequence, it precipitates and forms a stable colored band in a polyacrylamide gel. For detection of superoxide dismutase, the chromogen is incubated with a superoxide-generating system (as described above), and enzyme activity is measured, as before, by inhibition of color formation. (Thus, superoxide dismutase bands are visualized on gels as "negatives," colorless bands against a blue background.) With the xanthine/xanthine oxidase/O_2 system as the source of superoxide, the reduction of NBT is about 90% inhibitable by saturating amounts of superoxide dismutase (26). A variation on the NBT assay is to replace the xanthine/xanthine oxidase/O_2 system for superoxide generation by the direct addition of superoxide, as the crown ether-solubilized DMSO solution described earlier (12).

Tetranitromethane is reduced by superoxide to the nitroform anion radical, which can be detected spectroscopically ($\lambda_{max} = 350$ nm):

$$O_2{}^{\cdot-} + C(NO_2)_4 \rightarrow O_2 + C(NO_2)_3{}^-$$

The rate constant for this reaction is near the diffusion-controlled limit (27).

SIDEBAR: EPR SPIN TRAPPING

Another approach to detecting superoxide, electron paramagnetic resonance (EPR) spin trapping, constitutes a unique tool for the analysis of free radical processes in biochemical systems. Spin trapping provides qualitative and semiquantitative information about the kinds of reactive radicals formed in chemical systems. Free radicals are paramagnetic; that is, they align in a magnetic field. Just as in NMR (nuclear magnetic resonance), the different spin states of a paramagnetic molecule in a magnetic field are of different energies, and these energy differences can be measured by the resonant absorption of electromagnetic energy. This is the basis of EPR spectroscopy. In contrast to NMR, the energy differences involved in EPR are much larger, so EPR is inherently a very sensitive technique. Radical concentrations as low as 10^{-9} M may be detectable. Furthermore, diamagnetic molecules (those with no net spin) are EPR-silent. Thus, both in principle and in practice, a tiny population of free radicals can be studied by EPR even in the presence of a vastly greater number of nonradical molecules; this is the invariable situation in a biochemical system.

As with an NMR spectrum, the EPR spectrum provides detailed information about the structure of the molecules responsible for the signal. In the case of NMR, information is provided by the chemical shift values and spin–spin splitting (nucleus–nucleus magnetic interactions). In the case of EPR, information is provided by the g-value of the radical and by hyperfine splitting constants (electron–nucleus magnetic interactions). The interpretation of EPR spectra is discussed elsewhere (28).

For spectroscopic reasons that will not be discussed here, the superoxide radical cannot be detected directly by the EPR technique. In any event, its steady-state concentration is usually below that required for detection of radicals by EPR. In the EPR spin-trapping technique, the primary radical is captured by a diamagnetic molecule, the spin trap, to yield a relatively stable free radical (usually, a nitroxide), which can be detected by EPR:

Primary radical + Spin trap → Spin adduct

In favorable cases, the spectrum of the spin adduct (usually, a nitroxide radical) will be characteristic of the primary radical, and thereby allow its identification. Spin adducts can sometimes be identified by conventional chromatographic separation and mass spectrometric analysis (29).

Various classes of spin trap have been developed, including alkyl and aryl nitroso compounds and nitrones. A useful spin trap must meet many criteria, including (1) rapid reaction with the primary radical, (2) stability of the spin adduct, (3) absence of unproductive side reactions, (4) distinctive spectroscopic signature of the spin adducts, and (5) good solubility for use in biochemical studies. Inevitably, some of these attributes must be compromised.

The most useful spin traps for studies of reactive oxygen species, such as superoxide and hydroxyl radical, are dimethylpyrroline-*N*-oxide (DMPO) and PBN (phenyl-*tert*-butyl nitrone). DMPO reacts with superoxide to give a nitroxide spin adduct characterized by a six-line spectrum with distinctive hyperfine splitting constants (hfsc).

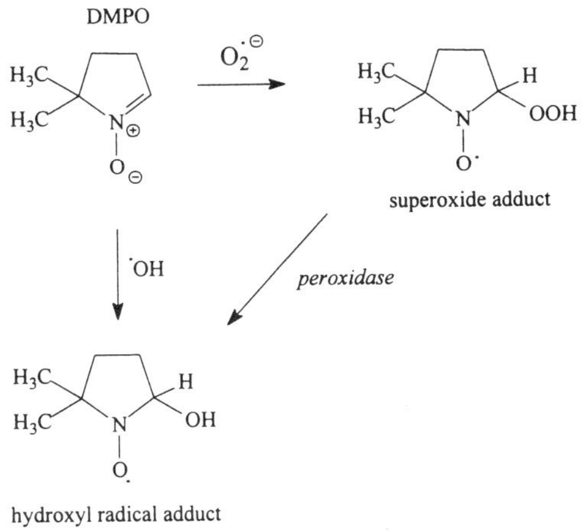

superoxide adduct

hydroxyl radical adduct

The presence of this signal, and its sensitivity to inhibition by superoxide dismutase, is excellent evidence for formation of superoxide, and the technique has been applied in many studies of biochemical and cellular systems suspected of generating oxygen radicals. Hydroxyl radical ($\cdot$OH) is also trapped by DMPO, and it yields an adduct with a distinctive four-line spectrum. (In the presence of $\cdot$OH scavengers, such as dimethyl sulfoxide or ethanol, the hydroxyl radical is converted to methyl or hydroxyethyl radicals, respectively, and these radicals can also be spin-trapped.)

Spin-trapping can also be conducted in vivo, by administering the spin trap to an experimental animal and collecting bile for spectroscopic analysis (30).

SUPEROXIDE DISMUTASE: ENZYME STRUCTURE—FORMS AND DISTRIBUTION

Three classes of superoxide dismutases can be distinguished on the basis of their metal content: Cu,Zn (the enzyme first isolated by McCord and Fridovich), Mn, and Fe. At first, the Cu,Zn enzyme was believed to be exclusively eukaryotic; then, several bacterial species turned out to possess Cu,Zn superoxide dismutase, including *Caulobacter crescentus*, *Brucella abortus*, and the human pathogen, *Legionella pneumophila* (31). Recently, a Cu,Zn superoxide dismutase was also found in *E. coli*; it had previously escaped notice because of its lability (32). The Mn and Fe enzymes are homologous in both sequence and structure, and they presumably evolved from a common progenitor. The Mn enzyme is found in many species of bacteria and in the mitochondria of eukaryotic cells. This distribution pattern lends support to the widely held view that eukaryotic mitochondria are evolved from prokaryotic cells which entered the progenitor eukaryotic cell as a symbiont. The Fe enzyme is found in bacteria and in a few families of higher plants, such as the ginkgo. In most other green plants, the chloroplasts contain Cu,Zn superoxide dismutase, and the mitochondria contain the Mn enzyme.

Virtually all oxygen-tolerant organisms possess some form of superoxide dismutase, as one would expect if the toxicity of reduced oxygen species is an inevitable challenge to aerobic life. However, a few anomalies have come to light. For example, the bacterium *Lactobacillus plantarum* has apparently substituted the accumulation of very high levels of Mn(II), which has weak superoxide dismutase activity, for the synthesis of superoxide dismutase enzyme. Nevertheless, the strong association between possession of superoxide dismutase and aerobiosis constitutes one of the clearest pieces of evidence for the role of superoxide in mediating oxygen toxicity.

Cu,Zn SUPEROXIDE DISMUTASE

The eukaryotic Cu,Zn superoxide dismutase can be purified from mammalian sources by treatment with ethanol/chloroform, which denatures and precipitates hemoglobin and other unwanted proteins. Cu,Zn superoxide dismutase is soluble in the organic phase; addition of acetone causes the enzyme to precipitate. Few other enzymes survive such a protocol. Ion-exchange and gel filtration chromatography are used for further purification.

Metal removal and reconstitution experiments have shown that the copper ion is essential for activity. Indeed, aqueous Cu(II) is an extremely effective catalyst of superoxide dismutation, but free copper ion probably cannot exist in the cell. The Zn-free enzyme has reduced, but still considerable, enzyme activity, so it is clear that the Cu ion undergoes the critical enzymatic redox-cycling [from Cu(II) to Cu(I)], while the Zn plays a secondary role (see below).

X-ray crystal structures have been obtained for both the bovine erythrocyte enzyme (33) and the recombinant human enzyme, expressed in yeast (34). The enzymes are homodimers of 151– (bovine) and 153–residue (human) subunits; each subunit contains one Cu and one Zn ion. Each subunit has a "β-barrel" design made up of eight antiparallel β-strands. The active site lies outside the barrel and is built from amino acids located in loops connecting the β-strands. The active site is located at the bottom of a channel, which is constructed as a sort of molecular funnel, leading to the Cu ion at the bottom of the channel. The enzyme protein appears to act as a sort of molecular lasso for pulling in superoxide anions. Although the net charge on the protein at physiological pH is negative (pI around 5.0), the active site is in a region of high electrostatic potential, due to the effects of lysine and arginine residues and the metal ions themselves. Tainer and colleagues have suggested that this "electrostatic facilitation" of superoxide binding is an important contributor to the extraordinarily high catalytic efficiency of the Cu,Zn enzyme. The second-order rate constant for reaction of superoxide with the enzyme is near the diffusion-controlled limit. This means that most of the collisions with the substrate are productive, even though the active site occupies only a fraction of the volume and solvent-exposed surface of the protein. Apparently, negative surface charges prevent unproductive collisions, and the positive potential in the channel pulls in the substrate. However, a full understanding of the electrostatic environment of the protein is still a formidable task, since one must consider interactions with solvent and salt counterions, which cannot be discerned from the X-ray crystal structure.

The copper ion is coordinated in a distorted square-planar geometry to the imidazole side-chain N atoms of four different histidine residues and is accessible to solvent. The Zn^{2+} ion is buried within the protein, inaccessible to solvent, and is approximately tetrahedral in coordination, with three histidine imidazole N ligands and one aspartate oxygen. Remarkably, one histidine residue bridges the copper and zinc ions, with one N liganded to each. No other protein is known to contain such an arrangement of metal ions. This coordination requires that the imidazole ring has lost both NH protons to form an imidazolate anion, which would normally require extremely basic conditions. The binding of the first metal ion must greatly reduce the pK for the second N, facilitating the binding of the second. This arrangement is probably of both structural and catalytic utility, although it must be remembered that the Zn ion is not essential for activity.

The catalytic mechanism proposed by Tainer et al. is shown below:

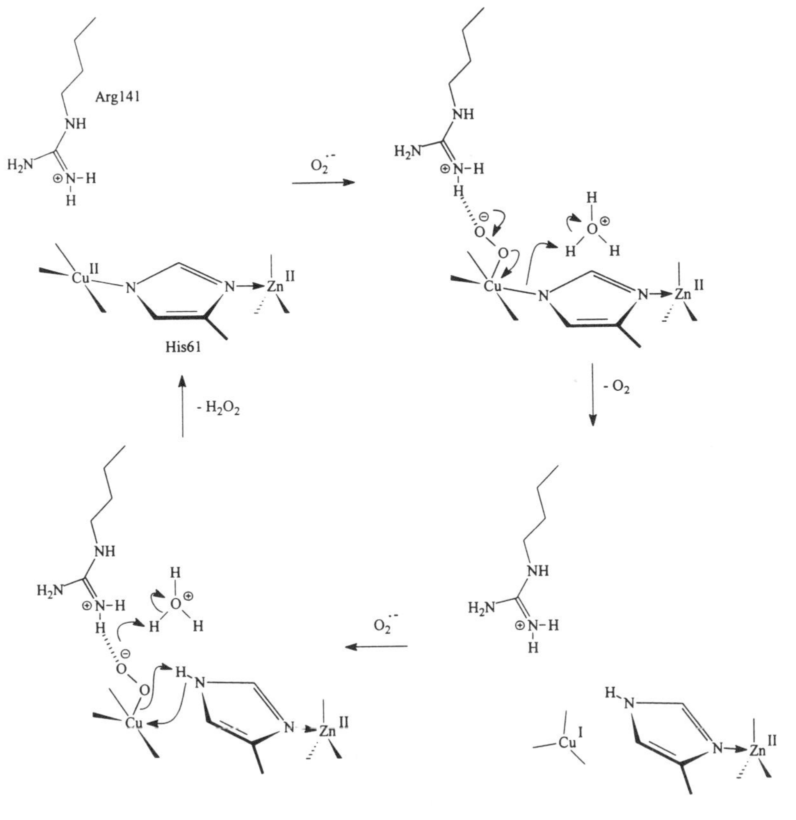

The participation of arginine-141 is supported by the results of site-directed mutagenesis experiments (see Chapter 2): Replacement of this residue by lysine reduces enzyme activity, and replacement by neutral amino acids abolishes activity. The ligiding of the superoxide anion to the Cu^{2+} is consistent with the geometry of the substrate channel, described above. In the first half of the reaction, superoxide reduces the Cu^{2+} center to Cu^+; the coordinate bond to the imidazolate anion breaks; the histidine residue rotates, to allow the Cu^+ to adopt a more favorable coordination geometry, and the highly basic imidazolate, freed from coordination to the cupric ion, abstracts a proton from the solvent. In the second half of the mechanism, a second molecule of superoxide coordinates to the cuprous ion, then reoxidizes it and abstracts the imidazole proton, returning the enzyme to its native state. The nascent HO_2^- anion is protonated by solvent to release H_2O_2.

A second mammalian Cu,Zn superoxide dismutase was discovered in 1982; this enzyme is secreted into blood plasma and is therefore known as *extracellular superoxide dismutase* (EC-SOD). The enzyme is a homotetramer; each subunit contains one Cu and one Zn ion, in an active site which is probably similar to that of the cytosolic Cu,Zn superoxide dismutase (35). However, the sequences of the two enzymes are very different and antibodies to one do not react with the other.

Mn AND Fe SUPEROXIDE DISMUTASES

These enzymes occur as dimers or, in some cases, tetramers, composed of subunits with about 190 amino acids; each subunit contains one metal ion. The Mn and Fe enzymes have very similar structures and have almost certainly evolved from a common precursor. The tertiary structure is unrelated to that of the Cu,Zn enzyme; each subunit is composed of two domains, one mainly α-helical and the other containing both α and β structure (36). The Mn(III) ion in the oxidized enzyme (*T. thermophilus*) is in a roughly trigonal bipyramidal coordination to three histidines, one aspartate, and a solvent water molecule, in a very hydrophobic local environment. Despite the very different tertiary structure of these enzymes, compared to the Cu,Zn superoxide dismutase, some features are familiar: The metal ion is located at the end of a funnel-like channel, and positive charges (lys and arg residues) appear to attract anions into the funnel. The metal-specificity of the Mn and Fe superoxide dismutases is an outstanding riddle. Neither the sequences nor the crystal structures display any obvious differences which could account for the specific binding of Mn by one protein and Fe by the other. Stallings et al. suggest that "initial binding (selection) of the metals [might occur] in partly folded structures." A functional hybrid enzyme (heterodimer) is observed on gel electropherograms; nevertheless, if one metal is replaced by the other in the homodimer, activity is lost (37)!

The Mn superoxide dismutase, but not the Fe superoxide dismutase, of *E. coli* binds to DNA in a sequence-independent manner (38). Steinman and colleagues suggested that the Mn enzyme acts as a "tethered antioxidant," specifically protecting DNA by remaining localized in its vicinity.

The structure of the human mitochondrial Mn superoxide dismutase, a tetrameric enzyme, has also been determined (39). The active site geometry is similar to that of the *T. thermophilus* enzyme, although the nature of the subunit–subunit packing interactions holding together the tetramer is different.

CLONING THE SUPEROXIDE DISMUTASE GENES IN *E. coli*

The Fe and Mn superoxide dismutases of *E. coli* are encoded by the genes *sodB* and *sodA*, respectively. These genes were first identified by Daniele Touati and colleagues, in Paris, in the mid-1980s. This breakthrough has allowed the role of the superoxide dismutase enzymes of this bacterium to be studied in greater detail than has been possible in any other organism. The cloning of the genes for Mn and Fe superoxide dismutase was accomplished by a screening approach (40). A bank of cosmid clones, representing the entire *E. coli* chromosome, was prepared. *Cosmids are hybrid vectors, assembled from plasmids and fragments of bacteriophage* λ, *including the cos sites recognized by the* λ *DNA-packaging enzyme machinery. Cosmid vectors can incorporate large pieces of foreign DNA (about 40 kbp); the recombinant cosmids are then carried as large plasmids in E. coli cells (41)*. The *E. coli* chromosome consists of about 4000 kbp; therefore, a bank of a few hundred cosmids is likely to represent most of the genes in the bacterium, so the number of clones which must be screened is manageable. Strains carrying these cosmids were screened on the basis of enzyme activity or reactivity (immunoprecipitation) with rabbit antibodies to the purified Mn or Fe superoxide dismutase proteins. Four hundred clones had to be screened to find one expressing increased Fe superoxide dismutase activity. Once the positive clones were identified, the *sodA* and *sodB* genes could be obtained by subcloning. Null mutants were prepared by fusing marker genes, such as *lacZ* and *kan* (kanamycin resistance) into the cloned genes, and these constructs were used to prepare chromosomal null mutants by homologous recombination.

SIDEBAR: GENE FUSIONS

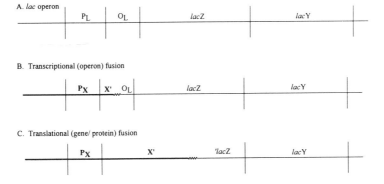

Genetic fusion technology is a very powerful tool for molecular analysis. The principle of the method is to replace a gene of interest by a reporter gene, such as *lacZ*, the *E. coli* gene encoding β-galactosidase. We can then use a standard assay for the activity of the reporter gene instead of the (possibly very difficult) assay for the replaced gene's product. Phage Mu derivatives have been constructed which transpose into the bacterial chromosome, carrying a selectable marker, and generating a fusion; these facilitate the isolation of the desired fusions (42, 43). Two classes of fusion can be constructed: *transcriptional* fusions (also called *operon* fusions) and *translational* fusions (also called *gene* fusions or *protein* fusions). A *transcriptional* fusion uses the entire *lacZ* gene, including its ribosome binding site (Shine–Dalgarno sequence) required for initiation of protein synthesis but separated from the *lac* control elements (promoter and operator). The fusion usually creates a null mutation in the gene (X) which it disrupts. If the fusion places *lacZ* downstream from the promoter for gene X, then the *lacZ* transcript and enzyme will be synthesized, but under the control of the normal regulatory machinery for gene X. Since β-galactosidase is easily assayed, this technique facilitates studies of gene regulation. The expression of β-galactosidase "reports" on the regulation of gene X in the wild-type cell. This approach was applied by Touati to study the regulation of *sodA* (44).

The inverse of this procedure is also useful: the structural gene for the enzyme of interest is stripped of its upstream regulatory sequences and fused to a well-characterized promoter, such as *lac* or *tac*. *tac* is a hybrid of the *trp* and *lac* promoters, and, like wild-type *lac*, it is induced by the lactose analogue IPTG (isopropyl β-D-thiogalactoside) (45). Such a fusion results in expression of the protein of interest under control of the *lac* promoter. The levels of the enzyme can then be modulated simply by varying the levels of IPTG added to the culture. In a recent application of this approach, the *sodA* and *sodB* genes were stripped of almost all noncoding sequences by restriction enzyme/exonuclease digestion and the "naked" structural genes were ligated into a plasmid vector, downstream of the *tac* promoter (46). These recombinant plasmids were then introduced into a *sodAsodB* mutant strain. Thus, the normal physiological control of the genes is eliminated, and enzyme expression levels can be manipulated experimentally.

The amino-terminal 26 amino acids of LacZ can be removed and replaced by other sequences (even hundreds of amino acids), without loss of β-galactosidase enzyme activity (47). This property of *lacZ* is exploited in the creation of *translational* (protein) fusions. In these fusions, part of the 5′ end of the coding sequence of *lacZ* is deleted, and the gene is thereby stripped of its translation start site. β-Galactosidase will only be expressed if the construct fuses, in the correct reading frame, to a chromosomal gene X. The product is a hybrid protein (X′-′LacZ), which will often be enzymatically active.

What has been learned about the biochemical function and regulation of superoxide dismutases in *E. coli*, using these molecular tools? The *sodAsodB* mutant, devoid of superoxide dismutase activity, is viable, but grows at only about half the rate of the wild-type or single mutants, in complete growth medium (48). In minimal medium (salts and glucose only), the double mutant does not grow at all, but supplementation with amino acids restores viability. Branched-chain amino acids (leucine, isoleucine, valine) are particularly important, because an enzyme in the biosynthetic pathway of these amino acids is highly sensitive to inactivation by superoxide. This enzyme is α,β-dihydroxy acid dehydratase, an Fe–S center-containing protein (49):

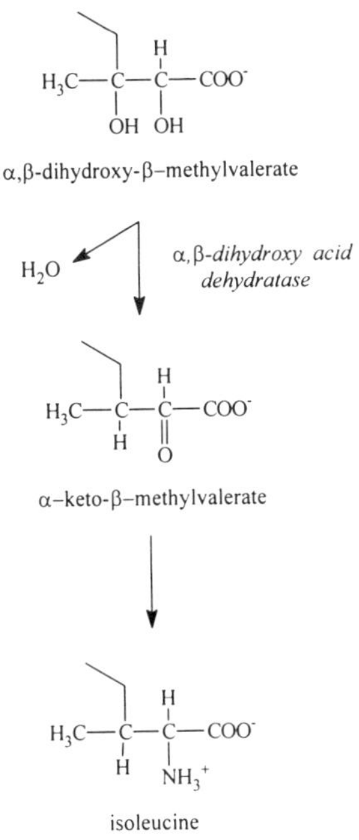

$$H_3C-\underset{\underset{OH}{|}}{C}-\underset{\underset{OH}{|}}{\overset{\overset{H}{|}}{C}}-COO^-$$

α,β-dihydroxy-β–methylvalerate

α,β-dihydroxy acid
dehydratase

H_2O

$$H_3C-\underset{\underset{H}{|}}{C}-\underset{\overset{\|}{O}}{\overset{\overset{H}{|}}{C}}-COO^-$$

α–keto-β–methylvalerate

$$H_3C-\underset{\underset{H}{|}}{C}-\underset{\underset{NH_3^+}{|}}{\overset{\overset{H}{|}}{C}}-COO^-$$

isoleucine

[Auxotrophies and impaired growth also characterize yeast mutants lacking cytoplasmic Cu,Zn superoxide dismutase or mitochondrial Mn superoxide dismutase (50).] The *sodAsodB* mutant shows a hypermutable phenotype (see table below). Spontaneous rates of forward mutation to trimethoprim resistance (a characteristic phenotype of thymine-requiring auxotrophic mutants) were studied (51).

	Thy⁻ Mutants per 10^7 Cells		
Strain Genotype	Air	Air + PQ[a]	N_2
Wild-type	20	19	15
sodB sodA	81	160	13
sodB sodA sodA⁺ (plasmid)	19	—	—
sodB sodA sodB⁺ (plasmid)	21	—	—

[a]PQ: paraquat, 200 μM.

The mutation rate is elevated in SOD⁻ cells; this elevation is eliminated by reintroduction of either *sodA* or *sodB* gene, via a plasmid, and also disappears when the cells are grown under anaerobic conditions. The addition of paraquat, to increase superoxide production, increases the mutation rate in the SOD⁻, but not in the wild type. These results are consistent with the idea that reactive oxygen species are potentially mutagenic and that superoxide dismutase activity inhibits this mutagenicity.

E. coli sodAsodB mutants are also sensitive to killing by the bactericidal proteins (complement system) present in human serum (52). This sensitivity is not due to generation of reactive oxygen species in the serum, since exogenous superoxide dismutase and catalase are not protective. Rather, it seems to reflect an inherent sensitivity of the mutant strain, resulting from the deleterious effects of elevated intracellular superoxide levels.

In view of the recent discovery of a third form of superoxide dismutase in *E. coli* (32), the interpretations of results obtained with the double mutants need to be reconsidered. For example, it is not clear that a truly SOD⁻ mutant strain will even be viable.

REGULATION OF SUPEROXIDE DISMUTASES IN *E. coli*

E. coli possesses two independently regulated catalases (see Chapter 5). The superoxide dismutases present an interesting comparison. Again, *E. coli* has two different enzymes. How are the levels of these enzymes controlled? The first studies to address these questions used biochemical analyses (activity-stained polyacrylamide gels) to measure the levels of each enzyme separately, under various conditions. Fridovich and colleagues established that the Fe superoxide dismutase is *constitutive*—that is, relatively insensitive to environmental conditions. This form of the enzyme is synthesized even under anaerobic conditions, and the level does not change greatly upon exposure to oxygen. In contrast, the Mn-containing enzyme is inducible by exposure of the cells to oxygen, and it reaches still higher levels with exposure to paraquat or high oxygen tension. This division of the enzymatic task between a constitutive and an inducible enzyme is also seen with the catalases, the terminal respiratory oxidases, and other *E. coli* enzyme systems. Since the catalytic properties and three-dimensional structures of the Mn-containing and Fe-containing superoxide dismutases are similar, differential regulation may be one of the most salient difference between the roles of the two enzymes. The inducibility of Mn-superoxide dismutase suggested that the enzyme may participate in the phenomenon of bacterial adaptation to oxidative stress (see Chapter 5).

SUPEROXIDE DISMUTASES IN THE FRUIT FLY, *Drosophila melanogaster*

Cu,Zn Superoxide Dismutase

The fruit fly *Drosophila melanogaster* provides an elegant system for the genetic and molecular analysis of the role of superoxide dismutase in a higher eukaryote. *Drosophila* Cu,Zn superoxide dismutase is a homodimer of 32-kD subunits, with extensive amino acid sequence homology to the enzymes from other species (53). The *Drosophila* enzyme was originally referred to as "tetrazolium oxidase," on the basis of its ability to block NBT reduction on electrophoresis gels (see above). Maximal levels of enzyme activity are reached in 5-day-old adults, and they persist through at least the midpoint of the adult life span.

Natural Allelic Variations

Studies of genetic variability in natural *Drosophila* populations have contributed greatly to our understanding of the mechanisms of evolutionary change. Theodosius Dobzhansky (Rockefeller University) was an early pioneer of such studies, beginning in the 1930s. Dobzhansky and his student Francisco Ayala discovered that two allozyme (allelic) variants, fast (Cu,Zn SOD^f) and slow (Cu,Zn SOD^s), are found in many natural *Drosophila* populations, at differing frequencies (54). The latter is less thermostable than the former, although it has a greater intrinsic specific activity (55). In fly populations from California, the two forms differ by a single amino acid: lys_{96} in Cu,Zn SOD^s is replaced by asn_{96} in Cu,Zn SOD^f. Two forms are also found in populations from Tunisia. In this case, the two forms differ at three sites: the same substitution (residue 96) which distinguishes the Californian strains, and two additional substitutions: Cu,Zn SOD^f has glu_{19} and ser_{100}; Cu,Zn SOD^s has pro_{19} and his_{100}. Comparison with the tertiary structure of the bovine enzyme (discussed above) indicates that the positions of all of these substitutions fall outside the domains of the protein which form the active site channel.

Recombination mapping (56) located the structural gene on the third chromosome, at 32.5 map units, and null alleles have been isolated (57). Phenotypic characterization of these null mutants elucidates the biological role of Cu,Zn superoxide dismutase (58). Homozygotes are viable as larvae and pupae, but die as young adults, with a mean adult life span of 11 days, versus about 60 days for the parental strain or for heterozygotes. Homozygotes are hypersensitive to paraquat, ionizing radiation, and hyperoxia. Males are sterile and have immobile spermatazoa; females are only weakly fertile. Females exhibit little increase in spontaneous germline mutation frequency, as measured by X-linked recessive lethal tests. This contrasts with the finding that Cu,Zn superoxide dismutase null mutants in yeast (59) and Fe superoxide dismutase null mutants in bacteria (60) show elevated spontaneous mutation frequencies under aerobic conditions. Either the lack of Cu,Zn superoxide dismutase in *Drosophila* null mutants does not significantly increase levels of oxidative DNA damage, or any such increased damage does not greatly exceed the DNA repair capacity.

The biological consequences of *elevated* levels of the enzyme have also been studied, through the use of genetic duplications of the Cu,Zn superoxide dismutase locus and of transgenics. Heterozygotes for a chromosome carrying a duplication of the Cu,Zn SOD locus express approximately 150% of normal enzyme activity and show increased resistance to ionizing radiation, but are *hypersensitive* to paraquat (61). The adult life span varies little in flies expressing approximately 50%, 100% and 150% of normal Cu,Zn superoxide dismutase activity, by virtue of possessing one, two or three doses, respectively, of the normal gene. Cu, Zn superoxide dismutase transgenics have been generated, by the use of P transposable element technology (62). P transposons encode a transposase enzyme, which specifically catalyzes the insertion of the transposon into random chromosomal sites. Because the transposase is synthesized only in germ cells, P transposons can be used to insert "passenger" genes into germ cell chromosomes, where they will be transmitted to, and expressed in, progeny, in typical Mendelian fashion.

Transgenic lines carrying native genomic Cu,Zn SOD genes, which supplement Cu,Zn superoxide dismutase activity to approximately 150% of normal, exhibit enhanced resistance to oxygen stress and only marginally increased adult life span (63). However, transgenic lines overexpressing both superoxide dismutase and catalase have recently been constructed and show a marked increase in life span (64). This result gives impressive support to the hypothesis that oxidative stress-induced damage is a major factor in aging.

The interaction of Cu,Zn superoxide dismutase with the radical scavenger uric acid (see above) has been investigated, through the use of *Drosophila* rosy (*ry*) mutants (65). The *ry* gene encodes the enzyme xanthine dehydrogenase (xanthine oxidase; see above). XDH-null *ry* mutants are devoid of urate and exhibit phenotypes indicative of oxidative damage (hypersensitivity to paraquat, hyperoxia, and ionizing radiation). They are temperature-sensitive lethals and have reduced adult life spans, but are otherwise viable, fertile, and robust under normal laboratory conditions. Cu,Zn superoxide dismutase-null; *ry* double mutants survive through embryonic and larval development, only to die in late metamorphosis. Similarly, null mutants of catalase, which are viable but exceptionally feeble as adults (66), are lethal in double mutant combination with Cu,Zn superoxide dismutase-null mutants.

The *Drosophila* Cu,Zn SOD gene and its mRNA have been sequenced (67). The *Drosophila* gene contains a single intron of 720 nucleotides between the codons specifying amino acid residues 22 and 23; this is analogous to the position of the first of the four introns in the human Cu,Zn SOD gene (68).

A Note on the Manganese Superoxide Dismutase in *Drosophila*

The biochemistry of Mn superoxide dismutase in *Drosophila* is virtually unknown, although the activity is detectable in native electrophoretic gels; the enzyme awaits thorough analysis and purification. No Mn superoxide dismutase mutants have yet been reported. Recently, however, Mn superoxide dismutase cDNA from *Drosophila* has been cloned and sequenced (69). The cDNA (803 nucleotides) carries an open reading frame which specifies a polypeptide of 228 amino acid residues, exhibiting >50% identity and >90% homology (identity or conservative substitutions) with Mn superoxide dismutase from both *C. elegans* and humans.

AMYOTROPHIC LATERAL SCLEROSIS AND SUPEROXIDE DISMUTASE

An extraordinary recent discovery in human genetics has focused new attention on the biochemistry of superoxide dismutase (70). The genetic mapping of the gene for familial amyotrophic lateral sclerosis (FALS) culminated in the identification of the gene responsible for the disease as SOD1, encoding Cu,Zn superoxide dismutase. FALS is the inherited form of ALS ("Lou Gehrig's disease"), a fatal degenerative disease which causes death of motor neurons, resulting in gradual loss of control over the muscles. Only about 10% of the cases of ALS are familial. A variety of SOD1 mutations were discovered in several different families affected by FALS. The SOD activity in red blood cells from affected individuals (heterozygotes) is less than half of the activity in normal controls (71). The mechanism leading to the selective loss of motor neurons is now the focus of intense research interest (72). The pace of new developments in this field is so fast that it is impossible to present a summary at the time of writing; a recent review is listed in note 73 to this chapter. Another recent study suggests that induction of apoptosis (programmed cell death; see Chapter 18) is promoted by FALS mutant forms of superoxide dismutase (74).

MECHANISMS OF SUPEROXIDE TOXICITY

The oxygen-sensitivity of superoxide dismutase null mutants, discussed above, is perhaps the strongest evidence for the toxicity of superoxide. The inhibition of enzymes such as aconitase provides an identifiable target for superoxide. But the question still remains: Why is superoxide toxic? What is the chemical basis of the observed biochemical effects? This has been a highly contentious question (75).

Superoxide anion is, perhaps disconcertingly, not very reactive. Superoxide can act as a reducing agent (as discussed earlier) or an oxidizing agent (oxidation of epinephrine, ascorbate, catecholamines, and other compounds). Superoxide can propagate autoxidation chain reactions, as discussed later in this chapter. The oxidation by superoxide of a ferrous iron in the [4Fe–4S] clusters of the enzymes α,β-dihydroxy acid dehydratase (see above) and aconitase (76) results in loss of catalytic activity. As a nucleophile, superoxide reacts with alkyl halides to give peroxides, and it also reacts with disulfides to form sulfinic and sulfonic acids (77).

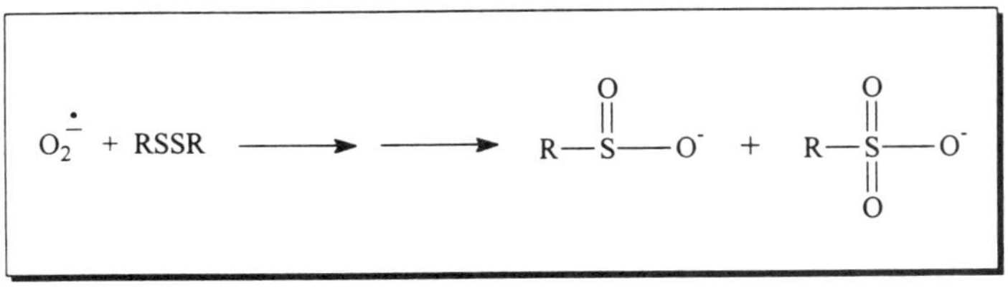

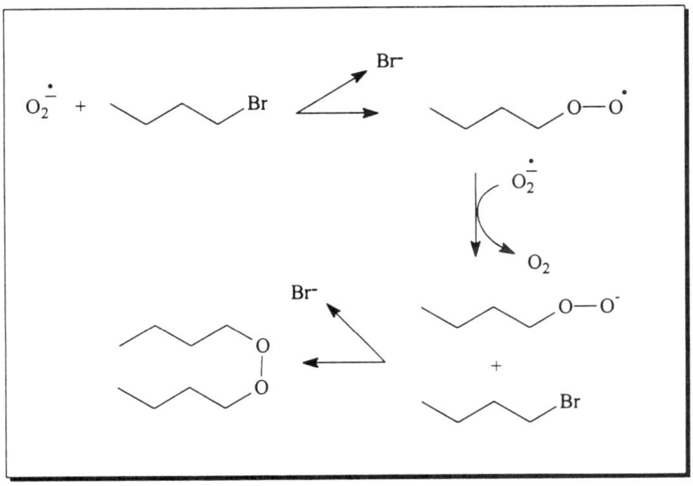

But reactions of this sort do not seem to fit with the concept of superoxide as a chemical agent of oxidant stress. On the other hand, sources of superoxide are also sources of hydrogen peroxide, via dismutation, and much attention has been focused on the possible interactions of these reduced oxygen products. The so-called Haber–Weiss stoichiometry:

$$O_2{}^{\cdot-} + H_2O_2 + H^+ \rightarrow O_2 + H_2O + OH^-$$

that is, one-electron reduction of hydrogen peroxide by superoxide, represents a source of the reactive hydroxyl radical. However, pulse radiolysis studies showed that this putative reaction does not occur at an appreciable rate. An alternative possibility is metal-catalyzed reduction of hydrogen peroxide, as follows:

$$O_2{}^{\cdot-} + Me^{n+} \rightarrow O_2 + Me^{(n-1)+}$$
$$Me^{(n-1)+} + H_2O_2 \rightarrow Me^{n+} + OH^- + OH^-$$

In this so-called metal-catalyzed Haber–Weiss reaction, a metal ion (e.g., Fe^{2+}) reduces hydrogen peroxide, and the role of superoxide is limited to that of a reducing agent. In fact, the second part of this reaction scheme, the reduction of hydrogen peroxide by ferrous iron, is well-precedented. As long ago as 1893, the English chemist Henry J. H. Fenton showed that ferrous iron plus hydrogen peroxide oxidized tartaric acid to dihydroxymaleic acid:

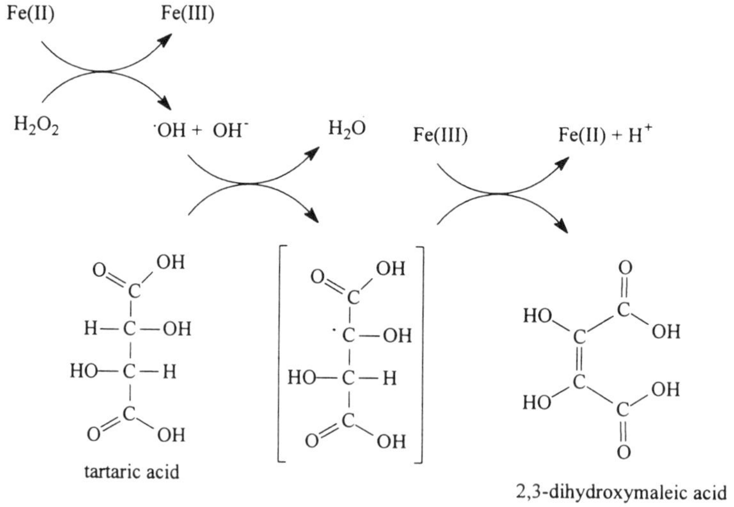

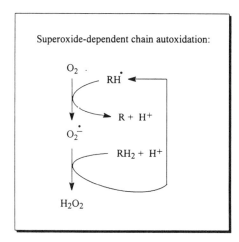

Fe(II)   Fe(III)

H_2O_2 $\cdot OH + OH^-$ H_2O Fe(III) $Fe(II) + H^+$

tartaric acid

2,3-dihydroxymaleic acid

Fenton later extended the use of this oxidizing system and developed several useful syntheses of carbohydrates by this route. The history and significance of Fenton's work has been reviewed recently (78). The possible involvement of hydroxyl radical in the mechanism of the Fenton reaction was first proposed in the 1940s. The biochemical significance of generation of hydroxyl radical by "Fenton chemistry" has been disputed, since free ferrous ion is probably not present in significant concentrations. [However, superoxide itself can cause the release of ferrous iron from the [4Fe–4S] clusters of some enzymes (79).]

An alternative hypothesis to account for the role of superoxide dismutase has been presented recently by Christine Winterbourn (80):

Superoxide-dependent chain autoxidation:

O_2

$RH^\bullet$

$R + H^+$

$O_2^{\cdot -}$

$RH_2 + H^+$

H_2O_2

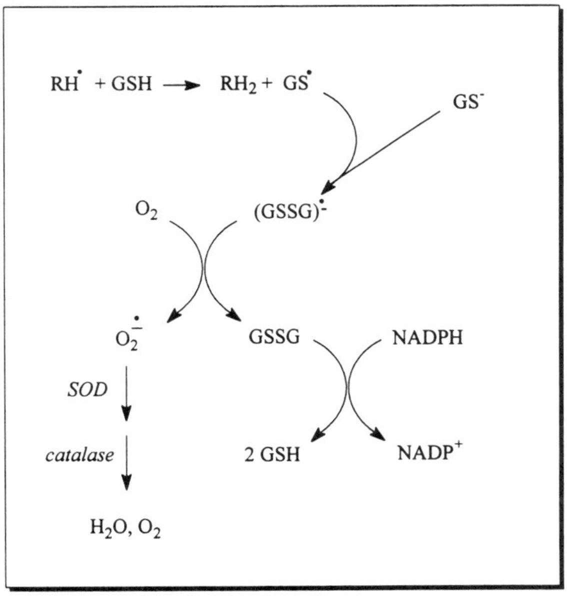

In this "radical sink" hypothesis, oxygen acts as the ultimate scavenger of many cellular radicals, via the action of reduced glutathione (γ-glutamylcysteinylglycine, GSH; see page 86 and Chapter 11):

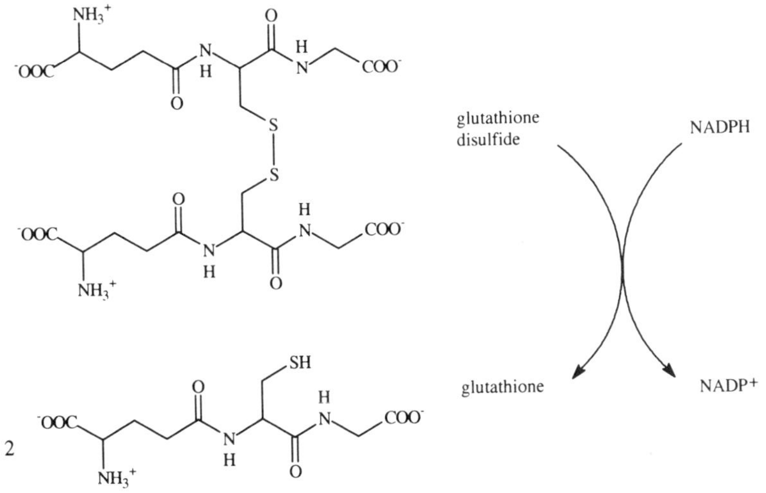

GSH repairs radicals (e.g., alkyl or alkoxyl radicals) by reduction:

$$R^\cdot + GSH \rightarrow RH + GS^\cdot$$

The product thiyl radical could, itself, propagate free radical damage, but is rapidly scavenged by a further molecule of glutathione anion:

$$GS^\cdot + GS^- \rightarrow (GSSG)^{\cdot\,-}$$

This reaction is feasible, since the pK_a of glutathione (8.8) allows a substantial concentration of the anion to exist at neutral pH, and pulse radiolysis studies have shown that the reaction is rapid. In turn, GSSG$^{\cdot-}$ rapidly, and irreversibly, reduces oxygen to super-oxide:

$$(GSSG)^{\cdot-} + O_2 \rightarrow GSSG + O_2^{\cdot-}$$

Glutathione disulfide is reduced by NADPH and the flavoenzyme glutathione reductase (81):

$$GSSG + NADPH \rightarrow 2GSH + NADP^+$$

while superoxide is detoxified by superoxide dismutase and catalases (see below):

$$2O_2^{\cdot-} + 2H^+ \rightarrow O_2 + H_2O_2$$
$$2H_2O_2 \rightarrow 2H_2O + O_2$$

Effectively, superoxide acts as the sink to which much or all of cellular radical generation is diverted; the combination of superoxide dismutase and catalase then disposes of the radical products. In this way, the cell uses glutathione as a general repair molecule for radical damages; the repair pathways converge on superoxide.

In the absence of superoxide dismutase, superoxide formation would impose oxidative stress on the cell; the ability of superoxide to propagate radical chain reactions means that a single superoxide molecule can produce many molecules of hydrogen peroxide. For example, consider the autoxidation of a hydroquinone or catecholamine, QH_2:

$$QH_2 + O_2^{\cdot-} + H^+ \rightarrow QH^\cdot + H_2O_2$$
$$QH^\cdot + O_2 \rightarrow Q + O_2^{\cdot-} + H^+$$
$$Net: \quad QH_2 + O_2 \rightarrow Q + H_2O_2$$

Oxidative stress and damage ensue from glutathione depletion and the accumulation of unrepaired radicals and hydrogen peroxide.

The "radical sink" idea links the roles of glutathione and superoxide dismutase, two key components of cellular defense against oxidative stress, and should provide a useful framework for future studies of the biochemistry of superoxide radical.

NOTES

1. Gerschman, R., Gilbert, D. L., Nye, S. W., Dwyer, P., and Fenn, W. O., Oxygen poisoning and X-irradiation: A mechanism in common, *Science* 119:623–626, 1954.
2. McCord, J. M., and Fridovich, I., Superoxide dismutase: The first twenty years (1968–1988), *Free Radic. Biol. Med.* 5:363–369, 1988.
3. Becker, B. F., Towards the physiological function of uric acid, *Free Radicals Biol. Med.* 14:615–631, 1993.
4. Horecker, B. L., and Heppel, L. A. The reduction of cytochrome c by xanthine oxidase, *J. Biol. Chem.* 178:683–690, 1949.
5. Weber, M. M., Lenhoff, H. M., and Kaplan, N. O., The reduction of cytochrome c and inorganic iron by flavin enzymes, *J. Biol. Chem.*, 220:93–104, 1956.
6. Fridovich, I., and Handler, P. Xanthine oxidase. V. Differential inhibition of the reduction of various electron acceptors, *J. Biol. Chem.* 237:916–921, 1962.
7. von Sonntag, C., *The Chemical Basis of Radiation Biology*, Taylor & Francis, London, 1987.
8. Schwarz, H. A., Free radicals generated by radiolysis of aqueous solutions, *J. Chem. Ed.* 58:101–105, 1981 (State of the Art Symposium: Radiation Chemistry).
9. McCord, J. M., and Fridovich, I. Superoxide dismutase: An enzymic function for erythrocuprein, *J. Biol. Chem.* 244:6049–6055, 1969.
10. Harcourt, A. V., On the peroxides of potassium and sodium, *J. Chem. Soc. (Lond.)* 14:267, 1861.

11. Neuman, E. W., Potassium superoxide and the three-electron bond, *J. Chem. Phys.* 2:31–33, 1934.

12. Valentine, J. S. and Curtis, A. B., A convenient preparation of solutions of superoxide anion and the reactions of superoxide anion with a copper(II) complex, *J. Am. Chem. Soc.* 97: 224–226, 1975.

13. Goldstein, S., Michel, C., Bors, W., Saran, M., and Czapski, G., A critical reevaluation of some assay methods for superoxide dismutase activity, *Free Radic. Biol. Med.* 4:295–303, 1988.

14. Klug, D., Fridovich, I., and Rabani, J., Pulse radiolysis investigation of superoxide disproportionation. Mechanism for bovine superoxide dismutase, *J. Am. Chem. Soc.* 95:2786–2791, 1973.

15. Asada, K., Kiso, K., and Yoshikawa, K. Univalent reduction of molecular oxygen by spinach chloroplasts on illumination, *J. Biol. Chem.* 249:2175–2181, 1974.

16. Asada, K., Production and scavenging of active oxygen in chloroplasts, in: *Molecular Biology of Free Radical Scavenging Systems*, J. G. Scandalios, Ed., Cold Spring Harbor Laboratory Press, Cold Spring Harbor, NY, 1992, pp. 173–192.

17. Hassan, H. M., and Fridovich, I., Paraquat and *Escherichia coli*: Mechanism of production of extracellular superoxide radical, *J. Biol. Chem.* 254:10846–10852, 1979.

18. Kappus, H., and Sies, H., Toxic drug effects associated with oxygen metabolism: Redox cycling and lipid peroxidation, *Experientia* 37:1233–1241, 1981.

19. Mason, R. P., Free radical intermediates in the metabolism of toxic chemicals, in: *Free Radicals in Biology*, Vol. 5, Pryor, W. A., Ed., Academic Press, New York, 1982, pp. 161–222.

20. Turner, C. E., Elsohly, M. A., Cheng, F. P., and Torres, L. M., Marijuana and paraquat, *JAMA* 240:1857, 1978.

21. Hassan, H. M., and Fridovich, I., Intracellular production of superoxide and of hydrogen peroxide by redox active compounds, *Arch. Biochem. Biophys.* 196:385–395, 1979.

22. Anraku, Y., and Gennis, R. B., The aerobic respiratory chain of *Escherichia coli*, *Trends Biochem. Sci.* 12:262–266, 1987.

23. Poole, R. K., and Ingeldew, W. J. Pathways of electrons to oxygen, in: *Escherichia coli and Salmonella typhimurium*, F. C. Neidhardt, Ed.), pp. 170–200, American Society for Microbiologists, Washington, D.C., 1987.

24. McManus, D. C., and Josephy, P. D., A new approach to measurement of redox-cycling activity in *Escherichia coli*, *Arch. Biochem. Biophys.* 304:367–370, 1993.

25. Kirby, T. W., and Fridovich, I., A picomolar spectrophotometric assay for superoxide dismutase, *Anal. Biochem.* 127:435–440, 1982.

26. Beauchamp, C., and Fridovich, I. Superoxide dismutase: Improved assays and an assay applicable to acrylamide gels, *Anal. Biochem.* 44:276–287, 1971.

27. Hodgson, E. K., and Fridovich, I., Reversal of the superoxide dismutase reaction, *Biochem. Biophys. Res. Commun.* 54:270–274, 1973.

28. Bunce, N. J., Introduction to the interpretation of electron spin resonance spectra of organic radicals, *J. Chem. Ed.* 64:907–914, 1987; Weil, J. A., Bolton, J. R., and Wertz, J. E., *Electron Paramagnetic Resonance: Elementary Theory and Practical Applications*, John Wiley & Sons, New York, 1994.

29. Iwahashi, H., Parker, C. E., Mason, R. P., and Tomer, K. B., Combined liquid chromatography/electron paramagnetic resonance spectrometry/electrospray ionization mass spectrometry for radical identification, *Anal. Chem.* 64:2244–2252, 1992.

30. Chamulitrat, W., Jordan, S. J., and Mason, R. P., Fatty acid radical formation in rats administered oxidized fatty acids: In vivo spin trapping study, *Arch. Biochem. Biophys.* 299:361–367, 1992; Mason, R. P., and Knecht, K. T., In vivo detection of radical adducts by electron spin resonance, *Methods Enzymol.* 233:112–117, 1994.

31. See, for example: Steinman, H. M., Function of periplasmic copper-zinc superoxide dismutase in *Caulobacter crescentus*, *J. Bacteriol.* 175:1198–1202, 1993.

32. Benov, L. T., and Fridovich, I., *Escherichia coli* expresses a copper- and zinc-containing superoxide dismutase, *J. Biol. Chem.* 269:25310–25314, 1994.

33. Tainer, J. A., Getzoff, E. D., Richardson, J. S., and Richardson, D. C. Structure and mechanism of copper, zinc superoxide dismutase, *Nature* 306:284–287, 1983.

34. Parge, H. E., Hallewell, R. A., and Tainer, J. A. Atomic structures of wild-type and thermostable recombinant human Cu,Zn superoxide dismutase, *Proc. Natl. Acad. Sci USA* 89:6109–6113, 1992.

35. Tibell, L., Aasa, R., and Marklund, S. L., Spectral and physical properties of human extracellular superoxide dismutase: A comparison with CuZn superoxide dismutase, *Arch. Biochem. Biophys.* 304:429–433, 1993.

36. Stallings, W. C., Bull, C., Fee, J. A., Lah, M. S., and Ludwig, M. L., Iron and manganese superoxide dismutases: Catalytic inferences from the structures, in *Molecular Biology of Free Radical Scavenging Systems*, J. G. Scandalios, Ed., Cold Spring Harbor Laboratory Press, Cold Spring Harbor, NY, 1992, pp. 193–211.

37. Beyer, W. F., Jr., and Fridovich, I., In vivo competition between iron and manganese for the active site region of the manganese superoxide dismutase of *Escherichia coli*, *J. Biol. Chem.* 266:303–308, 1991.

38. Steinman, H. M., Weinstein, L., and Brenowitz, M., The manganese superoxide dismutase of *Escherichia coli* K-12 associates with DNA, *J. Biol. Chem.* 269:28629–28634, 1994.

39. Borgstahl, G. E. O., Parge, H. E., Hickey, M. J., Beyer, W. F., Jr., Hallewell, R. A., and Tainer, J. A., The structure of human mitochondrial manganese superoxide dismutase reveals a novel tetrameric interface of two 4–helix bundles, *Cell* 71:107–116, 1992.

40. Touati, D., Cloning and mapping of the manganese superoxide dismutase gene (*sodA*) of *Escherichia coli* K-12, *J. Bacteriol.* 155:1078–1087, 1983; Sakamoto, H., and Touati, D., Cloning of the iron superoxide dismutase gene (*sodB*) in *Escherichia coli* K-12, *J. Bacteriol.* 159:418–420, 1984.

41. Watson, J. D., Gilman, M., Witkowski, J., and Zoller, M., *Recombinant DNA*, 2nd ed., W. H. Freeman, New York, 1992, pp. 126–127; Tabata, S., Higashitani, A., Takanami, N., Akiyama, K., Kohara, Y., Nishimura, Y., Yasuda, S., and Hirota, Y., Construction of an ordered cosmid collection of the *Escherichia coli* K-12 W3110 chromosome, *J. Bacteriol* 171:1214–1218, 1989.

42. Slauch, J. M., and Silhavy, T.J. Genetic fusions as experimental tools, *Methods Enzymol.* 204: 213–248, 1991.

43. Miller, J. H., *A Short Course in Bacterial Genetics*, Cold Spring Harbor Laboratory Press, Plainview, NY, 1992, pp. 385ff.

44. Touati, D., Transcriptional and posttranscriptional regulation of manganese superoxide dismutase biosynthesis in *Escherichia coli*, studied with operon and protein fusions, *J. Bacteriol.* 170:2511–2520, 1988.

45. Sambrook, J., Fritsch, E. F., and Maniatis, T., *Molecular Cloning: A Laboratory Manual*, 2nd ed., Cold Spring Harbor Laboratory Press, Cold Spring Harbor, NY, 1989, §17–13.

46. Hopkin, K. A., Papazian, M. A., and Steinman, H. M., Functional differences between manganese and iron superoxide dismutases in *Escherichia coli* K-12, *J. Biol. Chem.* 267:24253–24258, 1992.

47. Beckwith, J., The lactose operon, in: *Escherichia coli* and *Salmonella typhimurium: Cellular and Molecular Biology*, Vol. 2, F. C. Neidhardt, J. L. Ingraham, K. B. Low, B. Magasanik, M. Schaechter, and H. E. Umbarger (Eds.), American Society for Microbiology, Washington, D.C., 1987, pp. 1444–1452.

48. Carlioz, A., and Touati, D., Isolation of superoxide dismutase mutants in *Escherichia coli*: Is superoxide dismutase necessary for aerobic life? *EMBO J.*, 5:623–630, 1986.

49. Flint, D. H., and Emptage, M. H., Dihydroxy acid dehydratase—isolation, characterization as Fe–S proteins, and sensitivity to inactivation by oxygen radicals, In: *Biosynthesis of Branched-Chain Amino Acids*, Barak, Z., Chipman, D., and Schloss, J. V., Eds., Deerfield, Borch, and Balaban, Publishers, Philadelphia, 1990, pp. 285–314.

50. See review: Beyer, W., Imlay, J., and Fridovich, I., Superoxide dismutases, *Prog. Nucleic Acid Res. Mol. Biol.* 40:221–253, 1991.

51. Touati, D., and Farr, S. B., Elevated mutagenesis in bacterial mutants lacking superoxide dismutase, *Methods Enzymol.* 186:646–651, 1990.

52. McManus, D. C., and Josephy, P. D., Superoxide dismutase protects *Escherichia coli* against killing by human serum, *Arch. Biochem. Biophys.* 317:57–61, 1995.

53. Lee, Y. M., Friedman, D. J., and Ayala, F. J., Complete amino acid sequence of copper-zinc superoxide dismutase from *Drosophila melanogaster*, *Arch. Biochem. Biophys.* 241:577–589, 1985.

54. Ayala, F. J., Powell, J., and Dobzhansky, T., Polymorphisms in continental and island populations of *Drosophila willistoni*, *Proc. Natl. Acad. Sci. USA* 68:2480–2483, 1971.

55. Lee, Y. M., Misra, H. P., and Ayala, F. J., Superoxide dismutase in *Drosophila melanogaster*: Biochemical and structural characterization of allozyme variants, *Proc. Natl. Acad. Sci. USA* 78:2052–2055, 1981.

56. Suzuki, D. T., Griffiths, A. J. F., Miller, J. H., and Lewontin, R. C., *An Introduction to Genetic Analysis*, 4th ed., W. H. Freeman, New York, 1989; pp. 100 ff. and Fig. 5-14.

57. Campbell, S. D., Hilliker, A. J., and Phillips, J. P., Cytogenetic analysis of the cSOD microregion in *Drosophila melanogaster*, *Genetics* 112:205–215, 1986.

58. Phillips, J. P., Campbell, S. D., Michaud, D., Charbonneau, M., and Hilliker, A. J., A null mutation of superoxide dismutase in *Drosophila* confers hypersensitivity to paraquat and reduced longevity, *Proc. Natl. Acad. Sci. U.S.A.* 86:2761–2765, 1989.

59. Gralla, E. B., and Valentine, J. S., Null mutants of *Saccharomyces cerevisiae* Cu,Zn superoxide dismutase: Characterization and spontaneous mutation rates. *J. Bactertiol.* 173:5918–5920, 1991.

60. Touati, D., Molecular genetics of superoxide dismutases, *Free Radic. Biol. Med.* 5:393–402, 1988.

61. Staveley, B. E., Phillips, J. P., and Hilliker, A. J., Phenotypic consequences of copper/zinc superoxide dismutase overexpression in *Drosophila melanogaster*, *Genome* 33:867–872, 1991.

62. Lewin, B., *Genes IV*, Oxford University Press, New York, 1990, pp. 700–701.

63. Seto, N. O., Hayashi, S., and Tener, G. M., Overexpression of Cu–Zn superoxide dismutase in *Drosophila* does not affect life-span, *Proc. Natl. Acad. Sci. USA* 87:4270–4274, 1990.

64. Orr, W. C., and Sohal, R. S., Extension of life-span by overexpression of superoxide dismutase and catalase in *Drosophila melanogaster*, *Science* 263:1128–1130, 1994.

65. Hilliker, A. J., Duyf, B., Evans, D., and Phillips, J. P., Urate-null rosy mutants of *Drosophila melanogaster* are hypersensitive to oxygen stress, *Proc. Natl. Acad. Sci. USA* 89:4343–4347, 1992.

66. Orr, W. C., Arnold, L. A., and Sohal, R. S., Relationship between catalase activity, life span and some parameters associated with antioxidant defenses in *Drosophila melanogaster*, *Mech. Ageing Dev.* 63:287–296, 1992.

67. Seto, N. O. L., Hayashi, S., and Tener, G. M., The sequence of the Cu–Zn superoxide dismutase gene of *Drosophila*, *Nucleic Acids Res.* 15:10601–10601, 1987.

68. Levanon, D., Lieman-Hurwitz, J., Dafni, A., Wigderson, M., Sherman, L., Bernstein, Y., Laver-Rudich, Z., Danciger, E., Stein, O., and Groner, Y., Architecture and anatomy of the chromosomal locus in human chromosome 21 encoding the Cu/Zn superoxide dismutase, *EMBO J.* 4:77–84, 1985.

69. Duttaroy, A., Meidinger, R., Kirby, K., Carmichael, S., Hilliker, A., and Phillips, J., A manganese superoxide dismutase-encoding cDNA from *Drosophila melanogaster*, *Gene* 143:223–225, 1994.

70. Rosen, D. R., Siddique, T., Patterson, D., Figlewicz, D. A., Sapp, P., Hentati, A., Donaldson, D., Goto, J., O'Regan, J. P., Deng, H.-X., Rahmani, Z., Krizus, A., McKenna-Yasek, D., Cayabyab, A., Gaston, S. M., Berger, R., Tanzi, R. E., Halperin, J. J., Herzfeldt, B., Van den Bergh, R., Hung, W. Y., Bird, T., Deng, G., and Mulder, D. W., Mutations in Cu/Zn superoxide dismutase gene are associated with familial amyotrophic lateral sclerosis, *Nature* 362:59–62, 1993.

71. Deng, H.-X., Hentati, A., Tainer, J. A., Iqbal, Z., Cayabyab, A., Hung, W.-Y., Getzoff, E. D., Hu, P., Herzfeldt, B., Roos, R. P., Warner, C., Deng, G., Soriano, E., Smyth, C., Parge, H. E., Ahmed, A., Roses, A. D., Hallewell, R. A., Pericak-Vance, M. A., and Siddique, T., Amyotrophic lateral sclerosis and structural defects in Cu,Zn superoxide dismutase, *Science* 261:1047–1051, 1993.

72. Borchelt, D. R., Lee, M. K., Slunt, H. S., Guarnieri, M., Xu, Z.-S., Wong, P. C., Brown, R. H., Jr., Price, D. L., Sisodia, S. S., and Cleveland, D. W., Superoxide dismutase 1 with mutations

linked to familial amyotrophic lateral sclerosis possesses significant activity, *Proc. Natl. Acad. Sci. USA* 91:8292–8296, 1994.

73. Smith, R. G., and Appel, S. H., Molecular approaches to amyotrophic lateral sclerosis, *Annu. Rev. Med.* 46:133–145, 1995.

74. Rabizadeh, S., Gralla, E. B., Borchelt, D. R., Gwinn, R., Valentine, J. S., Sisodia, S., Wong, P., Lee, M., Hahn, H., and Bredesen, D. E., Mutations associated with amyotrophic lateral sclerosis convert superoxide dismutase from an antiapoptotic gene to a proapoptotic gene: Studies in yeast and neural cells, *Proc. Natl. Acad. Sci. USA* 92:3024–3028, 1995.

75. Fridovich, I., Superoxide radical and superoxide dismutases, *Annu. Rev. Biochem.* 64:97–112, 1995.

76. Gardner, P. R., and Fridovich, I., Superoxide sensitivity of the *Escherichia coli* aconitase, *J. Biol. Chem.* 266:19328–1933, 1991.

77. Afanas'ev, I. B., *Superoxide Ion: Chemistry and Biological Implications*, Vol. 1, CRC Press, Boca Raton, FL, 1989.

78. Koppenol, W. H., The centennial of the Fenton reaction, *Free Radic. Biol. Med.* 15:645–651, 1993.

79. Liochev, S. I., and Fridovich, I., The role of $O_2^{\cdot-}$ in the production of HO$^{\cdot}$: In vitro and in vivo, *Free Radic. Biol. Med.* 16:29–33, 1994.

80. Winterbourn, C. C. Superoxide as an intracellular radical sink, *Free Radic. Biol. Med.* 14:85–90, 1993.

81. Voet, D., and Voet, J. G., *Biochemistry*, 2nd ed., Wiley, New York, 1995, pp. 400–406.

5

HYDROGEN PEROXIDE, CATALASE, AND PEROXIDASES

Hydrogen peroxide can arise in the biological milieu either directly (e.g., as a product of oxygen reduction by certain oxidases) or indirectly, via the dismutation of superoxide. Hydrogen peroxide is removed by catalase or peroxidase:

$$Catalase: \quad H_2O_2 + H_2O_2 \rightarrow 2H_2O + O_2$$
$$Peroxidase: \quad H_2O_2 + AH_2 \rightarrow 2H_2O + A$$

Catalase is a special case of peroxidase, in which hydrogen peroxide acts as both oxidant and reductant in the reaction; peroxidases oxidize other organic or inorganic substrates.

The term *hydroperoxidase* refers collectively to peroxidases and catalases. Hydroperoxidases are very widely distributed in bacteria, yeast, plants, and animals (1), and they are probably ubiquitous in aerobic organisms. The study of catalase has occupied an important place in the development of biochemical science. Hydrogen peroxide was first prepared by the French chemist Thénard in the early nineteenth century. Thénard observed the characteristic bubbling of hydrogen peroxide solutions in the presence of animal tissues, due to the evolution of oxygen gas. His observation preceded, by many decades, the development of the enzyme concept. The isolation of catalases (from tobacco, yeast, and blood) was first attempted early in this century. (An early hypothesis held that hydrogen peroxide decomposition was a universal property of enzymes; the theory is long since discredited, but accounts for the peculiar name of the enzyme, which has remained in use.) In 1936, the prosthetic group of beef liver catalase was identified as heme; the enzyme was crystallized one year later.

CATALASE AND PEROXIDASE REACTION CYCLES

Following the pioneering spectroscopic studies of David Keilin, Britton Chance and colleagues (University of Pennsylvania) applied the new technique of fast-flow spectrophotometry to study the formation and decay of intermediates in the reaction cycles of catalase and peroxidases in the 1940s (2). The native state of catalase contains ferric (Fe^{3+}) heme. Chance identified, by optical spectroscopy, a short-lived oxidized intermediate form of the enzyme, which he named "Compound I":

$$Catalase (Fe^{3+}) + H_2O_2 \rightarrow Catalase\ Compound\ I\ (Fe^{5+}\ O^{2-}) + H_2O$$
$$Catalase\ Compound\ I + H_2O_2 \rightarrow Catalase\ (Fe^{3+}) + O_2 + H_2O$$

Compound I is formed upon interaction of the ferric enzyme with hydrogen peroxide, and it represents a form of the protein with a formal oxidation state of Fe^{5+}. In fact, it is probably better viewed as containing ferryl heme (Fe^{4+}) and a porphyrin π-cation radical (3). Compound I was the first enzyme–substrate complex to be detected spectroscopically; its existence confirmed the validity of the [ES] hypothesis of Michaelis and Menten, which was postulated from kinetic theory. The structure of compound I is also of interest as a paradigm for the structure of the catalytic intermediates of the heme enzyme cytochrome P-450 (see Chapter 14) and other metalloenzymes which interact with oxygen (4).

The reaction cycle of peroxidases also begins with Compound I formation. However, with most organic reducing substrates, the return to the resting (ferric) enzyme occurs via one-electron steps; the half-oxidized enzyme state is known as Compound II and has also been identified by optical spectroscopy.

Peroxidase (Fe^{3+}) + H_2O_2 → Peroxidase Compound I (Fe^{5+} O^{2-}) + H_2O

Peroxidase Compound I (Fe^{5+} O^{2-}) + RH_2 → Peroxidase Compound II (Fe^{4+}) + RH˙ + OH^-

Peroxidase Compound II (Fe^{4+}) + RH_2 → Peroxidase (Fe^{3+}) + RH˙ + H^+

Net: H_2O_2 + 2 RH_2 → 2 H_2O + 2 RH˙

The organic substrate is oxidized to a free radical. Substrate-derived radicals formed by peroxidases were first detected by Yamazaki and colleagues (5), using electron paramagnetic (spin) resonance spectroscopy (EPR); see Chapter 4. Typical peroxidases, such as horseradish peroxidase, can oxidize a wide variety of substrates, including ascorbate, hydroquinones, aminophenols, aromatic amine and diamines, and polycyclic aromatic hydrocarbons. In some cases, these oxidations generate reactive intermediates which may be of toxicological importance (6).

SIDEBAR: PROSTAGLANDIN H SYNTHASE

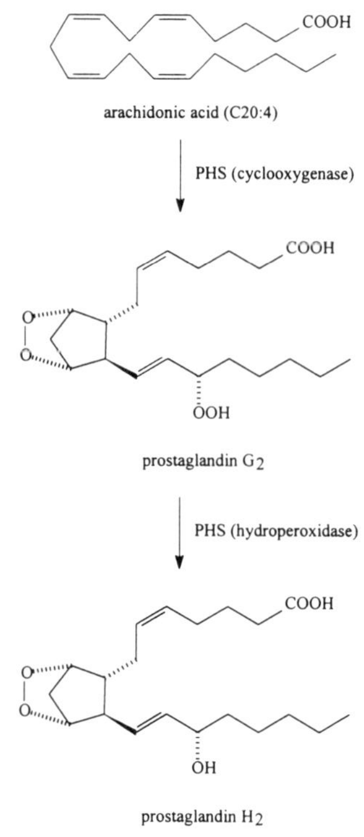

arachidonic acid (C20:4)

PHS (cyclooxygenase)

prostaglandin G₂

PHS (hydroperoxidase)

prostaglandin H₂

Prostaglandin H synthase (see also Chapter 7), the enzyme which catalyzes the first step in the biosynthesis of the prostaglandins from polyunsaturated fatty acids, has two activities: cyclooxygenase (conversion of arachidonic acid to PGG_2) and peroxidase (reduction of PGG_2 hydroperoxide to PGH_2 alcohol). PHS is an unusual peroxidase: The enzyme generates its own peroxide substrate, via the cyclooxygenase step, an enzyme-catalyzed lipid peroxidation reaction (7). PHS activity is found in many important target organs for chemical carcinogenesis, including the lung, kidney, skin, and bladder. The peroxidase activity of PHS may convert xenobiotic substrates, including aromatic amines and polycyclic aromatic hydrocarbons, into reactive intermediates in vivo (8).

Escherichia coli HYDROPEROXIDASES

Escherichia coli produces two hydroperoxidases, HPI and HPII (9), which differ in structural, kinetic, and regulatory properties. HPI is produced under both aerobic and anaerobic conditions and is induced when cells are exposed to hydrogen peroxide (10). HPII is produced at low levels when cultures are grown anaerobically, or are in exponential growth phase, but is the principal catalase in aerobic, stationary phase cultures. HPI is composed of four 80-kD subunits and contains two molecules of protoheme IX (one molecule per two subunits). HPII is composed of six identical 93-kD subunits (11) and contains one molecule of heme d per subunit. Heme d

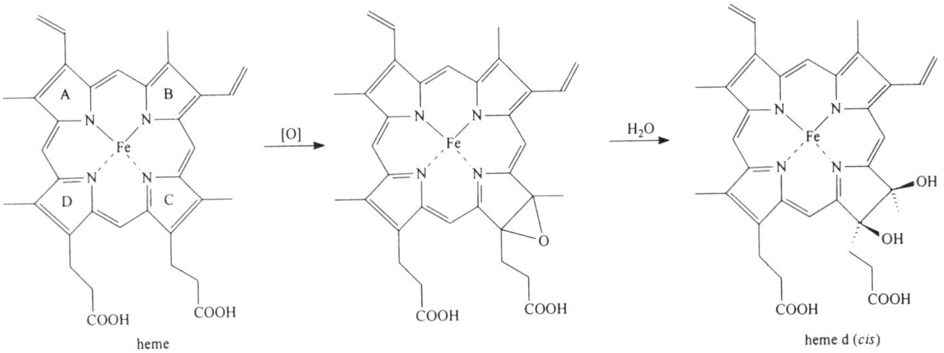

heme   heme d (*cis*)

is a modified form of heme, in which the C ring is oxidized to a dihydrodiol. Heme is incorporated into the enzyme at biosynthesis, and oxidation to heme d occurs during the first catalytic turnovers (12).

The availability of hydroperoxidase mutants has facilitated studies on the regulatory aspects of the two isozymes and has allowed isolation of the structural and regulatory genes that control their expression. Genetic screens to isolate catalase-deficient mutants are based on either (a) the phenotype of hydrogen peroxide sensitivity of cultures grown on Petri dishes (HPI-deficient mutants) or (b) a plate assay for catalase activity (HPII-deficient mutants). Wild-type *E. coli* colonies produce oxygen gas bubbles when flooded with a solution of hydrogen peroxide.

In the early 1980s, Peter Loewen (University of Manitoba) and co-workers, using the latter assay as a screen, identified *E. coli* mutants that do not produce gas; two genes (*katE* and *katF*) were responsible for synthesis of the major aerobically produced catalase, HPII. Both *katE* and *katF* have been cloned and sequenced (13). *katF* is a regulator of *katE*, the structural gene for HPII. Based on nucleic acid sequence homology and in vitro transcription assays using purified *katF*-regulated genes (14), KatF protein was identified as an alternative *sigma factor*, a subunit of RNA polymerase that directs the transcription of specific genes (see following section).

HPI is probably the most important cellular determinant for hydrogen peroxide resistance. Unlike HPII, HPI has both catalase and peroxidase activity (22). The structural gene for HPI, *katG*, has been mapped, cloned, and sequenced (23). HPI is part of a group of approximately 30 proteins that are induced when cells are exposed to hydrogen peroxide (see below).

Ma and Eaton (24) have recently shown that the protective action of bacterial catalase against hydrogen peroxide toxicity is only manifested at high bacterial cell concentrations. Since hydrogen peroxide is freely permeable to the bacterial cell wall, isolated *E. coli* cells are unable to generate an inside/outside concentration gradient of this oxidant. At low cell densities, catalase⁻ mutants are no more sensitive to hydrogen peroxide than are wild-type cells. However, colonies of catalase-producing cells (or dense suspension cultures) can exert a mass-action effect and can clear hydrogen peroxide from solutions (25); this effect protects the cells against hydrogen peroxide toxicity. Therefore, at high cell densities in culture, or in the case of colonial growth on plates, wild-type cells are much more resistant to hydrogen peroxide than are catalase⁻ mutants. This phenomenon illustrates the ability of colonial (or multicellular) aggregates to carry out homeostatic regulation of their milieu. Such considerations may help to explain the selective pressure leading to the evolution of multicellular organisms.

GLOBAL REGULATORY RESPONSES TO OXIDATIVE STRESS IN *E. coli* AND *S. typhimurium*

Bacteria respond to environmental stresses by regulation of gene transcription. Recent investigations have identified several global responses to stress: coordinated regulation of many genes at dispersed sites on the chromosome, collectively called a *regulon*. These regulons include the heat-shock response (15), the "adaptive response" to alkylating agents, and the SOS response to DNA damage (16). Regulon control plays a fundamental role in the physiology and ecology of bacteria, and analogous control circuits exist in eukaryotes.

In 1983, Demple and Halbrook (26) demonstrated the existence of an adaptive response to hydrogen peroxide. They showed that preexposure of *E. coli* to low concentrations (approximately 5–100 μM) of hydrogen peroxide resulted in greatly increased resistance to the toxicity of a subsequent challenge with a high level of hydrogen peroxide. This preexposure induces the expression of catalase HPI (but not SOD) in *E. coli*. The response is under the control of the *oxyR* gene; *oxyR*1 mutants constitutively overexpress a set of 8–10 H_2O_2-inducible proteins (including catalase HPI, alkyl hydroperoxide reductase, and gutathione reductase) and are H_2O_2-resistant. These effects are mediated biochemically by the oxidation of the OxyR protein, which alters its interaction with promoter targets (27). Under "nonstress" conditions, OxyR is not a transcriptional activator. However, under conditions of oxidative stress, signaled by the presence of hydrogen peroxide, the protein becomes oxidized, causing a conformational change in OxyR (28). This modified form activates transcription of the genes of the OxyR regulon. In the case of the *katG* gene, the transcription rate is 100-fold higher when OxyR is in the oxidized form. OxyR also regulates its own expression, by repressing transcription of the *oxyR* gene; both the reduced and oxidized forms are equally effective as autoregulators. As a consequence, the amount of OxyR produced in the cell is relatively constant and activation of the OxyR regulon is caused almost solely by oxidation of OxyR to the active form (29).

The levels of HPII in stationary cells are much higher than in exponentially growing cells (about 30-fold). Many other cellular proteins are also found in much greater amounts in stationary phase than in exponential cells. As a group, these proteins have been called pex (*post exponential*) phase proteins (17). Does the KatF protein control expression of these other post-exponential proteins? By comparing the two-dimensional protein profiles of *katF* mutants to those of wild-type cells, Lange and Hengge-Aronis (18) and Matin and co-workers (15) showed that up to 32 stationary-phase proteins are controlled by KatF protein (also called RpoS). While the functions of most of these proteins have not yet been identified, the few which have been characterized include the HPII catalase, the DNA repair enzyme exonuclease III (19), glycogen synthetase, trehalose synthesis functions, outer-membrane proteins, acid phosphatase, and virulence factors (20). The diversity of these activities may reflect the need for many housekeeping functions required to maintain cellular viability, even when the cells are growing slowly or not at all. *katF* mutants die rapidly once cultures reach plateau (stationary) growth phase.

What activates this postexponential phase regulon? Two possibilities are now being considered. Cells entering stationary phase begin to grow much more slowly, as the preferred carbon sources are depleted. Increase in expression of pex proteins may be intrinsically coupled to the reduction in growth rate that occurs as cells enter stationary phase. Consistent with this idea, some KatF-directed genes have consensus sequence "gear box" promoters, which vary in activity as a function of cellular growth rate. Another possibility is that an accumulating cellular metabolite serves as an inducing signal and turns on the KatF-directed regulon. Supporting this hypothesis, Schellhorn and Hassan (21) found that supernatants taken from early stationary phase cultures induce *katE* expression.

Paraquat (PQ^{2+}) and menadione, redox-cycling agents, induce the synthesis, in *E. coli*, of a distinct set of polypeptides (30, 31). Constitutive mutants (*soxR^c*) selected on the basis of menadione resistance are cross-resistant to other oxidants and also, surprisingly, to many antibacterial drugs, such as chloramphenicol. The mutants have elevated levels of 10 proteins, including the enzymes endonuclease IV (an enzyme that repairs various oxidant-induced DNA damages), G6PDH, Mn superoxide dismutase, and an oxidant-resistant fumarase. Deletion mutants of the *soxR* locus cannot induce G6PDH upon exposure to menadione, although the basal levels of the enzyme are unaffected by the elimination of *soxR*. The locus encodes two genes, *soxR* and *soxS*. The SoxR protein, which contains an iron–sulfur center, is the sensor of oxidative stress (32). SoxR activation leads to increased synthesis of SoxS, which, in turn, causes increased transcription of the genes of the regulon (33).

Global responses to oxidative stress may also exist in mammalian cells, but this field of study is still at a very early stage (34).

MAMMALIAN CATALASE

Mammalian catalase is a homotetrameric protein, with a native molecular weight of 240 kD. Each subunit has one heme group and one bound molecule of NADPH (35, 36). Indeed, catalase is the major reservoir for erythrocyte NADPH. Catalase is found in erythrocyte cytosol; in liver and other tissues, catalase is localized in subcellular organelles called *peroxisomes*. The localization of catalase in peroxisomes may reflect the local production of large amount of hydrogen peroxide in these organelles.

The X-ray crystal structure of bovine liver catalase has been determined (37), and the gene encoding the enzyme has been cloned and sequenced from many sources, including humans (38).

The physiological role of catalase is elucidated by examination of another inborn error of metabolism: acatalasemia (39). Acatalasemia was discovered by a Japanese otolaryngologist, Shigeo Takahara (Okayama University Medical School). He routinely applied hydrogen peroxide solution as an antiseptic during oral surgery. One day in 1946, he undertook surgery on a girl suffering from oral gangrene. When he applied hydrogen peroxide to the wound, he was astonished to observe the patient's gums turning brown-black. Upon investigation, blood samples from four of the seven siblings in the family showed the same peculiar reaction to hydrogen peroxide, and they failed to "fizz" from the evolution of oxygen.

To date, extensive screening studies in Japan have uncovered a total of about 90 cases of congenital acatalasemia. A few cases have also been discovered in Peruvians with Japanese ancestry, as well as in Switzerland, but acatalasemia is clearly an extremely rare condition. The oral gangrene which led to the original discovery of acatalasemia is, in fact, a common symptom of the condition and is now known as *Takahara's disease*. The lesions apparently result from the effects of hydrogen peroxide production by the metabolic action of bacteria, such as *Streptococcus*, normally found on the gums. Aside from this symptom, however, acatalasemic individuals seem to get along normally and live full life spans. About half of the patients do not even manifest Takahara's disease.

The Japanese acatalasemics show a very small residual catalase activity in the blood and in some tissues (a few percent of normal activity, or less), and this residual enzyme appeared electrophoretically normal. But Northern blots of mRNA from cultured patient fibroblasts, probed with the cDNA for human catalase, revealed that almost no catalase mRNA was present. Genomic cloning of the mutant gene identified the molecular cause of acatalasemia as a G:C → A:T base substitution (transition mutation) at a splice site in an intron. Evidently, the splice site mutation prevents the successful processing of the catalase mRNA. [Interestingly, normal levels of mRNA were reported in Swiss acatalasemics, so a structural (exon) mutation would appear to be involved in these cases, which obviously arose independently.]

GLUTATHIONE PEROXIDASE

The observation that the clinical consequences of acatalasemia are minor leads one to suspect that some other enzyme can substitute for catalase and remove endogenous hydrogen peroxide. One alternative route for hydrogen peroxide reduction is the glutathione-dependent pathway. *Glutathione* is an essential component of antioxidant defense in eukaryotic cells (see Chapter 11). Red blood cells contain about 3 mM glutathione.

Glutathione peroxidase catalyzes the following reactions:

$$H_2O_2 + 2GSH \rightarrow 2H_2O + GSSG$$

$$ROOH + 2GSH \rightarrow ROH + H_2O + GSSG$$

Glutathione peroxidase is a remarkable enzyme: It incorporates a residue of *selenocysteine* at the active site. Selenocysteine is coded by the codon UGA, which is usually a stop codon (*opal*). (This codon also does "double duty" as a tryptophan codon in mitochondria.) The residue is incorporated by a specific selenocysteine tRNA (40). (Some isozymes of glutathione transferase also catalyze this reaction and are referred to as selenium–independent glutathione peroxidases—see Chapter 11.)

One form of selenium-dependent glutathione peroxidase was discovered in erythrocytes and has since been identified in many cell types. This "classical" glutathione peroxidase is a tetramer of 17-kD subunits. Three additional selenium-dependent glutathione peroxidases have been characterized. One is highly active with phospholipid hydroperoxides and consequently appears to be particularly important in protection against lipid peroxidation. Another enzyme has been isolated from blood plasma. The enzyme most recently discovered is a distinct intracellular selenium-dependent glutathione peroxidase. Experiments with cells in tissue culture have demonstrated that transfection of glutathione peroxidase cDNA causes increased intracellular enzyme activity and concomitant increased resistance to H_2O_2, organic hydroperoxides, or prooxidants, such as the cytostatic drug doxorubicin (see Chapter 11).

Glutathione reductase, a flavoenzyme, maintains glutathione in the reduced state:

$$GSSG + NADPH \rightarrow 2GSH + NADP^+$$

The crystal structure and catalytic mechanism of this enzyme are discussed in Chapter 11. Cellular glutathione is maintained highly reduced, at the expense of NADPH from the pentose phosphate pathway.

Whether glutathione peroxidase or catalase plays the major role in scavenging erythrocyte hydrogen peroxide remains controversial, but it appears that both enzyme systems participate (41, 42).

NOTES

1. Everse, J., Everse, K. E., and Grisham, M. B., Eds., *Peroxidases in Chemistry and Biology*, CRC Press, Boca Raton, FL, 1991.
2. Saunders, B. C., Holmes-Siedle, A. G., and Stark, B. P., *Peroxidase: The Properties and Uses of a Versatile Enzyme and of Some Related Catalysts*, Butterworths, London, 1964.
3. Chuang, W.-J., and Van Wart, H. E., Resonance Raman spectra of horseradish peroxidase and bovine liver catalase compound I species, *J. Biol. Chem.* 267:13292–13301, 1992.
4. Karlin, K. D., Metalloenzymes, structural motifs, and inorganic models, *Science* 261:701–708, 1993.
5. Yamazaki, I., Mason, H. S., and Piette, L., Identification by electron paramagnetic resonance spectroscopy of free radicals generated during peroxidase oxidations, *J. Biol. Chem.* 235:2444–2449, 1960.
6. Aust, S. D., Chignell, C. F., Bray, T. M., Kalyanaraman, B., and Mason, R. P., Free radicals in toxicology, *Toxicol. Appl. Pharmacol.* 120:168–78, 1993.
7. Boyd, J. A., Prostaglandin H synthase, *Methods Enzymol.* 186:283–287, 1990.
8. Eling, T. E., and Curtis, J. F., Xenobiotic metabolism by prostaglandin H synthase, *Pharmacol. Ther.* 53:261–273, 1992.
9. Loewen, P. C., Isolation of catalase-deficient *Escherichia coli* mutants and genetic mapping of *katE*, a locus that affects catalase activity, *J. Bacteriol.* 157:622–626, 1984; Loewen, P. C., and Triggs, B. L., Genetic mapping of *katF*, a locus that with *katE* affects the synthesis of a second catalase species in *Escherichia coli*, *J. Bacteriol.* 160:668–675, 1984; Loewen, P. C., Triggs, B. L., George, C. S., and Hrabarchuk, B., Genetic mapping of *katG*, a locus that affects synthesis of the bi-functional catalase-peroxidase hydroperoxidase I in *Escherichia coli*. *J. Bacteriol.* 162:661–667, 1985.
10. Loewen, P. C., Switala, J., and Triggs-Raine, B. L., Catalases HPI and HPII in *Escherichia coli* are induced independently, *Arch. Biochem. Biophys.* 243:144–149, 1985.
11. Loewen, P. C., and Switala, J., Purification and characterization of catalase HPII from *Escherichia coli* K-12, *Biochem. Cell. Biol.* 64:638–646, 1986.
12. Loewen, P. C., Switala, J., Von Ossowski, I., Hillar, A., Christie, A., Tattrie, B., and Nicholls,

P., Catalase HPII of *Escherichia coli* catalyzes the conversion of protoheme to *cis*-heme d, *Biochemistry* 32:10159–10164, 1993.

13. Mulvey, M. R., and Loewen, P. C., Nucleotide sequence of *katF* of *Escherichia coli* suggest KatF protein is a novel σ transcription factor, *Nucleic Acids Res.* 17:9979–9991, 1989; von Ossowski, I., Mulvey, M. R., Leco, P. A., Borys, A., and Loewen, P. C., Nucleotide sequence of *Escherichia coli katE*, which encodes catalase HPII, *J. Bacteriol.* 173:514–520, 1990.

14. Tanaka, K., Takayanagi, Y., Fujita, N., Ishihama, A., and Takahashi, H., Heterogeneity of principal σ factor of *Escherichia coli*: The rpoS gene product, σ^{38}, is the second principal σ factor of RNA polymerase in stationary-phase *Escherichia coli*, *Proc. Natl. Acad. Sci. U.S.A.* 90:3511–3515, 1993.

15. Yura, T., Nagai, H., and Mori, H., Regulation of the heat-shock response in bacteria, *Annu. Rev. Microbiol.* 47:321–350, 1993.

16. Witkin, E. M., RecA protein in the SOS response: Milestones and mysteries, *Biochimie* 73:133–141, 1991.

17. McCann, M. P., Kidwell, J. P., and Matin, A., The putative σ factor KatF has a central role in development of starvation-mediated general resistance in *Escherichia coli*, *J. Bacteriol.* 173:4188–4194, 1991.

18. Lange, R., and Hengge-Aronis, R., Identification of a central regulator of stationary-phase gene expression in *Escherichia coli*, *Mol. Microbiol.* 5:49–59, 1991.

19. Sak, B.D., Eisenstark, A., and Touati, D., Exonuclease II and the catalase hydroperoxidase II of *Escherichia coli* are both regulated by the *katF* product, *Proc. Natl. Acad. Sci. U.S.A.* 86:3271–3275, 1989.

20. Fang, F. C., Libby, S. J., Buchmeier, N. A., Loewen, P. C., Switala, J., Harwood, J., and Guiney, D.G, The alternative σ factor KatF (RpoS) regulates *Salmonella* virulence, *Proc. Natl. Acad. Sci. U.S.A.* 89:11978–11982, 1992.

21. Schellhorn, H. E., and Hassan, H. M., Transcriptional regulation of *katE* in *Escherichia coli* K-12, *J. Bacteriol.* 170:4286–4292, 1988.

22. Claiborne, A., and Fridovich, I., Purification of the *o*-dianisidine peroxidase from *Escherichia coli* B, *J. Biol. Chem.* 254:4245–4252, 1979.

23. Triggs-Raine, B. L., Doble, B. W., Mulvey, M. R., Sorby, P. A., and Loewen, P. C., Nucleotide sequence of *katG* encoding catalase HPI of *Escherichia coli*, *J. Bacteriol.* 170:4415–4419, 1988.

24. Ma, M., and Eaton, J. W., Multicellular oxidant defense in unicellular organisms, *Proc. Natl. Acad. Sci. U.S.A.* 89:7924–7928, 1992.

25. DeBruin, L. S., and Josephy, P. D., Dichlorobenzidine–DNA binding catalyzed by peroxidative activation in *Salmonella typhimurium*, *Arch. Biochem. Biophys.* 269:25–31, 1989.

26. Demple, B., and Halbrook, J., Inducible repair of oxidative DNA damage in *Escherichia coli*, *Nature* 304:466–468, 1983.

27. Storz, G., Tartaglia, L. A., and Ames, B. N., Transcriptional regulation of oxidative stress inducible genes: Direct activation by oxidation, *Science* 248:189–194, 1990; Storz, G., and Altuvia, S., OxyR regulon, *Methods Enzymol.* 234:217–223, 1994.

28. Toledano, M. B., Kullik, I., Trinh, F., Baird, P. T., Schneider, T. D., and Storz, G., Redox-dependent shift of OxyR–DNA contacts along an extended DNA-binding site: A mechanism for differential promoter selection, *Cell* 78:897–909, 1994.

29. Toledano, M. B., Kullik, I., Trinh, F., Baird, P. T., Schneider, T. D., and Storz, G., Redox-dependent shift of OxyR–DNA contacts along an extended DNA-binding site: A mechanism for differential promoter selection, *Cell* 78:897–909, 1994.

30. Greenberg, J. T., and Demple, B., A global response induced in *Escherichia coli* by redox-cycling agents overlaps with that induced by peroxide stress, *J. Bacteriol.* 171:3933–3939, 1989.

31. Demple, B., Regulation of bacterial oxidative stress genes, *Annu. Rev. Genet.* 25:315–337, 1991.

32. Hidalgo, E., and Demple, B., An iron–sulfur center essential for transcriptional activation by the redox-sensing SoxR protein, *EMBO J.* 13:138–146, 1994.

33. Nunoshiba, T., Hidalgo, E., Cuevas, C. F. A., and Demple, B., Two-stage control of an oxidative stress regulon: The *Escherichia coli* SoxR protein triggers redox-inducible expression of the *soxS* regulatory gene, *J. Bacteriol.* 174:6054–6060, 1992; Nunoshiba, T., Hidalgo, E., Li,

Z., and Demple, B., Negative autoregulation by the *Escherichia coli* SoxS protein: A dampening mechanism for the *soxRS* redox stress response, *J. Bacteriol.* 175:7492–7494, 1993.

34. Kullik, I., and Storz, G., Transcriptional regulators of the oxidative stress response in prokaryotes and eukaryotes, *Redox Report* 1:23–29, 1994.

35. Kirkman, H. N., and Gaetani, G. F., Catalase: A tetrameric enzyme with four tightly bound molecules of NADPH, *Proc. Natl. Acad. Sci. U.S.A.* 81:4343–4347, 1984.

36. Jouve, H. M., Gouet, P., Boudjada, N., Buisson, G., Kahn, R., and Duee, E., Crystallization and crystal packing of *Proteus mirabilis* PR catalase, *J. Mol. Biol.* 221:1075–1077, 1991.

37. Reid, T. J., Murthy, M. R. N., Sicignano, A., Tanaka, N., Musick, W. D., and Rossman, M. G., Structure and heme environment of beef liver catalase at 2.5Å resolution, *Proc. Natl. Acad. Sci. U.S.A.* 78:4767–4771, 1981.

38. Korneluk, R. G., Quan, F., Lewis, W. H., Gusie, K. S., Willard, H. F., Holmes, M. T., and Gravel, R. A., Isolation of human fibroblast catalase cDNA clones, *J. Biol. Chem.* 259:13819–13823, 1984.

39. Ogata, M., Acatalasemia, *Hum. Genet.* 86:331–340, 1991.

40. Chambers, I., and Harrison, P. R., A new puzzle in selenoprotein biosynthesis: Selenocysteine seems to be encoded by the 'stop' codon, UGA, *Trends Biochem. Sci.* 12:255–256, 1987; Hatfield, D., and Diamond, A., UGA: A split personality in the universal genetic code, *Trends Genet.* 9:69–70, 1993.

41. Eaton, J. W., Hallaway, P. E., and Agar, N. S., Erythrocyte glutathione: A dispensable oxidant defense?, in: *The Red Cell: Seventh Ann Arbor Conference*, G. J. Brewer, Ed., Alan R. Liss, New York, 1989, pp. 23–38.

42. Gaetani, G. F., Kirkman, H. N., Mangerini, R., and Ferraris, A. M., Importance of catalase in the disposal of hydrogen peroxide within human erythrocytes, *Blood* 84:325–330, 1994.

6

THE RESPIRATORY BURST

PHAGOCYTOSIS

Nature has evolved effective enzymatic defenses against the toxicity of reactive oxygen species, as described in Chapters 4 and 5. Nature has also learned how to exploit this toxicity as a defensive component of the immune system. Phagocytic white blood cells (neutrophils, monocytes, macrophages) deliberately generate large amounts of superoxide and other oxidants, and they use these species to kill microorganisms. In this section, we will discuss this process, known as the *respiratory burst*. The biochemistry of this immune defense mechanism illuminates the mechanisms of oxygen toxicity, and it also has important implications in medicine.

The idea that white blood cells engulf and digest invading microorganisms was first propounded by the Russian zoologist Metchnikov (1845–1916), who shared the Nobel Prize in Medicine (with Paul Ehrlich) in 1908. The process of phagocytosis is triggered when phagocytic cells encounter foreign antigens, such as the surface antigens of microorganisms, which have been recognized and "tagged" by circulating antibodies (opsonization).* The phagocyte, in turn, recognizes the opsonic factors, surrounds and engulfs the invader, and wraps it in the phagocyte's plasma membrane. The membrane closes around the engulfed particle, forming a phagocytic *vacuole*.

A complex series of cellular biochemical events accompanies phagocytosis and our understanding of these events is still far from complete. Because of the vital role of phagocytosis in the immune response, this is a field of intense scientific effort. Some aspects of the response are becoming clear, especially the critical role played by the enzyme system known as the *phagocyte NADPH oxidase* or *respiratory burst oxidase*; we will focus on this enzyme (1).

The first evidence that unusual biochemical events were occurring in the phagocyte came from the observation, in 1933, that neutrophils undergo an increase in oxygen consumption within a few seconds of activation by exposure to opsonized antigens. This *respiratory burst* response can be measured in vitro by manometric (or, later, electrochemical) measurements of oxygen consumption by suspensions of isolated white blood cells challenged with antigenic materials, such as opsonized zymosan (yeast). The remarkable nature of the increased metabolic activity in phagocytes was first appreciated by Sbarra and Karnovsky in 1959 (2). They realized that, upon stimulation with antigens, the respiration rate of the neutrophil increases to as much as 100-fold above the basal level. They also tested the effect of typical chemical inhibitors of respiration, such as cyanide and azide; surprisingly, these inhibitors were ineffective. Clearly, the burst is *not* due simply to an increase in the rate of normal cellular respiration; rather, it is a specific metabolic response to the task of phagocytosis.

*See special issue, "Phagocytosis," *Trends Cell Biol.* 5(3), March 1995.

In a mitochondrial respiratory electron transport chain, of course, water is the product of oxygen reduction. Only very small amounts of reactive oxygen intermediates are formed, in the absence of exogenous redox-cycling agents (see Chapter 4). However, in the 1960s, hydrogen peroxide was detected as a product of the respiratory burst. The discovery of superoxide dismutase raised the obvious question: Is superoxide the primary product of the burst?

Bernard Babior and colleagues at Scripps Research Institute, La Jolla, California, demonstrated the production of superoxide by activated neutrophils in the 1970s (3). The key to success was the ability to recover respiratory burst activity in a cell-free system, the plasma membrane fraction of homogenized zymosan-activated neutrophils. In the intact cell, of course, common assays for superoxide (such as the superoxide dismutase-inhibitable reduction of cytochrome c) are not readily applicable. In 1987, the same research group achieved the reconstitution of the oxidase activity as a soluble system, comprising a mixture of cytosol and deoxycholate-solubilized membrane preparation from human neutrophils (4). More recently, considerable progress has been made in (a) purifying the many protein components involved in the respiratory burst and (b) cloning the cDNA sequences for these proteins (5, 6).

STOICHIOMETRY OF THE OXIDASE

The first, deceptively simple question in the study of this or any other enzyme is to establish the net stoichiometry of the reaction. What substrate is consumed, and what products are formed? The identity of the source of reducing equivalents for the oxidase remained controversial until the development of the reconstituted cell-free systems, but it then became clear that NADPH is the substrate of choice: The K_M values are about 40 μM and 2 mM for NADPH and NADH, respectively. Consistent with this interpretation, the pentose phosphate pathway is activated during the respiratory burst to maintain the supply of NADPH, and a severe deficiency of glucose-6-phosphate dehydrogenase (see Chapter 8) compromises the ability to induce the respiratory burst (see chronic granulomatous disease, below).

The determination of the reaction *products* is more difficult, since the putative products $O_2^{\cdot-}$ and H_2O_2 are both rapidly decomposed by superoxide dismutase and peroxidase/catalase, respectively. The detection of superoxide radical [by methods such as spin trapping (see sidebar on page 62) or cytochrome c reduction, discussed earlier] does not necessarily prove that superoxide is the only, or even the most important, product of oxygen reduction. As already discussed, the quantitative measurement of superoxide formation in intact cells is difficult or impossible. Studies with disrupted cells or solubilized enzyme preparations will always be somewhat suspect, since one may argue that the process of disruption has affected the result. Investigators have attempted to calculate the ratios among (a) oxygen consumed [measured with the polarographic Clark oxygen electrode (7)], (b) NADPH consumed, and (c) $O_2^{\cdot-}$ or H_2O_2 formed. These ratios measure the univalent flux of reducing equivalents—that is, the fraction of oxygen molecules reduced to $O_2^{\cdot-}$ rather than to water. If we assume that $O_2^{\cdot-}$ is the only product formed by the enzyme, then we can expect the following ratios, depending on the experimental system studied:

1. *If all the superoxide is trapped and detected* (e.g., as reduced cytochrome c):

$$1NADPH \rightarrow 2e^- \rightarrow 2O_2^{\cdot-} \rightarrow 2cyt.\ c\ (Fe^{2+})$$

(1NADPH oxidized to 2O_2 consumed).

2. *If $O_2{}^{\cdot-}$ is allowed to dismutate* (whether spontaneously or enzyme-catalyzed), *but catalase is absent*:

$$1NADPH \rightarrow 2e^- \rightarrow 2O_2{}^{\cdot-} \rightarrow 1H_2O_2 + 1O_2$$

(1NADPH oxidized to 1O_2 consumed; the second O_2 is recovered unchanged).

3. *If $O_2{}^{\cdot-}$ is allowed to dismutate and catalase is present*:

$$1NADPH \rightarrow 2e^- \rightarrow 2O_2{}^{\cdot-} \rightarrow 1H_2O_2 + 1O_2 \text{ and } 1H_2O_2 \rightarrow {}^1/_2O_2 + 1H_2O$$

$$\textit{Net:} \quad 1NADPH \rightarrow 2e^- \rightarrow 2O_2{}^{\cdot-} \rightarrow 1{}^1/_2O_2 + 1H_2O$$

(1NADPH oxidized to ${}^1/_2O_2$ consumed).

We shall not consider all the (sometimes conflicting) data which have been gathered, using various enzyme preparations and various assays; the student is referred to the recent reviews and the primary literature for further details (8). The consensus suggests that $O_2{}^{\cdot-}$ is a major, if not the exclusive, primary product of oxygen reduction by the NADPH oxidase. In other words, the net stoichiometry of the enzyme is

$$NADPH + 2O_2 \rightarrow NADP^+ + H^+ + 2O_2{}^{\cdot-}$$

MYELOPEROXIDASE

The neutrophil contains several types of *granules*. Upon stimulation of the phagocyte, the primary (or azurophilic) granules migrate to, and fuse with, the phagosome and release their contents into the vacuole. The granules deliver the enzyme *myeloperoxidase* (Greek *myelo* = bone marrow), which uses H_2O_2, produced from the respiratory burst (via superoxide dismutation) to oxidize halide ions (chloride and bromide) to hypohalites:

$$H_2O_2 + X^- \rightarrow HOX + OH^- \qquad (X = Cl \text{ or } Br)$$

Myeloperoxidase (9) is therefore an unusual form of peroxidase, which accepts halide ions as reducing substrates. The product is hypohalous acid (HOX $\rightleftarrows$ OX$^-$), a very potent oxidant (household bleach is sodium hypochlorite, NaOCl).

REACTIVE NITROGEN INTERMEDIATES

In addition to the reactive oxygen intermediates discussed above, macrophages also produce nitric oxide NO via the enzyme nitric oxide synthase (10, 11; also see Chapter 11). NO, a free radical, is the progenitor of a series of products referred to as reactive nitrogen intermediates (12). In aqueous solution, NO rapidly reacts with oxygen, giving (via nitrogen dioxide) nitrite and nitrate:

$$2NO + O_2 \rightarrow 2NO_2 \rightarrow NO_3^- + NO_2^-$$

NO also reacts rapidly with superoxide, forming the peroxynitrite anion (NO + $O_2{}^{\cdot-} \rightarrow$ ONOO$^-$), which can give rise to hydroxyl radical:

$$ONOO^- + H^+ \rightarrow ONOOH \rightarrow {}^{\cdot}OH + NO_2$$

There is no simple way to sort out which of these species is chiefly responsible for killing the phagocytosed microorganism.

COMPONENTS OF THE PHAGOCYTE NADPH OXIDASE

A. W. Segal and colleagues first highlighted the importance of the presence, in neutrophils and other phagocytes, of a very unusual membrane-bound cytochrome, which has been called cytochrome b_{-245} or cytochrome b_{558} (13). The former name identifies the remarkably low redox potential of the protein, $\Delta E_0' = -0.245$ V. This low potential implies that the reduced enzyme is a powerful reductant, well matched to the reduction potential of the $O_2/O_2^{\cdot-}$ couple (-0.33 V). The latter name identifies the unusual optical absorption spectrum of the cytochrome, with an α-band peak at 558 nm. The protein has been studied by biochemical and molecular biological techniques (14). It is composed of two subunits, in contrast to typical mammalian cytochrome b proteins, such as cytochrome b_5 (see Chapter 8), which are single-subunit. The components of cytochrome b_{558}

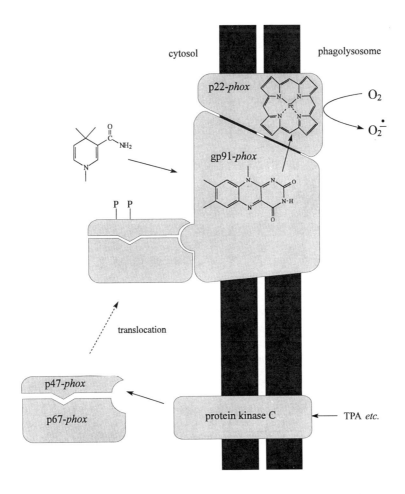

are a smaller subunit (p22^{phox}), $M_r = 22$ kD, and a larger subunit (gp91^{phox}), $M_r = 91$ kD (15). The larger subunit is an extensively glycosylated 56-kD polypeptide.

Activation of the oxidase following stimulation of the cell is a very complex process and is far from being completely understood. The burst can be activated, in intact neutrophils, by many agents: opsonized foreign microorganisms or zymosan (yeast prepara-tion); the *chemotactic peptide N*-formylmethionyl-leucyl-phenylalanine (fMLP), which carries the *N*-formylmethionyl group characteristic of bacterial proteins; and phorbol myristate acetate (PMA). PMA is a natural product isolated from croton oil, the oil of the *Euphorbia* plant. PMA activates protein kinase C, a component of the inositol–phospho-lipid signal transduction system (16), which is responsible for transmitting information from the cell surface receptors into the interior of the cell, to trigger the burst response.

The discovery that respiratory burst in neutrophil homogenates could be activated by arachidonic acid and other anionic lipids allowed investigators to begin purifying (and cloning) each of the protein components of this complex system. Activation requires the participation of at least two soluble proteins (p47^{phox} and p67^{phox}) and a cytosolic G pro-tein [guanine nucleotide-binding protein; (17)] called p21^{rac}. p47^{phox} and p67^{phox} probably interact via their *SH3 domains*. SH3 (*src* homology region) domains are structural "mod-ules" found in a variety of proteins, especially ones involved in membrane signal transduc-tion processes; the domains can be identified by sequence homology searches, but their func-tional significance is still not understood (18). The components of the respiratory burst oxidase remain separate until activation occurs, and then they assemble with cytochrome b$_{558}$ at the membrane. As Babior and Woodman observed, this "fail-safe" system is remi-niscent of storing the component parts of nuclear weapons in separate places, until the phago-cyte "detonates"—a process which is cytosuicidal, as well as bactericidal (19).

These accessory proteins are required for activation of oxidase activity, but they are probably not involved as redox components. Rather, it appears that the oxidase protein cytochrome b$_{558}$ itself acts as a flavin-binding dehydrogenase, a heme-containing cy-tochrome, and an oxidase. In other words, a single protein mediates electron flow from NADPH to oxygen. Further biochemical analysis is required to test this model.

CHRONIC GRANULOMATOUS DISEASE

The clearest demonstration of the importance of the respiratory burst, and a powerful tool for its molecular analysis, is the condition known as *chronic granulomatous disease* (GCD) a rare, severe, inherited immune disorder (20). *The diagnostic feature of this disease is the inability of neutrophils to generate a respiratory burst.* This is readily evaluated in vitro by using a histochemical stain based on the superoxide-dependent reduction of ni-tro blue tetrazolium to formazan (see Chapter 4). CGD patients suffer recurrent, chronic infections, beginning in infancy, and many patients die from untreatable bouts of bacter-ial or fungal infections. Many different microorganisms cause disease in CGD patients, including *Staphylococcus aureus*, *Pseudomonas*, fungi such as *Aspergillus* and *Candida*, and *Mycobacterium tuberculosis*. Infections occur in the lungs, lymph nodes, liver, and other organs. The disease can be managed, in many cases, by antibiotic therapy; γ-inter-feron treatment has also shown promise (20). In some cases, bone marrow replacement has been attempted.

More than half of CGD cases are transmitted as a sex-linked recessive Mendelian char-acteristic (as with glucose-6-phosphate dehydrogenase deficiency; see Chapter 8). The gene for the gp91^{phox} subunit of cytochrome b$_{558}$ is on the X chromosome. As with glu-cose-6-phosphate dehydrogenase deficiency, females carriers are *mosaics*, containing two populations of white cells. (Oxidase^{+} and oxidase^{-} cells can easily be identified follow-ing staining with nitro blue tetrazolium.) Since the proteins necessary for reconstitution of oxidase activity have been purified and cloned (see above), biochemical and molecular biological analyses of the genetic defects are possible. Less frequent autosomal mutations also cause the CGD phenotype; these are associated with mutations in the genes for $p21^{phox}$, $p47^{phox}$, $p67^{phox}$, and possibly other proteins. As in any chain, any single weak link causes a break—that is, a nonfunctional respiratory burst. Indeed, in severe cases of glucose-6-phosphate dehydrogenase deficiency, CGD symptoms are sometimes observed: The supply of NADPH to the oxidase becomes rate-limiting. These individuals are also subject to hemolytic anemia.

An animal model of the human disease has recently been established by the application of transgenic animal technology (see Chapter 2). A mouse strain bearing a disrupted gene for $p47^{phox}$ was constructed; homozygous animals display all the symptoms of the human disease (21).

NOTES

1. Segal, A. W., and Abo, A., The biochemical basis of the NADPH oxidase of phagocytes, *Trends Biochem. Sci.* 18:43–47, 1993; Babior, B. M., The respiratory burst oxidase, *Adv. Enzymol.* 65:49–95, 1992; Jesaitis, A. J., and Dratz, E. A., Eds., *The Molecular Basis of Oxidative Damage by Leukocytes*, CRC Press, Boca Raton, FL, 1992.

2. Sbarra, A. J., and Karnovsky, M. L., The biochemical basis of phagocytosis. I. Metabolic changes during the ingestion of particles by polymorphonuclear leukocytes, *J. Biol. Chem.* 234:1355–1362, 1959.

3. Babior, B. M., Kipnes, R. S., and Curnutte, J. T., Biological defense mechanisms. The production by leukocytes of superoxide, a potential bactericidal agent, *J. Clin. Invest.* 52:741–744, 1973.

4. Curnutte, J. T., Kuver, R., and Babior, B. M., Activation of the respiratory burst oxidase in a fully soluble system from human neutrophils, *J. Biol. Chem.* 262:6450–6452, 1987.

5. Hamers, M. N., and Roos, D., Oxidative stress in human neutrophilic granulocytes: Host defence and self-defence, in: *Oxidative Stress*, H. Sies, Ed., Academic Press, London, 1985, pp. 351–381.

6. Berton, G., Dusi, S., and Bellavite, P., The respiratory burst of phagocytes, in: *The Respiratory Burst and Its Physiological Significance*, A. J. Sbarra, and R. R. Strauss, Eds., Plenum Press, New York, 1988, pp. 33–52.

7. Holme, D. J., and Peck, H., *Analytical Biochemistry*, 2nd ed., Longman, New York, 1993, p. 188.

8. Borregaard, N., The respiratory burst: An overview, in: *The Respiratory Burst and Its Physiological Significance*, A. J. Sbarra and R. R. Strauss, Eds., Plenum Press, New York, 1988, pp. 1–31.

9. Andersen, M. R., Atkin, C. L., and Eyre, H. J., Intact form of myeloperoxidase from normal human neutrophils, *Arch. Biochem. Biophys.* 214:273–283, 1982; Johnson, K., Gemperlein, I., Hudson, S., Shane, S., and Rovera, G., Complete nucleotide sequence of the human myeloperoxidase gene, *Nucleic Acids Res.* 17:7985–7986, 1989.

10. McCall, T. B., Boughton-Smith, N. K., Palmer, R. M. J., Whittle, B. J. R., and Moncada, S., Synthesis of nitric oxide from L-arginine by neutrophils; release and interaction with superoxide anion, *Biochem. J.* 261:293–296, 1989; Prince, R. C., and Gunson, D. E., Rising interest in nitric oxide synthase, *Trends Biochem. Sci.* 18:35–36, 1993.

11. Cochrane, C. G., and Gimbrone, M. A., Jr., *Biological Oxidants: Generation and Injurious Consequences*, Academic Press, New York, 1992.

12. Klebanoff, S. J., Reactive nitrogen intermediates and antimicrobial activity: Role of nitrite, *Free Radic. Biol. Med.* 14:351–360, 1993.

13. Segal, A. W., and Jones, O. T. G., Novel cytochrome b system in phagocytic vacuoles of human granulocytes, *Nature* 276:515–517, 1978.

14. Segal, A. W., West, I., Wientjes, F., Nugent, J. H. A., Chavan, A. J., Haley, B., Garcia, R. C.,

Rosen, H., and Scrace, G., Cytochrome b$_{-245}$ is a flavocytochrome containing FAD and the NADPH-binding site of the microbicidal oxidase of phagocytes, *Biochem. J.* 284:781–788, 1992.

15. Umeki, S., Mechanisms for the activation/electron transfer of neutrophil NADPH–oxidase complex and molecular pathology of chronic granulomatous disease, *Ann. Hematol.* 68:267–277, 1994.

16. Moran, L. A., Scrimgeour, K. G., Horton, H. R., Ochs, R. S., and Rawn, J. D., *Biochemistry*, 2nd ed., Neil Patterson Publishers, Englewood Cliffs, NJ, 1994, pp. 12.42ff.

17. Moran, L. A., Scrimgeour, K. G., Horton, H. R., Ochs, R. S., and Rawn, J. D., *Biochemistry*, 2nd ed., Neil Patterson Publishers, Englewood Cliffs, NJ, 1994, pp. 12.38ff.

18. Mayer, B. J., and Baltimore, D., Signalling through SH2 and SH3 domains, *Trends Cell Biol.* 3:8–13, 1993.

19. Babior, B. M., and Woodman, R. C., Chronic granulomatous disease, *Semin. Hematol.* 27:247–259, 1990.

20. Thrasher, A. J., Keep, N. H., Wientjes, F., and Segal, A. W., Chronic granulomatous disease, *Biochim. Biophys. Acta* 1227:1–24, 1994.

21. Jackson, S. H., Gallin, J. I., and Holland, S. M., The p47*phox* mouse knock-out model of chronic granulomatous disease, *J. Exp. Med.* 182:751–758, 1995.

7

LIPID PEROXIDATION

Free radicals, generated by a variety of processes, can attack target biomolecules to manifest their toxic actions. These targets include proteins (1) (especially the thiol groups of cysteine residues), DNA and RNA bases, and cholesterol in lipoprotein complexes. The polyunsaturated fatty acyl (PUFA) chains of phospholipids in biological membranes are particularly susceptible to oxidative damage by free radicals. Uncontrolled lipid peroxidation is a toxic process resulting in the deterioration of biological membranes. However, *the same chemical processes are harnessed for the biosynthesis of important biologically active compounds, the eicosanoids (prostaglandins, leukotrienes, and related compounds).* In this latter case, the peroxidation process is enzyme-catalyzed. The biochemistry of PUFA peroxidation is the focus of this chapter.

(The term *peroxidation* usually refers to the incorporation of molecular oxygen into polyunsaturated fatty acids (PUFAs) of biological membranes. In studies of chemical model systems, the term *autoxidation* is generally employed.)

The biological sources of reactive oxygen species, which can initiate peroxidation processes, are discussed elsewhere in this text. Among the significant sources are normal aerobic metabolism (discussed in Chapter 4) and the activity of phagocytic polymorphonuclear leukocytes, lymphocytes, and macrophages, in response to infection (Chapter 6). Phagocytic cells can also attack lipid-rich atherosclerotic plaques. The generation of reactive oxygen species plays a major role in the pathology of ischemia/reperfusion events, in which the supply of blood and oxygen to an organ is temporarily cut off, as can occur during a stroke, heart attack, or organ transplantation surgery. When the blood supply is restored, oxidative species are generated as a result of the activation of oxidase activities, and this *reperfusion injury* can damage the affected organ or tissue (2).

As discussed earlier, exogenous agents (xenobiotics), such as CCl_4, ethanol, paraquat, and menadione, can also cause the generation of $O_2^{\cdot-}$ and $OH^{\cdot}$. Drugs such as acetaminophen, adriamycin, bleomycin, primaquine, cyclosporin A, and halothane can generate toxicologically significant free radicals under conditions of drug overdose or in idiosyncratic reactions in susceptible patients (3).

MECHANISMS AND PRODUCTS OF LIPID PEROXIDATION

Lipid peroxidation proceeds by a free-radical chain reaction mechanism. Thus, a single initiating event can trigger the peroxidation of a large number of target molecules. Peroxidation produces a vast array of isolable lipid degradation products, and the elucidation of the chemical steps involved is still incomplete. However, many important features are now understood.

The primary products of peroxidation of PUFAs are produced via the free-radical mechanism shown below:

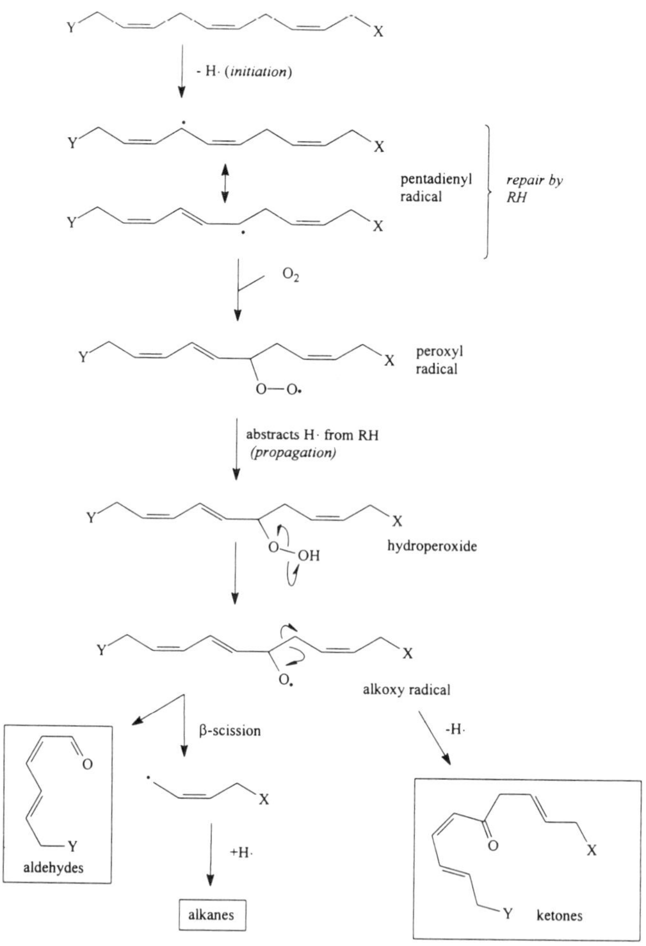

Formation of the primary conjugated hydroperoxides and major secondary products of the peroxidation of a PUFA.

Initiation involves the abstraction of a hydrogen atom from the PUFA by the oxidizing free radical: RH → R$^{\cdot}$. The ease of formation of the initial lipid radical product is controlled by the bond dissociation energy (BDE) of the C−H bond involved. Since *bis*-allylic C−H bonds are relatively weak (~314 kJ/mol) compared to monoallylic C−H bonds (~368 kJ/mol) (4), *the methylene-bridged double bonds of common PUFA molecules (such as linoleic, linolenic, and arachidonic acids) are much more easily oxidized than are monounsaturated fatty acids.* As detailed below, the chain reaction is propagated by the rapid reaction of the carbon-centred *pentadienyl radical* with molecular oxygen, yielding a peroxyl radical: R$^{\cdot}$ + O_2 → ROO$^{\cdot}$; the product radical acts as an initiator, abstracting H$^{\cdot}$ from another PUFA: ROO$^{\cdot}$ + RH → ROOH + R$^{\cdot}$. [Hydrogen abstraction from the O−H bond of preformed hydroperoxides is relatively difficult (BDE ~376 kJ/mol) and is of negligible importance.] The chain reaction terminates by the combination of any two free radicals to form various nonradical products, especially by the process ROO$^{\cdot}$ + ROO$^{\cdot}$ → nonradical products.

Alternatively, the radical chain reaction may be broken by the action of *antioxidants*, such as the lipid-soluble phenolic compounds vitamin E (tocopherol) and the synthetic preservatives BHA (*tert*-butyl hydroxyanisole) and BHT (di-*tert*-butyl hydroxytoluene):

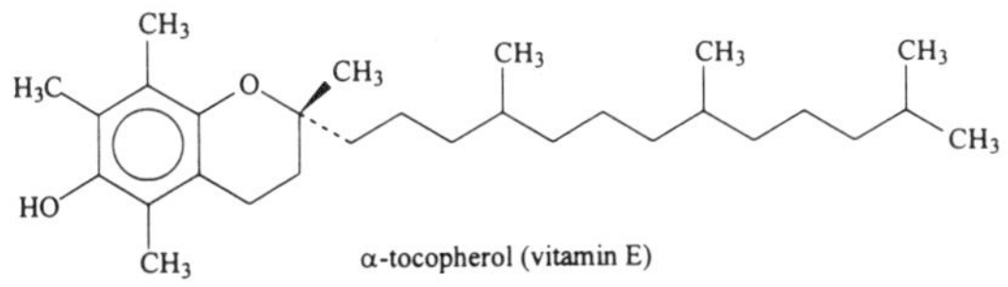

α-tocopherol (vitamin E)

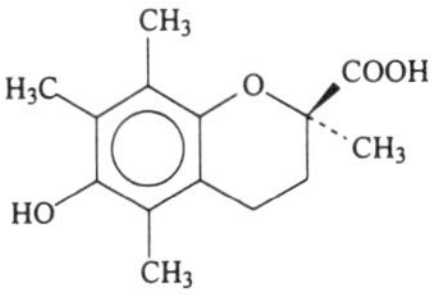

Trolox

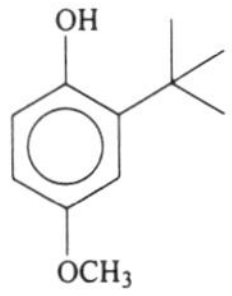

BHA (butylated hydroxyanisole)

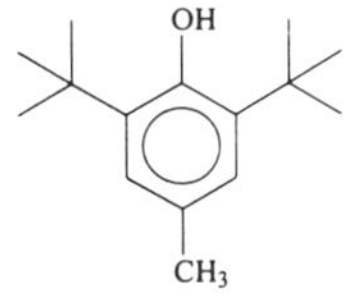

BHT (butylated hydroxytoluene)

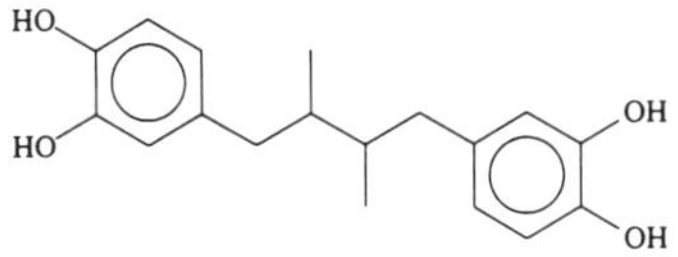

NDGA (nordihydroguaiaretic acid)

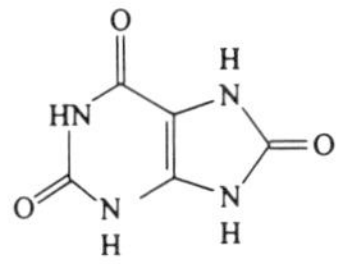

uric acid

An antioxidant repairs the free radical by reduction: $ROO^{.} + ArOH \rightarrow ROOH + ArO^{.}$. The product phenolic radical is resonance-stabilized and insufficiently reactive to participate in further H-abstraction reactions.

The free-radical mechanism displayed on page 98 shows the formation of the primary conjugated hydroperoxides and the major secondary products resulting from the peroxidation of a PUFA (5). The pentadienyl radical generated in the initiation reaction can be viewed as a resonance hybrid of forms with the unpaired electron centred on one of three carbon atoms. The forms in which the two double bonds are conjugated are the more important contributors. The pentadienyl radical reacts with O_2 in a rapid (essentially diffusion-controlled) reaction. The lipid peroxyl radical can then abstract a hydrogen atom from another PUFA to form a metastable, conjugated lipid hydroperoxide and another fatty acyl free radical.

The second phase of the lipid peroxidation process converts the primary hydroperoxides into more stable end products. Homolytic splitting of the hydroperoxide forms the very reactive $HO^{.}$ radical and a lipid alkoxy radical. This step may be catalyzed by Fe^{2+}. The $HO^{.}$ radical can further propagate the lipid peroxidation chain-reaction; thus, iron catalysis of hydroperoxide cleavage can amplify the effects of lipid peroxidation.

Alkoxy radicals are highly reactive analogues of the hydroxyl radical. Abstraction of a hydrogen atom from water forms another $HO^{.}$ radical plus an acyl alcohol; abstraction from a fatty acyl moiety (R'') leads to a branched fatty acyl ether ($R-O-R'$). The alkoxy radical can also undergo β-scission to form a shortened fatty acyl aldehyde and an alkyl radical, which can, in turn, abstract yet another hydrogen atom to form an alkane. Pentane and ethane are common products of lipid peroxidation of ω-6 and ω-3 fatty acids, respectively. A common fatty acyl aldehyde detected in peroxidized biological membranes is the chemically reactive and cytotoxic 4-hydroxynonenal:

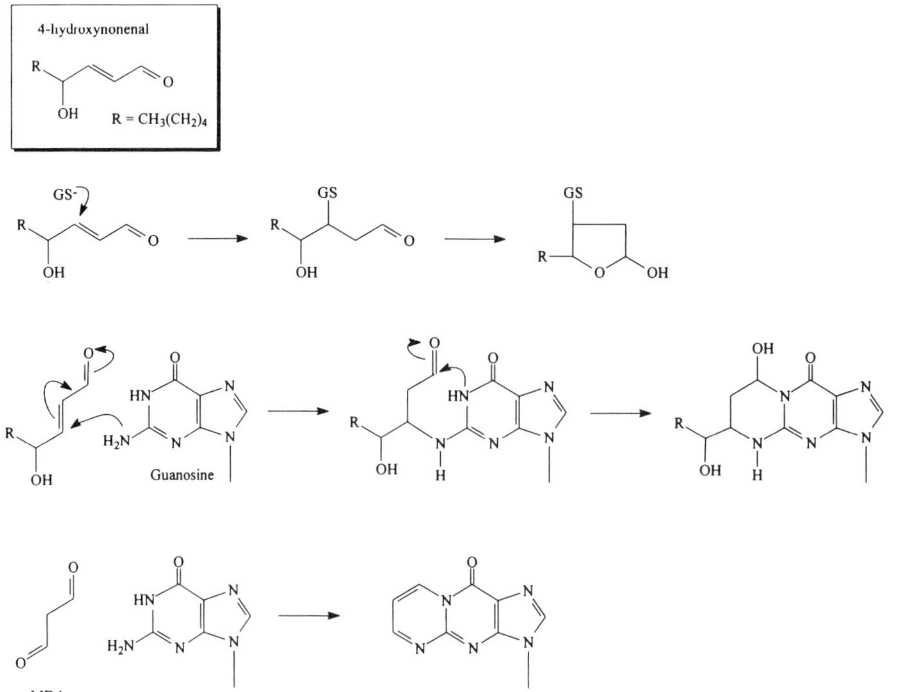

4-hydroxynonenal

R = CH$_3$(CH$_2$)$_4$

GS$^-$

GS

GS

Guanosine

OH

MDA

4-Hydroxynonenal reacts with nucleophiles, such as glutathione, and forms cyclic adducts with guanosine residues in DNA (6). The fatty acyl aldehydes can be oxidized to fatty acyl carboxylic acids or subjected to further free-radical attack. Finally, the alkoxy radical can lose a methinyl hydrogen atom and form a fatty acyl ketone.

Additional secondary products have been observed following the peroxidation of PUFA with more than two double bonds. Triene and tetraene fatty acids yield monocyclic peroxides, serial cyclic products, and bicyclic endoperoxides (7). Malonaldehyde (malondialdehyde, propanedial, MDA), an end product of the peroxidation of arachidonic acid (20:4Ω6) and other PUFAs, is a DNA-reactive compound (see scheme above) and is often used as a chemical marker of lipid peroxidation (see the next section). The mechanism of MDA formation is not entirely understood. MDA is probably derived from a cyclic peroxide (endoperoxide) precursor:

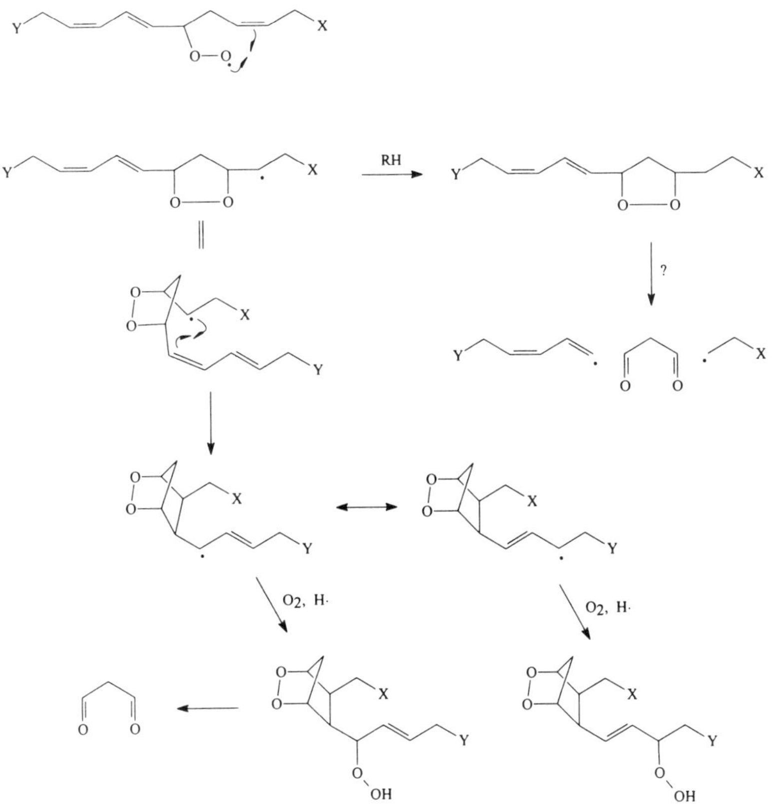

Pathway for the conversion of linolenate (18:3Ω6) to endoperoxides, the postulated precursors of MDA. X and Y are $-(CH_2)_3CO_2^-$ and $-C_4H_9$, respectively. The analogous reaction of prostaglandin synthesis is shown on page 82.

This mechanism is similar to the enzymatic mechanism of prostaglandin formation, catalyzed by the enzyme prostaglandin H synthase. Prostaglandin G_2 is the precursor of the prostaglandins, which are short-lived, potent intercellular messengers (autocoids) that regulate vasoconstriction/vasodilatation, platelet aggregation, and inflammation (8). The enzymatic process gives rise to a single product, with regio- and stereospecificity. In contrast, the nonenzymatic process gives rise to a wide range of isomers.

The action of *lipoxygenase* enzymes generates another series of biologically active peroxidized fatty acid derivatives, hydroperoxides, and alcohols known as HPETEs (hydroperoxyeicosatetraenoic acids) and HETES (hydroxyeicosatetraenoic acids):

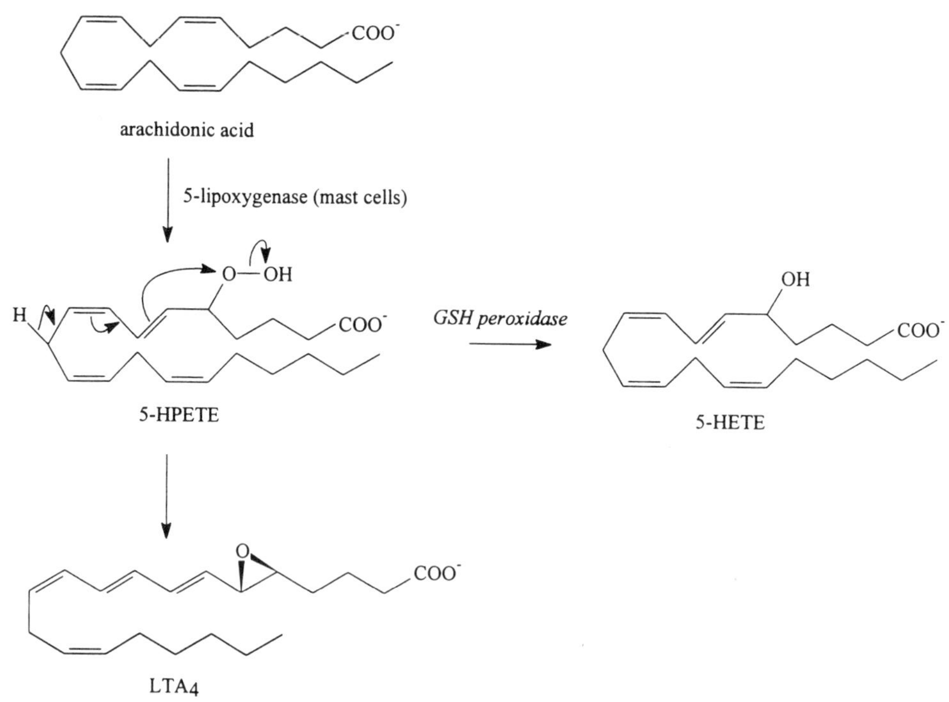

arachidonic acid

5-lipoxygenase (mast cells)

5-HPETE

GSH peroxidase

5-HETE

LTA₄

Again, the enzymatic process is under regio- and stereospecific control. 5-HPETE is the precursor of the leukotrienes; see Chapter 11 (9).

METHODS OF ASSESSMENT OF LIPID PEROXIDATION

Several methods have been developed for the evaluation of lipid peroxidation. Oxygen uptake can be used to measure peroxidation kinetics in vitro, but is, of course, not applicable to the assessment of the extent of existing peroxidation in a biological sample.

Even in cases of extensive lipid peroxidation, the primary products may be difficult to detect, due to their rapid conversion to secondary metabolites or removal by the cellular defense mechanisms. Thus one usually relies on the detection of the secondary products of lipid peroxidation. Among the methods which have been used (10) are measurements of the formation of (a) conjugated dienes, by UV absorption at 232 nm; (b) lipid hydroperoxides, by high-pressure liquid chromatography and chemiluminescence detection; and (c) alkanes (e.g., ethane, pentane) by gas chromatography/mass spectrometry.

By far the most popular of these methods, in both chemical and biological systems, is the thiobarbituric acid (TBA) reactivity test (11). This test is based on the condensation of one molecule of MDA with two molecules of TBA under acidic conditions:

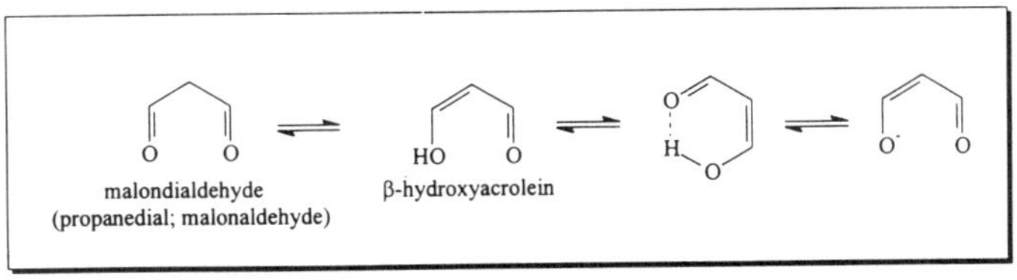

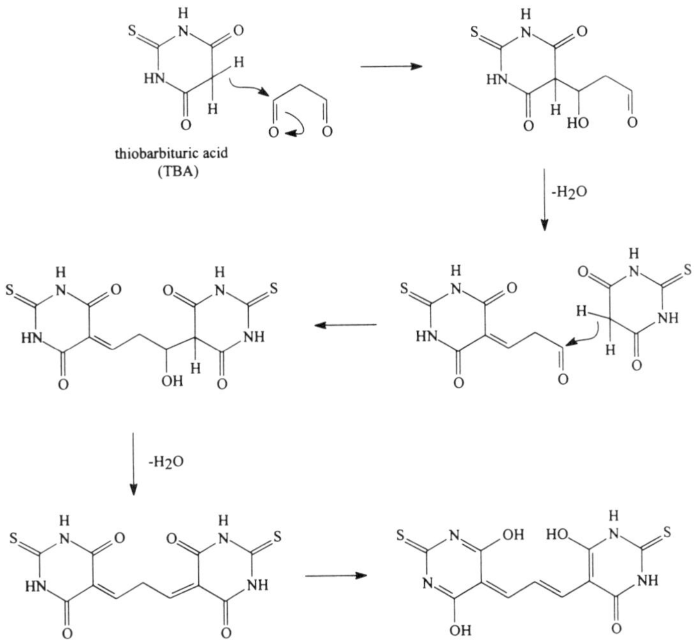

The condensation of malonaldehyde (MDA) with 2-thiobarbituric acid (TBA) yields the red pigment detectable at 532 nm.

The product is a red pigment, measured on the basis of its visible light absorption at 532 nm. The validity of this method rests on the assumptions that the MDA formed during the TBA assay is diagnostic of the presence and amount of peroxides, and that a quantitative relationship exists between the extent of lipid peroxidation and the MDA detected. (The TBA adducts formed by carbonyl compounds other than MDA have low absorption coefficients at 532 nm.)

CONSEQUENCES OF LIPID PEROXIDATION

Lipid peroxidation results in the shortening of the fatty acyl chains, formation of polar and/or charged acyl aldehydes, alcohols, ketones, and carboxylic acids and of branched fatty acyl ethers. Much of the early investigation of the peroxidation process was carried out by food scientists, since the peroxidation of lipids is responsible for the deterioration (rancidity) of lipid-rich foods, such as butter. The recognition of the role of lipid peroxidation in pathological and toxicological processes developed more recently (12).

Lipid peroxidation distorts the structure of the lipid bilayer and compromises its integrity and impermeability. Living cells maintain huge electrolyte concentration gradients. For example, typical intracellular Na^+ concentrations are about 10 mM, while extracellular (e.g., plasma) Na^+ concentration is about 145 mM. Intracellular K^+, on the other hand, is 140 mM, while extracellular K^+ is 5 mM. These gradients provide a source of free energy for transport processes which control cell turgor and allow active transport of metabolites. One of the primary biological effects of lipid peroxidation is membrane leakage: efflux of K^+, influx of Na^+, and concomitant influx of water into the cell.

The damaged cells swell up (cytotoxic edema) and may burst, and energy-requiring ionic pumps, such as the Na^+/K^+ ATPase, are activated, in an attempt to restore the normal ionic balance. Both the cell swelling and the bioenergetic deterioration have been observed in tissue culture, in perfused organ systems, and within the intact body by magnetic resonance imaging and spectroscopy techniques (13).

NOTES

1. Dean, R. T., Gieseg, S., and Davies, M. J., Reactive species and their accumulation on radical-damaged proteins, *Trends Biochem. Sci.* 18:437–441, 1993.
2. Hearse, D.J., and Bolli, R., Reperfusion injury: Manifestations, mechanisms, and clinical relevance, *Cardiovasc. Res.* 26:101–108, 1992.
3. Kamiyama, T., Sato, C., Liu, J., Tajiri, K., Miyakawa, H., and Marumo, F., Role of lipid peroxidation in acetaminophen-induced hepatotoxicity: Comparison with carbon tetrachloride, *Toxicol. Lett.* 66:7–12, 1993; Nordmann, R., Ribière, C., and Rouach, H., Implication of free radical mechanisms in ethanol-induced cellular injury, *Free Radic. Biol. Med.* 12:219–240, 1992.
4. Gardner, H. W., Oxygen radical chemistry of polyunsaturated fatty acids, *Free Radic. Biol. Med.* 7:65–86, 1989.
5. Porter, N. A., Mechanisms for the autoxidation of polyunsaturated lipids, *Acc. Chem. Res.* 19:262–268, 1986; Frankel, E. N., Secondary products of lipid oxidation, *Chem. Phys. Lipids* 44:73–85, 1987.
6. Esterbauer, H., Schaur, R. J., and Zollner, H., Chemistry and biochemistry of 4-hydroxynonenal, malonaldehyde and related aldehydes, *Free Radic. Biol. Med.* 11:81–128, 1991.
7. Porter, N.A., Chemistry of lipid peroxidation, *Methods Enzymol.* 105:273–282, 1984.
8. Lehninger, A. L., Nelson, D. L., and Cox, M. M., *Principles of Biochemistry*, 2nd ed., Worth Publishers, New York, 1993, p. 656.
9. Lehninger, A. L., Nelson, D. L., and Cox, M. M., *Principles of Biochemistry*, 2nd ed., Worth Publishers, New York, 1993, p. 658.
10. Slater, T. F., Overview of methods used for detecting lipid peroxidation, *Methods Enzymol.* 105:283–293, 1984.
11. Janero, D. R., Malonaldehyde and thiobarbituric acid-reactivity as diagnostic indices of lipid peroxidation and peroxidative tissue injury, *Free Radic. Biol. Med.* 9:515–540, 1990.
12. Nigam, S. K., McBrien, D. C. H., and Slater, T. F. (eds.), *Eicosanoids, Lipid Peroxidation, and Cancer*, Springer, Berlin, 1988.
13. Locke, S. J., and Brauer, M., The response of the rat liver in situ to bromobenzene—In vivo proton magnetic resonance imaging and ^{31}P magnetic resonance spectroscopy studies, *Toxicol. Appl. Pharmacol.* 110:416–428, 1991.

8

OXIDATIVE STRESS IN THE ERYTHROCYTE

What happens to a mammalian cell when it encounters oxidative stress conditions, imposed by exposure to chemical oxidants or drugs? The human erythrocyte, or red blood cell, provides a valuable model system for examining this question (1). An erythrocyte is a "bag of hemoglobin": A lipid bilayer membrane encloses a cytosol which is about 40% hemoglobin by weight; most of the remainder is water. Nevertheless, as we shall see, other enzymes and substrates are of critical importance. The red cell—which was regarded by early microscopists, almost contemptuously, as devoid of interest—is now understood to be "a tiny dynamo" of biochemical activity (2).

Why is the mammalian red blood cell such a rewarding system to study? Mature mammalian erythrocytes are non-nucleated (unlike those of birds) and devoid of organelles, so they represent one of the simplest cell types for biochemical study. [Erythrocytes are derived from nucleated precursor (stem) cells in the bone marrow. Immature erythrocytes, known as *reticulocytes*, comprise about 1% of the circulating population; these cells still contain ribosomes and synthesize hemoglobin. The ribosomes are lost as the reticulocyte matures into the erythrocyte.] Red blood cells are easily obtained and, because of their high buoyant density, can be isolated free of other blood cells by differential centrifugation on density gradients (e.g., Ficoll). Furthermore, damage to erythrocytes is a serious medical problem, resulting in anemia and kidney damage, and is easily diagnosed by the release of hemoglobin in the urine. Since analysis of blood biochemistry is a routine component of medical diagnosis, many inborn errors of metabolism which affect the blood, and especially the erythrocyte, are known. These "natural experiments" provide important clues to the metabolic roles of individual enzymes and the structural roles of individual amino acids in hemoglobin and other proteins.

Why is the erythrocyte particularly susceptible to oxidant stress? The oxygen-binding protein *hemoglobin* constitutes more than 90% of erythrocyte protein. Indeed, hemoglobin is packed so tightly into the cell that, in the case of sickle-cell anemia, it can aggregate and distort the shape of the entire cell. The erythrocyte probably encounters higher oxygen tensions than any other cell in the body, other than the cells of the lung. Most drugs and toxicants enter the body via the blood, and thus the erythrocyte cannot avoid exposure to xenobiotics. Since the mature erythrocyte is non-nucleated, protein synthesis cannot be carried out, and thus protein damage inevitably results in loss of cell function. Indeed, the red blood cell lives in the circulation for a few months, at most, before being removed in the spleen and degraded.

What are the targets for oxidative damage to the red blood cell? First, hemoglobin itself is susceptible. The oxygen-carrying capacity of hemoglobin is due to the ability of the ferrous iron center in the heme prosthetic group to coordinate molecular oxygen *without undergoing complete electron transfer*:

$$Fe^{2+} + O_2 \rightleftharpoons Fe^{2+}O_2 \text{ (fast)} \rightarrow Fe^{3+} + O_2^{\cdot-} \text{ (slow)}$$

Native hemoglobin is ferrous, Fe^{2+}; ferric heme, the usual oxidation state of most other heme proteins, is ineffective as an oxygen carrier. Hemoglobin repeatedly binds and releases oxygen *without* undergoing chemical oxidation. Nevertheless, hemoglobin does become oxidized to the ferric form at a measurable rate (3). Ferric hemoglobin (i.e., at least one of the four heme groups oxidized) is known as *methemoglobin* (the prefix *met-* meaning beyond, as in *metaphysics*). In a healthy individual, about 1% of total hemoglobin is methemoglobin.

Since the circulation time of a red blood cell from the lungs to the tissues, and back to the lungs, occurs in a few seconds, but the lifetime of the cell is about 140 days, biochemical mechanisms must exist to deal with methemoglobin formation. Here, we will discuss these pathways, as an illustration of the control of oxidative stress. We will also consider the consequences of failure of these systems, induced by exposure to xenobiotics.

Besides hemoglobin, other enzymes and proteins in the erythrocyte are potential targets for oxidative damage. The membrane of the erythrocyte is composed primarily of phospholipid and protein; it combines great mechanical strength, required to remain intact throughout its traverse of the circulatory system, with the fluidity required to maintain the rheological properties of the blood. Damage to the membrane lipids or proteins may lead, for example, to inactivation of the Na^+/K^+ ATPase (Na^+/K^+ pump), which plays a critical role in regulating cytosolic ionic composition and cell volume. Disruption of the membrane of the erythrocyte, a possible consequence of severe oxidative stress, causes release of the hemoglobin into the blood plasma; such *hemolysis* is potentially fatal, since plasma hemoglobin interferes with the function of the kidneys.

SIDEBAR: HEMOGLOBIN STRUCTURE; COOPERATIVE BINDING OF OXYGEN

The oxidation state of hemoglobin can be measured spectrophotometrically; oxyhemoglobin gives the red color of arteries, while deoxyhemoglobin gives the characteristic color of veins (usually referred to as "blue," but perhaps "dark purple-brown" is a more accurate description). If we vary the oxygen concentration in a cuvette containing a sample of red blood cells and measure the blue-to-red transition spectrophotometrically, we can determine the relationship between oxygen concentration and binding to hemoglobin. [In practice, one varies the partial pressure of the oxygen in the gas phase, and so the independent variable is pO_2 (mm Hg).] We usually call this relationship the "kinetics" of binding, by analogy to the Michaelis–Menten curves of enzyme kinetics, although it is actually a thermodynamic (chemical equilibrium) relationship.

For normal hemoglobin, such a plot of fractional saturation (% oxyhemoglobin) versus partial pressure of oxygen has a characteristic sigmoidal shape. [The degree of cooperativity can be estimated by the use of the "Hill plot" (4).] Such behavior cannot be accounted for by a simple binding equilibrium of the form

$$P + O_2 \rightleftharpoons P{\cdot}O_2 \qquad K_{eq} = [P{\cdot}O_2]/[P][O_2]$$

This simple scheme leads directly to a curve with the same shape as the Michaelis–Menten equation. *The sigmoidal behavior of hemoglobin reflects its cooperative binding of four oxygen molecules, and this in turn reflects its quaternary structure, a tetramer of four protein chains.* The binding of oxygen to the heme group of one protein subunit alters the affinity of oxygen binding to the other subunits.

The chemical mechanism of hemoglobin cooperativity is subtle and extraordinary (5). The heme groups themselves are buried within each of the four protein subunits, and hence the oxygen-binding sites cannot interact directly. Instead, the conformation of the protein subunit serves as the messenger, carrying information about oxygen-binding status from one subunit to the others. This transmission is based upon the delicate interplay between oxygen binding to the heme groups, the motions of the alpha helices adjacent to the hemes, and the many contacts at the α_1–β_2 interface between globin subunits (6). Hemoglobin cooperativity is a consequence of the shift of the protein from one conformation ("T") to a different conformation upon oxygen binding. The work of Perutz and colleagues has elucidated the structures of these two states. Oxygen binding to the heme groups is coupled to (a) the motions of the α-helices adjacent to the hemes and (b) changes in the interactions at the α_1–β_2 interfaces between globin subunits (7). Hemoglobin is finely balanced or poised between the two conformations, and the small enthalpic contribution of oxygen binding is sufficient to cause the global transition from "T" to "R." Note that the "R" and "T" designations are *not equivalent* to "oxy" and "deoxy." Rather, they refer to two distinct conformations of the protein. The "R" state is *favored* upon binding of oxygen to the heme, but, in principle, both oxy- and deoxyhemoglobin can undergo the R–T transition (8).

The analogy of a teeter-totter is apt:

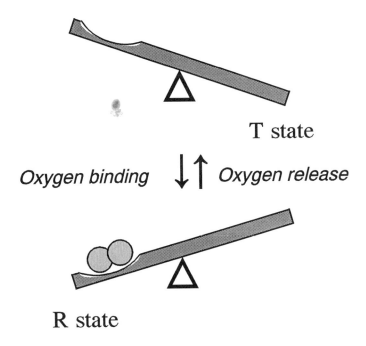

In the absence of oxygen, one state ("T") is slightly more favorable, but the protein can still flip into the "R" state occasionally, because the energy difference between the states is small. Nevertheless, the conformations are very different, just as the "left-up" and "left-down" states of a teeter-totter are distinct, if the ends are marked somehow. Oxygen binding shifts the "T" to "R" equilibrium drastically, just as the addition of a very small weight shifts a teeter-totter. The effects of allosteric effectors, such as 2,3-*bis*-phosphoglycerate, H^+, Cl^-, and CO_2, can all be viewed as analogous to "hanging" small additional weights onto the "T" side. Although their chemical mechanisms are distinct, they all act by shifting the "R" $\rightleftharpoons$ "T" equilibrium.

An excellent illustration of the importance of the cooperative shift from "T" to "R" is provided by the recent crystallization of deoxyhemoglobin in the presence of polyethylene glycol. Previously obtained crystals of deoxyhemoglobin, of course, shattered upon oxygenation, due to the "T" to "R" transition. The polyethylene glycol-induced crystals yield a "T" form which is unable to relax to the "R" state upon oxygenation, due to the constraints of the crystal lattice, but which remains intact (9). "T" state crystals of hemoglobin bind oxygen noncooperatively (Hill coefficient of exactly 1.0).

OXYGEN BINDING TO MYOGLOBIN AND HEMOGLOBIN

The physiological significance of the cooperative transition in hemoglobin can be seen from a comparison of the oxygen-binding curves of hemoglobin and myoglobin:

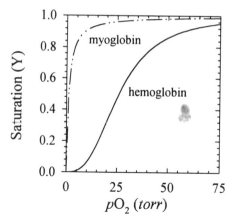

The oxygen-binding curve of myoglobin is hyperbolic, whereas that of hemoglobin is sigmoidal. Effectively, hemoglobin acts as a low-oxygen-affinity receptor at low oxygen partial pressures, and then it "switches" into a high-oxygen-affinity receptor at high oxygen partial pressures. This "switch" results from the cooperative transition of all subunits in the quaternary structure from the "R" to the "T" state, which occurs following oxygen binding to the first one or two subunit hemes. The fractional saturation, Y, changes abruptly over the physiological range of oxygen partial pressures: Hemoglobin "loads up" with oxygen in the lungs ($pO_2 \approx 100$ torr) and "unloads" in the tissues, where the partial pressure is much lower ($pO_2 \approx 25$ torr). In contrast, myoglobin would retain the bound O_2, even at tissue pO_2, and would be ineffective as an O_2 carrier.

ANALYTICAL DETERMINATION OF METHEMOGLOBIN

Since the absorbance spectrum of the heme group is substantially shifted by the binding of axial ligands, the spectrum of hemoglobin protein also exhibits characteristic changes. These shifts allow the analytical determination of methemoglobin and other binding states.

Hb Form	β Band	α Band
Deoxy		555
$Hb^{2+}O_2$	541	577
$Hb^{2+}CO$	540	569
Hb^{3+} (pH 6.4)	500	630 (weak)
$Hb^{3+}CN^-$		540

Reduction of methemoglobin to hemoglobin can be followed by monitoring the disappearance of methemoglobin (630 nm) or the appearance of oxyhemoglobin (577 nm) (10).

What is the biological effect of methemoglobin formation? *The consequences of partial conversion of hemoglobin heme to the ferric form* (e.g., 33% methemoglobin) *are much more profound than the effect of loss of an equivalent amount of protein* (in anemia, for example, with a 33% reduction in the number of circulating red blood cells). If, on average, one heme subunit in three is oxidized to the ferric state, then most of the (tetrameric) hemoglobin molecules will contain *at least one* ferric subunit. The ferric subunit is unable to bind oxygen; therefore, this protein subunit is virtually unable to undergo the transition to the "R" form. Since the transition is highly cooperative, the restriction of one subunit to the "T" form locks the entire protein into the "T" form and severely reduces the oxygen affinity of the entire hemoglobin molecule. The analogous effect occurs with carbon monoxide poisoning (CO–heme formation), which locks the hemoglobin molecule into the "R" state and severely impairs the ability of hemoglobin to release oxygen in the tissues.

HEMOGLOBIN MUTANTS

Hundreds of mutant forms of hemoglobin α and β chains have been discovered by the analysis of human blood samples by electrophoresis. Many different forms of hemoglobin M have been found; these are mutants in which the ferric heme state is favored. The clinical severity of such mutations varies. In a typical hemoglobin M, "hemoglobin Boston," the distal histidine of the α chain is replaced by tyrosine. This alters the protein conformation, freezing it into the "T" state. In hemoglobin M "Milwaukee," a valine near the β-chain heme iron is replaced by glutamate, which forms a sixth ligand to the heme iron and stabilizes the ferric oxidation state.

Mutations affecting components of the enzymatic systems responsible for methemoglobin reduction also lead to congenital methemoglobinemia. These conditions will be discussed later.

CHEMICAL INDUCTION OF METHEMOGLOBIN

A remarkably wide variety of chemical agents can induce methemoglobin formation. Some agents [e.g., ferricyanide, $Fe(CN)_6^{3-}$] are only active when added directly to hemoglobin in vitro: The negatively charged complex ion is unable to cross the erythrocyte cell membrane. Other agents—for example, nitrobenzene—are only active in vivo; metabolic bioactivation converts these agents into the species responsible for methemoglobin formation. Nitrite (NO_2^-), N-hydroxyarylamines, and hydrogen peroxide are active both in vivo and in vitro. Several of these agents can be clinically significant. For example, exposure to nitrate fertilizers can be high in agricultural areas, notably in children drinking well-water; the nitrate can be reduced to nitrite by intestinal microflora. Nitrite is used per se as a preservative for meat. An outbreak of acquired methemoglobinemia in Dublin, Ireland, was traced to the application of excessive nitrite to pork by the local butcher (11). Acquired methemoglobinemia can also be induced by various drugs; some examples are given later.

In view of the diversity of the chemical structures of methemoglobinemia-inducing agents, one should not expect that a single mechanism accounts for their activities. The list includes both oxidizing (ferricyanide, hydrogen peroxide) and reducing (nitrite, N-hydroxyarylamines) compounds. In only a few cases has a reasonably complete understanding of the mechanism of hemoglobin oxidation been achieved.

MECHANISMS OF METHEMOGLOBIN FORMATION

The simplest interpretation of the mechanism of hemoglobin oxidation, given earlier, is one-electron transfer from dioxygen to iron: $Fe^{2+} O_2 \rightarrow Fe^{3+} + O_2^{\cdot-}$. However, this is clearly not the whole story. Hemoglobin is a tetramer of heme-containing subunits, so the complete stoichiometry of oxidation should account for all four. Also, the fate of the superoxide product of the first step must be considered. In the erythrocyte, superoxide dismutase and catalase (or glutathione peroxidase) will convert $O_2^{\cdot-}$ to oxygen and water. In a model system of pure hemoglobin, the involvement of $O_2^{\cdot-}$ and hydrogen peroxide in methemoglobin formation can be studied by adding back superoxide dismutase and catalase. Such experiments have been carried out (12), and they were interpreted according to the following scheme for autoxidation of pure hemoglobin:

$$Fe^{2+}O_2 \rightarrow Fe^{3+} + O_2^{\cdot-} \tag{1}$$

$$Fe^{2+}O_2 + O_2^{\cdot-} + 2H^+ \rightarrow Fe^{3+} + O_2 + H_2O_2 \tag{2}$$

$$Fe^{2+}O_2 + H_2O_2 \rightarrow Fe^{3+} + OH^- + HO\cdot + O_2 \tag{3}$$

$$Fe^{2+}O_2 + HO\cdot \rightarrow Fe^{3+} + OH^- + O_2 \tag{4}$$

Net: $4(Fe^{2+}O_2) + 2H^+ \rightarrow 4Fe^{3+} + 2OH^- + 3O_2$

The first step is the one-electron transfer reaction. In step 2, the superoxide anion and the heme iron reduce the heme-bound dioxygen to hydrogen peroxide, yielding ferric heme and dioxygen. This process, whereby a reducing agent (in this case, superoxide) generates methemoglobin and hydrogen peroxide, by unleashing the oxidizing power of the hemoglobin-bound oxygen molecule, is very significant: It demonstrates that *a reducing species can cause oxidative stress*. This mechanism underlies the apparently paradoxical methemoglobin induction by reducing species, such as nitrite and many drugs (13); see below. Step 3 is a form of Fenton chemistry: production of hydroxyl radical from hydrogen peroxide and ferrous iron. In step 4, this hydroxyl radical oxidizes one more ferrous heme unit.

These results, obtained with purified hemoglobin solutions, illustrate the potential for hemoglobin autoxidation to generate all the reactive species ($O_2^{\cdot-}$, H_2O_2, $HO\cdot$) associated with radiation damage and oxidative stress. In the intact red cell, these species will either participate in hemoglobin oxidation (as shown above), be detoxified by antioxidant enzymes and metabolic antioxidants, or lead to oxidative damage of other red cell constituents, including the cell membrane.

CONGENITAL METHEMOGLOBINEMIA

Rare individuals are congenitally cyanotic, with much-elevated levels of methemoglobin, even in the absence of exposure to xenobiotic chemicals. This condition, congenital methemoglobinemia, may be caused by mutations (hemoglobin M) in the gene for hemoglobin α or β chains, as mentioned earlier. In addition, defects in the enzymes of methemoglobin reduction (see below) can cause congenital methemoglobinemia. These enzymes include NADH-methemoglobin reductase, cytochrome b_5, and possibly others (14). Analysis of red cells from such patients has been critical for elucidation of the metabolic pathways of methemoglobin reduction in normal individuals, as discussed in the following sections. This is another illustration of the principle that evidence from the study of genetic diseases can tell us a great deal about normal metabolic processes.

METABOLIC REDUCTION OF METHEMOGLOBIN

Since autoxidation of hemoglobin is unavoidable, even in the absence of xenobiotic stress, and hemoglobin cannot be replaced by the red cell, methemoglobin must be reduced enzymatically back to the ferrous state. In addition, the superoxide flux generated by autoxidation must be dealt with, or oxidative stress will destroy vital cellular functions, such as membrane integrity (15). Both of these metabolic challenges require reducing power. Let us examine how each challenge is met by the erythrocyte.

The red blood cell (like the brain) relies almost exclusively on blood glucose for energy. It has no mitochondria, and therefore it cannot utilize the Krebs cycle. Of course, this greatly limits the energy-generating capacity of the cell, since oxidative phosphorylation cannot occur. Glucose metabolism takes place by glycolysis (Embden–Meyerhof pathway) to pyruvate or by the hexose monophosphate shunt pathway (see figure, p. 116).

What does this imply for generation of reducing power? Glycolysis, from glucose to lactate, is a redox-balanced process; glucose is split into two three-carbon fragments. The NADH generated by glyceraldehyde-3-phosphate dehydrogenase is consumed by lactate dehydrogenase (reduction of pyruvate to lactate). This is the standard route of anaerobic glycolysis. On the other hand, if another mechanism exists for regeneration of NAD^+ from NADH, then glycolysis can terminate at pyruvate. The reduction of methemoglobin provides such an avenue. NADH is the main source of reducing equivalents for regeneration of ferrous hemoglobin from methemoglobin.

CYTOCHROME b_5 AND NADH-CYTOCHROME b_5 REDUCTASE: THE METHEMOGLOBIN REDUCTASE TEAM

The Irish physiologist Q. H. Gibson observed that red cells treated with amyl nitrite reduced the resulting methemoglobin when subsequently incubated with glucose (16). (The measurement of methemoglobin reduction was performed by measuring the binding of CO to the ferrous product, using a mercury manometer—a reminder that important science can sometimes be done without fancy equipment!) Cells from an individual with congenital methemoglobinemia failed to do so. Iodoacetic acid, a well-known glycolytic inhibitor, stopped the glucose-dependent reduction observed in the normal cells. Lactate could also drive the reduction, and the lactate-dependent reaction was iodoacetate-insensitive. This evidence was consistent with an NADH-dependent process, since iodoacetate inhibits glyceraldehyde-phosphate dehydrogenase, the NADH-generating step in glycolysis. Lactate dehydrogenase, acting in the reverse direction to glycolysis, also generates NADH, but is insensitive to iodoacetate.

The NADH-dependent reduction of methemoglobin was first demonstrated in a cell-free system by Scott and Griffith in 1959 (17). Their pioneering work was simple in design, but incisive, and the paper deserves careful study. NADH-methemoglobin reductase activity could, in principle, be assayed directly by monitoring NADH-dependent reduction of methemoglobin. However, in those days, scanning spectrophotometers were still rare. Furthermore, the presence of many other absorbing species in a crude red blood cell hemolysate (osmotically ruptured cells) could interfere with the measurement. Therefore, a simple colorimetric assay was devised. The artificial electron acceptor dichloroindophenol (DCIP) is purple in its oxidized form and is colorless in the reduced "leuco" form. DCIP rapidly redox-equilibrates with the hemoglobin/methemoglobin couple, so reduction of DCIP (600 nm) can be used to monitor methemoglobin reduction. Nitrite-treated hemolyzate from normal individuals catalyzed the NADH-dependent reduction of DCIP. Nitrite-treated hemolyzate from persons with congenital methemoglobinemia did not do so. The enzyme catalyzing the observed NADH-dependent reduction of DCIP was named diaphorase.

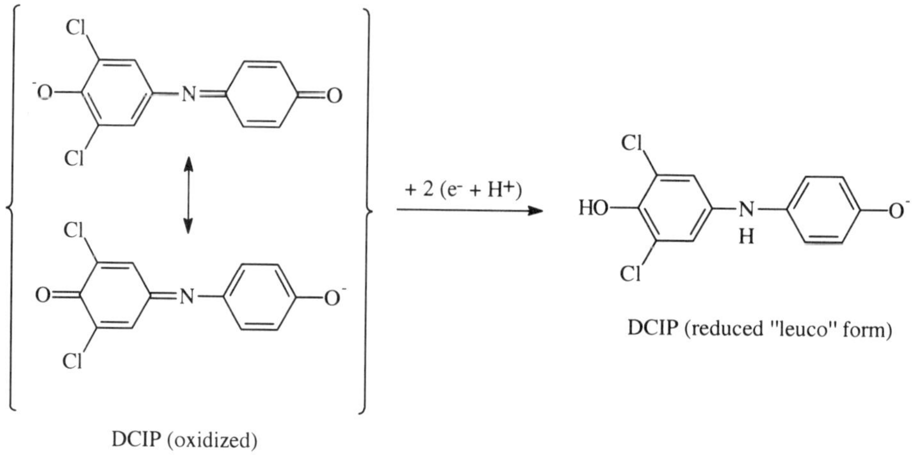

DCIP (oxidized)

DCIP (reduced "leuco" form)

The key breakthrough in elucidation of the enzymology of methemoglobin reduction was the discovery that cytochrome b_5 is an intermediary electron carrier (18). The enzyme which accepts electrons from NADH was then named as NADH-cytochrome b_5 reductase, rather than "diaphorase," the old term for an enzyme capable of reducing dyes (19). Reducing equivalents from NADH are carried through an electron-transport chain, via the flavoprotein (NADH-cytochrome b_5 reductase) and the cytochrome (b_5), to methemoglobin as the terminal electron acceptor:

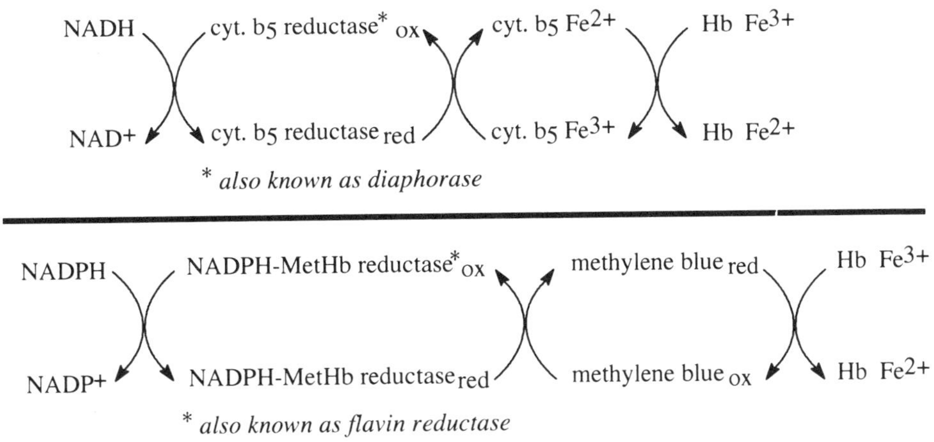

NADH $\quad$ cyt. b5 reductase* ox $\quad$ cyt. b5 Fe^{2+} $\quad$ Hb Fe^{3+}

NAD+ $\quad$ cyt. b5 reductase red $\quad$ cyt. b5 Fe^{3+} $\quad$ Hb Fe^{2+}

also known as diaphorase

NADPH $\quad$ NADPH-MetHb reductase* ox $\quad$ methylene blue red $\quad$ Hb Fe^{3+}

NADP+ $\quad$ NADPH-MetHb reductase red $\quad$ methylene blue ox $\quad$ Hb Fe^{2+}

also known as flavin reductase

The pathways of methemoglobin reduction: NADH-dependent and NADPH-dependent (dormant).

(See discussion of electron transport chains in Chapter 3.)

A spectroscopically similar cytochrome b_5 was already known to be involved in the hepatic microsomal electron-transfer system responsible for the synthesis of unsaturated fatty acids. In that system, too, electrons are transferred to cytochrome b_5 from NADH via a flavoprotein, NADH-dependent cytochrome b_5 reductase. [These enzymes are integral membrane proteins of the endoplasmic reticulum (microsomes) and also contribute to the catalytic activity of cytochrome P-450. We will return to a discussion of their roles in the chapter on cytochrome P-450.] The erythrocyte cytochrome b_5 and cytochrome b_5 reductase are, of course, cytosolic enzymes. What is the relationship between the microsomal and soluble b_5 systems?

Hultquist et al. (20) "postulated . . . that these cytoplasmic redox proteins of the erythrocyte are derived from corresponding membranous proteins of the endoplasmic reticulum of immature erythroid cells during erythroid maturation. The consequence of such proteolysis would be the conversion of a microsomal enzyme system which desaturates fatty acids to a cytoplasmic system which has the role of reducing methemoglobin."

Has nature found two very different roles for a single enzyme system? This hypothesis was strengthened by the discovery, in 1975, of a more severe form of congenital methemoglobinemia with NADH-cytochrome b_5 reductase deficiency. In this form, the patients were not only cyanotic but also suffered severe neurological problems and mental retardation. *This form of the disease affected not only the methemoglobin reductase (as in the milder form of the defect) but also the microsomal fatty acid desaturase in other tissues and cells (e.g., leukocytes).*

Decisive progress in characterization of NADH-cytochrome b_5 reductase was made by Yubisui et al. (21) in Japan, who purified the erythrocyte NADH-cytochrome b_5 reductase and used the partial amino acid sequence as a basis for cloning its cDNA and genomic sequence. The erythrocyte enzyme is composed of 275 amino acid residues (31 kD), whereas the microsomal enzyme has an additional 25 amino acid residue N-terminal membrane-binding *signal sequence* [see section on UDPGT in Chapter 10 for discussion of membrane proteins, signal sequences, and signal recognition particles (SRPs)]. It seems very likely that a single gene encodes both the cytosolic and microsomal forms of the protein.

To obtain recombinant human NADH-cytochrome b_5 reductase from a bacterial system, part of the cDNA for the enzyme was incorporated into a pUC13-derived plasmid vector. Since the erythrocyte form's N-terminal amino acid is phenylalanine, the protein cannot be expressed per se in *E. coli*: Bacterial translation always begins at an AUG (*N*-formylmethionine) codon. A recombinant protein was designed, such that the desired protein could be recovered by the action of a sequence-specific protease, α-thrombin. The cDNA was digested with *Xho*I, which cuts the sequence at the position of codons 10–11 of the erythrocyte form of the protein. The resulting fragment was ligated with a synthetic oligonucleotide fragment, encoding part of the *lacZ* gene and the proteolytic recognition sequence of α-thrombin (Ala-Pro-Arg). This sequence was then fused into the *lacZ* gene of pUC13:

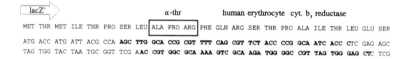

The plasmid was transformed into *E. coli*, and the expressed fusion protein (7% of the total bacterial protein) was purified. The fusion protein was treated with α-thrombin to release the recombinant human erythrocyte NADH-cytochrome b_5 reductase. The resulting protein had full enzymatic activity and kinetic properties similar to those of the erythrocyte protein.

In the case of cytochrome b_5, the situation is similar: one gene encodes both the soluble erythrocyte form and the membrane-bound hepatic microsomal form (22). The liver form has 134 residues; the erythrocyte form has only 98. But in this case the microsomal protein does not have an N-terminal signal sequence; instead, it has a C-terminal membrane-binding domain, which is absent in the reticulocyte form of the enzyme. The hydrophilic, soluble N-terminal domain of the enzyme is enzymatically active. In the reticulocyte, this domain is released by cathepsin proteolysis (see below). Proteolytic release of the active, soluble domain can also be achieved by trypsin treatment; the crystal structure of the tryptic product has been determined (23). The heme group is held within a crevice formed by a bundle of four α-helices (24).

In the hepatocyte, transport of the microsomal form to the endoplasmic reticulum occurs by a poorly understood, SRP-independent (25) mechanism, which requires a specific short sequence within the C-terminal domain (26). The topology of membrane insertion of microsomal cytochrome b_5 is not understood; the crystal structure of the soluble form does not address this question. In one proposed model, a hydrophobic segment of the C-terminal domain penetrates only one side of the lipid bilayer leaflet (27).

How is the proteolytic conversion of the microsomal to the erythrocyte forms carried out? Hultquist et al. (20) have recently addressed this problem by a painstaking biochemical approach. Membrane fraction was prepared from rabbit reticulocytes; these cells are expected to be a good source of the activity, since they are in the process of maturation into the final erythrocytic form. The putative protease was solubilized by treatment with CHAPS detergent. Activity was measured by using PAGE to monitor the conversion of purified microsomal cytochrome b_5 into the soluble form. Anion exchange chromatography on DE-52 cellulose and affinity chromatography on pepstatin-aminohexyl Sepharose yielded a partially purified preparation. Characterization of the 45-kD enzyme, by immunological and chemical approaches, confirmed the identification of the protease as *cathepsin D*. Cathepsins are typical degradative proteases found in lysosomes and are active at low pH. Pepstatin A is a peptide inhibitor of proteases, including cathepsins; it is often used to inhibit proteolysis during protein purifications. In this protocol, the protease was suspected to be a cathepsin, and thus matrix-bound pepstatin was used for affinity chromatography of the enzyme.

NADPH-DEPENDENT REDUCTION OF METHEMOGLOBIN

About 10% of the flux of glucose catabolism in the red blood cell occurs via the pentose phosphate pathway (29). The oxidative steps of the pathway (catalyzed by glucose-6-phosphate dehydrogenase and 6-phosphogluconate dehydrogenase) generate NADPH. (Glucose-6-phosphate dehydrogenase deficiency, a very common inborn error of metabolism leading to lowered synthesis of NADPH, is discussed on p. 118.) In the red cell, the pathway operates primarily to generate NADPH; the carbohydrate product of the oxidative reactions, ribulose-5-phosphate, is converted to fructose-6-phosphate and glyceraldehyde-3-phosphate, which reenter the glycolytic pathway to pyruvate (30).

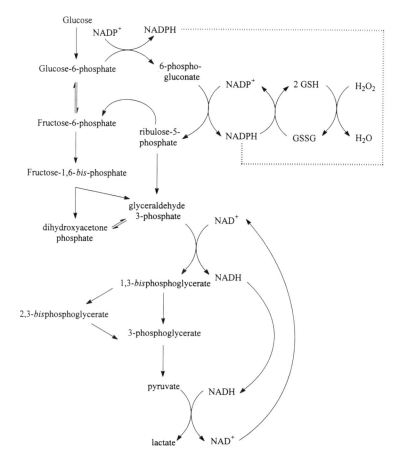

Glucose catabolism in the red blood cell.

Red cell NADPH maintains glutathione in the reduced form (p. 75). NADPH can also support the reduction of methemoglobin. This *NADPH-dependent* activity is apparently "dormant" under normal circumstances. However, the treatment of red cells with certain redox-active dyes stimulates this pathway (figure, p. 113) by facilitating intermolecular electron transfer processes. The best-known agent (first used by Warburg in 1930) is *methylene blue*:

methylene blue; λ_{max}=609, 668 nm.

$2 (H^+ + e^-)$

colourless (*leuco*) reduced form

Methylene blue can penetrate the erythrocyte membrane and is clinically useful for treatment of methemoglobinemia. In a peculiar twist, cyanotic "blue" methemoglobinemic patients can be restored to a healthy pink by treatment with this intensely blue dye (31, 32)!

The cytosolic NADPH-methemoglobin reductase has been purified to near-homogeneity (33). The enzyme is an unusual green protein, with an M_r of 26 kD; it binds porphyrins and fatty acids with high affinity. The enzyme's biological role remains a mystery, but it is probably *not* methemoglobin reduction, judging by the very slow rate at which NADPH supports this process (even in the presence of methylene blue). Congenital deficiency of the enzyme is not associated with methemoglobinemia. Also, the protein is present in many cells and tissues, other than the erythrocyte. Quandt and Hultquist recently cloned and sequenced the cDNA encoding the (bovine) enzyme (34). The enzyme catalyzes the reduction of flavins as well as methemoglobin, and is now commonly named "flavin reductase." With the molecular characterization of the protein and gene, further progress toward understanding its biological significance can be anticipated.

MECHANISMS OF INDUCTION OF METHEMOGLOBIN BY XENOBIOTICS

As was pointed out earlier, the chemistry of hemoglobin autoxidation is complex, and reduced oxygen species propagate the reaction. The chemistry of xenobiotic-induced methemoglobin formation is also complex. One of the few reagents which oxidizes hemoglobin stoichiometrically is ferricyanide. One equivalent of ferricyanide oxidizes one heme moiety in a simple second-order process. However, ferricyanide is neither active in vivo nor of toxicological significance.

The overall stoichiometry of nitrite-induced methemoglobin formation can be represented as

$$4Hb^{2+}O_2 + 4ONO^- + 4H^+ \rightarrow 4Hb^{3+} + 4NO_3^- + O_2 + 2H_2O$$

Both nitrite and heme are oxidized; the ultimate oxidant is not the xenobiotic, but dioxygen itself. The kinetics of the process are characterized by an initial lag phase and a subsequent autocatalytic phase (35).

Many drugs have been observed to cause methemoglobinemia, at least in occasional susceptible individuals. In many cases, such as with the common anesthetics benzocaine and lidocaine, the mechanisms remain obscure. In the following pages, I will discuss a few examples for which the mechanistic basis is at least partly understood.

PHENYLHYDRAZINE; HEINZ BODIES

Phenylhydrazine (phenyl-NH-NH$_2$) was used in the experimental induction of methemoglobinemia in the nineteenth century. In 1890 the German physician Heinz noted that red cells from guinea pigs treated with acetylphenylhydrazine acquired an unusual appearance under the microscope: The cells accumulated a number of very dense granules, now known as *Heinz bodies*. These granules are aggregates composed of degraded, insoluble pigments derived from hemoglobin oxidation. Methemoglobinemia does not necessarily lead to Heinz body accumulation, but many agents cause both effects.

Heinz bodies interfere with red cell fluidity and function, and they mark the cell for repair or elimination by the spleen (36):

The [Heinz body] inclusion is removed at the wall of the splenic sinus. . . . Cells . . . enter the sinuses by squeezing through slits between the endothelial "staves" of the sinus "barrel". The

Heinz body is a hard little "clinker" and, although the easily deformable red cell slithers into the sinus, it stops when the rigid inclusion stops. . . . At this juncture, the red cell simply amputates its inclusion body and proceeds into the splenic vein. The Heinz body, sheathed in red cell membrane, is ingested by a phagocyte. This *pitting function* of the spleen [is] reminiscent of . . . squeezing the pits out of cherries. . . .

Oddly, the spleen of the cat is ineffective at "pitting," and Heinz bodies are commonly observed in the red blood cells of healthy cats; the biological significance of this peculiarity is still obscure (37).

Primaquine and related antimalarial drugs, synthetic analogues of the natural product *quinine* (see structures, p. 119) increase oxidative stress in the red blood cell, probably by oxidizing hemoglobin (38):

$$Fe^{2+}O_2 + \text{Primaquine radical} \rightarrow Fe^{3+} + O_2 + \text{Primaquine (reduced)}$$

Metabolites of primaquine, such as 5-hydroxyprimaquine and the dimer, 5,5-diprimaquine, are even more effective than the parent drug at inducing methemoglobin formation and may be the more important species, in vivo (39).

The malaria parasite probably succumbs to a level of oxidative stress which the red cell can tolerate: This may explain the therapeutic activity of these drugs. (But, antimalarial drugs may have other mechanisms of action as well; see below). However, many individuals are primaquine-sensitive and are susceptible to severe hemolytic anemia following administration of the drug. This phenomenon was discovered in dramatic fashion when large numbers of U.S. soldiers were given primaquine, as a routine prophylactic treatment, during the war in Korea (after 1951). The primaquine-sensitivity occurred mainly in personnel of black African or Mediterranean ethnic origin. An intensive research effort culminated in the discovery that primaquine-sensitive individuals are deficient in glucose-6-phosphate dehydrogenase activity (40). This research project was carried out under the aegis of the U.S. Army, and it relied on the participation of volunteers from the Stateville Penitentiary near Chicago, both as experimental subjects and as research assistants. The extraordinary history of this enterprise has been related by Beutler (41).

GLUCOSE-6-PHOSPHATE DEHYDROGENASE DEFICIENCY

This enzyme deficiency is probably the most common "genetic disease" in the world, affecting at least 100 million people (42, 43). But it is misleading to call it a disease; the deficiency is a genetic polymorphism, including many allelic forms of the gene encoding the enzyme and conferring selective advantages or disadvantages in particular environments. While diminished glucose-6-phosphate dehydrogenase (G6PD) enzyme activity predisposes to primaquine-induced hemolytic anemia, it protects against infection by the malaria parasite.

G6PD is a dimeric or tetrameric protein composed of 515-amino-acid subunits. The G6PD gene is located on the long arm of the X-chromosome, so the phenotype is sex-linked. G6PD deficiency in females provides the textbook illustration of the phenomenon of X-chromosome *mosaicism* (as discussed for chronic granulomatous disease; see p. 94 (44). During development of the female embryo, one X-chromosome in each cell is inactivated (chosen, apparently, at random). As a consequence, female heterozygotes contain two distinct populations of red cells, with either deficient or normal levels of G6PD. Since the G6PD-deficient cells are sensitive to hemolysis, such individuals often show clinical symptoms of G6PD deficiency. Males have only one X-chromosome and are therefore necessarily homozygous and symptomatic.

The molecular basis of the G6PD polymorphism was studied phenotypically (enzyme assays) in the 1950s and at the protein sequence level in the 1960s. Several forms of the enzyme were identified. The cDNA for the G6PD gene was cloned in 1981, and much has subsequently been learned about the polymorphism at the nucleic acid sequence level. Recently, the PCR technique has been used to obtain genomic sequences, circumventing the difficulties of obtaining cDNA (43).

More than 10% of the male African-American population is G6PD type A(−). In these individuals, the enzyme is destabilized, and older red cells have very low enzyme activity. These cells are differentially sensitive to drug-induced hemolysis. The A(−) form appears to have arisen from a previous variant, A(+), which is even more common in male African-Americans. A(+) is enzymatically normal, but electrophoretically distinguishable: The mutation is A → G at position 376 of the coding sequence, causing substitution of negatively charged aspartic acid for neutral asparagine. Two forms of A(−) have been distinguished by DNA sequencing. In one form, the A(+) mutation is accompanied by the mutation G → A at position 202 (val → met). In other forms, the A(+) mutation is accompanied by other mutations which lead to a similar phenotype.

Another common G6PD variant is found mainly in populations living near the Mediterranean Sea, as well as among Sephardic Jews. The incidence of G6PD deficiency among Iraqi Jews was reported to be almost 25%. G6PD Mediterranean individuals are usually asymptomatic, but exposure to oxidant drugs can trigger severe, even fatal, hemolysis.

Favism (45) is an acute hemolytic anemia which occurs following ingestion of the Mediterranean broad bean (*Vicia faba*). This bean is a common foodstuff in Italy, Greece, and Middle Eastern countries. Again, only certain individuals are sensitive, and glucose-6-phosphate dehydrogenase deficiency is an important (but not the only) contributing factor. Reputedly, Pythagoras advised his followers to avoid the fava bean—perhaps an indication that this biochemical problem was appreciated in antiquity. The active constituent of the bean is believed to be the glycoside *divicine*, among other components (46). The action of bacteria in the digestive tract hydrolyzes divicine to the active aglycone:

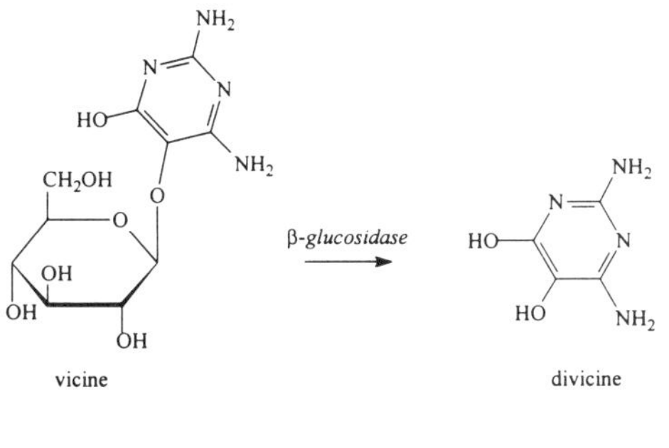

vicine   divicine

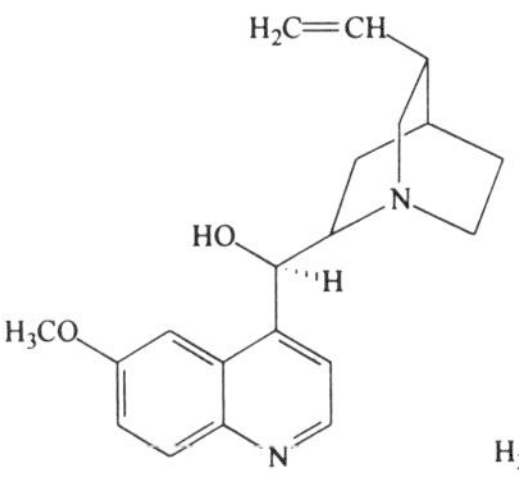

quinine 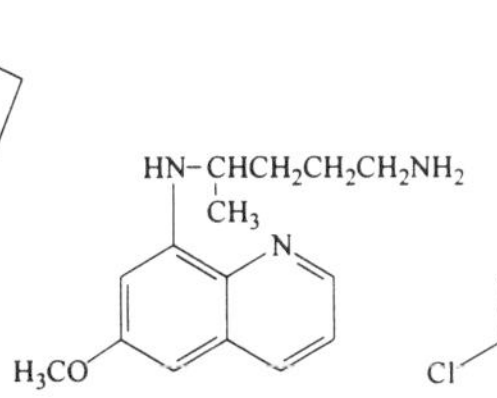   primaquine 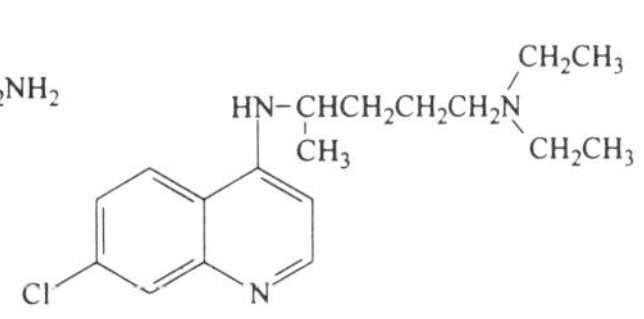   chloroquine

It seems paradoxical that glucose-6-phosphate dehydrogenase deficiency should be common in the same semitropical countries where fava beans are regularly consumed. Since enzyme-deficient individuals are particularly susceptible to favism, the diet should have selected against the enzyme defect. However, *vicine itself has antimalarial activity*, and "a staple diet of fava beans may have been the equivalent of a regular intake of pro-phylactic doses of antimalarial drugs over many generations" (47). The pathogen and the diet have probably both acted as important selective pressures on the gene pool.

What is the biochemical basis for the oxidant sensitivity of glucose-6-phosphate dehy-drogenase-deficient cells? Impairment of NADPH generation would be expected to cause depletion of reduced glutathione and reduced ability to scavenge superoxide and hydro-gen peroxide. In addition, erythrocyte catalase contains bound NADPH (as mentioned above), which protects the enzyme against peroxide-induced inactivation. Reduced cata-lase activity in glucose-6-phosphate dehydrogenase-deficient cells may be the critical fac-tor in oxidant sensitivity (48).

MALARIA

Malaria is one of the most prevalent parasitic diseases in the world, and over 200 million people suffer from its effects (49). At least one million die of the disease annually. Most of these people live in the tropical countries of Africa, South America, and Asia, although malaria was even endemic in Canada and Siberia at one time. The word "malaria" is de-rived from the Italian "bad air"—the common explanation of its etiology, in the days be-fore the infectious theory of diseases was accepted.

Malaria is a parasitic infection by protozoa of the genus *Plasmodium*, transmitted be-tween human individuals by the bite of the anopheline mosquito, in which the parasite undergoes sexual development. Several different species of parasite are known, and they produce characteristic forms of the disease. *Plasmodium falciparum* is the most debili-tating species and is often fatal. Infections with *Plasmodium vivax* are generally less se-vere. The parasite undergoes a complex life cycle, multiplying in both the liver and ery-throcyte.

As with other parasitic diseases (e.g., schistosomiasis, onchocerciasis, Chagas' disease, sleeping sickness), effective chemotherapy is difficult. The similarity between the me-tabolism of the parasite and that of the human host frustrates most attempts to design se-lective chemical agents.

OXIDATIVE STRESS AND MALARIA

Several lines of evidence support the view that oxidative stress can play a significant role in the treatment of malaria; nevertheless, the connection remains controversial (50, 51). In tissue culture, the malaria parasite grows best at low partial pressures of oxygen (about 2%). Indeed, laboratory culture of the parasite was very difficult until this oxygen-sensi-tivity was appreciated. The metabolic basis of this sensitivity is unclear, but it may be re-lated to the problem of dealing with the heme released by catabolism of hemoglobin (see below). The malaria parasite is also sensitive to many pro-oxidant drugs, such as phenyl-hydrazine, divicine, alloxan, and the Chinese traditional medicine qinghaosu. Many anti-malarial drugs (e.g., chloroquine, dapsone) induce red cell oxidative stress, methemoglo-binemia, glutathione depletion, and hemolysis. These drugs act, at least in part, by depleting GSH and placing increased oxidative stress on the parasite. Of course, most of these drugs also place this stress on the erythrocyte, leading to hemolysis in susceptible individuals (see above).

The geographical distributions of many of the inborn errors of red cell metabolism and variant hemoglobins (e.g., G-6-P dehydrogenase deficiency, sickle-cell anemia, thalassemias) correlate strikingly with malaria incidence, as was first pointed out by J. B. S. Haldane. He hypothesized that these alleles persist because the heterozygotes (carriers) are relatively resistant to malaria infection. Indeed, in one study, parasite growth in G6PD-deficient red blood cells (both Mediterranean and African types) was found to be impaired (52). Malaria is such a common disease in many of these regions that it may be one of the strongest selective pressures on the human population.

Other mechanisms of antimalarial drug action may also be important. The malaria parasite, growing in the red blood cell, derives most of its nutrient by catabolism of hemoglobin within specialized acid food vacuoles (53). Just as with the cells of the spleen (see above), the parasite must find a way to dispose of the heme moieties released by catabolism of the apoprotein. Lacking heme oxygenase activity (see Chapter 10), the parasite produces a *heme polymerase*, which catalyzes the polymerization of heme to form the insoluble pigment *hemozoin*. Chloroquine is an effective inhibitor of this enzyme, and this inhibition may be the chief reason for its effectiveness (54).

NOTES

1. Stern, A., Red cell oxidative damage, in: *Oxidative Stress*, H. Sies, Ed., Academic Press, London, 1985, pp. 331–349.
2. Beutler, E., The red cell: A tiny dynamo, in: *Blood, Pure and Eloquent*, M. M. Wintrobe, Ed., McGraw-Hill, New York, 1980, pp. 141–168.
3. Winterbourn, C. C., Oxidative reactions of hemoglobin, *Methods Enzymol.* 186:265–272, 1990.
4. Fersht, A., *Enzyme Structure and Mechanism*, 2nd ed., W. H. Freeman, New York, 1985, pp. 272–283.
5. Dickerson, R. E., and Geis, I., *Hemoglobin: Structure, Function, Evolution, and Pathology*, Benjamin/Cummings, Menlo Park, CA, 1983.
6. Fersht, A., *Enzyme Structure and Mechanism*, 2nd ed., W. H. Freeman, New York, 1985; pp. 278–281; Voet, D., and Voet, J. G., *Biochemistry*, 2nd ed., Wiley, New York, 1995, pp. 227–233.
7. Perutz, M. F., *Protein Structure: New Approaches to Therapy and Disease*, W. H. Freeman, New York, 1992.
8. Josephy, P. D., Haemoglobin and cooperativity, *Biochem. Ed.* 20:91–93, 1992.
9. Mozzarelli, A., Rivetti, C., Rossi, G. L., Henry, E. R., and Eaton, W. A., Crystals of haemoglobin with the T quaternary structure bind oxygen noncooperatively with no Bohr effect, *Nature* 351:416–419, 1991.
10. See ref. 3.
11. Walley, T., and Flanagan, M., Nitrite-induced methemoglobinemia, *Postgrad. Med. J.* 63:643–644, 1987.
12. Watkins, J. A., Kawanishi, S., and Caughey, W. S., Autoxidation reactions of hemoglobin A free from other red cell components: a minimal mechanism, *Biochem. Biophys. Res. Commun.* 132:742–748, 1985.
13. Castro, C. E., Wade, R. S., and Belser, N. O., Conversion of oxyhemoglobin to methemoglobin by organic and inorganic reductants, *Biochemistry* 17:225–231, 1978; French, C. L., Yaun, S. S., Baldwin, L. A., Leonard, D. A., Zhao, X. Q., and Calabrese, E. J., Potency ranking of methemoglobin-forming agents, *J. Appl. Toxicol.* 15:167–174, 1995.
14. Hegesh, E., Hegesh, J., and Kaftory, A., Congenital methemoglobinemia with a deficiency of cytochrome b_5, *N. Engl. J. Med.* 314:757–761, 1986.

15. Stern, A., Red cell oxidative damage, in: *Oxidative Stress*, H. Sies, Ed., Academic Press, 1985, pp. 331–349.

16. Gibson, Q. H., The reduction of methemoglobin in red blood cells and studies on the cause of idiopathic methemoglobinemia, *Biochem. J.* 42:13–23, 1948.

17. Scott, E. M., and Griffith, I. V., The enzymic defect of hereditary methemoglobinemia: Diaphorase, *Biochim. Biophys. Acta* 34:584–586, 1959.

18. Hultquist, D. E., and Passon, P. G., Catalysis of methaemoglobin reduction by erythrocyte cytochrome b₅ and cytochrome b₅ reductase, *Nature New Biol.* 229:252–254, 1971.

19. Cadenas, E., Antioxidant and prooxidant functions of DT-diaphorase in quinone metabolism, *Biochem. Pharmacol.* 49:127–140, 1995.

20. Hultquist, D. E., Rodriguez, C., and Schafer, D. A., Cathepsin D in erythroid cells, in: *The Red Cell: Seventh Ann Arbor Conference*, G. J. Brewer, Ed., Alan R. Liss, New York, 1989, pp. 93–106.

21. Shirabe, K., Yubisui, T., and Takeshita, M., Expression of human erythrocyte NADH-cytochrome b5 reductase as an alpha-thrombin–cleavable fused protein in *Escherichia coli, Biochim. Biophys. Acta* 1008:189–192, 1989; Shirabe, K., Fujimoto, Y., Yubisui, T., and Takeshita, M., An in-frame deletion of codon 298 of the NADH-cytochrome b5 reductase gene results in hereditary methemoglobinemia type II (generalized type). A functional implication for the role of the COOH-terminal region of the enzyme, *J. Biol. Chem.* 269:5952–5957, 1994.

22. Giordano, S. J., and Steggles, A. W., The human liver and reticulocyte cytochrome b₅ mRNAs are products from a single gene, *Biochem. Biophys. Res. Commun.* 178:38–44, 1991.

23. Mathews, F. S., Levine, M., and Argos, P., The structure of calf liver cytochrome b₅ at 2.8 Å resolution, *Nature New Biol.* 233:15–16, 1971.

24. Branden, C., and Tooze, J., *Introduction to Protein Structure*, Garland Publishers, New York, 1991, pp. 153–154.

25. Moran, L. A., Scrimgeour, K. G., Horton, H. R., Ochs, R. S., and Rawn, J. D., Biochemistry, 2nd ed., Neil Patterson Publishers, Englewood Cliffs, NJ, 1994, pp. 30.37–30.42.

26. Mitoma, J.-y., and Ito, A., The carboxy-terminal 10 amino acid residues of cytochrome b₅ are necessary for its targeting to the endoplasmic reticulum, *EMBO J.* 11:4197–4203, 1992.

27. Voet, D., and Voet, J. G., *Biochemistry*, 2nd ed., Wiley, New York, 1995, Figure 11-24, p. 294.

28. Li, X. R., Giordano, S. J., Yoo, M., and Streggles, A. W., The isolation and characterization of the human cytochrome b5 gene, *Biochem. Biophys. Res. Commun.* 209:894 900, 1995.

29. Palsson, B. O., Narang, A., and Joshi, A., Computer model of human erythrocyte metabolism, in: *The Red Cell: Seventh Ann Arbor Conference*, G. J. Brewer, Ed., Alan R. Liss, New York, 1989, pp. 133–154.

30. Stryer, L., *Biochemistry*, 4th ed., W. H. Freeman, New York, 1995, p. 565.

31. Smith, R. P., Toxic responses of the blood, in: *Casarett and Doull's Toxicology*, 3rd ed., C. D. Klaassen, M. O. Amdur, and J. Doull, Ed., Macmillan, New York, 1986, p. 237.

32. Harvey, J. W., and Keitt, A. S., Studies of the efficacy and potential hazards of methylene blue therapy in aniline-induced methaemoglobinaemia, *Br. J. Haematol.* 54:29–41, 1983.

33. Xu, F., Quandt, K. S., and Hultquist, D. E., Characterization of NADPH-dependent methemoglobin reductase as a heme-binding protein in erythrocytes and liver, *Proc. Natl. Acad. Sci. U.S.A.*, 89:2130–2134, 1992.

34. Quandt, K. S., and Hultquist, D. E., Flavin reductase: Sequence of cDNA from bovine liver and tissue distribution, *Proc. Natl. Acad. Sci. USA* 91:9322–9326, 1994.

35. Spagnuolo, C., Rinelli, P., Coletta, M., Chiancone, E., and Ascoli, F., Oxidation reactions of human oxyhemoglobin with nitrite: A reexamination, *Biochim. Biophys. Acta* 911:59–65, 1987.

36. Crosby, W. H., The Spleen, in: *Blood, Pure and Eloquent*, M. M. Wintrobe, Ed., McGraw-Hill, New York, 1980, p. 120.

37. Christopher, M. M., Perman, V., and Eaton, J. W., Contribution of propylene glycol-induced Heinz body formation to anemia in cats, *J. Am. Vet. Med. Assoc.*, 194:1045–1056, 1989.

38. Watkins, J. A., Kawanishi, S., and Caughey, W. S., Autoxidation reactions of hemoglobin A free from other red cell components: A minimal mechanism, *Biochem. Biophys. Res. Commun.* 132:742–748, 1985.

39. Da Silva Morais, M., and Augusto, A., Peroxidation of the antimalarial drug primaquine: characterization of a benzidine-like metabolite with methaemoglobin-forming activity, *Xenobiotica* 23:133–139, 1993.

40. Carson, P. E., Flanagan, C. L., Ickes, C. E., Alving, A. S., Enzymatic deficiency in primaquine-sensitive erythrocytes, *Science* 124:484–485, 1956.

41. See ref. 2.

42. Senozan, N. M., and Thielman, C. A., Glucose-6–phosphate dehydrogenase deficiency: An inherited ailment that affects 100 million people, *J. Chem. Ed.* 68:7–10, 1991.

43. Beutler, E., Kuhl, W., Gelbart, T., and Forman, L., DNA sequence abnormalities of human glucose-6-phosphate dehydrogenase variants, *J. Biol. Chem.* 266:4145–4150, 1991.

44. Suzuki, D. T., Griffiths, A. J. F., Miller, J. H., and Lewontin, R. C., *An Introduction to Genetic Analysis*, 4th ed., W. H. Freeman, New York, 1989, pp. 379ff.

45. Shibamoto, T., and Bjeldanes, L. F., *Introduction to Food Toxicology*, Academic Press, New York, 1993, pp. 74–75.

46. McMillan, D. C., Schey, K. L., Meier, G. P., and Jollow, D. J., Chemical analysis and hemolytic activity of the fava bean aglycon divicine, *Chem. Res. Toxicol.* 6:439–444, 1993.

47. Clark, I. A., and Cowden, W. B., Antimalarials, in: *Oxidative Stress*, H. Sies, Ed., Academic Press, New York, 1985, pp. 131–149.

48. Scott, M. D., Wagner, T. C., and Chiu, D. T.-Y., Decreased catalase activity is the underlying mechanism of oxidant susceptibility in glucose-6–phosphate dehydrogenase-deficient erythrocytes, *Biochim. Biophys. Acta* 1181:163–168, 1993.

49. Miller, L. H., The challenge of malaria, *Science* 257: 36–37, 1992.

50. Clark, I. A., Chaudhri, G., and Cowden, W. B., Some roles of free radicals in malaria, *Free Radic. Biol. Med.* 6:315–321, 1989.

51. Hunt, N. H., and Stocker, R., Oxidative stress and the redox status of malaria-infected erythrocytes, *Blood Cells* 16:499–526, 1990.

52. Roth, E., Jr., and Schulman, S., The adaptation of *Plasmodium falciparum* to oxidative stress in G6PD deficient human erythrocytes, *Br. J. Haematol.* 70:363–367, 1988.

53. Goldberg, D.E., Plasmodial hemoglobin degradation: An ordered pathway in a specialized organelle, *Infect. Agents Dis.* 1:207–211, 1992.

54. Slater, A. F. G., and Cerami, A., Inhibition by chloroquine of a novel haem polymerase enzyme activity in malaria trophozoites, *Nature* 355:167–169, 1992.

9

INTRODUCTION TO XENOBIOTIC METABOLISM

THE ENZYMOLOGY OF XENOBIOTIC BIOTRANSFORMATION: MULTIPLE SUBSTRATES AND MULTIPLE ENZYMES

The student of biochemistry is taught, early on, that enzymes differ from conventional chemical catalysts: Each enzyme is highly specific for one substrate (or, at most, a few similar substrates). Enzymes can be named systematically, based on the reactions which they catalyze. Even slight chemical modification of the substrate, such as deletion of a methylene unit from an alkyl chain, converts a substrate into a competitive inhibitor. For example, malonate (HOOC-CH$_2$-COOH) is a close chemical analogue of succinate (HOOC-CH$_2$-CH$_2$-COOH), and malonate is a competitive inhibitor of the citric acid cycle enzyme succinate dehydrogenase. Typically, enzymes have very high catalytic efficiencies, reflected in low values of K_M (i.e., tight binding of substrate) and high values of k_{cat} (turnover number).

However, as our understanding of biochemistry has deepened, this simple scheme has broken down in several ways. First, the application of techniques for the high-resolution purification of proteins (especially electrophoresis and isoelectric focusing) revealed that enzyme preparations previously regarded as pure were, in fact, heterogenous mixtures of similar but distinct proteins. *Isozymes* are multiple forms of an enzyme catalyzing a given reaction. In some cases, these proteins are posttranslationally modified products of a single gene sequence. In other cases, they are products of distinct, but homologous, genes. The multiple forms of lactate dehydrogenase and hexokinase are well-known examples of isozyme diversity in intermediary metabolism.

Second, many enzymes act on multiple substrates. Hexokinase also serves as an example of this kind of complexity: Even a single form of hexokinase, purified to homogeneity, can still accept a variety of substrates (in this case, different hexose sugars) as substrates.

Researchers in molecular toxicology are often asked: Why do animals possess enzymes which can metabolize xenobiotics (foreign compounds, such as plant secondary metabolites, drugs, and pesticides), including synthetic compounds which do not exist in nature? In attempting to answer this fundamental question, we should first observe that the natural world is, in fact, filled with hazardous chemicals of biological origin. Some animals and many plants produce natural product toxins as defence mechanisms. Many important drugs are either natural products or their synthetic analogues. Animals have evolved in response to strong selective pressure for protection against these toxic natural products. The enzymatic biotransformation of xenobiotics facilitates their elimination from the body. In the absence of such processes, lipophilic xenobiotics would be cleared extremely slowly; their toxic actions would be of prolonged duration following exposure. With repeated exposures, they would accumulate in the tissues, reaching toxic levels. Organisms—especially herbivorous animals, which consume a wide variety of plant materials, often laden with unusual natural products and toxic secondary metabolites—must carry out the metabolic transformation of a tremendously diverse spectrum of foreign compounds.

Furthermore, the distinction between the metabolism of xenobiotics and of endogenous compounds no longer seems as clear as was once thought. Many endogenous substrates of "xenobiotic biotransformation enzymes" have been identified. For example, cytochromes P-450 and sulfotransferases play key roles in the metabolism of steroids; UDP-glucuronosyltransferases conjugate bilirubin. Researchers continue to debate whether these enzymes evolved primarily for the detoxication of xenobiotics, and were then adapted to the metabolism of endogenous compounds, or vice versa; probably, both functions co-evolved (1).

No organism has the genetic or metabolic capacity to produce tens of thousands of distinct enzymes so as to detoxify an equal number of foreign compounds in the diet. And, as a species' environment changes, how can individuals respond to the challenges of new compounds encountered in the diet? Clearly, another strategy is needed if an organism is to deal with the witches' brew of toxic natural products in its environment, let alone the myriad new substances introduced by modern chemical technology.

We can begin to understand nature's solution to this challenge if we consider the relationship between catalytic *specificity* and *efficiency*. The enzymes of intermediary metabolism are both highly efficient (high turnover numbers and enormous rate enhancements relative to the uncatalyzed reactions) and highly substrate-specific. High catalytic efficiency demands a precise chemical fit between the substrate and enzyme, and this fit, in turn, dictates stringent substrate specificity. In contrast, *many of the enzymes of xenobiotic metabolism are characterized by broad substrate specificity and relatively low catalytic efficiency.* These enzymes represent a metabolic compromise: The ability to metabolize diverse substances is achieved at the cost of reduced precision of substrate binding to the enzyme.

How can enzymes of low catalytic efficiency carry out the vital task of eliminating toxic compounds from the body? Several additional features of the biochemistry of biotransformation help to explain this. *Many of the enzymes are present in very large amounts.* For example, in the liver, cytochromes P-450, the key enzymes of phase I biotransformation, are the predominant proteins of the endoplasmic reticulum, and glutathione transferases are the most abundant proteins in the cytosol. A large amount of versatile (but low-efficiency) catalyst substitutes for a small amount of highly efficient catalyst. Many of the enzymes of biotransformation have diverged evolutionarily into *large families of enzymes with overlapping substrate specificities.* Each form carries out the same general reaction (e.g., acetylation) but handles slightly different groups of substrates. Many xenobiotics are encountered only occasionally, and in relatively low concentrations (e.g., toxic plant alkaloids, ingested when a particular foodstuff is consumed). In such cases, only a small amount of compound must be metabolized. This contrasts with the continuous large fluxes of material through the central pathways of intermediary metabolism.

The production of the enzymes of xenobiotic biotransformation can be regulated at the transcriptional, translational, and posttranslational levels. Therefore, *continued exposure of the organism to specific chemicals may induce the synthesis of greatly elevated levels of particular forms* of biotransformation enzymes. In some (but not all) instances, the induced forms carry out the metabolism of the inducing agent itself. This mechanism allows the organism to adapt to a chronic exposure to a toxicant or pollutant. A well-known example is the induction of ethanol-metabolizing systems in chronic alcoholics. As we will see later, many instances of enzyme induction following repeated human exposure to drugs or toxicants have been identified.

These phenomena—broad substrate specificities and existence of isozymes—frustrate our attempts to assign unambiguous names to specific enzymes, based on their catalytic activities. For example, suppose we attempt to characterize the forms of UDP-glucuronosyltransferase. Each form catalyzes the same general reaction, glucuronide formation. If we assay the glucuronidation of a particular substrate, say morphine, we will probably identify the enzyme of interest as *morphine UDP-glucuronosyltransferase*. Purification of this activity may well yield several distinct proteins: Multiple enzymes get one name, perhaps distinguished by an appended number. If we choose another substrate, say, *para*-nitrophenol, we will isolate several more enzyme proteins, which may or may not be distinct from the morphine enzymes. Thus, if morphine UDP-glucuronosyltransferase turns out to be identical to *para*-nitrophenol UDP-glucuronosyltransferase, one enzyme gets multiple names. Frequently, assay substrates are chosen for analytical convenience rather than physiological significance, so enzyme names may be of little physiological significance.

When an experimental protocol has been developed for the purification of the individual members of a class of enzymes, it may be possible to isolate a large number of isozyme forms without even using an enzyme assay. Such a protocol might involve a particular protein purification technique (such as isoelectric focusing or affinity chromatography) or be based on the physicochemical properties of the enzyme proteins (such as thermal stability). In such a case, the enzymes are likely to be named forms I, II, III, and IV in one laboratory ... and forms c, d, b, and a in another! Another common approach is to use treatment with specific chemical agents to induce the proliferation of a particular isozyme, which is then named after the inducing agent. Thus we speak of cytochromes P-450 as phenobarbital-inducible (P-450$_{PB}$) versus 3-methylcholanthrene-inducible (P-450$_{MC}$). Sometimes enzyme forms are distinguished on the basis of their physical or spectroscopic characteristics (e.g., cytochrome P-450 versus cytochrome P-448, whose reduced-CO complexes absorb ultraviolet (UV) light at the designated wavelengths). In these instances, the substrates of the enzymes may be unknown.

The advent of microsequencing methods for proteins (2) and DNA, and the resulting explosive growth of protein and gene sequence data, has opened a new era in analysis of enzyme structure and function and provides a new tool for the classification of proteins based on sequence homologies and evolutionary relationships. Using these methods, isozymes can be grouped into families and subfamilies based on amino acid sequence, rather than catalytic properties. This systematic approach promises to be less ambiguous than earlier phenomenological approaches. Sequence-based classifications can clarify the relationships between enzymes isolated from different species. For example, we now recognize that the cytochrome P-450 forms originally classified as c (rat), P$_1$ (mouse), and LM$_6$ (rabbit) are related; each has been reclassified as form P-4501A1 (see Chapter 14). Sequence comparisons can also reveal unexpected similarities between isozymes with markedly different catalytic activities. On the other hand, sequence-based nomenclature tends to obscure biological function; to a nonexpert in the field, the designation "dimethylnitrosamine demethylase" is biochemically more informative than "P-4502E1." And the development of sequence-based nomenclature for some families of enzymes is still at an early stage. We shall use systematic, sequence-based names wherever it is helpful to do so.

CONJUGATION REACTIONS

Xenobiotics enter the body through various routes—orally, through the skin or the lungs, directly injected—and they leave through various routes—urine, faeces, sweat, exhaled air. For many compounds, the urine and the bile (feces) are the most important routes. Most environmentally persistent toxic chemicals are hydrophobic, and this property facilitates transport across biological membranes and absorption into the body.

> The leperous distilment; whose effect
> Holds such an enmity with blood of man
> That swift as quicksilver it courses through
> The natural gates and alleys of the body ...
> *Hamlet*, I:5

Urine is formed by the ultrafiltration of the blood in the kidneys, accompanied by the selective readsorption of solutes, either by active transport or passive diffusion. Lipophilic compounds tend to be passively readsorbed. Similarly, lipophilic compounds are readsorbed by the liver during the process of formation and secretion of bile. Thus, *compounds which are readily absorbed or readsorbed tend to be poorly excreted*. As we have already noted, this is characteristic of most persistent toxicants. This conundrum is solved by metabolic transformation: *Most lipophilic drugs and toxicants are transformed into water-soluble conjugates*, which are readily excreted.

This process of conjugation is often referred to as "Phase II" biotransformation, as distinguished from the oxidative, reductive, or hydrolytic reactions of Phase I. However, this term is misleading, since many compounds can undergo conjugative "Phase II" reactions directly, without prior "Phase I" metabolism. Perhaps it is more instructive to group several of these reactions together as *synthetic conjugations*.* In these enzymatic reactions, xenobiotics are modified by linkage to endogenous metabolites, often leading to a more water-soluble product (3). In addition, some of the functional groups used in conjugation, such as the carboxylic acid functionality of glucuronic acid, are recognized by specific organic anion active transport systems in the liver and kidney, which facilitate excretion into the bile and urine, respectively.

With the exception of glutathione conjugation (considered separately in Chapter 11), *the conjugating group is introduced via an electrophilic activated donor*. These donors can then react with nucleophilic centers in xenobiotic substrates, such as oxygen in hydroxyl groups and nitrogen in amines. Before we examine these reactions, let us consider each of these activated donors.

ACTIVATED DONORS

UDP-Glucuronic Acid

Conjugation of lipophilic compounds to a sugar derivative (glycosidation) usually results in a great increase in water-solubility. For example, nucleosides are water-soluble glycosides of the hydrophobic bases in nucleic acids. Glucuronic acid is the sugar commonly used for the glycosidation of xenobiotics by mammals, and UDP-glucuronic acid is the activated donor of this sugar moiety (see Table 9.1). UDP-glucuronic acid is derived from UDP-glucose, which is the proximate substrate for glycogen synthesis, the primary route for storage of carbohydrate as polysaccharide.

---

*For this reason, we eschew the often-heard expression "metabolic breakdown" of a drug or toxicant. Almost invariably, the metabolic process is one of biochemical *synthesis*, not "breakdown": The metabolites are of higher molecular weight than the original toxicant.

Table 9.1. Selected Enzymes of Xenobiotic Conjugation

Reaction	Enzyme	Cellular Compartment	Activated Donor
Glucuronidation	UDP-glucuronosyltransferase	Microsomal	UDP-glucuronic acid
Sulfation	Sulfotransferase	Cytosolic[a]	3'-Phosphoadenosine-5'-phosphosulfate
Methylation	Methyltransferase	Cytosolic[a]	S-Adenosylmethionine
Acetylation	Acetyltransferase	Cytosolic	S-Acetylcoenzyme A

[a]Some microsomal forms also exist.

The sugar phosphate moieties required for the assembly of polysaccharides (e.g., glycogen) are first coupled to the high-energy compound UTP, and pyrophosphate (PP_i) is released; the subsequent energetically favorable hydrolysis of PP_i to inorganic phosphate provides an additional driving force for the coupling reaction:

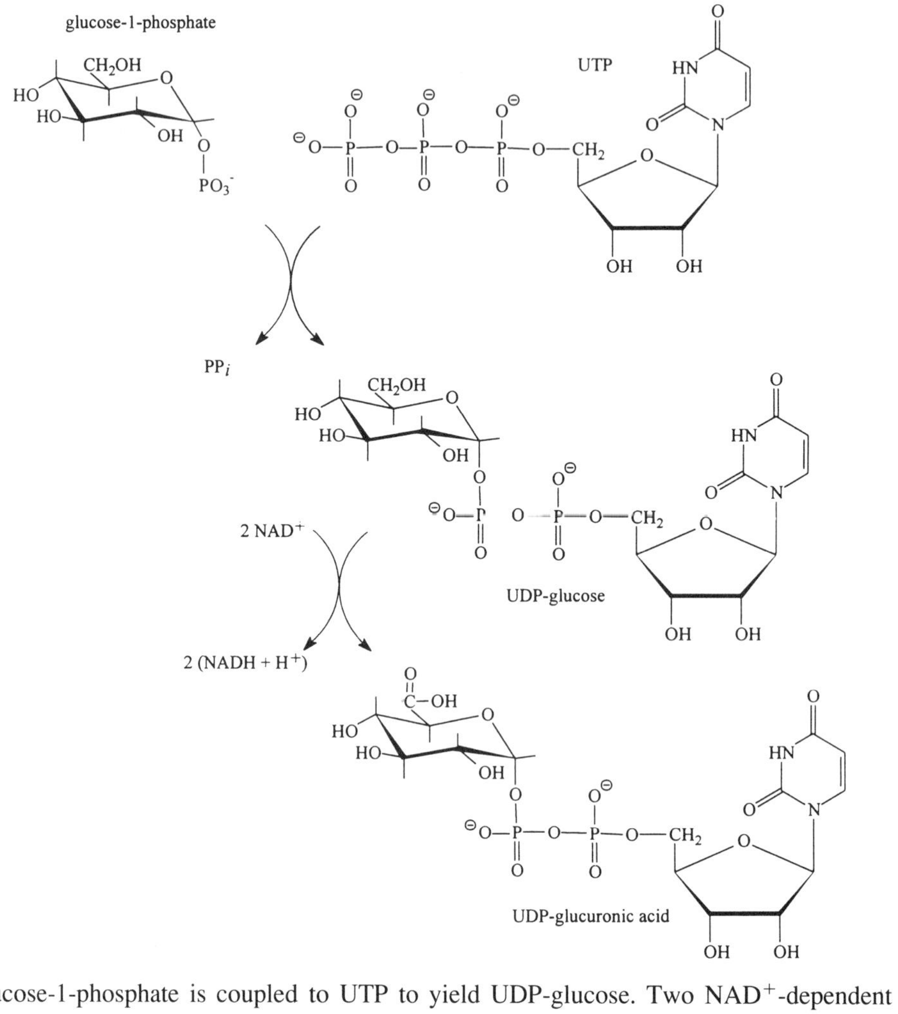

Glucose-1-phosphate is coupled to UTP to yield UDP-glucose. Two NAD^+-dependent oxidations of UDP-glucose yield the sugar acid *glucuronic acid*, in the form of UDP-glucuronic acid (UDPGA).

3'-Phosphoadenosine-5'-Phosphosulfate

The identity of "activated sulfate," the metabolic donor of sulfate groups, was elucidated by the work of Lipmann (best known for his development of the concept of ATP as the cell's energy currency) and others, in the late 1950s. 3'-Phosphoadenosine-5'-phospho-sulfate is synthesized from ATP and inorganic sulfate:*

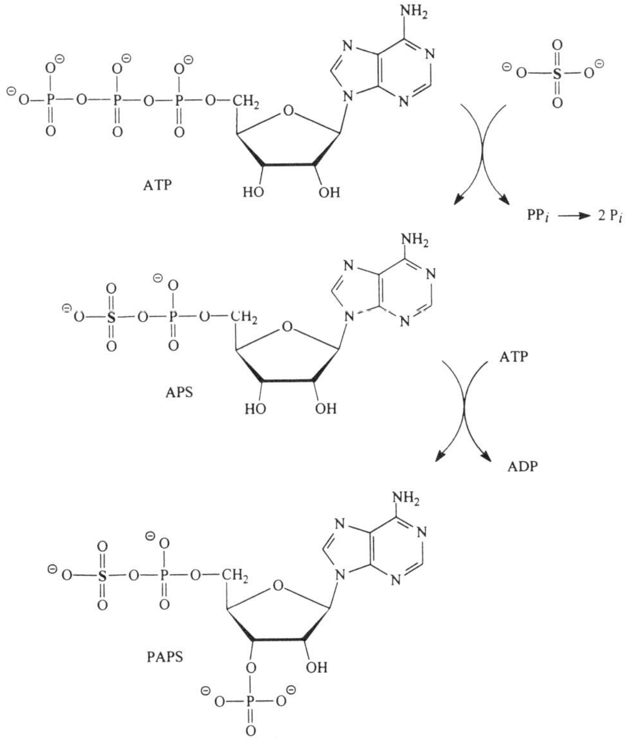

ATP

HO   OH

PP$_i$ $\longrightarrow$ 2 P$_i$

APS

HO   OH

ATP

ADP

PAPS

OH

Sulfate is activated by linkage to the 5' α-phosphate group of adenylate, giving adenylyl sulfate (APS). The $\Delta G^{0'}$ for this reaction is highly positive; even coupling to the subsequent hydrolysis of pyrophosphate is insufficient to drive the overall process forward (4). Therefore, in a second step, an additional molecule of ATP is used to phosphorylate the 3'-OH of APS, yielding PAPS. This second phosphorylation uses a high-energy phosphate anhydride (ATP) to produce a low-energy phosphate ester (3'-phosphate of PAPS), and thus it is energetically favorable. This second phosphorylation provides thermodynamic power which drives the first step to completion. Following transfer of the sulfate moiety to an acceptor (see below), the product 3'-phosphoadenosine-5'-phosphate is cleaved to inorganic phosphate and AMP.

The body's reserves of free sulfate are limited; the serum sulfate concentration in humans is about 0.3 mM. Administration of sulfotransferase substrates, such as acetaminophen, can cause a substantial transient drop in serum sulfate. The sulfate level is restored by catabolism of sulfated polysaccharides, such as chondroitin and keratan, glycosaminoglycans of the extracellular matrix. *Brachymorphic* (Greek: *short shape*) mice have short legs and tails, resulting from defective formation of cartilage glycosaminoglycans, such as chondroitin sulfate. The trait is due to a single recessive gene which results in reduced formation of PAPS (5) and these mice also have diminished capacity for sulfation of xenobiotics.

*The synthesis of PAPS in *Escherichia coli* is catalyzed by enzymes encoded by genes of the sulfate activation operon. The first step, APS synthesis, is catalyzed by ATP sulfurylase, an enzyme composed of two subunits, the product of the *cysD* and *cysN* genes. APS activation to PAPS, the second step, is catalyzed by APS kinase, the product of the *cysC* gene.

SIDEBAR: SULFATE, SULFITE, THIOSULFATE, AND CYANIDE TOXICITY

Bisulfite (HSO_3^-) is used as an antioxidant and food preservative; for example, many wines are treated with bisulfite. Sulfur dioxide (SO_2) is a significant air pollutant in industrialized areas, formed especially by the combustion of sulfur-rich coal. These species contain sulfur in the $+4$ oxidation state, and they exist in equilibrium with sulfite (SO_3^{2-}) in aqueous solution. In mammals, sulfite is detoxified by oxidation to sulfate, catalyzed by the enzyme *sulfite oxidase* (6):

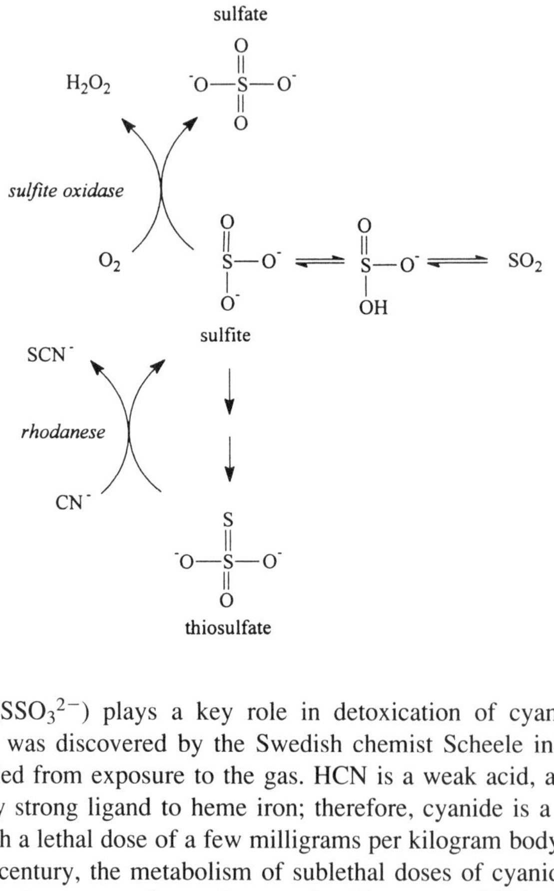

Thiosulfate (SSO_3^{2-}) plays a key role in detoxication of cyanide. Hydrogen cyanide (HCN) was discovered by the Swedish chemist Scheele in the eighteenth century, who died from exposure to the gas. HCN is a weak acid, and cyanide ion (CN^-) is a very strong ligand to heme iron; therefore, cyanide is a potent respiratory poison, with a lethal dose of a few milligrams per kilogram body weight. In the late nineteenth century, the metabolism of sublethal doses of cyanide was studied, and the major product excreted was shown to be thiocyanate, SCN^-. This metabolic process, which detoxifies cyanide, is catalyzed by the ubiquitous enzyme rhodanese (the name derives from "rhodanic acid," an old term for thiocyanate). Rhodanese transfers sulfur from various donors to cyanide; the most important appears to be thiosulfate. The availability of thiosulfate limits the action of rhodanese; thus, cyanide poisoning can be treated by administration of thiosulfate.

It is unclear whether detoxication of cyanide is the primary physiological role of rhodanese. The enzyme's presence in mitochondria suggests a possible respiratory function. However, cyanide is released by the hydrolysis of *cyanogenic glycosides*, such as amygdalin, found in apricot pits:

Cyanogenic glycosides

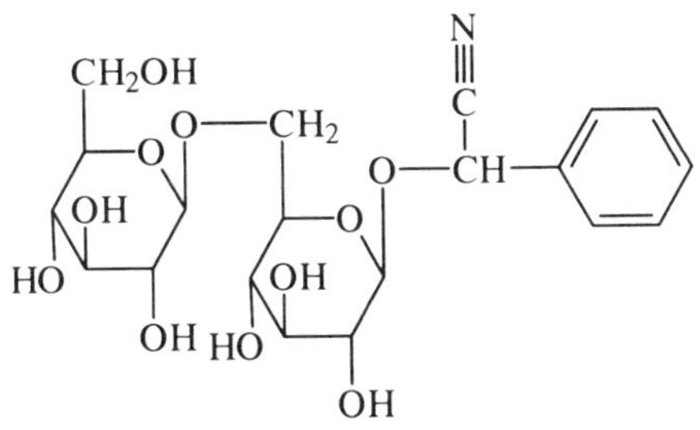

amygdalin

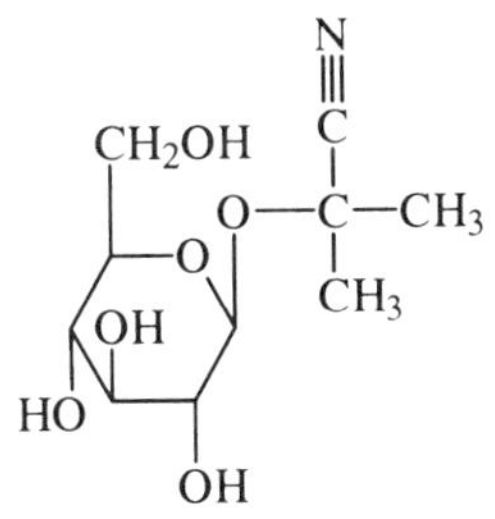

linamarin

Bitter almonds contain enough amygdalin to produce 250 mg HCN per 100 g seeds. Cassava root, a staple starch crop in Africa, also contains significant amounts of cyanogenic glycosides and is traditionally processed by chopping the root under running water to wash away the cyanogens (7). Perhaps, defense against cyanide toxicity has evolved under the evolutionary pressure of exposure to such natural product toxins.

S-Adenosylmethionine

S-Adenosylmethionine (SAM or Ado-Met) is a donor of methyl groups in intermediary metabolism. SAM (8) is produced by enzyme-catalyzed nucleophilic attack of the sulfur atom of methionine on the 5′ carbon of ATP. In this unusual reaction, the three phosphate groups of ATP are released, as P_i and PP_i; the latter is subsequently hydrolyzed to $2P_i$. Thus, the complete hydrolysis of ATP to adenosine + $3P_i$ is used to drive the formation of SAM.

The sulfur atom in SAM is a positively charged *sulfonium ion*. The configuration at the sulfur atom is approximately tetrahedral, and only a single enantiomer is formed. The positive charge on the SAM sulfonium ion gives the methyl group carbocation character; a nucleophile will displace adenosylhomocysteine (the leaving group) in an S_N2 reaction:

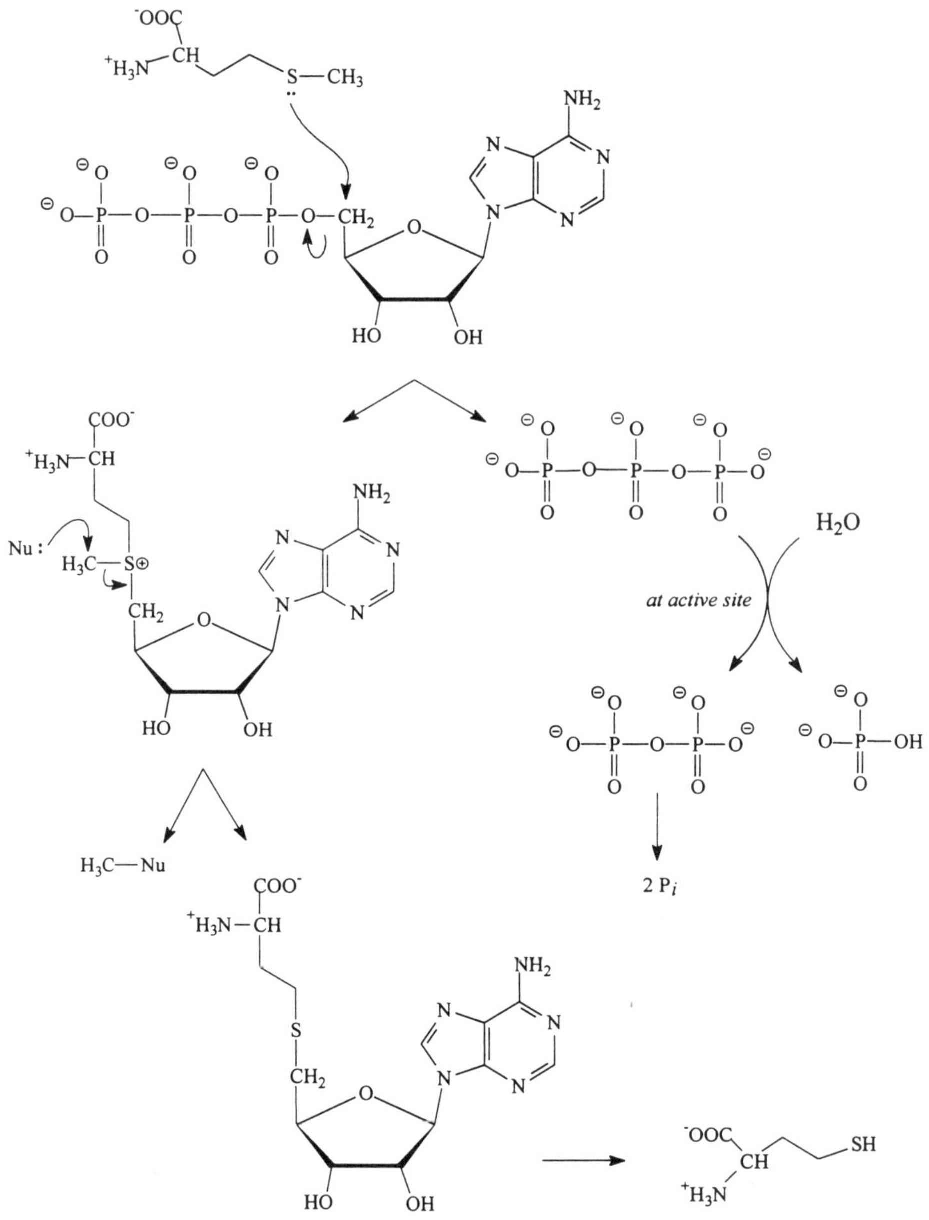

SAM is the prototypical *alkylating agent*. As we will see later (p. 282) uncontrolled alkylation can wreak havoc in the cell, particularly by covalent modification of nucleophilic sites in DNA. The detectable level of biological methylation damage observed in the absence of xenobiotic alkylating agents may result, in part, from nonenzymatic chemistry of SAM.

SAM serves as a substrate for enzyme-catalyzed methylation reactions in drug metabolism and biosynthesis, including the formation of 5-methylcytosine residues in DNA. The enzymology of drug methylation will not be discussed further in this text; interested readers are referred to a recent review (9).

Acetyl CoA

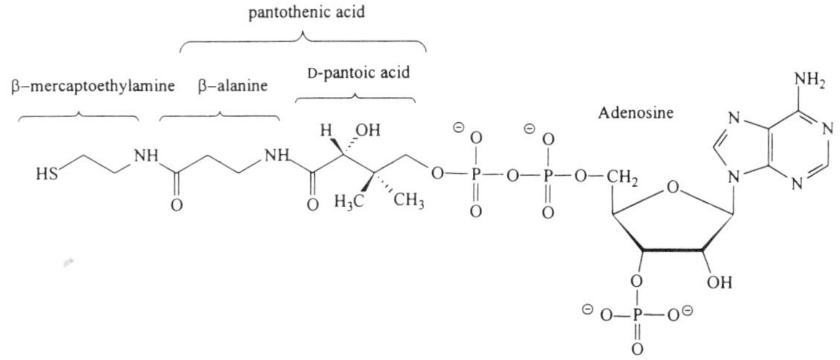

Coenzyme A (CoASII) is the ubiquitous metabolic carrier of two-carbon acetyl units. Acetyl CoA (CoASAc) molecules are generated by glycolysis or fatty acid β-oxidation and are the "feedstock" for energy generation in the citric acid cycle. The hydrolysis of the "high-energy" thioester linkage drives the condensation reactions of citrate synthase (feeding the citric acid cycle) and fatty acid synthesis, as well as the acetylation of nucleophilic heteroatoms in xenobiotics. To carry out an acetylation, an organic chemist would choose an acyl chloride or acid anhydride, using halide ion or carboxylate anion as the leaving group in a solvent such as pyridine. Why has nature chosen coenzyme A, a thioester, rather than an analogous oxygen ester? Oxygen esters hydrolyze spontaneously in aqueous solution; thioesters are much more stable. As with the choice of phosphoanhydrides (ATP) as the cell's energy currency, the elegance lies in the selection of reagents which are reactive enough for facile biotransformation but stable enough that reaction requires enzymatic catalysis. Also, thiolate anion (RS^-) is a much better leaving group than alkoxide anion (RO^-) (10), so the carbonyl carbon atom of a thioester is activated toward reactions with nucleophiles. This reactivity is the key to the mechanism of the N-acetyltransferase reaction (Chapter 12).

NOTES

1. See, for example, Nebert, D. W., Drug-metabolizing enzymes in ligand-modulated transcription, *Biochem. Pharmacol.*, 47:25–37, 1994.
2. Patterson, S. D., From electrophoretically separated protein to identification: Strategies for sequence and mass analysis, *Anal. Biochem.* 221:1–15, 1994.
3. Jakoby, W. B., Ed., *Enzymatic Basis of Detoxication*, Vol. II, Academic Press, New York, 1980.
4. Metzler, D. E., *Biochemistry: The Chemical Reactions of Living Cells*, Academic Press, New York, 1977, pp. 636–637.
5. Sugahara, K., and Schwartz, N. B., Defect in 3'-phosphoadenosine-5'-phosphosulfate synthesis in brachymorphic mice. I. Characterization of the defect, *Arch. Biochem. Biophys.* 214:589–601, 1982.
6. Garrett, R. M., Bellissimo, D. B., and Rajagopalan, K. V., Molecular cloning of human liver sulfite oxidase, *Biochim. Biophys. Acta* 1262:147–149, 1995.
7. Shibamoto, T., and Bjeldanes, L. F., *Introduction to Food Toxicology*, Academic Press, New York, 1993, pp. 71–72.
8. Stryer, L., *Biochemistry*, 4th ed., W. H. Freeman, New York, 1995, pp. 721–723.
9. Weinshilboum, R. M., Methylation pharmacogenetics: Thiopurine methyltransferase as a model system, *Xenobiotica* 22:1055–1071, 1992.
10. Rawn, J. D., *Biochemistry*, Harper & Row, New York, 1983, pp. 397ff.

10

GLUCURONIDE FORMATION

Glucuronic acid conjugation is one of the most important pathways for biotransformation of many foreign substances, ranging from alkaloids (e.g., morphine—see below) to pollutants [e.g., hydroxylated metabolites of polycyclic aromatic hydrocarbons (1)] to chemotherapeutic drugs [e.g., azidothymidine (2)]. In addition, several endogenous lipophilic compounds—especially, bilirubin and various steroid hormones—are metabolized by UDP-glucuronosyltransferase-catalyzed glucuronidation. Glucuronidation is a specific example of glycosidation—sugar conjugation. We refer to the nonsugar substrate as an *aglycone* (Greek, "without sugar"); the product is a *glycoside*.

Glucuronidation proceeds by the enzyme-catalyzed attack of a nucleophile (typically, hydroxyl or amino functions) on the C-1-oxygen bond of UDP-glucuronate:

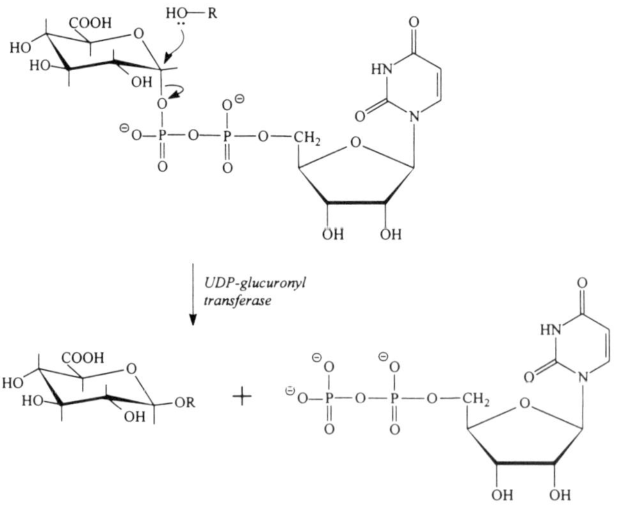

UDP is the leaving group in this S_N2-type displacement reaction; the reaction proceeds with inversion of optical configuration at the asymmetric carbon atom. Thus, UDPGA has α configuration, but the product glycoside is β (3). Some typical glucuronides are shown:

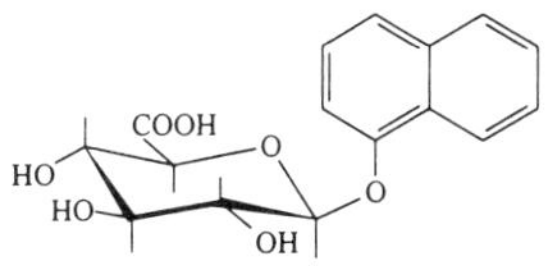

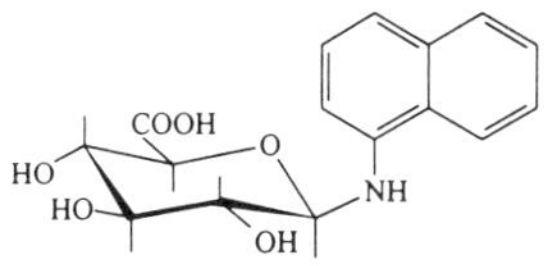

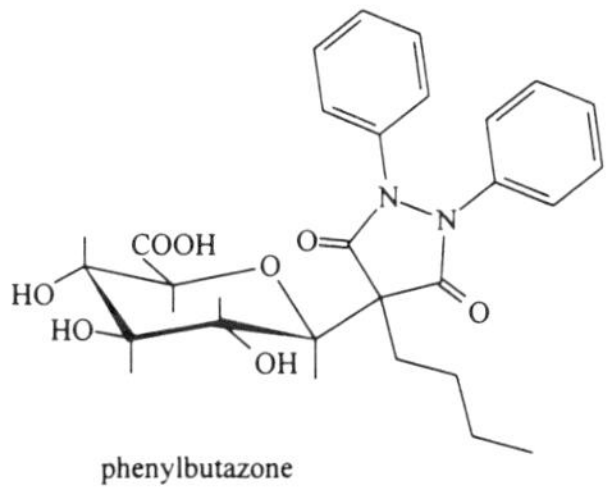

phenylbutazone

The most common glucuronides are formed at the nucleophilic oxygens of hydroxyl or carboxylic acid groups (yielding ether or ester glucuronides, respectively), amino nitrogen, or sulfur. A unique example of a C-glucuronide has been observed with the drug phenylbutazone. In this case the central carbon atom of the β-diketone unit of the heterocyclic ring is nucleophilic, since the carbanion is stabilized by resonance.*

Another unusual glucuronidation reaction is the formation of O-glucuronide conjugates of arylhydroxylamines and arylhydroxamic acids, the N-oxidized forms of aromatic amines and amides, respectively. In contrast to the usual pattern of glucuronidation leading to detoxification, *these metabolites are reactive electrophiles*, believed to play a role in the bioactivation of the carcinogenic aromatic amines and amides.

HEME CATABOLISM

Before examining the glucuronidation of xenobiotics, we will discuss the degradation of heme, an important example of the role of glucuronidation in the metabolism of endogenous metabolites. As described in an earlier chapter, human red blood cells have a lifetime of a few months. Red blood cells are turned over at a rate of several million cells per second. The catabolism of the hemoglobin of the red cells removed from circulation generates several hundred milligrams of heme per day. Free heme is toxic (perhaps because it is a good catalyst of oxygen radical production) and must be catabolized. Heme oxygenase is a microsomal enzyme found in the macrophage, hepatocyte, and spleen cell. All these cells are involved in the breakdown of aged or damaged red cells (see Chapter 8). The enzyme binds heme with 1:1 stoichiometry (4), and it catalyzes the remarkable process illustrated below:

*See, Richter, W. J., et al., *Helv. Chim. Acta* 58:2512–2517, 1975; the nucleophilicity of β-dicarbonyls is exploited in synthetic reactions such as the malonic ester synthesis.

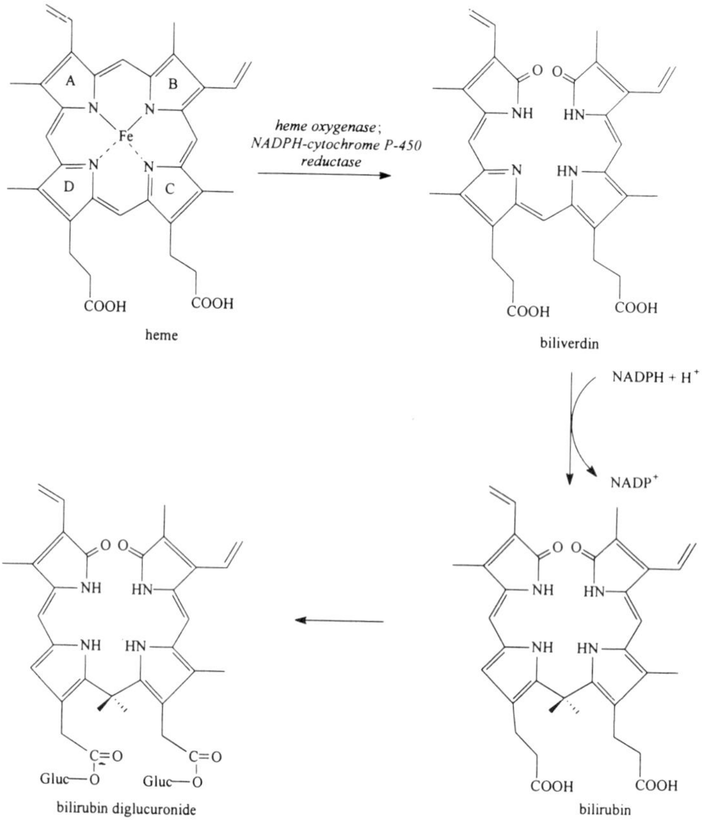
A
B
C
D
Fe
N
COOH
COOH
heme
heme oxygenase;
NADPH-cytochrome P-450
reductase
O
NH
HN
biliverdin
NADPH + H+
NADP+
bilirubin
C=O
Gluc—O
bilirubin diglucuronide

Although the mechanism is far from fully understood, a tentative scheme is presented below:

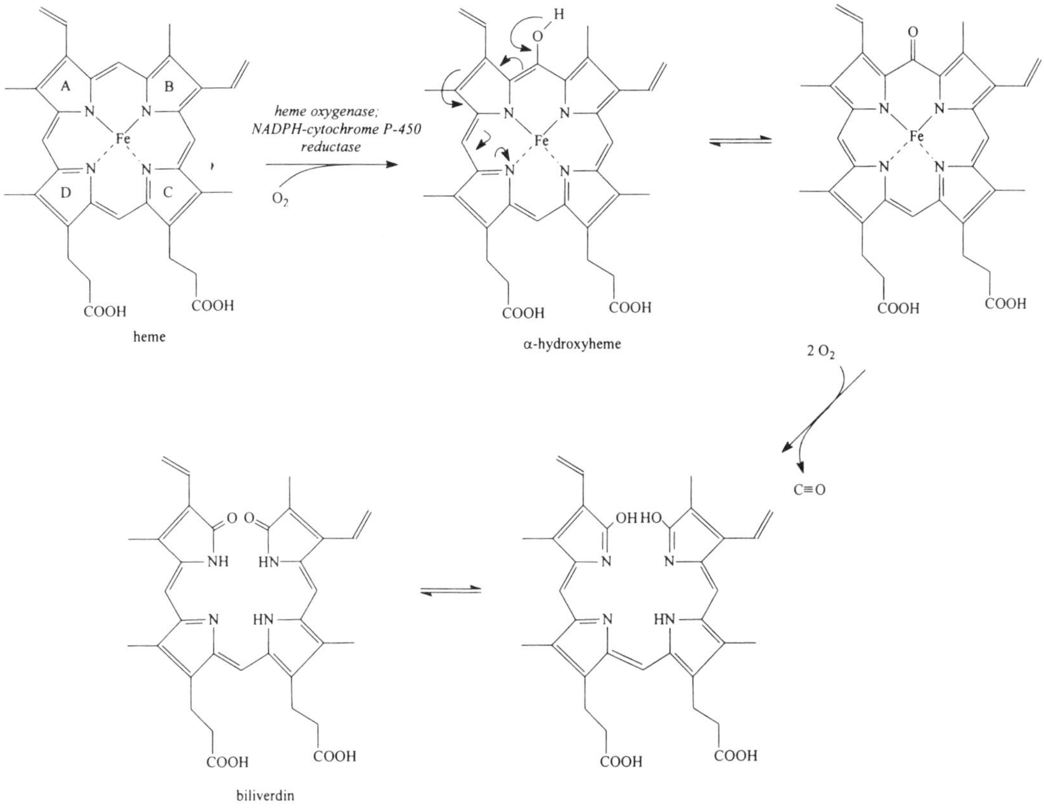

heme

heme oxygenase;
NADPH-cytochrome P-450
reductase

O_2

α-hydroxyheme

$2 O_2$

$C \equiv O$

biliverdin

Molecular oxygen is required and is incorporated into the substrate: The CO and carbonyl oxygen atoms are all O_2-derived, as deduced by experiments with ^{18}O-labeling. In the first stage, the heme ring is regiospecifically hydroxylated to give α-hydroxyheme (5), which is in tautomeric equilibrium with the keto form, as illustrated. This reaction requires molecular oxygen and two reducing equivalents, supplied by NADPH-cytochrome P-450 reductase. Thus, heme oxygenase resembles cytochrome P-450, another microsomal hydroxylase (discussed in Chapter 14). Two isozymes of human heme oxygenase have been cloned. One form is constitutive, and the other is induced by environmental stresses, including heat shock and heavy metal exposure (6).

Hydroxylation disrupts the conjugation of the porphyrin π-system, and it renders the A and B rings more "pyrrole-like" and susceptible to further oxidation. In the subsequent, poorly understood steps, two additional moles of molecular oxygen are consumed, and *the bridging methene carbon of the porphyrin ring is released as carbon monoxide.* This extraordinary reaction is the only metabolic source of carbon monoxide in the body. Indeed, a person's rate of heme catabolism can be determined from the measurement of CO in the exhaled breath.

The product of the heme oxygenase-catalyzed reaction is the conjugated, blue-green compound *biliverdin*. (Biliverdin is the blue pigment of a robin's egg.) In humans, biliverdin is reduced at the γ-carbon, to give *bilirubin*. This reduction breaks the conjugated π-system into two halves and therefore shifts the absorbance band to shorter wavelengths: Bilirubin is red-orange colored. The catabolic progression from heme to biliverdin to bilirubin can be seen in the changing appearance of a healing bruise.*

Surprisingly, in view of its many hydrogen-bond forming functionalities, bilirubin is very lipophilic and is insoluble in water or methanol (7). This phenomenon is due to the formation of strong *intramolecular* hydrogen bonds, as shown below:

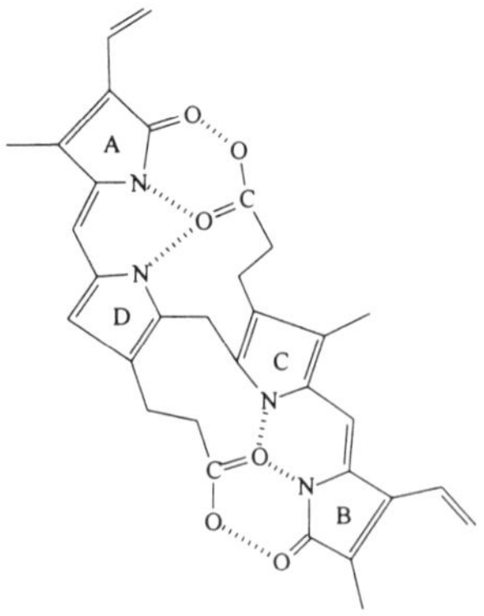

Lightner and McDonagh have pointed out that, of the four isomers which would result from heme cleavage at the α, β, γ, or δ methene bridges, natural bilirubin is the only insoluble compound. Bilirubin is toxic at high levels, and it cannot be excreted without further conjugative metabolism (see below); birds and reptiles excrete biliverdin directly, without reduction to bilirubin. Why, then, do mammals synthesize bilirubin, which accumulates to levels of 10 μM or higher in the plasma? Bilirubin, like many other lipophilic substances, does not circulate as a free species in the plasma, but is bound with high affinity by plasma proteins, especially serum albumin. Polyunsaturated fatty acids, which are particularly prone to autoxidation (see Chapter 7), are also carried on albumin, and bilirubin acts as an antioxidant, inhibiting this deterioration (8, 9).

In some situations, accumulation of bilirubin to plasma levels over about 200 μM exhausts the binding capacity of serum albumin and leads to bilirubin toxicity. The mechanisms of this toxicity are still only poorly understood, but bilirubin crosses the *blood–brain barrier* and enters the central nervous system; brain damage (encephalopathy) is the major symptom.

The plasma concentration of bilirubin is limited by glucuronic acid conjugation, catalyzed by *bilirubin-UDP-glucuronosyltransferase*. Both monoglucuronides (C and D ring propionates) are formed, as well as a diglucuronide:

---

* Mistress Quickly: . . . one of them . . . is beaten black and blue . . .
   Falstaff: What tell'st thou me of black and blue?
   I was beaten myself into all of the colours of the rainbow . . .
                                   The Merry Wives of Windsor, IV:5

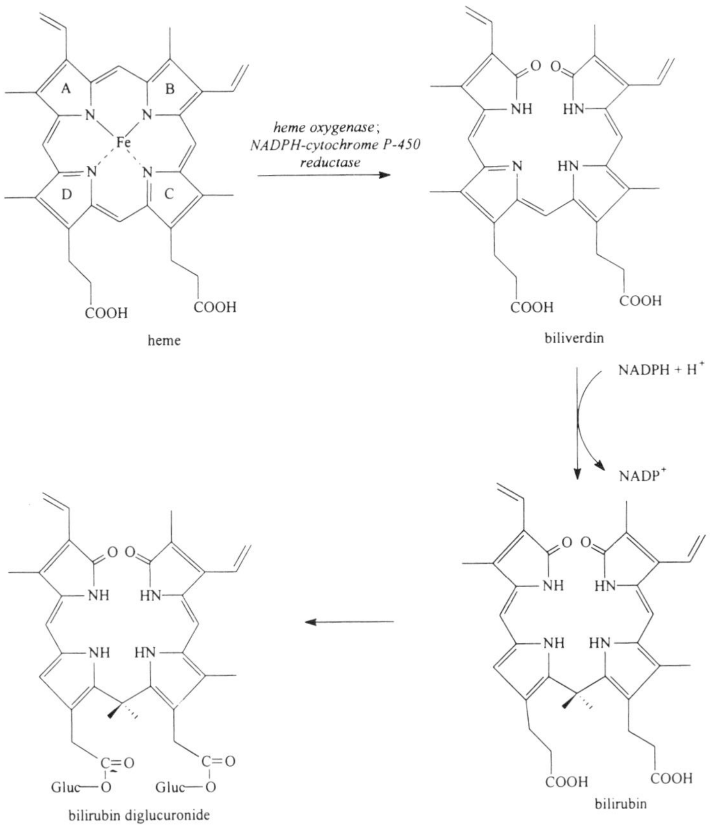

A single enzyme carries out both glucuronidation steps (10). All of these conjugates are water-soluble and readily excreted.

JAUNDICE

Excessive accumulation of bilirubin leads to the condition known as *jaundice*. The name is etymologically related to the French *jaune* (yellow), and it attests to the characteristic buildup of yellow bilirubin, particularly noticeable in the whites of the eyes. Jaundice may result from liver damage, which impairs glucuronidation. Another well-known syndrome is *neonatal jaundice*. The fetus can pass bilirubin transplacentally, relying on the maternal liver and kidneys for glucuronidation. Newborn infants are suddenly deprived of this resource. Bilirubin-UDP-glucuronosyltransferase activity is low in newborns. Enzyme activity usually reaches adequate levels within a few weeks of birth, but in some infants (especially premature deliveries) the jaundice becomes severe. A simple and effective treatment is *phototherapy* (7). An English nurse first observed that the yellowish skin of jaundiced newborns became bleached upon exposure to sunlight. Indeed, bilirubin is photochemically converted to more soluble and readily excreted products. Phototherapy of jaundiced newborns by exposure to fluorescent light is now routine in maternity wards.

The low UDPGT activity in newborns also has implications for drug therapy. The antibacterial drug chloramphenicol is sometimes administered to newborns, for treatment of ampicillin-resistant *Haemophilus influenzae* and other infections. Initially, a repeat dosage regimen based on experience with older children was used. Glucuronidation is the major metabolic pathway for chloramphenicol elimination. Because newborns have little chloramphenicol glucuronidation activity, repeated doses of the drug were not cleared from the body, and the drug built up to toxic (in some cases, fatal) levels. It is now recommended that serum levels should be monitored when low-birth-weight infants are treated with chloramphenicol (11). (How should the drug dosage schedule be modified in this situation? The *first* dose must *not* be changed, since plasma levels adequate for therapeutic effect must be achieved. Subsequent doses should be reduced or delayed, to accommodate the reduced rate of metabolic clearance.)

Biliary excretion of bilirubin is an important route of elimination; the compound's name reflects its presence in bile. In the intestinal tract, bacterial metabolism (β-glucuronidase) releases the glucuronic acid moieties. Presumably, the bacteria are chiefly concerned with liberating sugars, which they can use as foodstuff. But, at the same time, bilirubin is re-formed. In the reducing environment of the intestine, further bacterial metabolism converts bilirubin into stercobilin, a fecal pigment, and urobilinogen:

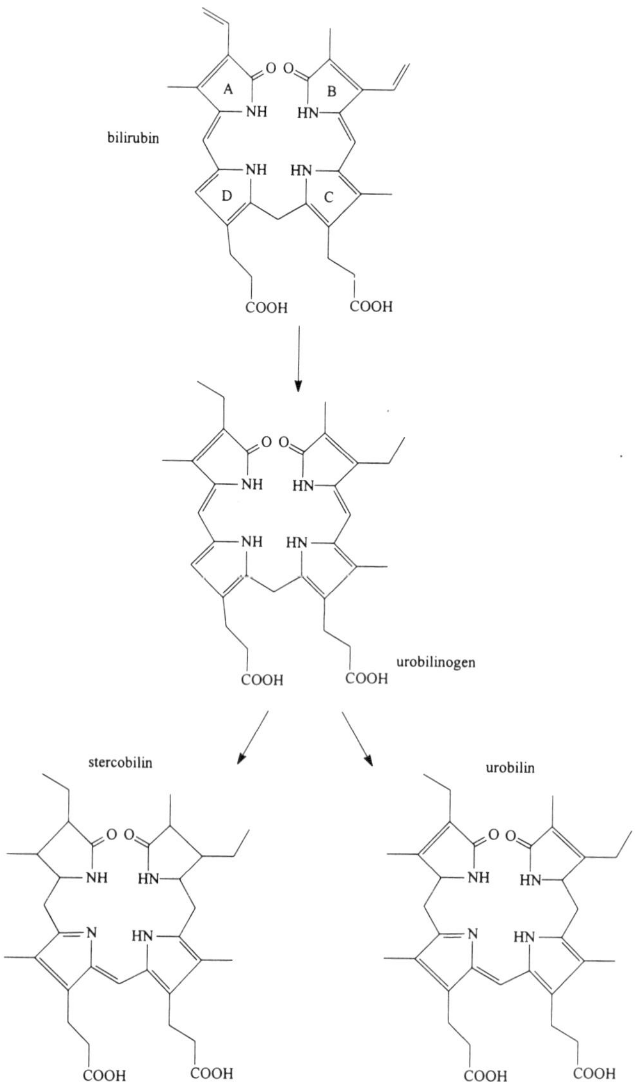

Urobilinogen, in particular, is readily readsorbed through the intestinal wall, and it returns to the blood. This process of conjugation, intestinal hydrolysis, and reabsorption, is referred to as *enterohepatic circulation*. This phenomenon occurs with many drugs, and it prolongs their lifetime in the circulation. Urobilinogen is reoxidized to urobilin in the kidney; urobilin is the major component giving urine its characteristic yellow color. What a diverse family of colored products arises from the heme of our red blood cells!

DRUG GLUCURONIDATION: MORPHINE

Morphine is the major narcotic alkaloid of the opium poppy. Glucuronidation is an important biotransformation route for this natural product opiate. Morphine has two hydroxyl groups; one is phenolic and the other is secondary aliphatic:

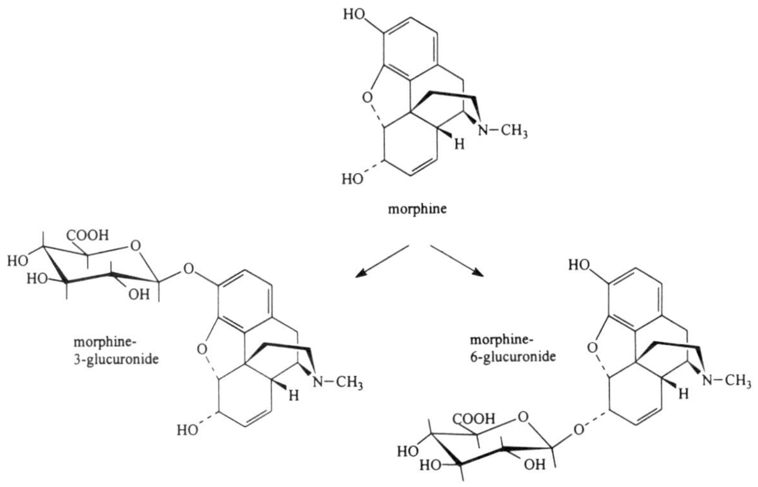

Morphine is rapidly metabolized by glucuronidation at either the 3- or the 6-position (see scheme); the 3-glucuronide is the major metabolite (12). (Synthetic acetylation of both groups, which blocks this route of elimination, yields diacetylmorphine, better known as *heroin*.) Opiates are therapeutically valuable for the treatment of severe pain, and of course they are major drugs of abuse. The complex pharmacological actions of opiates are mediated through several classes of cellular opioid receptor proteins in neural and other tissues. The opiates are *agonists* which bind to these receptors; the endogenous agonists are apparently the peptides known as *enkephalins* (13).

UDP-GLUCURONOSYLTRANSFERASES

Now let us turn our attention to the enzymes which catalyze glucuronic acid conjugations, UDP-glucuronosyltransferases (14–16). The enzyme activity can be measured by (a) incubating the enzyme preparation with an appropriate substrate and UDP-glucuronic acid and (b) monitoring either the formation of the glycoside product or the disappearance of the aglycone substrate. In some cases the aglycone and glycoside can be separated by organic extraction of the aglycone; either the substrate or product is quantitated by absorbance or fluorescence. In other cases the glycoside and aglycone are separated by thin-layer chromatography or other techniques, before quantitation. The chromatographic approach provides for confirmation of the identity of the glycoside; in rare cases, multiple glycosidations occur with a single substrate, and the products can be separated chromatographically. UDP-glucuronic acid, radiolabeled in the sugar moiety, is available, and this allows detection and quantitation of the glycosides by scintillation counting.

The lability and difficulty of purification of UDP-glucuronosyltransferases hampered their characterization, but the application of improved biochemical techniques for enzyme purification, along with improved molecular biological methods, has allowed great progress to be made in the last few years (17, 18). Emulgen 911 has been the detergent of choice for solubilization without loss of activity. Affinity chromatography on UDP-hexanolamine Sepharose 4B is effective for purification. UDP is the product of the reaction catalyzed by the enzyme; presumably, UDP binds to the conserved UDPGA binding site (see below).

All known UDP-glucuronosyltransferases are integral membrane proteins (M_r = 50–60 kD) of the endoplasmic reticulum. Integral membrane proteins are anchored in the membrane by at least one embedded α-helical segment. These α-helices are, of course, composed largely of hydrophobic residues. Some proteins have multiple membrane-spanning helices. Some proteins with a single membrane-spanning helix are oriented with their N-terminus inside the lumen of the endoplasmic reticulum and C-terminus on the cytoplasmic side (Type I); other proteins have the opposite orientation (Type II) (19, 20). *Protein topology is determined by primary sequence motifs, which interact with the enzymatic machinery responsible for delivery of the protein to the endoplasmic reticulum (ER) and translocation into the membrane in the appropriate orientation.* These sequences are not identical among different proteins, but they share certain homologies, or common features, especially with regard to the charge and polarity of the amino acid residues in the sequences.

Proteins destined for the ER (or other membranous organelles) usually bear an N-terminal *signal sequence*. Typically, several polar residues occur near the N-terminus, followed by a dozen or more hydrophobic residues. Since proteins are synthesized from the N-terminal end, the hydrophobic signal sequence extends from the ribosome early in the process of translation. The signal sequence is recognized by a *signal recognition particle* (SRP) riboprotein complex, which binds to an SRP receptor in the ER membrane. The receptor helps lead the nascent polypeptide chain into the membrane. Polypeptide translation is completed, and in many cases the membrane-embedded signal sequence is then cleaved by proteolysis [catalyzed by *signal peptidase* (21)]. The new N-terminus of the mature protein is exposed in the lumen. [More extensive discussions of this process are presented in other texts (22).] Therefore, such cleaved proteins are always of Type I, as defined above. All known UDP-glucuronosyl transferases fall into this class.

The sequence of one isozyme of human bilirubin-UDP-glucuronosyltransferase, deduced from the cDNA, is shown below (23). Cleaved signal sequences do not adhere to a simple consensus sequence, but some of the characteristic features are seen in the HUG-Br1 sequence: a basic residue near the amino terminal (arg-9); a highly hydrophobic core of 10–15 residues (pro-10 to leu-20); and a cleavage site for signal peptidase, with small neutral residues, particularly alanine, at positions 1 and 3 with respect to the cleavage site, located about five residues past the hydrophobic core (ser-his-ala 25–27).

What stops the growing protein chain from passing completely into the lumen of the ER? Another sequence motif, known as the *stop-transfer signal* or *anchor sequence*, calls the halt by remaining embedded in the membrane. The common theme appears to be a hydrophobic (α-helix-forming) stretch, with polar, charged residues on either end and greater positive charge on the C-terminal end. In the HUG-Br1 protein sequence, note the hydrophobicity of the core of the stop-transfer signal (val-ile-gly-phe-leu-leu-ala-val-val-leu-thr-val-ala-phe-ile-thr-phe; 491–507) and the very high density of positive charge (lys and arg residues) near the C-terminal.

```
start
MAVESQGGRP LVLGLLLCVL GPVVSHAGKI LLIPVDGSHW LSMLGAIQQL        50
           memb. ins. signal

QQRGHEIVVL APDASLYIRD GAFYTLKTYP VPFQREDVKE SFVSLGHNVF       100


ENDSFLQRVI KTYKKIKKDS AMLLSGCSHL LHNKELMASL AESSFDVMLT       150


DPFLPCSPIV AQYLSLPTVF FLHALPCSLE FEATQCPNPF SYVPRPLSSH       200


SDHMTFLQRV KNMLIAFSQN FLCDVVYSPY ATLASEFLQR EVTVQDLLSS       250


ASVWLFRSDF VKDYPRPIMP NMVFVGGINC LHQNPLSQEF EAYINASGEH       300
                                 →seq. = HUG-Br2

GIVVFSLGSM VSEIPEKKAM AIADALGKIP QTVLWRYTGT RPSNLANNTI       350


LVKWLPQNDL LGHPMTRAFI THAGSHGVYE SICNGVPMVM MPLFGDQMDN       400
                      putative UDPGA binding site

AKRMETKGAG VTLNVLEMTS EDLENALKAV INDKSYKENI MRLSSLHKDR       450

                                 probe region
PVEPLDLAVF WVEFVMRHKG APHLRPAAHD LTWYQYHSLD VIGFLLAVVL       500
                                            stop-transfer

TVAFITFKCC AYGYRKCLGK KGRVKKAHKS KTH                         533
signal                highly basic region
```

HUG-Br1 (UGT1A) protein sequence, derived from sequence of the cDNA. The cDNA was cloned on the basis of hybridization to a 51-base-pair probe corresponding to the sequence HDLTWFQYHSLDVIGFL, which is highly conserved among UDP-glucuronosyltransferase sequences. This probe sequence is found at residues 478–495, and it has tyrosine rather than phenylalanine at the sixth position. Potential N-linked glycosylation sites (NXS or NXT) are indicated. From residue 285 on, the sequence is identical to that of another isozyme, HUG-Br2 (UGT1D). The significance of this identity is discussed later. See text for explanation of other sequence features.

Although no high-resolution crystal structure data is available for UDP-glucuronosyl-transferase enzymes, a simple model can be drawn, based on sequence analysis and physicochemical studies (see next page):

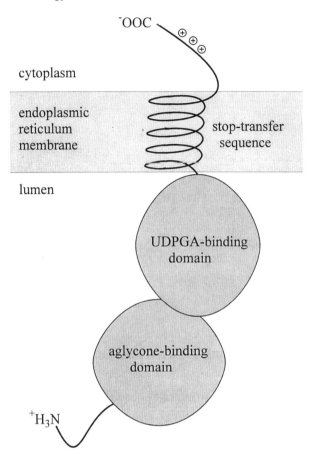

Model of the structure of a typical UDP-glucuronosyltransferase enzyme protein. [Based on Tephly and Burchell (14).]

The protein is, of course, embedded in the ER membrane by the hydrophobic portion of the stop-transfer sequence near the C-terminus. Two domains form the large lumenal portion of the protein. A hydrophilic region of highly conserved residues occurs in the vicinity of residues 365–420 of known UDP-glucuronosyltransferase sequences (24); this region shows homologies with proteins such as β-galactosidase, pyruvate kinase, xylose transport protein, and pyrophosphatase, proteins which bind nucleotides, sugars, or phosphates. This C-terminal domain probably contains the UDPGA-binding site.

SIDEBAR: COMPARTMENTALIZATION OF GLUCURONIDATION

Glucuronidation occurs in the lumen of the endoplasmic reticulum. However, UDPGA is formed in the cytosol, and aglycone substrates (xenobiotics or endogenous substrates, such as bilirubin) reach the ER through the cytosol. This topology implies the existence of multiple transporters. Presumably, the ER membrane must incorporate transporters (channels or carriers) for aglycones (possibly several different transporters corresponding to different classes) and UDPGA. Furthermore, the products of the glucuronidation reaction must be exported to the cytosol and, in the case of glucuronides, to the bile or bloodstream for excretion. Thus, additional transporters are needed for UMP and phosphate (the products of UDP hydrolysis) and for the polar glucuronides. Very little is yet known about these carriers.

The less-conserved N-terminal domain B contains the aglycone binding site. This hypothesis was first verified by construction of chimeric proteins (24). The cDNAS for two different forms of rat liver UDP-glucuronosyltransferase were studied: One form (Tr-4) glucuronidates the 17-β-hydroxyl group of the steroid hormone testosterone as a preferred substrate, and the other (Tr-3) glucuronidates the 3-α-hydroxyl group of etiocholanolone, a pyrogenic steroid metabolite:

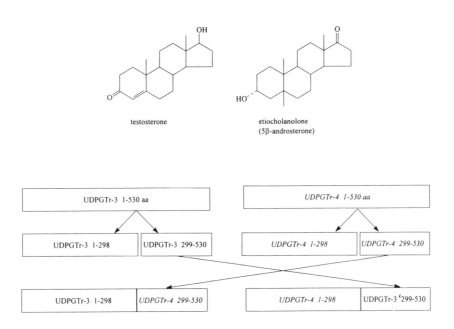

The cDNAs for these proteins, carried on expression plasmids, were cut at a *Sac*I restriction site common to both genes. The appropriate fragments were purified on agarose gels, recovered, and ligated together in order to make chimeric genes and, hence, proteins.

The chimeric constructs were transfected into COS cells, which produced the desired chimeric proteins. The enzymatic activities of the proteins were measured by incubating aliquots of homogenate preparation from the transfected COS cells with steroid substrate and radiolabeled UDPGA; the product ^{14}C-glucuronides were separated by thin-layer chromatography and detected by autoradiography. Both chimeric proteins were enzymatically active, and they displayed *the substrate specificities of the parent protein contributing the N-terminal section* (roughly, domain B). This result supports the hypothesis that the N-terminal domain determines substrate specificity.

FAMILIES OF UDP-GLUCURONOSYLTRANSFERASE ENZYMES

Preliminary classifications of the known UDP-glucuronosyltransferase forms, as well as schemes for systematic, sequence-based nomenclature, have recently been published (15). The *UGT1* family comprises genes for isozymes inducible by the chlorinated compound TCDD (enzyme induction is discussed in more detail in Chapter 14). The *UGT2* family isozymes are constitutive or, in one case, inducible by phenobarbital. Proteins from the two distinct families are less than 50% homologous at the amino acid sequence level; within each family, protein sequences are about 60% homologous or more. The study of the correlation of substrate specificities with gene sequences is at a very early stage. The *UGT1* family (see below for further discussion) includes enzymes which glucuronidate 4-nitrophenol, halogenated phenols, bilirubin, and so on. The *UGT2* family includes the rat hepatic forms Tr-2, Tr-3, and Tr-4, which *O*-glucuronidate hydroxysteroids and *N*-glucuronidate the carcinogen β-naphthylamine. One particularly interesting subfamily of *UGT2* includes proteins specifically expressed in the olfactory epithelium; these enzymes may play a major role in termination of odorant signals, by glucuronidating (and hence inactivating) hydroxyl-containing odorant molecules, such as eugenol (the scent of cloves), borneol, and 4-hydroxybiphenyl (25). This action prevents the odorant from continuing to stimulate the receptor cells and may also protect the brain from exposure to airborne toxicants.

GENETIC UDP-GLUCURONOSYLTRANSFERASE DEFICIENCY CONDITIONS

Since UDP-glucuronosyltransferase enzymes are responsible for bilirubin conjugation, inborn errors of metabolism affecting these enzymes might be manifested as hereditary jaundice. Indeed, such conditions are known. In the most severe case, known as *Crigler–Najjar syndrome*, bilirubin-UDP-glucuronosyltransferase activity is greatly reduced or undetectable. On the other hand, *para*-nitrophenol glucuronidation is normal. Clearly, not every UDPGT isozyme is affected. Ida Owens (of the National Institute of Child Health and Human Development, Bethesda, MD) and colleagues have recently identified one mutation responsible for Crigler–Najjar syndrome, a deletion mutation in exon 1 of the *UGT1* gene locus (see below).

A much more common, but less serious, condition is known as *Gilbert's syndrome*. This appears to be a mild deficiency in glucuronidation activity, with elevated levels of plasma bilirubin. About 5% of the North American population is believed to be affected, but the syndrome is usually asymptomatic (26). The molecular basis of Gilbert's syndrome is now being characterized; several missense mutations have been identified in the bilirubin UDPGT gene (27). In cases requiring treatment, phenobarbital administration is an option, since the drug induces glucuronidation activity.

An *animal model* of inherited UDP-glucuronosyltransferase deficiency also exists. In 1934, C. H. Gunn (of the Dominion Experimental Fox Ranch in Prince Edward Island, Canada) observed three yellowish, jaundiced pups among a litter of 13 borne by a laboratory rat of the Wistar inbred strain. The jaundice was inherited as a recessive Mendelian trait; Gunn wrote that his work gave "new evidence for the single gene theory of a syndrome," and he rightly suspected that a single enzyme was deficient. These animals are the progenitors of a strain now known as the "Gunn rat" (28).

In the 1950s the biochemical basis of this mutation was shown to be the absence of bilirubin–UDPGT activity. (UDPGA synthesis is not deficient.) The Gunn rat is also deficient in glucuronidation of phenolic compounds, an activity associated with the 3-methylcholanthrene-inducible form of UDPGT. *The bilirubin UDPGT and 3-methyl-cholan-threne-inducible UDPGTs are distinct enzyme proteins.* How can a single mutation inactivate two different forms of UDPGT? Recent molecular studies (29) have identified the rat cDNAs for these two forms of UDPGT (bilirubin UDPGT and 3-methylcholanthrene-inducible UDPGT). *The cDNAs are identical over a 913-base-pair region at their 3' ends, encoding the C-terminal portions of the two proteins, but have different 5' regions, encoding different N-terminal domains.*

When the Gunn rat strain was examined, a −1-base-pair frameshift mutation was detected in codon 414; this mutation creates a TGA ("opal") termination codon at codon 416. Therefore the C-terminal domain is truncated prematurely; 115 residues are lost. The cDNAS for both the bilirubin and 3-methylcholanthrene-inducible forms of UDPGT from the Gunn strain bear the same mutation. *Both enzyme forms are derived from a single gene, whose mRNA is subjected to alternative splicing.* The same phenomenon is also observed with the human genes for enzymes HUG-Br1 (*UGT1A*) and HUG-Br2 (*UGT1D*), as noted on the sequence of the former gene; see below). The primary mRNA transcript is a *complex transcript*, which produces at least two different mature mRNAs and, therefore, two different proteins (27), by alternative choice of splice sites.

Feline species also have a very poor capacity for glucuronidation of phenolic compounds, although they can glucuronidate bilirubin satisfactorily. (The feline enzymes and genes of glucuronidation have not yet been analyzed in detail.) Consequently, cats tend to excrete drugs as sulfate conjugates rather than as glucuronides. This peculiarity of drug biotransformation has to be considered in veterinary pharmacological practice (31).

THE UGT1 GENE CLUSTER

The UDPGT enzymes comprise an aglycone-binding domain and a UDPGT-binding domain. These domains can, in some cases, be switched between cDNAs in recombinant DNA experiments, and the analysis of cDNA sequences suggests that nature, too, has played this game. The recent cloning of the chromosomal DNA sequence and the analysis of the exon–intron structure of the genes for the human UGT1 family (32) proved the existence of such an "exon shuffling" (33) arrangement: The exons coding for the UDPGA-binding domains of these enzymes are matched with exons coding for aglycone-binding domains of the protein. In this remarkable genetic system, at least six different exon 1 "cassettes" are positioned, at almost regular intervals, over a range of 85 kb, upstream from a set of four closely spaced exons (2–5):

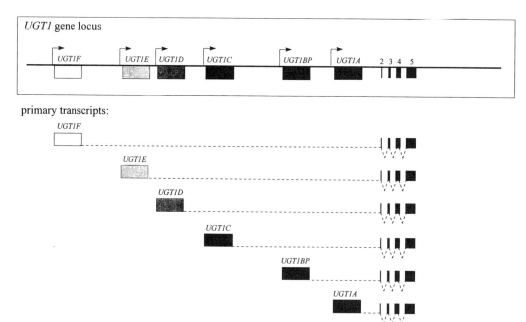

Each of the six forms of exon 1 has a transcriptional promoter sequence, translation start, and coding sequence, and each terminates with a splice donor site. The first splice acceptor site is located at the beginning of exon 2. Thus, six or more primary transcripts are possible, and each is spliced to give a message containing one of the six forms of exon 1 and exons 2–5.

What proteins are synthesized from these six messages? Hybridization to cDNA probes revealed that *UGT1A*, *UGT1D*, and *UGT1F* correspond to HUG-Br1, HUG-Br2 (bilirubin UDPGTs), and HLUGP1 (a phenol UDPGT), respectively. *UGT1C* and *UGT1E* are highly homologous to *UGT1D*, but the substrate specificities of these enzymes are not yet known. *UGT1BP* contains a −1 frameshift mutation and appears to be a pseudogene, not yielding a functional protein product (at least, in the individual genomic library studied). Presumably, one of the coding exon 1s was the progenitor of this complex genetic locus, and additional exon 1s arose by a process of gene duplication and subsequent divergent evolution. Further analysis will clarify the relationship between these exons and the human genetic defects of glucuronidation.

CHEMICAL ANALYSIS OF GLUCURONIDES AND OTHER POLAR CONJUGATES

Finally, we return to the chemical aspects of glucuronidation and consider the techniques for the analysis and identification of glucuronide metabolites. Extraction of glucuronides from biological fluids and chromatographic separation (especially by gas chromatography) are difficult, due to their high polarity and low volatility. However, enzymatic hydrolysis of the conjugates, liberating the aglycones, can often be achieved. The aglycones of the glucuronide conjugates are then analyzed. β-Glucuronidase from *E. coli* is commonly used for this purpose. The same difficulties arise in the analysis of sulfates (see Chapter 11). In this case the enzyme *arylsulfatase* (from the snail *Helix pomatia*) is often capable of releasing the parent compound. Of course, since enzyme treatment converts the conjugate to the parent compound, the conjugate must be determined as the difference between the amounts of parent compound present in the sample, before and after enzyme treatment. Some conjugates may fail to be cleaved, and the yield of aglycone will be less than 100%. These considerations limit the sensitivity of detection.

More recently, mass spectrometry methods have been developed for the analysis of glucuronide conjugates, without prior hydrolysis (34). Chemical (ammonia) ionization, fast atom bombardment, and laser desorption ionization techniques have been applied successfully. For example, fast atom bombardment ionization was used recently to establish the structure of the ether glucuronide metabolite of the antischizophrenic drug fluphenazine (35).

NOTES

1. Mackenzie, P. I., Rodbourn, L., and Iyanagi, T., Glucuronidation of carcinogen metabolites by complementary DNA-expressed uridine 5′-diphosphate glucuronosyltransferases, *Cancer Res.* 53:1529–1533, 1993.
2. Mulder, G. J., Glucuronidation and its role in regulation of biological activity of drugs, *Annu. Rev. Pharmacol. Toxicol.* 32:25–49, 1992.
3. Note that this mechanism is fundamentally different from that of the superficially analogous reactions catalyzed by glycogen phosphorylase and glycogen synthase, in which the α configuration of the anomeric hydroxyl group is retained, not inverted. The latter reactions probably proceed via oxonium ion intermediates (S_N1 mechanism).
4. Takahashi, S., Wang, J., Rousseau, D. L., Ishikawa, K., Yoshida, T., Host, J. R., and Ikeda-Saito, M., Heme–heme oxygenase complex. Structure of the catalytic site and its implication for oxygen activation, *J. Biol. Chem.* 269:1010–1014, 1994.
5. Kikuchi, G., and Yoshida, T., Function and induction of the microsomal heme oxygenase, *Mol. Cell. Biochem.* 53/4:163–183, 1983.
6. Shibahara, S., Yoshizawa, M., Suzuki, H., Takeda, K., Meguro, K., and Endo, K., Functional analysis of cDNAs for two types of human heme oxygenase and evidence for their separate regulation, *J. Biochem. (Tokyo)* 113:214–218, 1993.
7. Lightner, D. A., and McDonagh, A. F., Molecular mechanisms of phototherapy for neonatal jaundice, *Acc. Chem. Res.* 17:417–424, 1984; McDonagh, A. F., and Lightner, D. A., 'Like a shrivelled blood orange'—bilirubin, jaundice, and phototherapy, *Pediatrics* 75:443–455, 1985.
8. Stocker, R., Glazer, A. N., and Ames, B. N., Antioxidant activity of albumin-bound bilirubin, *Proc. Natl. Acad. Sci. U.S.A.* 84:5918–5922, 1987.
9. Stocker, R., Yamamoto, Y., McDonagh, A. F., Glazer, A. N., and Ames, B. N., Bilirubin is an antioxidant of possible physiological importance, *Science* 235:1043–1046, 1987.
10. Crawford, J. M., Ransil, B. J., Narciso, J. P., and Gollan, J. L., Hepatic microsomal bilirubin UDP-glucuronosyltransferase: The kinetics of bilirubin mono- and diglucuronide synthesis, *J. Biol. Chem.* 267:16943–16950, 1992.
11. Glazer, J. P., Danish, M. A., Plotkin, S. A., and Yaffe, S. J., Disposition of chloramphenicol in low birth weight infants, *Pediatrics* 66:573–578, 1980.
12. Mulder, G. J., Pharmacological effects of drug conjugates: Is morphine 6–glucuronide an exception?, *Trends Pharmacol. Sci.* 13:302–304, 1992.
13. Devlin, T. M., Ed., *Textbook of Biochemistry with Clinical Correlations*, 3rd ed., Wiley-Liss, New York, 1992, p. 861.
14. Tephly, T. R., and Burchell, B., UDP-glucuronosyltransferases: A family of detoxifying enzymes, *Trends Pharmacol. Sci.* 11:276–279, 1990.
15. Burchell, B., Nebert, D. W., Nelson, D. R., Bock, K. W., Iyanagi, T., Jansen, P. L. M., Lancet, D., Mulder, G. J., Roy Chowdhury, J., Siest, G., Tephly, T. R., and MacKenzie, P. I., The UDP-glucuronosyltransferase gene superfamily: Suggested nomenclature based on evolutionary divergence, *DNA Cell Biol.* 10:487–494, 1991; Tukey, R. H., and Johnson, E. F., Molecular as-

pects of regulation and structure of the drug-metabolizing enzymes, In: *Principles of Drug Action: The Basis of Pharmacology*, 3rd ed, W. B. Pratt and P. Taylor, Eds., Churchill Livingstone, New York, 1990, pp. 423–467.

16. Burchell, B., Coughtrie, M. W., and Jansen, P. L., Function and regulation of UDP-glucuronosyltransferase genes in health and liver disease: report of the Seventh International Workshop on Glucuronidation, September 1993, Pitlochry, Scotland, *Hepatology* 20:1622–1630, 1994.

17. Reviewed in: Tephly, T. R., Isolation and purification of UDP-glucuronosyltransferases, *Chem. Res. Toxicol.* 3:509–516, 1990.

18. Mackenzie, P. I., Rat liver UDP-glucuronosyltransferase: Sequence and expression of a cDNA encoding a phenobarbital-inducible form, *J. Biol. Chem.* 261:6119–6125, 1986; Mackenzie, P. I., Rat liver UDP-glucuronosyltransferase: Identification of cDNAs encoding two enzymes which glucuronidate testosterone, dihydrotestosterone, and β-estradiol, *J. Biol. Chem.* 262:9744–9749, 1987.

19. Stryer, L., *Biochemistry*, 4th ed., W. H. Freeman, New York, 1995, Fig. 35-9, pp. 912–918.

20. Schatz, G., and Dobberstein, B., Common principles of protein translocation across membranes, *Science* 271:1519–1526, 1996.

21. Dalbey, R. E., and von Heijne, G., Signal peptidases in prokaryotes and eukaryotes—a new protease family, *Trends Biochem. Sci.* 17:474–478, 1992.

22. Lewin, B., *Genes V*, Oxford University Press, Oxford, 1994, pp. 282ff; Voet, D., and Voet, J.G., *Biochemistry*, 2nd ed., Wiley, New York, 1995, pp. 306–312.

23. Ritter, J. K., Crawford, J., and Owens, I. S., Cloning of two human liver bilirubin UDP-glucuronosyltransferase cDNAs with expression in COS-1 cells, *J. Biol. Chem.* 266:1043–1047, 1991.

24. MacKenzie, P. I., Expression of chimeric cDNAs in cell culture defines a region of UDP-glucuronosyltransferase involved in substrate selection, *J. Biol. Chem.* 265:3432–3435, 1990.

25. Lazard, D., Zupko, K., Poria, Y., Nef, P., Lazarovits, J., Horn, S., Khen, M., and Lancet, D., Odorant signal termination by olfactory UDP glucuronosyl transferase, *Nature* 349:790–793, 1991.

26. de Morais, S. M. F., Uetrecht, J. P., and Wells, P. G., Decreased glucuronidation and increased bioactivation of acetaminophen in Gilbert's syndrome, *Gastroenterology* 102:577–586, 1992.

27. Aono, S., Adachi, Y., Uyama, E., Yamada, Y., Keino, H., Nanno, T., Koiwai, O., and Sato, H., Analysis of genes for bilirubin UDP-glucuronosyltransferase in Gilbert's syndrome, *Lancet* 345:958–959, 1995.

28. Gunn, C. K., Hereditary acholuric jaundice in the rat, *Can. Med. Assoc. J.* 50:230–237, 1944.

29. Iyanagi, T., Watanabe, T., and Uchiyama, Y., The 3–methylcholanthrene-inducible UDP-glucuronosyltransferase deficiency in the hyperbilirubinemic rat (Gunn rat) is caused by a -1 frameshift mutation, *J. Biol. Chem.* 264:21302–21307, 1989; Sato, H., Aono, S., Kashiwamata, S., and Koiwai, O., Genetic defect of bilirubin UDP-glucuronosyltransferase in the hyperbilirubinemic Gunn rat, *Biochem. Biophys. Res. Commun.* 177:1161–1164, 1991; Iyanagi, T., Molecular basis of multiple UDP-glucuronosyltransferase isoenzyme deficiencies in the hyperbilirubinemic rat (Gunn rat), *J. Biol. Chem.* 266:24048–24052, 1991; Ishii, Y., Tsuruda, K., Tanaka, M., and Oguri, K., Purification of a phenobarbital-inducible morphine UDP-glucuronyltransferase isoform, absent from Gunn rat liver, *Arch. Biochem. Biophys.* 315:345–351, 1994.

30. Lehninger, A. L., Nelson, D. L., and Cox, M. M., *Principles of Biochemistry*, 2nd ed., Worth Publishers, New York, 1993, pp. 873–874.

31. Sherding, R. G., *The Cat: Diseases and Clinical Management*, 2nd ed., Churchill Livingstone, New York, 1994.

32. Ritter, J. K., Chen, F., Sheen, Y. Y., Tran, H. M., Kimura, S., Yeatman, M. T., and Owens, I. S., A novel complex locus *UGT1* encodes human bilirubin, phenol, and other UDP-glucuronosyltransferase isozymes with identical carboxyl termini, *J. Biol. Chem.* 267:3257–3261, 1992.

33. Lewin, B., *Genes V*, Oxford University Press, 1994, pp. 688–689.

34. Fenselau, C., Analysis of glucuronides using condensed phase ionization techniques, in: *Mass Spectrometry in the Health and Life Sciences*, A. L. Burlingame and N. Castagnoli, Jr., Eds., Elsevier, Amsterdam, 1985, pp. 321–331.

35. Jackson, C.-J. C., Hubbard, J. W., and Midha, K. K., Biosynthesis and characterization of glucuronide metabolites of fluphenazine: 7-Hydroxyfluphenazine glucuronide and fluphenazine glucuronide, *Xenobiotica* 21:383–393, 1991.

11

GLUTATHIONE AND DETOXICATION

Glutathione (GSH), the tripeptide γ-L-glutamyl-L-cysteinylglycine, plays a central role in the biotransformation and elimination of xenobiotics and in the defense of the cell against oxidative stress (see Chapter 4). GSH

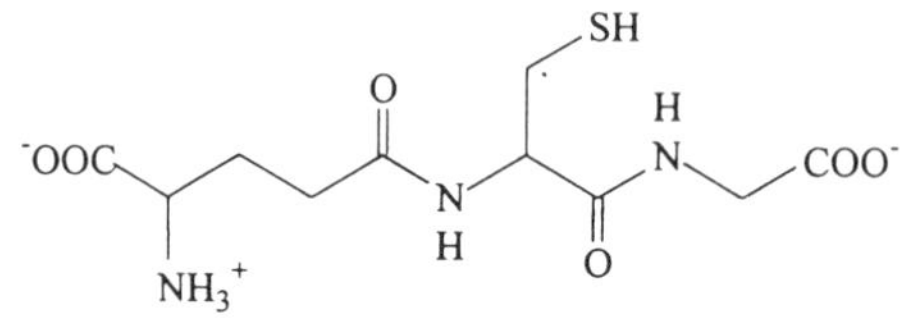

occurs intracellularly, at high concentrations, in essentially all aerobic organisms (1). Note the unusual γ-peptide linkage; the presence of the γ-glutamyl moiety and the free α-carboxylate group prevents the hydrolysis of GSH by cellular peptidases that degrade other small peptides.* GSH is the most abundant cellular low-molecular-mass thiol;† human erythrocytes contain 2 mM GSH and hepatocytes, greater than 10 mM. [In certain plants, such as the mung bean (*Phaseolus aureus*), the similar compound *homoglutathione* (γ-L-glutamyl-L-cysteinyl-β-alanine)

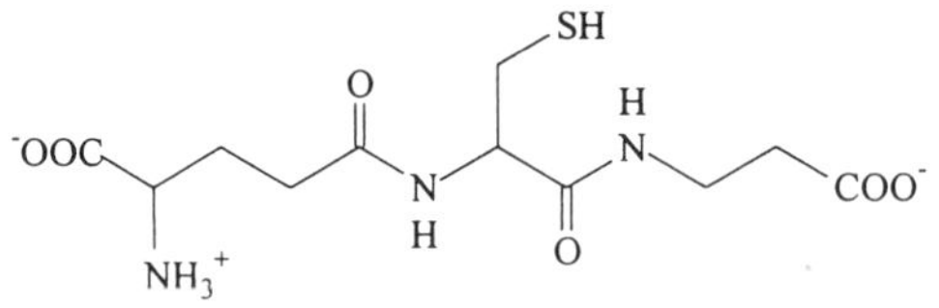

replaces GSH as the most abundant thiol. Functionally, this replacement seems to make little difference.]

Many of the reactions of GSH involve the reactive sulfhydryl group, −SH. The cloud of electrons surrounding the nucleus of the sulfur atom is highly polarizable, making the sulfhydryl group a good *nucleophile* for reaction with electrophilic chemical compounds. Its ability to donate electrons to other compounds also makes it a good *reductant*. The combination of its abundance in aerobic organisms and the chemical properties of its

---

*The γ-glutamyl group can be removed by the action of the enzyme γ-glutamyltranspeptidase, using, as acceptor, the amino group of a free amino acid, or certain other nucleophiles (including water). γ-Glutamyl transpeptidase is found in the cell membrane; the transpeptidation reaction is involved in a series of reactions which transport amino acids into cells, a process called the γ-*glutamyl cycle*.
†Or nonprotein sulfhydryl, NPSH.

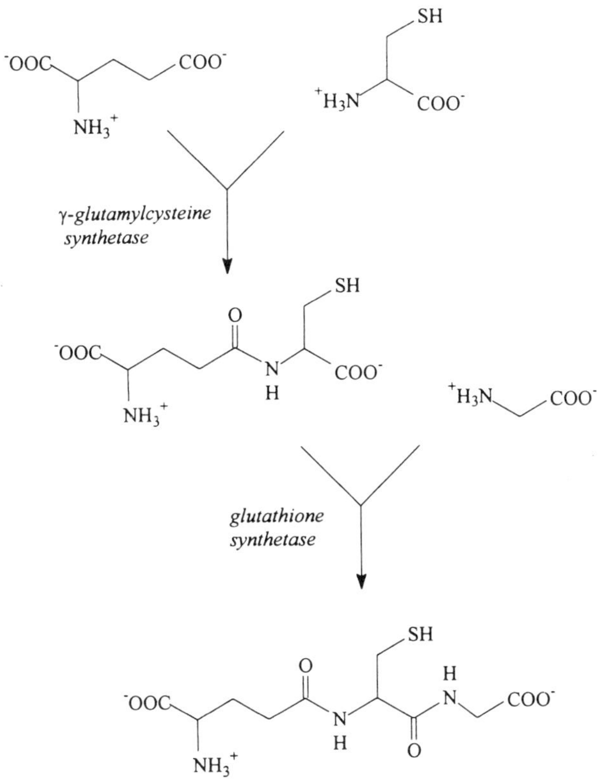

glutathione

sulfhydryl group support the view that GSH arose in biochemical evolution as a protectant against reactive oxygen species and the electrophilic compounds generated by oxidative processes in the organism as well as in its environment.

BIOSYNTHESIS OF GLUTATHIONE

The biosynthesis of GSH does not occur by the same route as protein synthesis, but is catalyzed by two specific enzymes (2). In the first reaction, γ-L-glutamyl-L-cysteine is formed from its constituent amino acids, in a reaction catalyzed by *γ-glutamylcysteine synthetase*. The dipeptide is then linked to glycine by the action of *glutathione synthetase*. Both of these steps require ATP and Mg^{2+}. γ-Glutamylcysteine synthetase is subject to negative feedback regulation by GSH, thereby preventing excess production of GSH or accumulation of the intermediate, γ-glutamylcysteine. If the conversion of γ-glutamylcysteine to GSH is impaired, an alternative reaction predominates: conversion to 5-oxoproline, catalyzed by *γ-glutamylcyclotransferase*:

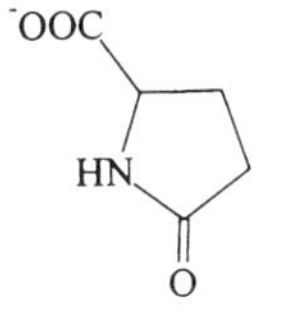

5-oxoproline 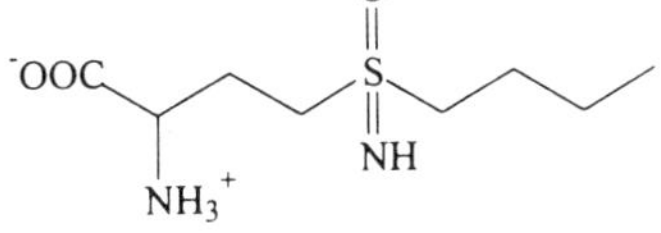   buthionine sulfoximine (BSO)

Excessive production of 5-oxoproline occurs in cases of hereditary deficiency of glu-tathione synthetase and is characterized by 5-oxoprolinuria, chronic metabolic acidosis, and neurological disturbances.

The biosynthesis of GSH can be inhibited by buthionine sulfoximine (BSO), an in-hibitor with structural similarity to an activated intermediate in the reaction catalyzed by γ-glutamylcysteine synthetase (2). In experimental systems, suppression of intracellular GSH concentrations by BSO has been shown to make cells more sensitive to ionizing ra-diation and to certain cytostatic drugs. This sensitization is currently being explored for clinical use in cancer therapy. A limitation of this approach is that both normal and tu-mor cells may be affected and that toxic effects on normal tissues may be more impor-tant than the advantage of making tumor cells more susceptible to treatment. One way of circumventing this problem is to make use of localized irradiation or topical application of cytostatic drugs in order to limit toxic effects on normal tissues.

GLUTATHIONE REDUCTASE

A major role of GSH is to provide protection against oxidative stress and chemical oxi-dants, including free radicals, that occur in biological systems (3). Numerous reactions involve GSH as a reductant, and in most cases GSH is converted into its oxidized disul-fide form, GSSG.*

The enzyme responsible for reduction of GSSG is named *glutathione reductase*, an in-tracellular enzyme occurring as ubiquitously as GSH itself. The human enzyme has been investigated in great detail, and its properties seem to be representative of those of the en-zyme from higher eukaryotes (4). The reaction catalyzed is (see p. 75):

$$GSSG + NADPH + H^+ \rightarrow 2\ GSH + NADP^+$$

The enzyme has high specificity toward both disulfide and pyridine nucleotide sub-strates. Among naturally occurring disulfides, only some mixed disulfides of GSH and related low-M_r thiols serve as alternative substrates, and the low activities observed are probably not of physiological relevance. Similarly, glutathione reductase has no bio-logically significant activity with NADH as an alternative reducing substrate. Glu-tathione reductase consists of two identical subunits, and the binding sites for GSSG are located at the interface between the two subunits (4, 5). Each subunit has a distinct domain with a binding site for NADPH. The pyridine nucleotide is bound in an orien-tation such that the nicotinamide moiety, which carries the reducing equivalents, reaches into the center of the enzyme molecule in a direction toward the GSSG-binding site. The reducing equivalents from NADPH are transferred via two redox-active functional groups of the enzyme, namely, FAD and a disulfide formed by two cysteine residues of the protein. Thus, the electrons originating from NADPH are conducted via FAD to the protein disulfide in order to reach GSSG. The reduction of GSSG actually involves two separate steps. The first leads to release of one GSH molecule, with concomitant formation of a mixed disulfide between one of the redox-active cysteine residues of the active site and the other GS− half of the GSSG molecule. The second partial reaction consists of an intramolecular thiol–disulfide interchange reaction, which releases the second GSH molecule from the intermediate mixed disulfide in the active site. The in-

*GSSG should be referred to as *glutathione disulfide* rather than *oxidized glutathione*, because the latter desig-nation has no precise meaning. Mixed disulfides of GSH (GSSR), sulfinic (GSO_2H) and sulfonic (GSO_3H) acids of GSH, and S-sulfoglutathione ($GSSO_3H$) are other forms of "oxidized glutathione" that occur in biological systems.

teraction between the enzyme and GSSG has similarities to other disulfide reductions catalyzed by redox-active proteins such as thioltransferase and thioredoxin (3). The prosthetic group FAD, which serves as a physical barrier between the GSSG- and NADPH-binding sites, provides the electrochemical coupling between the redox chemistry of NADPH and the disulfide reduction.

GLUTATHIONE AS A REDUCTANT

GSH serves as a reductant for various molecules of biological significance, especially those containing scissile sulfur–sulfur or oxygen–oxygen bonds (disulfides and peroxides, respectively). We will consider these in turn.

Disulfides are formed from low-molecular-mass thiols, polypeptides, and proteins. Intracellular redox conditions are normally such that thiols (RSH) are maintained largely in the reduced form, even if oxidative processes generate a flux of disulfides (RSSR). The reduction of disulfides takes place via thiol–disulfide interchange with GSH, with the intermediate formation of a mixed disulfide (GSSR) (3).

$$GSH + RSSR \rightarrow GSSR + RSH$$
$$\underline{GSSR + GSH \rightarrow GSSG + RSH}$$
$$RSSR + 2\,GSH \rightarrow 2\,RSH + GSSG$$

Thus, a disulfide is converted into the corresponding thiol at the expense of reducing equivalents derived from two GSH molecules. The GSSG formed is reduced by the reaction catalyzed by glutathione reductase: $GSSG + NADPH + H^+ \rightarrow 2\ GSH + NADPH^+$, thereby coupling the reduction of disulfides to the reducing equivalents of the pyridine nucleotide pool.

Both of the consecutive thiol–disulfide interchange reactions are catalyzed by thioltransferase, a cytosolic protein of M_r 11 kD (6). The enzyme has a broad substrate specificity and is active with naturally occurring disulfides (such as cystine and coenzyme A disulfide) and their mixed disulfides with GSH. Even disulfide bonds in proteins may be reduced in the same manner, provided that they are not sterically hindered (7). Many enzymes require reduced sulfhydryl groups for activity and are reversibly activated/inactivated by thiol/disulfide interconversion.

In the endoplasmic reticulum of eukaryotic cells, however, the glutathione redox equilibrium is shifted; the ratio of GSH to GSSG may be only about 1:1. This conclusion is based on a study of a synthetic cysteine-containing peptide, which was designed to be glycosylated, and thereby trapped, within the endoplasmic reticulum (ER) (8). This more oxidized state of the ER may be required for formation of protein disulfide bonds.

In addition, S-sulfo-substituted thiols, such as the naturally occurring S-sulfoglutathione ($GSSO_3^-$), are reduced via a thioltransferase catalyzed reaction:

$$GSH + GSSO_3^- \rightarrow GSSG + HSO_3^-$$

Thus, thioltransferase-catalyzed reactions serve to maintain cysteine, coenzyme A, and other important cellular thiols in their reduced state.

Hydrogen peroxide (H_2O_2) is produced as a byproduct of cellular respiration, cytochrome P-450-catalyzed reactions, and other oxidative processes linked to oxygen metabolism (see Chapters 4 and 5). Organic hydroperoxides (ROOH) are formed endogenously by lipid peroxidation and oxidative damage to nucleic acids and also occur in food. Reduction of hydroperoxides is catalyzed by selenium-dependent glutathione peroxidases (see Chapter 5).

CONJUGATION REACTIONS

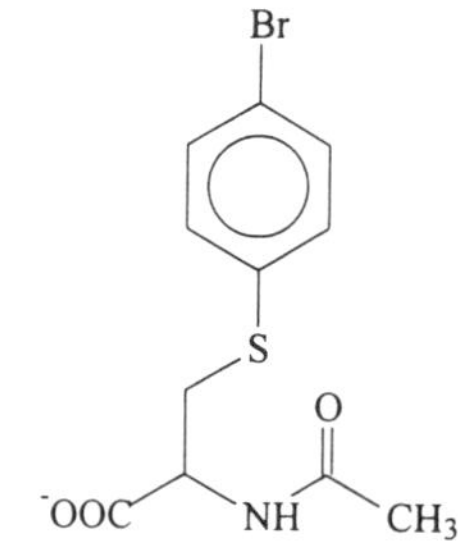

N-acetyl-S-(p-bromophenyl)cysteine

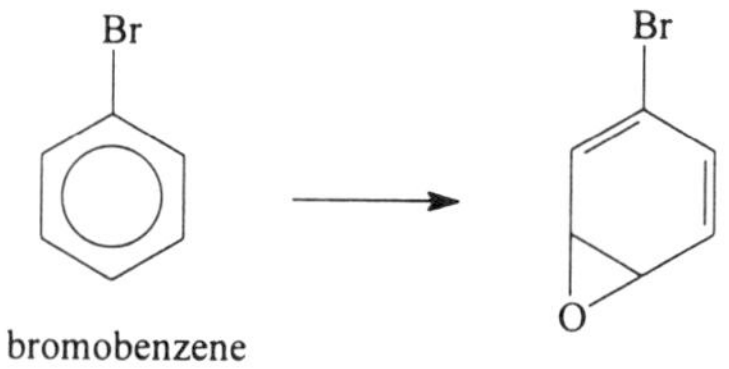

bromobenzene

1-bromo-3,4-dihydro-
3,4-oxybenzene

In 1879, *N*-acetyl-*S*-*p*-bromophenyl-cysteine was isolated from the urine of dogs that had been fed bromobenzene. This metabolite is an example of *mercapturic acids* [*N*-acetyl-*S*-(substituted)-cysteines], so named because, upon treatment with alkali, they decompose to odoriferous mercaptans (thiols). By the late 1950s, it became clear that mercapturates derive from GSH conjugation. In the case of bromobenzene, the aromatic hydrocarbon is epoxidized to 1-bromo-3,4-dihydro-3,4-oxybenzene (see Chapter 14). This reactive epoxide reacts with the thiol group of GSH. The epoxide and the GSH conjugate are unstable because the aromatic character of the benzene ring has been destroyed. Aromaticity and stability are regained by spontaneous elimination of water;

The GSH conjugate is subsequently transformed by the action of γ-glutamyltranspepti-dase and dipeptidase, to give the corresponding cysteine conjugate:

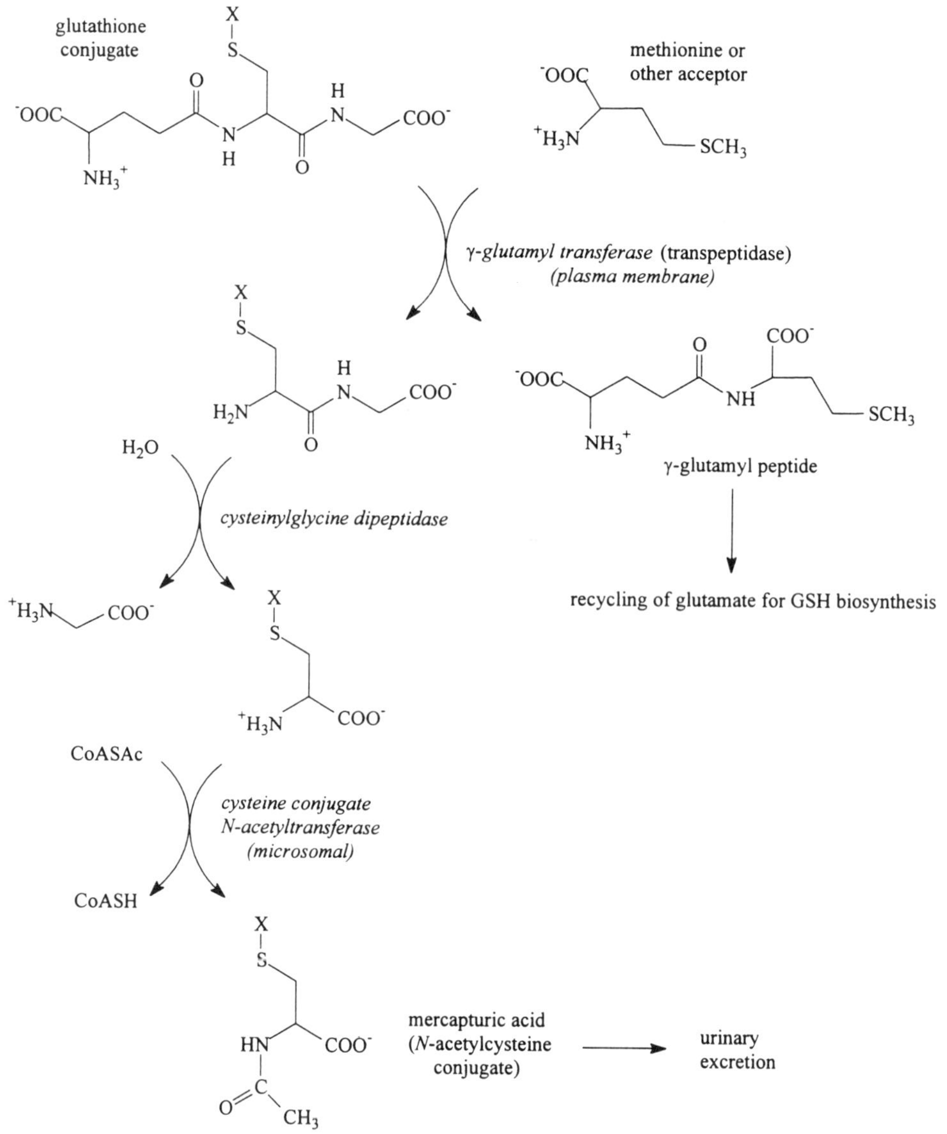

The final step in mercapturic acid formation is the acetylation of the amino group of cysteine. The last process requires acetyl-coenzyme A and an N-acetyltransferase.*

GLUTATHIONE TRANSFERASES

Glutathione transferases (GST) catalyze the conjugation of GSH with a very broad range of electrophilic chemical compounds (9). Electrophiles are often cytotoxic, mutagenic, and carcinogenic; the GSTs constitute the major defense system against hazardous electrophiles. The enzymes have been found in all aerobic organisms investigated and they occur in high concentrations in mammalian tissues. For example, up to 5% of the cytosolic protein in human liver comprises GSTs, and their content in rat liver may exceed

*The mercapturate-forming enzyme is unrelated to the aromatic amine N-acetyltransferase discussed in Chapter 12.

10%. The GSTs can be classified into cytosolic (soluble) enzymes and membrane-bound (microsomal) enzymes. Microsomal GST is localized in the endoplasmic reticulum and the outer mitochondrial membrane, where it may represent 3–4% of the total protein.

In addition to the GSTs with broad substrate specificities, which are considered as detoxication enzymes, a membrane-bound GST enzyme catalyzes the conjugation of GSH with the epoxide leukotriene A_4 to yield the GSH conjugate leukotriene C_4:

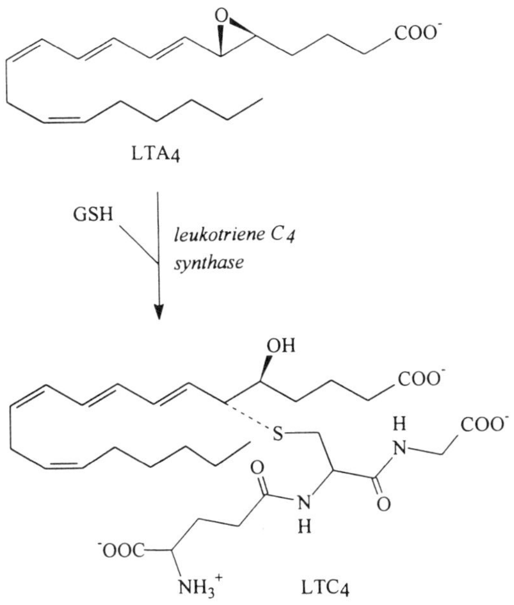

This enzyme, leukotriene C_4 synthase, is distinctly different from other microsomal GSTs (10). Leukotriene C_4 and its metabolites, leukotrienes D_4 and E_4, are important mediators of pathophysiological reactions in asthma and inflammatory processes. The substrate specificity of leukotriene C_4 synthase appears to be limited to leukotriene A_4 and some closely related epoxides of polyunsaturated fatty acids. The tissue distribution of the enzyme is different from that of the microsomal GST; pronounced enzyme activity has been detected only in cells known to produce leukotriene C_4 and its congeners.

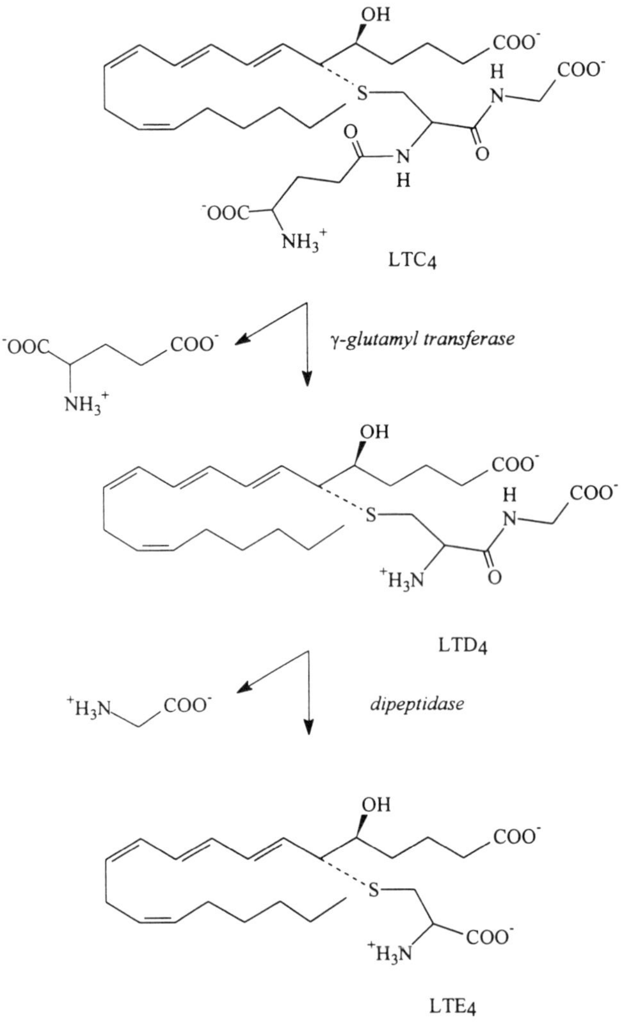

THE DISCOVERY OF GLUTATHIONE TRANSFERASES

The earliest reports on enzyme-catalyzed GSH conjugation reactions date back to 1961, when crude preparations from rat liver were observed to catalyze nucleophilic substitution reactions of aromatic halogen compounds, such as 3,4-dichloro-1-nitrobenzene and bromosulfophthalein. The range of organic compounds recognized as substrates for GSTs rapidly expanded as novel electrophilic substances were analyzed. Glutathione transferases were first purified on the basis of their capacity to bind lipophilic compounds, such as bilirubin. The identity of these binding proteins, called "ligandins," with forms of glutathione transferase, was soon recognized (11).

GLUTATHIONE TRANSFERASES: ASSAY

GSTs have evolved, under selective pressure, to catalyze the inactivation of noxious electrophilic substances, some of which occur naturally in biological systems. These substrates include epoxides, activated alkenes, and organic hydroperoxides, which are inevitably generated when organic molecules are exposed to molecular oxygen. Since the enzyme accepts many different substrates, it can be assayed in many ways.

A convenient, although nonphysiological, substrate is 1-chloro-2,4-dinitrobenzene:

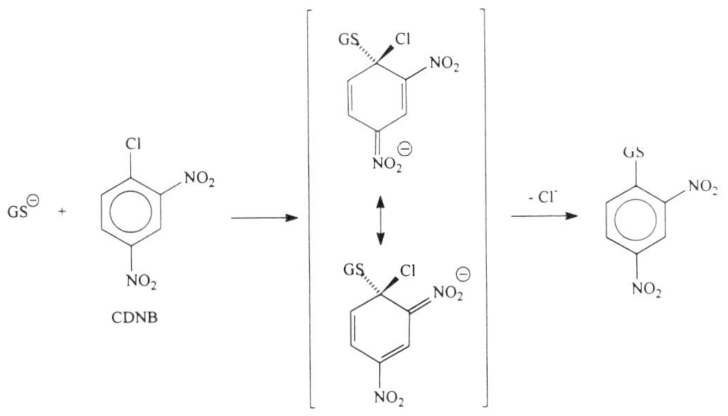

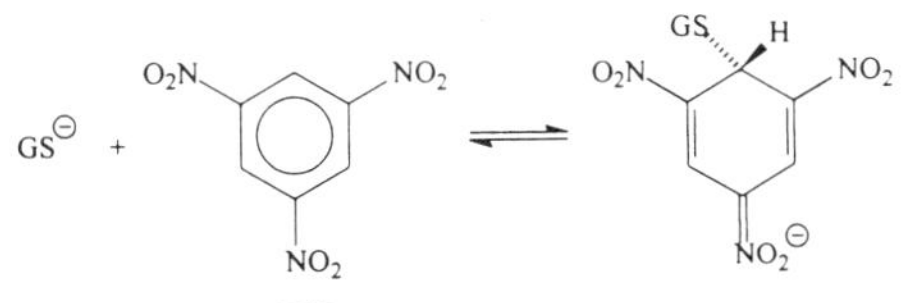

The formation of the GSH conjugate of CDNB can be measured spectrophotometrically; this is the most common method for measurement of GST activity. However, some GSTs have very low activity with CDNB; also, the significant nonenzymatic reaction rate limits the sensitivity.

The reaction between GSH and CDNB is a nucleophilic aromatic substitution. These processes involve the formation of an intermediate known as a *Meisenheimer complex*, after the chemist who first isolated such complexes in the early years of the twentieth century. The formation of the anionic complex is facilitated by the stabilizing effect of the electron-withdrawing nitro groups. The formation of the deep-red anion complex of GS⁻ and trinitrobenzene (TNB) is reversible; the complex does not form product, since the chloride leaving group is absent. This complex is a transition-state analogue for the GST reaction and is an inhibitor of GST activity. Recently, the crystal structure of a Mu-class GST complex with this transition-state analogue has been solved (12).

Many other GST substrates have chromophores that allow spectrophotometric assay of enzyme activity. In some cases, GSTs also catalyze reductive reactions in which GSH is oxidized to GSSG. An important example is the reduction of hydroperoxides:

$$ROOH + 2GSH \rightarrow ROH + H_2O + GSSG$$

(the non-selenium glutathione peroxidase reaction). Such reactions can be coupled to the glutathione reductase-catalyzed reduction of GSSG and monitored by following the oxidation of NADPH at 340 nm.

However, for a large number of reactions catalyzed by GSTs, simple spectrophotometric assays are not available, and one must separate the substrates and products by chromatography, electrophoresis, or solvent partitioning. High-performance liquid chromatography (HPLC) is often used. Radioactively labeled GSH or xenobiotic substrate can be employed. As with any reaction, one can measure product formation or reactant disappearance. Consumption of GSH is common to all reactions catalyzed by GSTs, but measurements based on product formation are preferable.

GLUTATHIONE TRANSFERASES: PURIFICATION

GSTs can be purified to homogeneity by ion-exchange chromatography, gel filtration, and other traditional purification methods. However, most GST isoenzymes* bind to immobilized GSH derivatives and can be purified by affinity chromatography (13). Suitable affinity matrices include S-hexylglutathione-Sepharose and glutathione-Sepharose:

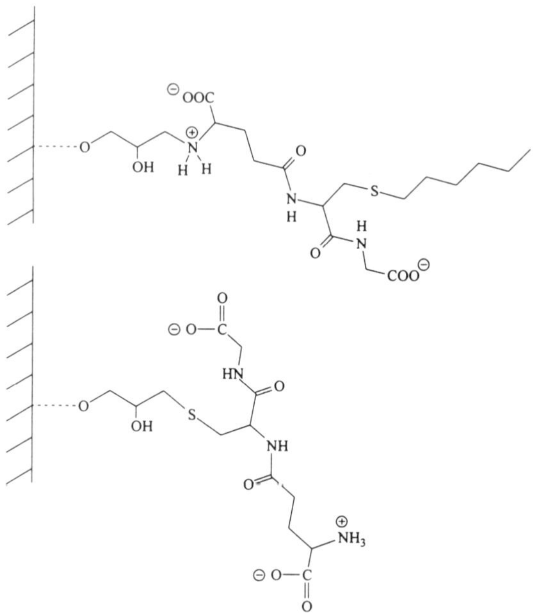

Under favorable conditions, a single step of affinity purification may isolate the GSTs from essentially all other proteins in the sample.† The different isoenzymes can be separated by means of a high-resolution technique, such as chromatofocusing or preparative isoelectric focusing. For analytical purposes, high-performance liquid chromatography has proved useful for separation and quantitation of the different GST subunits.

GLUTATHIONE TRANSFERASES: CLASSIFICATION AND NOMENCLATURE

The existence of multiple forms of GST was discovered in the 1960s by Eric Boyland and co-workers in England. As with other enzymes of biotransformation, the classification and nomenclature of GSTs developed haphazardly. One approach is classification on the basis of substrate specificity. However, once highly purified samples of different isoenzymes had been obtained, it became clear that the substrate specificities for different forms of

---

*Affinity ligands for class Theta and microsomal GSTs have not yet been identified.
†The simplicity of this purification is exploited in the GST fusion method described in Chapter 1.

GST are overlapping. Therefore, unambiguous classification on this basis is impossible. (Nevertheless, substrate specificity is the criterion by which leukotriene C_4 synthase is identified.)

In the early 1980s, the quaternary structure of cytosolic GSTs was elucidated: The enzymes occur as binary combinations of subunits, including both homodimers and heterodimers (14). This finding led to a rational nomenclature: The isoenzyme name reflects the subunit composition. Most recently, distinct classes of GST have been assigned on the basis of primary (protein or DNA) sequence data: Alpha, Mu, Pi, and Theta.* Thus, human GST A1-1 denotes the homodimeric isoenzyme composed of two copies of subunit 1 from the Alpha class. GST A1-2 is a heterodimeric isoenzyme composed of subunits 1 and 2 from the Alpha class, and so on. The properties of the human GST enzymes are discussed in a recent comprehensive review (15).

Within each of the four classes, Alpha, Mu, Pi, and Theta, members are >50% sequence identical (usually >70%), irrespective of the mammalian species from which the enzyme is isolated. Sequences from different classes are usually <30% identical in primary structure. The microsomal GST, on the other hand, shows no structural similarity with any of the cytosolic enzymes.

The GSTs in biological species phylogenetically distant from mammals do not have a generally accepted classification. However, the mammalian class Theta enzymes appear to be most similar to the ancestral form of GST.

Similarity in primary structure among the members of a class of GSTs explains why polyclonal antibodies often display cross-reactivity with isozymes of the same class. Antibodies raised against an enzyme within a given class do not cross-react with GSTs from other classes.

Is there any correlation between isozyme class (sequence) and catalytic activity? Using a pattern recognition approach, based on multivariate analysis, Mannervik et al. (16) demonstrated that substrate-specificity data and inhibition parameters can be correlated with the sequence-based classification. For example, high activity with organic hydroperoxides is expressed by certain class Alpha enzymes; with epoxides, by some class Mu enzymes; and with activated alkenes, by some class Pi enzymes. However, definite predictions of activity based on sequence cannot be made. Indeed, site-directed mutagenesis experiments show that even single-point mutations in the active site may drastically alter the substrate specificity of a given enzyme.

Several nomenclature systems for designation of the GST isozymes have been used in parallel (17). A new system, based on the assignment of the different enzyme forms into the classes Alpha (A), Mu (M), Pi (P), and Theta (T), has recently been introduced for the human enzymes (18); similar systems for other species, such as rat and mouse, are in preparation. The cytosolic GSTs are dimeric proteins, and each of the subunits is given a number within the class to which it belongs. Thus the human class Alpha GST composed of two copies of subunit 1 is denoted GST A1-1; the related heterodimeric isoenzyme composed of subunits 1 and 2 is denoted GST A1-2. The class Mu enzyme GST M1-1 displays a genetic polymorphism (see above), and the two common allelic variants, which differ in a single amino acid residue (number 173), are distinguished by a lowercase letter: M1a (Lys 173) and M1b (Asn 173). The two variant subunits give rise to three isozymes; since a positive residue (Lys) is substituted for a neutral one (Asn), the forms are distinguishable by electrophoresis; they are named GST M1a-1a, GST M1a-1b, and GST M1b-1b. The membrane-bound GST (microsomal GST) isolated from the endoplasmic reticulum is a trimeric protein, structurally unrelated to the cytosolic enzymes.

---

*The names of the Greek letters are written in full, in Roman characters.

GLUTATHIONE TRANSFERASES: STRUCTURE

As mentioned, GST molecules are composed of subunits; the cytosolic enzymes are dimers of approximately 25-kD subunits; microsomal GST is a trimer of 17-kD subunits. The functional properties (catalytic efficiency with different substrates; inhibition characteristics) of a given subunit in a cytosolic GST dimer are little influenced by the nature of the neighboring subunit, whether identical or nonidentical (14, 19).

The three-dimensional structures of representatives of classes Alpha, Mu, and Pi GSTs have been determined by X-ray crystallography in recent years (20) (see Figure 11.1).

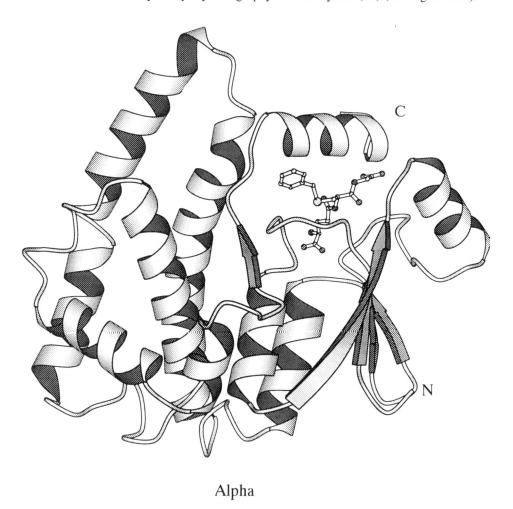

Alpha

Figure 11.1. X-ray crystal structures of three GST enzyme subunits, representing the Alpha, Mu, and Pi classes of enzymes. Coils represent α-helices and arrows represent β-strands. The bound ligands (Alpha: S-benzylglutathione; Mu: reduced glutathione; Pi: S-hexylglutathione) are represented as ball-and-stick structures. The amino (N) and carboxyl (C) termini are indicated.

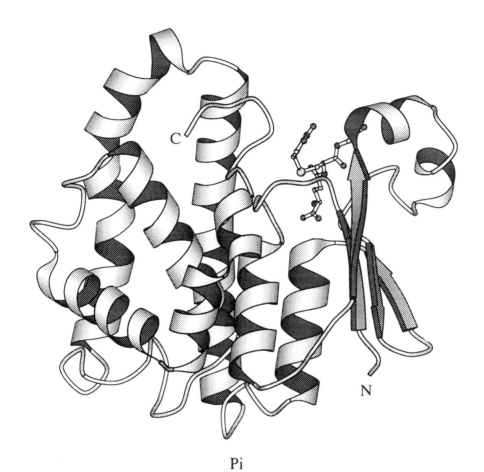

Pi

Figure 11.1. (Continued).

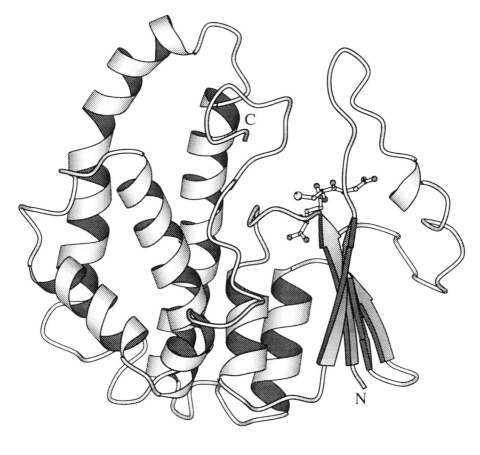

Mu

Figure 11.1. (Continued).

The fold of the polypeptide chain of a subunit is very similar for all three structures, but significant changes occur in the active site region (21). The two protein subunits of the enzyme are related to one another by a two-fold symmetry axis and each subunit contains an active site. The two active sites are 15–20 Å apart, and ligands bound in one active site are, therefore, not close to a ligand bound to the other site (in the neighboring subunit). The γ-glutamyl portion of GSH bound to the active site of one subunit interacts with an aspartic acid residue in the neighboring subunit, via an ionic bond; the functional significance of this interaction is not known.

An individual GST subunit is built of two domains. The N-terminal domain comprises approximately the first 80 residues and is an α/β-structure.* This domain harbors the GSH-binding site ("G-site"). The protein-substrate interactions which bind GSH to the G-site are illustrated schematically in the following scheme.†

*See C. Branden and J. Tooze, *Introduction to Protein Structure*, Garland Publishing, New York, 1991, Chapter 4.
†Adapted from B. Mannervik and M. Widersten, Human glutathione transferases: Classification, tissue distribution, structure, and functional properties, in: *Advances in Drug Metabolism in Man*, G. M. Pacifici and G. N. Fracchia, Eds., European Commission, Luxembourg, 1995, pp. 407–459.

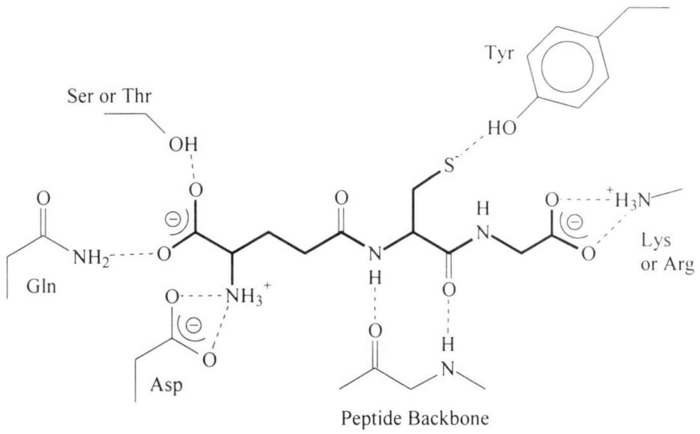

Peptide Backbone

GLUTATHIONE TRANSFERASES: BIOCHEMICAL EVOLUTION

GSH is ubiquitous among aerobic organisms, but does not generally occur in anaerobic microorganisms; the distribution of GSH-linked enzymes may be expected to follow that of GSH (22). One may conclude that GSH and GSH-dependent enzymes arose at the time, in evolutionary history, when oxygen first became abundant in the atmosphere. A common feature of GSH-dependent enzymes is the specific binding of the GSH molecule. Perhaps, the evolution of the enzyme proteins has involved the shuffling of a GSH binding domain with other protein domain structures, conferring diverse catalytic activities to the combined molecule. Structural evidence for this hypothesis derives from X-ray diffraction analysis of GSH transferases, glutathione peroxidase, and glutaredoxin, all of which have a similar polypeptide fold in the portion of the protein that interacts with GSH (21).

At the level of evolution of individual isoenzymes within an enzyme family, novel forms may have arisen by recombination of segments of DNA encoding limited parts of the protein structure. In the case of GSTs, *exon shuffling* and *gene conversion* have been proposed as mechanisms for generation of novel substrate specificities. Exon shuffling refers to the hypothesis that existing proteins evolved from combinations of a limited "universe" of exons via exchange of the corresponding DNA coding sequences. Gene conversion occurs when a segment of one gene replaces the corresponding segment of a related gene (nonreciprocal recombination) (23).

GLUTATHIONE TRANSFERASES: CATALYTIC MECHANISM

The common denominator in GST-catalyzed reactions is nucleophilic attack of the sulfur atom of GSH on the electrophilic second substrate. This attack is facilitated by ionization of GSH to its thiolate form. The pK_a value for the thiol group of the enzyme-bound GSH is estimated as less than 7.0, versus 9.2 for GSH in aqueous solution. Therefore, enzyme-bound GSH is largely ionized. The thiolate anion is stabilized by a hydrogen bond from the phenolic hydroxyl group of a tyrosine residue in the active site. This tyrosine residue, close to the N-terminus, is conserved among the known GST structures of classes Alpha, Mu, and Pi. In the class Alpha enzymes, an additional hydrogen bond is contributed by a conserved active-site arginine residue. Since the dissociation constant for the binary enzyme–GSH complex (approximately 0.1 mM) is at least an order of magnitude lower than the intracellular concentration of GSH, the enzymes should be almost saturated with GSH in the cell.* Exposure to the toxic elec-trophilic substrate probably occurs only transiently; in this scenario, the enzymes are predominantly idle, but loaded with GSH in the thiolate form and ready to attack elec-trophiles that they may encounter. The detailed mechanism by which GSH is ionized upon binding to the enzyme is not clear, but the phenolic hydroxyl of the active-site ty-rosine residue has a pK_a value of 8 to 8.5, which is lower than that of free tyrosine by approximately 2 units. Dipole moments of helices pointing toward the active-site tyro-sine may contribute to the stabilization of the phenolate form of the tyrosine side chain and the thiolate form of enzyme-bound GSH.

The enzyme contributes to catalysis not only by activating the thiol group, but also by positioning the tripeptide in a favorable orientation with respect to the second substrate. Binding of GSH involves interactions with amino acid side chains as well as peptide bonds of the main chain. The interactions with the second substrate are less clearly defined. Apart from the proximity effect caused by specific binding, little is known about the role of the enzyme (if any) in activating the electrophile for reaction with GSH. However, in the case of a class Mu enzyme, a second tyrosine residue in the active side-region can do-nate a hydrogen bond to free electron pairs in the electrophilic substrate or in a transi-tion-state structure. Such hydrogen bonding to the oxirane function of epoxides may ex-plain the characteristically high activity of class Mu enzymes with epoxides (24).

GLUTATHIONE TRANSFERASES: TISSUE DISTRIBUTION

The expression of GST isoenzymes is differential: Isoenzyme profiles generally differ from tissue to tissue. Since the enzymes have different substrate specificities, the occur-rence of a given enzyme form will influence the cellular capacity for inactivating elec-trophilic toxic chemicals. The absence of particular isoenzymes in the cells may predis-pose tissues for organ-selective toxicity. For example, absence of class Mu GSTs, which generally have high activity with epoxides, may render an organ susceptible to the toxic effects of this class of compounds.

GLUTATHIONE TRANSFERASES: HUMAN POLYMORPHISMS

In 1980, Mannervik and co-workers discovered a previously unknown form of GST with distinctive catalytic properties. The enzyme was first named GST μ but is now referred to as GST M1-1. A striking genetic polymorphism exists: Only approximately 50% of the population possess this gene (25). This distribution appears to apply to populations throughout the world. The gene for the enzyme subunit GST M1 resides in a cluster of genes on human chromosome 1. The *GST M1* gene is flanked by the genes for the related Mu class subunits GST M4 and M2, on one side, and GST M3 and M5, on the other side (26). Possibly, the *GST M1* gene originated in a neighboring gene and was created by a gene conversion event. Epidemiological studies indicate that individuals lacking GST M1-1 (GST M1 null phenotype) are at higher risk of cancers in certain organ sites than are individuals expressing the enzyme. For example, a recent study in Kitakyushu, Japan, re-ported an elevated frequency of the null phenotype among patients with urothelial cancer compared to healthy controls (27).

---

*Theta class GSTs display a low affinity for GSH and are probably not fully saturated at physiological con-centrations of GSH.

A polymorphism in the expression of human Theta-class GSTs also exists; its biological significance remains to be explored.

GLUTATHIONE TRANSFERASE: INDUCTION

GSTs can be induced by a variety of chemical compounds, including conventional inducers of drug-metabolizing enzymes, such as phenobarbital, 3-methylcholanthrene, and TCDD.

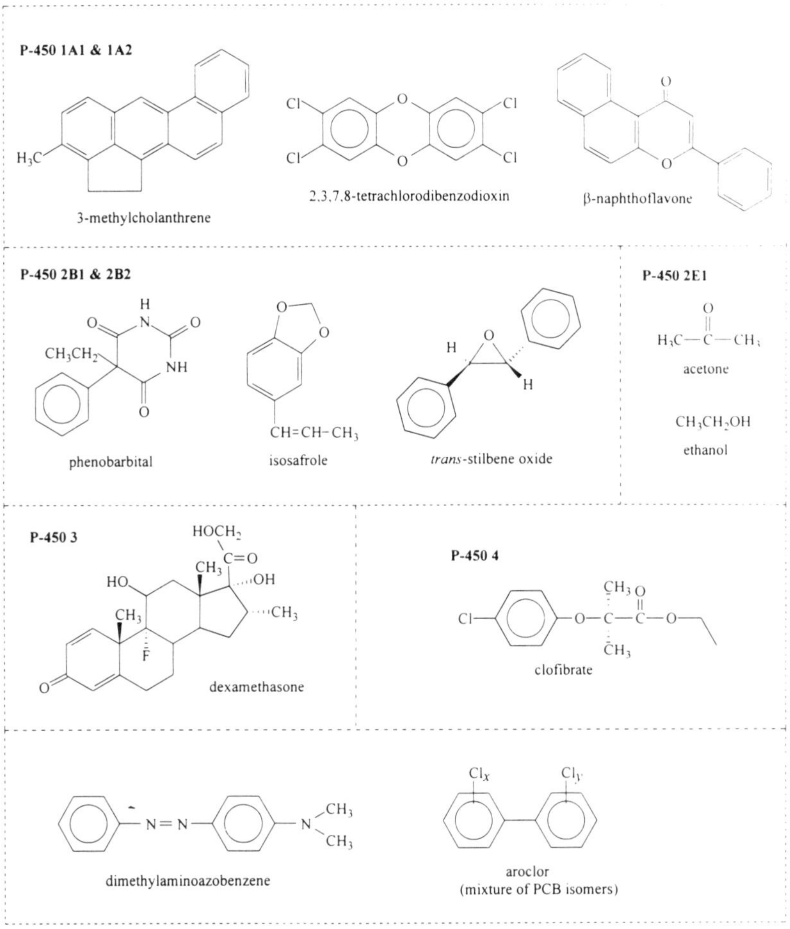

(most P-450 inducers are discussed in Chapter 14). Only certain forms of GST are induced by a given compound. The regulation of gene expression differs from one species to another, and it is not clear to what extent the knowledge about induction of GST genes in the rat and the mouse is applicable to the human counterparts. However, inducibility of the enzymes appears to be a common feature and has been observed in many species, including plants.

Notably, electrophilic substrates for the enzymes are often effective inducers (transcriptional activators) of GST genes. Therefore, exposure to such compounds induces the synthesis of enzymes that catalyze their detoxication. In many cases, novel isoenzymes that are not expressed constitutively appear following administration of the inducer. The induction is reversible and the concentration of an induced enzyme returns to its original level after removal of the inducing substance. By this device, the cellular enzyme concentrations may be adjusted to the current requirements. Induction will be considered again in the chapter on cytochrome P-450 (Chapter 14).

GLUTATHIONE TRANSFERASE: HORMONAL CONTROL OF EXPRESSION

The transcription of GST genes is affected by hormones and other physiological regulatory factors. Surgical removal of endocrine glands causes alterations in the relative amounts of different forms of GST in various organs. A particularly striking example is the regulation of the class Pi GST in mouse liver.* Adult male mice express this enzyme as one of the major hepatic forms, whereas females and young males have approximately tenfold lower cytosolic concentrations of this enzyme (28). When the young males reach puberty, the class Pi GST level increases to the high levels of adult males. Castration of adult males reduces the enzyme concentration to the juvenile levels, and administration of testosterone brings the concentration up to adult levels.

Similarly, hypophysectomy of rats causes dramatic changes in the adrenal glands (29), with pronounced induction of a class Alpha enzyme (GST 8-8) with characteristically high activity toward 4-hydroxyalkenals (see Chapter 7). Regulatory effects of growth hormone and thyroxine have been demonstrated in adrenal glands as well as in the liver.

Studies of animals or cells in tissue culture have demonstrated that other regulatory substances, such as interferon and retinoic acid, may also affect the cellular concentrations of GSTs, in an isoenzyme-specific manner. In studies of the nucleotide sequences of genes for GSTs, genetic elements known to bind transcription factors linked to glucocorticoids and retinoic acid have been found.

The intracellular concentration of GST isoenzymes may vary with different phases of the cell cycle, but the physiological significance of the variations is not yet clear.

THE BIOLOGICAL FUNCTION OF GLUTATHIONE TRANSFERASES

The occurrence of substrates for GSTs is linked to oxygen metabolism. Many of the important electrophilic groups of substrate molecules, including epoxide, activated alkene, and hydroperoxy groups, may arise by oxidative processes in the cell. The detoxication mechanisms have to be very general in order for cells to cope with the myriad of toxic molecules that can arise from endogenous and exogenous compounds. As with cytochrome P-450, this may be a reason why multiple isoenzymes of GST, with overlapping substrate specificities, have evolved.

XENOBIOTIC METABOLISM BY GLUTATHIONE CONJUGATION: EXAMPLES

A few examples of xenobiotics, including synthetic compounds, metabolized by GSH conjugation are given here.

Styrene is used in large quantities (millions of tons per year) for plastic manufacturing. Styrene is epoxidized by the cytochrome P-450 system, and styrene-7,8-oxide

---

*Normal hepatocytes of rat or human origin do not express significant amounts of the class Pi GST.

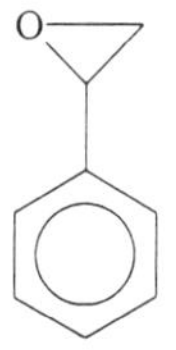

styrene 7,8-oxide

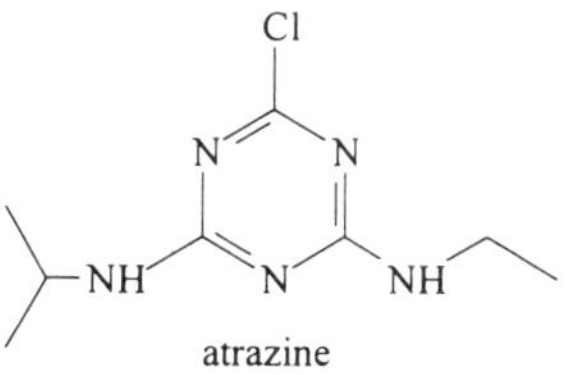

atrazine

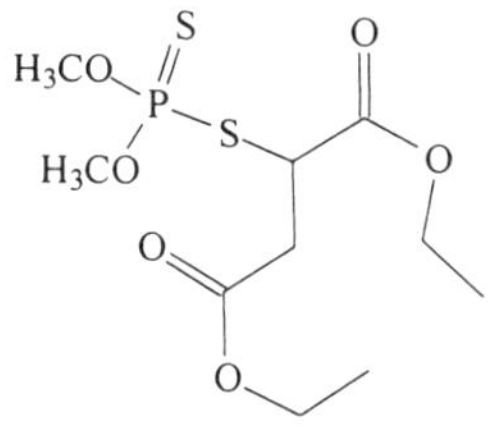

malathion

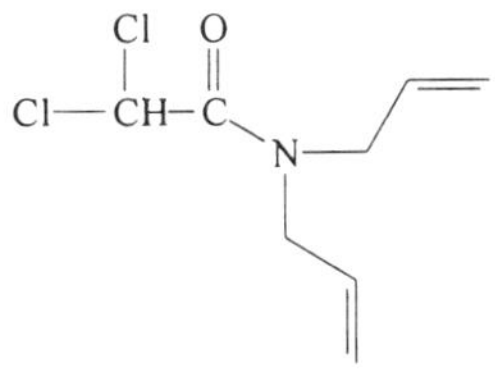

N,N-diallyl-2,2-dichloro-
acetamide

is a mutagenic and carcinogenic metabolite. The benzylic carbon atom of styrene oxide is optically active. Four distinct GSH conjugates (two pairs of enantiomers) can be formed by attack of GSH at either carbon (7 or 8) of the epoxide ring of either stereoisomer (30) (analogous to the four forms of BPDE; see Chapter 19).

The metabolism of the polycyclic aromatic hydrocarbon carcinogen benzo[a]pyrene is discussed in detail in Chapter 19. The ultimate carcinogen is believed to be the 7,8-dihydrodiol-9,10-epoxide (BPDE; see Chapter 19), which binds to guanine residues in DNA. Of the four diastereomeric forms of BPDE, (+) anti-BPDE has the highest carcinogenicity. This stereoisomer is a substrate for class Pi GSTs (31), and studies with isolated hepatocytes have shown that most of the carcinogen dose may be conjugated to GSH and detoxified. The polymorphic human GST M1-1 is also active with BPDE and other epoxide derivatives of benzo[a]pyrene.

Aflatoxin B_1 is a potent hepatocarcinogen produced by the mold *Aspergillus flavus*, which grows on peanuts and grains stored under warm, humid conditions (32). Dietary exposure to aflatoxin is probably a major cause of liver cancer in parts of China and Africa. Aflatoxin B_1 is activated to the ultimate carcinogen, the *exo*-8,9-epoxide,

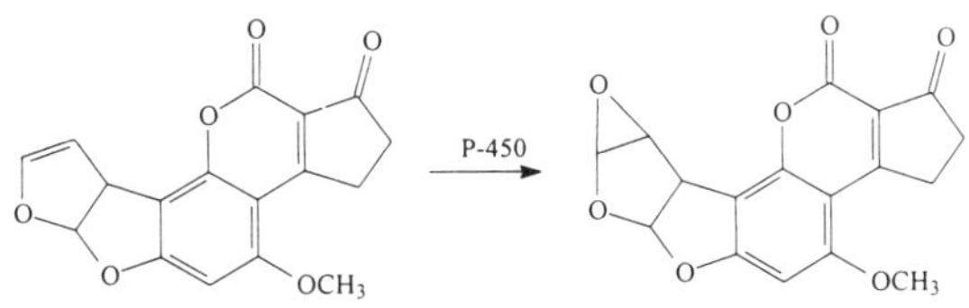

Aflatoxin B_1 AFB$_1$-2,3-oxide

through cytochrome-P-450-mediated oxygenation. A class Alpha GST found in the mouse catalyzes the inactivation of the carcinogen, but rats do not constitutively express an enzyme with a corresponding activity (33). This probably accounts for the much greater sensitivity to aflatoxin hepatocarcinogenesis of rats, compared to mice.

Paracetamol (acetaminophen; Tylenol) is a very widely used analgesic and antipyretic drug. Although safe at therapeutic doses, paracetamol overdose is a common accidental poisoning and is also sometimes used in attempted suicide. Overdose toxicity is due to hepatotoxicity. The mechanism of paracetamol hepatotoxicity has been studied intensively. Paracetamol is metabolized to *N*-acetyl-*p*-benzoquinoneimine. This compound, and other quinones, form GSH conjugates (34) by a Michael addition mechanism (35):

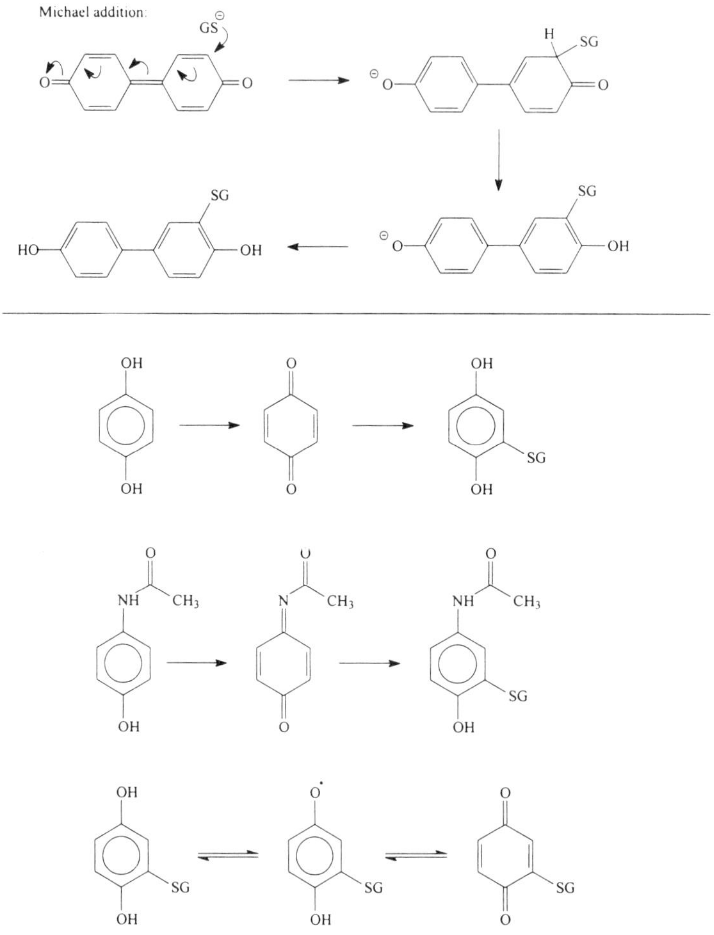

At high paracetamol doses, cells become completely depleted of GSH, and the activated paracetamol binds covalently to protein. The major protein target is the thiol group of cysteine residues (36). In experimental animals, the time course of liver damage following drug administration indicates that injury follows GSH depletion (37). Administration of N-acetyl-L-cysteine, which replenishes GSH stores, protects against paracetamol toxicity (38).

GLUTATHIONE TRANSFERASES AND DRUG RESISTANCE

Some agricultural herbicides may be inactivated by GST-catalyzed GSH conjugation. A typical example is the triazine *atrazine* [2-chloro-4-(ethylamino)-6-(isopropylamino)-*s*-triazine; (39)], which is used for postemergence control of weeds in corn and other crops (see structure in preceding section). Seeds of the crop to be cultivated can be treated with a "safener," or antidote, to increase subsequent resistance to the herbicide. In the case of corn (maize, *Zea mays*), the safener *N,N*-diallyl-2,2-dichloroacetamide (see structure in preceding section) induces the expression of a novel form of GST, which is undetectable in the untreated seedlings. This is a typical case of acquisition of increased resistance against xenobiotics effected by increased intracellular concentrations of a form of GST.

Insects treated with insecticides can also develop resistance against the toxic agent, by production of increased concentrations of GST. *Malathion* (see structure in preceding section) can be inactivated by glutathione-dependent *O*-demethylation, and GSTs contribute to resistance. Similar studies on animals or animal cells in tissue culture have demonstrated that GSTs are inducible by a wide range of chemical substances of greater or lower toxicity.

ANTICANCER DRUG RESISTANCE; ALKYLATING AGENTS

Alkylating agents are reactive electrophiles which can cause the replacement of a hydrogen atom by an alkyl substituent. As such, alkylating agents are of importance as synthetic reagents; they also comprise a large family of important therapeutic agents.

"Mustard" alkylating agents derive their name from the chemical warfare agent, mustard gas (*bis*-(2-chloroethyl)sulfide), which was used by the German army during World War I and by the Iraqi military in the war with Iran during the 1980s. The presence of the lone pair electrons on the central sulfur atom facilitates the loss of Cl^- to yield an electrophilic cation. Mustard gas exposure can rapidly cause lethal lung damage. The analogous nitrogen mustards are also potent alkylating agents. Mustard gas was studied as a chemotherapeutic agent against experimental rat tumors in the 1930s, but its toxicity precluded clinical use. The introduction of the nitrogen mustard methyl-*bis*-(2-chloroethyl)amine as an anticancer agent in the 1940s marked the beginning of modern chemotherapy for cancer. Many other valuable drugs were developed from this lead, including melphalan and chlorambucil (40). Nitrosoureas were first recognized as therapeutically useful alkylating agents as a result of the program of random screening by the U.S. National Cancer Institute, which identified the activity of *N*-methyl-*N*-nitrosourea. Development of this lead compound led to more useful agents, such as *bis*-1,3-(2-chloroethyl)-1-nitrosourea (BCNU) (41, 42):

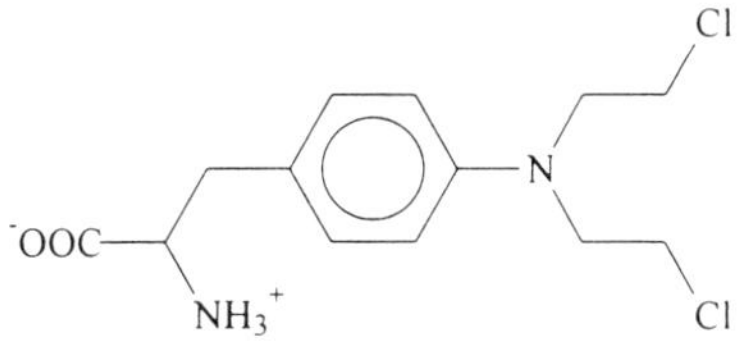

melphalan (phenylalanine mustard)

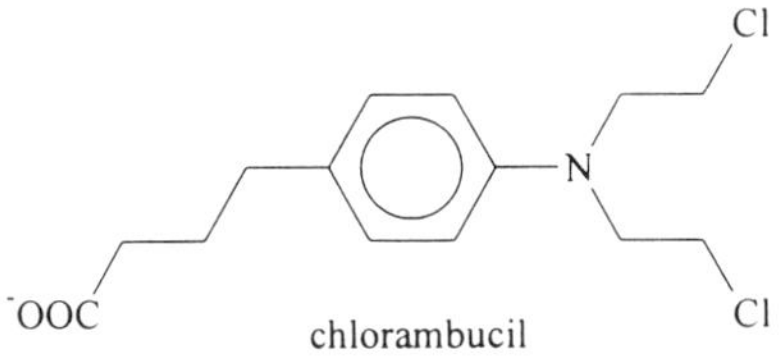

chlorambucil

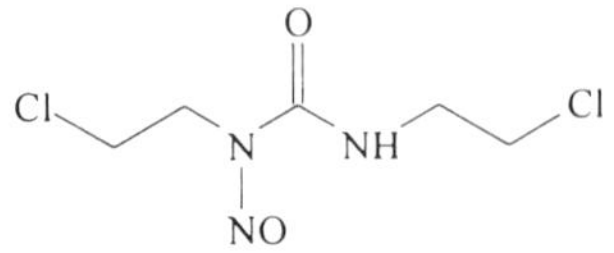

BCNU (*bis*-1,3-(2-chloroethyl)-1-nitrosourea)

$$ClCH_2CH_2SCH_2CH_2Cl$$

bis-chloroethyl sulfide

All of these agents induce covalent damage to biological macromolecules; presumably, the basis of their chemotherapeutic action is a rather nonselective activity against rapidly dividing cells. The bifunctional agents, such as the mustards and platinum compounds [e.g., cisplatin (*cis*-diamminedichloroplatinum(II)) (43)],

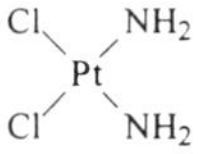

cisplatin

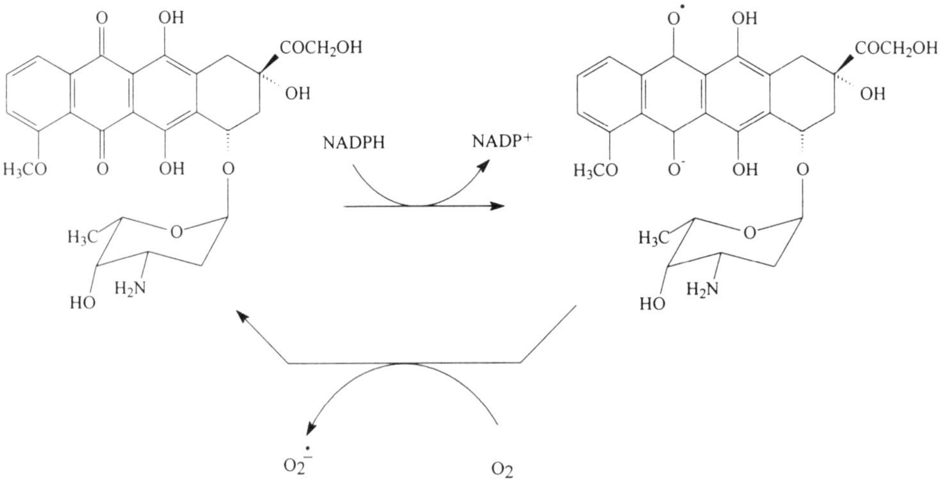

can cause covalent crosslinking of the polynucleotide strands of DNA. Not surprisingly, all of these electrophilic agents can react with GSH, and GSH conjugation may play an important role in their pharmacology. GSH interferes with DNA modification by reacting with the electrophilic functional groups of the drugs. Administration of BSO, which inhibits GSH biosynthesis and therefore lowers the intracellular concentration of GSH, makes tumor cells more sensitive to treatment with these agents.

The cytotoxic effects of anthraquinone drugs, such as adriamycin and doxorubicin [see preceding scheme (44)], probably result from the generation of free radicals and reactive oxygen species by redox cycling mechanisms [(45); see Chapter 4). GSH may counteract toxicity by scavenging free radicals and by reducing hydroperoxides. Although the role of GSH in the inactivation of cytostatic drugs is well established, the contribution of GSTs has been more difficult to assess. In vitro experiments with purified GSTs have demonstrated low but significant enzymatic activities with certain cytostatic drugs. In the case of the human enzymes, the class Alpha GST A1-1 is active with chlorambucil and melphalan, and the class Mu GST M3-3 has activity with BCNU. The low catalytic activity has raised questions about the relative importance of the enzyme-catalyzed and spontaneous reactions. The evidence for an important role of the enzymes includes the observation that tumor cells often express high intracellular concentrations of GSTs, which may compensate for the intrinsically low catalytic activities. Furthermore, acquisition of increased drug resistance is often linked to elevated levels of particular isoenzymes, and in some cases these same enzymes have been found to display catalytic activity with the cytostatic drug under consideration. Transfection of cDNA encoding particular GSTs into tumor cells in vitro provides increased intracellular concentrations of the corresponding enzymes and collateral increase in drug resistance. These findings also support the notion that GSTs contribute to cellular inactivation of cytostatic drugs.

Propenal (*acrolein*) is formed in the metabolic activation of the chemotherapeutic drug *cyclophosphamide*. (Lipid peroxidation also generates propenal and propenedial; see Chapter 7.) Cyclophosphamide is hydroxylated by certain isoenzymes of cytochrome P-450 (46) and acrolein is released when the ultimate cytostatic metabolite, phosphorodiamidate mustard, is formed:

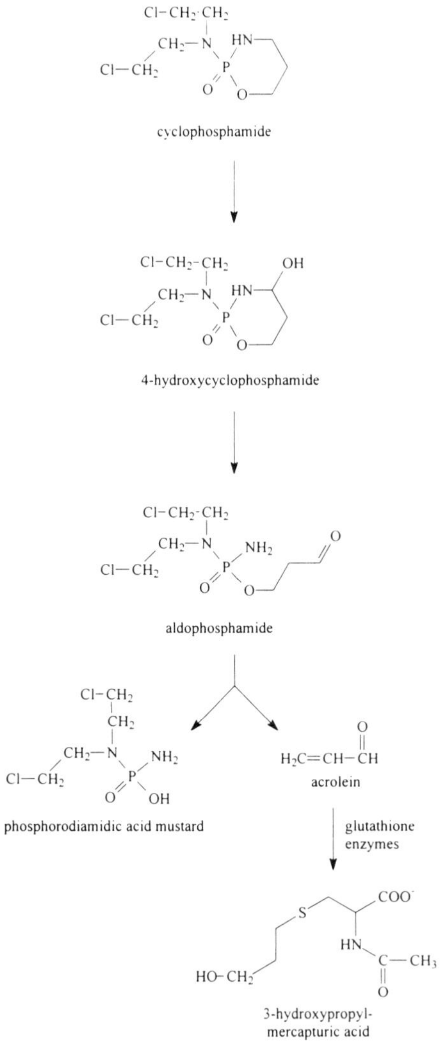

cyclophosphamide

4-hydroxycyclophosphamide

aldophosphamide

phosphorodiamidic acid mustard

$H_2C=CH-CH$
O
acrolein

glutathione
enzymes

3-hydroxypropyl-
mercapturic acid

Base propenals are formed from DNA by chain-breaking radical reactions, and they are formed as products of radiation damage and from the action of the drug *bleomycin* (47):

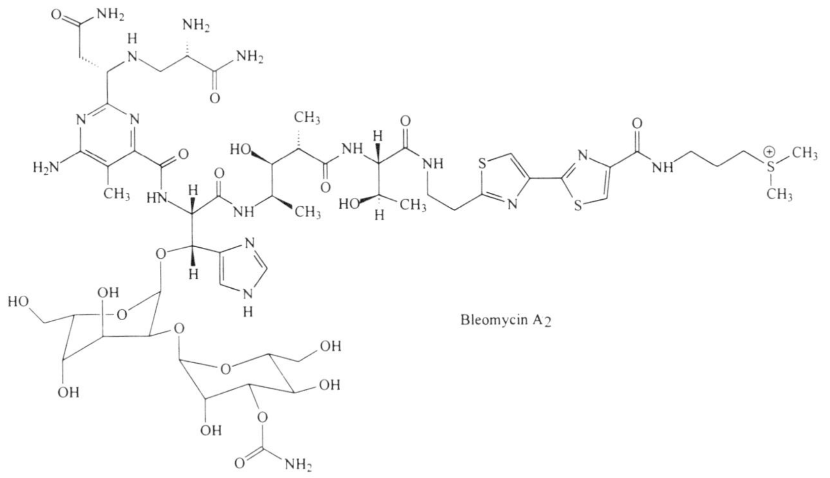

Bleomycin A₂

Propenal and base propenals are cytotoxic compounds that react with DNA and proteins. Both acrolein and the base propenals are among the best substrates known for human GST P1-1, and the enzyme may have evolved to achieve high catalytic efficiency for this group of cytotoxic substances (48). GSTs from other classes also display activity with propenal derivatives, but with considerably lower catalytic efficiencies; an exception is rat GST 8-8 (class Alpha), which is also the most efficient isoenzyme with 4-hydroxyalkenals.

In the presence of molecular oxygen, cells are constantly exposed to free radicals generated by oxidative processes. Lipid peroxidation (see Chapter 7) can give rise to reactive alkenes, such as the α,β-unsaturated carbonyl species. GSTs catalyze the inactivation not only of propenal derivatives but of a whole range of related electrophilic substances, and thus provide protection against their toxic effects (49).

TOXICATION OF XENOBIOTICS BY GLUTATHIONE CONJUGATION

The majority of GSH-linked reactions serve the function of detoxication, but in a limited number of cases, toxicity is increased by formation of a GSH conjugate (50). Let us examine some of these remarkable bioactivations.

1,2-Dibromoethane (ethylene dibromide; EDB) is a volatile compound used as a fumigant and insecticide. The reaction of GSH with vicinal dihaloalkanes such as EDB, catalyzed by GSTs, forms S-(2-haloethyl) conjugates. *These species are sulfur "half-mustards"* (having one chlorinated group rather than two, as in mustard gas). Thus, "lethal synthesis" has taken place, forming a mutagenic and nephrotoxic alkylating agent. The activation of EDB has been elucidated by F. P. Guengerich and colleagues at Vanderbilt University, Tennessee; the EDB-derived DNA adducts have been isolated and characterized. The EDB–GSH conjugate cyclizes to form a strongly alkylating episulfonium ion, which binds to DNA and other cellular targets (51):

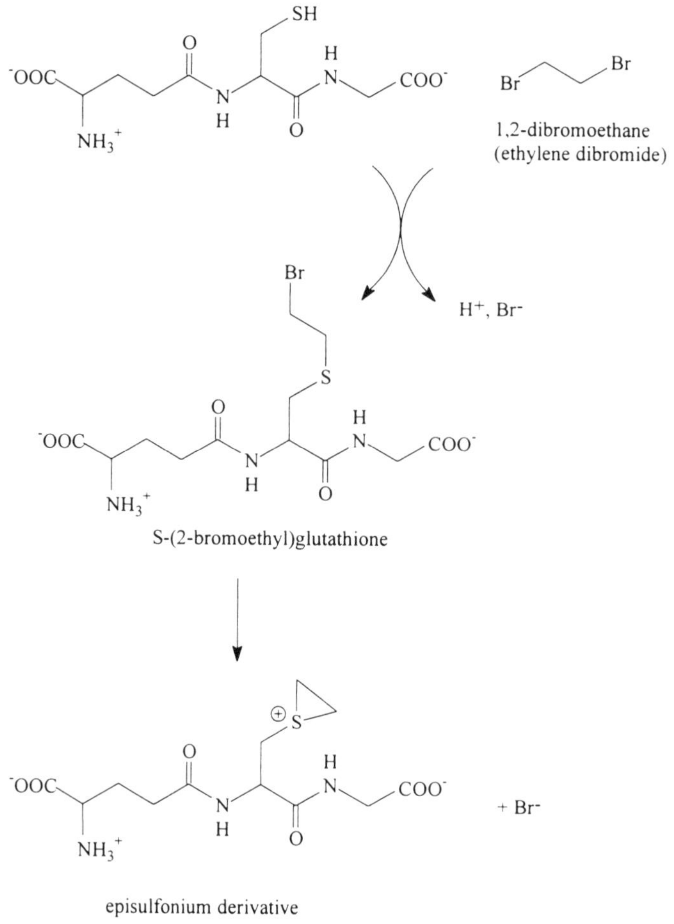
1,2-dibromoethane
(ethylene dibromide)
H+, Br-
S-(2-bromoethyl)glutathione
+ Br-
episulfonium derivative

Although dichloromethane (methylene chloride, a common industrial and laboratory solvent) is far less toxic than carbon tetrachloride or chloroform, its reaction with GSH yields formaldehyde via an intermediate *S*-(chloromethyl)glutathione:

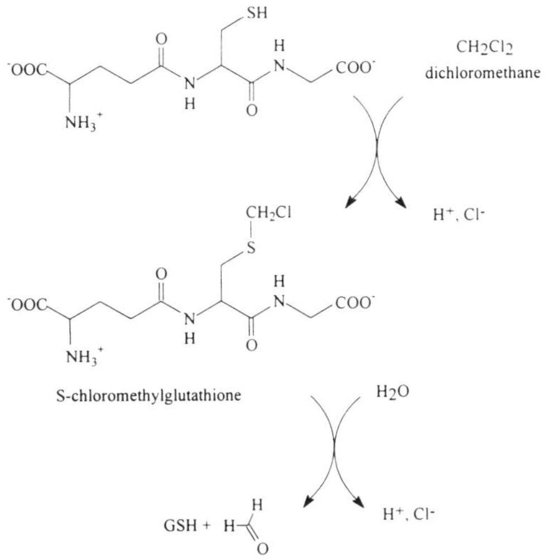

SH

O H

$^-$OOC N N COO$^-$

H

NH$_3$$^+$ O

CH$_2$Cl$_2$
dichloromethane

H$^+$, Cl$^-$

CH$_2$Cl

S

O H

$^-$OOC N N COO$^-$

H

NH$_3$$^+$ O

S-chloromethylglutathione

H$_2$O

H

GSH + H

O

H$^+$, Cl$^-$

Both the GSH conjugate and formaldehyde are reactive and potentially tumorigenic.

Trichloroethylene was once used as an industrial solvent for the extraction of oil from soybean meal. The protein-rich residue was used as cattle feed, until the realization that it induced lethal aplastic anemia in the animals. The toxic agent was isolated and characterized (52) as S-(1,2-dichlorovinyl)-L-cysteine (DCVC) formed by the reaction of the solvent with cysteine residues of the soy protein. (DCVC is also a potent nephrotoxin in rodents.) Chlorinated alkenes, such as trichloroethylene and hexachloro-1,3-butadiene (53), are conjugated to GSH; hepatic microsomal GST catalyzes the conjugation. The action of γ-glutamyltranspeptidase and dipeptidase (the metabolic pathway leading to mercapturic acid formation) form the corresponding cysteine S-conjugates. However, rather than simply being N-acetylated and excreted (see above), the cysteine conjugate is a substrate for the kidney enzyme *cysteine conjugate β-lyase*. This enzyme is pyridoxal phosphate-dependent (54). The chemistry of the reaction is shown below (55):

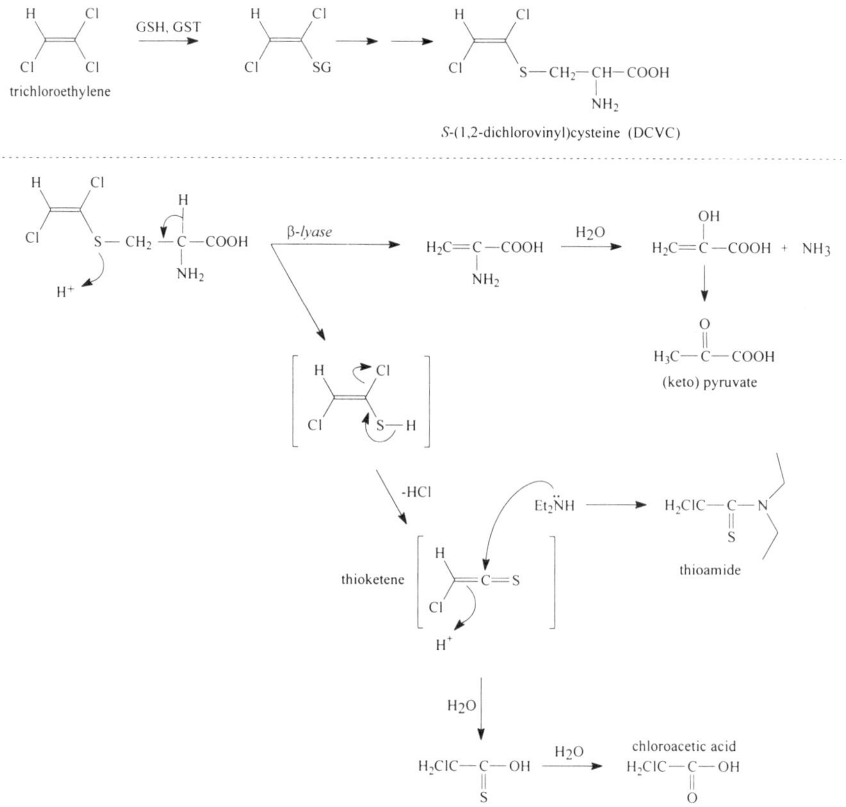

trichloroethylene

GSH, GST

S-(1,2-dichlorovinyl)cysteine (DCVC)

S—CH₂—CH—COOH
       |
      NH₂

β-lyase

H₂C=C—COOH
       |
      NH₂

H₂O

$H_2C=C-COOH$ OH   + NH₃

H₃C—C—COOH
     ‖
     O
(keto) pyruvate

H⁺

[thioketene]

-HCl

Et₂N̈H

H₂ClC—C—N
       ‖
       S
thioamide

H⁺

H₂O

H₂ClC—C—OH
       ‖
       S

H₂O

chloroacetic acid
H₂ClC—C—OH
       ‖
       O

Bioactivation of S-(1,2-dichlorovinyl)-L-cysteine. DCVC is formed by the processing of the glutathione conjugate of trichloroethylene, catalyzed by γ-glutamyltranspeptidase and dipeptidase. The resulting cysteine conjugate is metabolized by cysteine conjugate β-lyase. (Lyases are enzymes that catalyze group eliminations, yielding double bonds.) In this case, the C—S bond β to the cysteine α carbon is broken. The amino acid product hydrolyzes to pyruvate and ammonia. The thiol product loses HCl, generating the reactive chlorothioketene. This species cannot be isolated; its hydrolysis yields, ultimately, chloroacetic acid. Alternatively, the thioketene can be trapped with a nucleophile, such as diethylamine, to give an isolable product (in this case, a thioamide).

The product is a *thioketene* (or, possibly, a closely related species). Thioketenes, like the oxygen analogues, ketenes, are strongly electrophilic agents. The parent molecule, thioketene ($H_2C=C=S$), is unstable, but some hindered analogues, such as di-*tert*-butylthioketene, have been characterized at room temperature (56).

Hydroquinones (see scheme on page 172) and aminophenols, upon oxidation, may give rise to GSH conjugates. The conjugates can undergo redox cycling (see Chapter 4) and consequently give rise to semiquinones, which may initiate radical reactions and consequent oxidative tissue damage. The oxidized counterparts are quinones, which also may cause alkylation of cellular targets.

GLUTATHIONE AND NITRIC OXIDE

The remarkable biological roles of nitric oxide (NO) have been the focus of intense research interest in recent years (57); see Chapter 6. NO is an important biological signal molecule, which is generated directly in certain cells by the action of the enzyme nitric oxide synthase on arginine (58). NO regulates the action of guanylate cyclase and thereby stimulates pharmacological responses, such as the relaxation of vascular smooth muscle. As this muscle relaxes, the blood vessel which it surrounds dilates and blood pressure drops. This action of NO probably explains the long-known pharmacological activity of glyceryltrinitrate (nitroglycerin), a coronary vasodilator, which releases NO in vivo (59).

Organic nitrites and nitrates react with GSH to form *S-nitrosoglutathione* (GSNO). *S*-Nitrosothiols (also called *thionitrites*: $R-S-N=O$, the esters of thionitrous acid, $H-S-N=O$) are isolable, but unstable, compounds; their thermal decomposition gives thiyl radicals (RS$^{\cdot}$) and nitric oxide (NO) (60). *S*-Nitrosothiols, like NO, have vasodilator activity.

MANIPULATION OF GLUTATHIONE TRANSFERASES IN TUMOR CELLS

As noted earlier, cellular resistance to certain drugs can be decreased by lowering the intracellular concentration of GSH. Such sensitization of cells may also affect enzyme-catalyzed drug inactivation, provided that the relevant enzymes are not still saturated with GSH at the lowered GSH concentration. In other words, the effect of an altered GSH concentration will depend on the value of the GSH concentration relative to the corresponding Michaelis constant for the enzyme-catalyzed reaction.

Nevertheless, a more direct way of affecting the rate of an enzyme-catalyzed reaction is to regulate the enzyme activity. Decreased intracellular enzyme activity may be obtained by administration of reversible or irreversible inhibitors or by lowering the concentration of enzyme protein in the target cells. A straightforward method is to administer enzyme inhibitors. Such attempts at *modulating* enzyme activity have been shown to sensitize tumor cells in vitro to treatment with various cytostatic drugs. Several compounds that inhibit GSTs (see below) are effective, but it is not clear that the effect is specific for GSTs and not due to interaction with other GSH-linked enzymes or other unrelated proteins. Modulation is currently considered a promising approach to increase the efficacy of anticancer drugs. In the case that drug resistance can be ascribed to overexpression of a particular enzyme (e.g., a certain isoenzyme of GST), administration of an isoenzyme-specific inhibitor might sensitize a tumor to treatment. Development of such inhibitors is a goal of drug design (61).

Intracellular levels of resistance factors might also be lowered by administration of antisense oligonucleotide derivatives. The antisense molecule is expected to hybridize with specific mRNAs, thereby inhibiting translation as well as increasing the rate of degradation of the mRNA.

Finally, an alternative approach to exploit tumor-specific expression of GSTs in tumor cells is the use of prodrugs that can be activated by the enzyme, expressed at high levels in the tumor. Such "mechanism-based" or "suicide" inhibition exploits the catalytic potential of the enzyme to generate toxic compounds in situ. Release of alkylating agents from glutathione-based prodrugs has been demonstrated recently (62).

INHIBITION OF GLUTATHIONE TRANSFERASES

The recent interest in the role of GSTs in drug resistance has stimulated efforts to identify compounds that can serve as reversible inhibitors or irreversible inactivators of the enzymes.

In a heterodimeric isozyme of cytosolic GSTs, a given subunit is inhibited to the same extent, irrespective of the nature of the neighboring subunit. In particular, a catalytic activity characteristic for one subunit may be selectively inhibited without affecting the activity of the neighboring subunit.

Rational design of GST inhibitors, based on structural similarities to the GSH molecule, has been attempted. Such inhibitors would, of course, be targeted to the G-site and compete with GSH, thereby inhibiting the enzymatic reaction. S-Alkyl GSH derivatives are competitive inhibitors, and they display increased effectiveness with increasing chain length of the S-substituent. Apparently, the S-alkyl group binds to the adjacent hydrophobic H-site of the enzyme, increasing the affinity of the inhibitor for the enzyme.

A serious limitation for the application of inhibitors based on the GSH structure is that GSH does not freely permeate cell membranes, and only a very limited number of cell types have a transport system for uptake of GSH. In order to circumvent this problem, the two carboxyl groups of GSH have been esterified with alcohols such as ethanol. By blocking the negatively charged carboxylate groups, the molecule is made more lipid-soluble than GSH. The compound is more easily taken up by cells, and the ester bonds of the carboxyl groups may be hydrolyzed by intracellular esterases.

In the search for inhibitors, a very wide range of chemical compounds have been investigated (14). For clinical trials aimed at overcoming drug resistance caused by GSTs, particular interest has been directed to compounds that have already been used as drugs, for other applications. By this approach, substances that have already been checked for possible side effects could be accepted for adjuvant treatment during chemotherapy, without having to be subjected to time-consuming toxicological evaluation.

Among such compounds, ethacrynic acid, a diuretic drug, has already been subjected to clinical trial. The compound is a good inhibitor for all GSTs so far investigated, and may also serve as an alternative substrate, in particular for class Pi enzymes (63). In the case of human GST A1-1, the structure of the enzyme-inhibitor complex has been determined by X-ray crystallography (64):

ethacrynic
acid

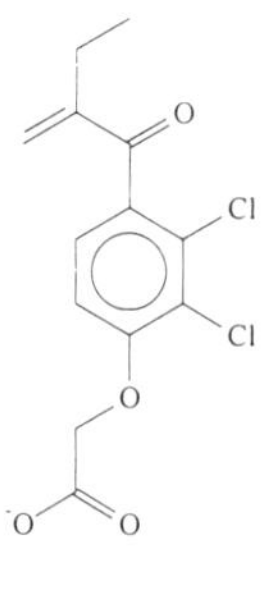

NOTES

1. Larsson, A., Orrenius, S., Holmgren, A., and Mannervik B., Eds., *Functions of Glutathione. Biochemical, Physiological, Toxicological and Clinical Aspects*, Raven Press, New York, 1983; Dolphin, D., Poulson, R., and Avramović, O., Eds., *Glutathione. Chemical, Biochemical, and Medical Aspects*, Parts A and B, Vol. 3, in the series *Coenzymes and Cofactors*, John Wiley & Sons, New York, 1989; Taniguchi, N., Higashi, T., Sakamoto, Y., and Meister, A., Eds. *Glutathione Centennial. Molecular Perspectives and Clinical Implications*, Academic Press, San Diego, 1989; Reed, D. J., Glutathione: Toxicological implications, *Annu. Rev. Pharmacol. Toxicol.* 30:603–631, 1990.

2. Meister, A., Metabolism and function of glutathione, in: *Glutathione: Chemical, Biochemical*

and Medical Aspects, D. Dolphin, R. Poulson, and O. Avramović, Eds., John Wiley & Sons, New York, 1989, Part A, pp. 367–474.

3. Mannervik, B., Carlberg, I., and Larson, K., Glutathione: General review of mechanism of action, in: *Glutathione: Chemical, Biochemical and Medical Aspects*, D. Dolphin, R. Poulson, and O. Avramović, Eds., John Wiley & Sons, New York, 1989, Part A, pp. 475–516.

4. Schirmer, R. H., Krauth-Siegel, R. L., and Schulz, G. E., Glutathione reductase, in: *Glutathione: Chemical, Biochemical and Medical Aspects*, D. Dolphin, R. Poulson, and O. Avramović, Eds., John Wiley & Sons, New York, 1989, Part A, pp. 553–596.

5. Voet, D., and Voet, J. G., *Biochemistry*, 2nd ed., Wiley, New York, 1995, pp. 400–407.

6. Askelöf, P., Axelsson, K., Eriksson, S., and Mannervik, B., Mechanism of action of enzymes catalyzing thiol-disulfide interchange thiol transferases rather than transhydrogenases, *FEBS Lett.* 38:263–267, 1974; Mieyal, J. J., Starke, D. W., Gravina, S. A., Dothey, C., and Chung, J. S., Thioltransferase in human red blood cells: purification and properties, *Biochemistry* 30:6088–6097, 1991; Wells, W. W., Yang, Y., Deits, T. L., and Gan, Z. R., Thioltransferases, *Adv. Enzymol.* 66:149–201, 1993.

7. Mannervik, B., Axelsson, K., Sundewall, A.-C., and Holmgren, A., Relative contributions of thioltransferase- and thioredoxin-dependent systems in reduction of low-molecular-mass and protein disulphides, *Biochem. J.* 213:519–523, 1983.

8. Hwang, C., Sinskey, A. J., and Lodish, H. F., Oxidized redox state of glutathione in the endoplasmic reticulum, *Science* 257:1496–1502, 1992.

9. Sies, H., and Ketterer, B., Eds., *Glutathione Conjugation. Mechanisms and Biological Significance*, Academic Press, San Diego, 1988; Tew, K. D., Pickett, C. B., Mantle, T. J., Mannervik, B., and Hayes, J. D., Eds., *Structure and Function of Glutathione Transferases*, CRC Press, Boca Raton, FL, 1993; Chasseaud, L. F., The role of glutathione and glutathione-*S*-transferases in the metabolism of chemical carcinogens and other electrophilic agents, *Adv. Cancer Res.* 29:175–274, 1979.

10. Söderström, M., Hammarström, S., and Mannervik, B., Leukotriene C synthase in mouse mastocytoma cells. An enzyme distinct from cytosolic and microsomal glutathione transferases, *Biochem. J.* 250:713–718, 1988; Nicholson, D. W., Ambereen, A., Klemba, M. W., Munday, N. A., Zamboni, R. J., and Ford-Hutchinson, A. W., Human leukotriene C_4 synthase expression in dimethyl sulfoxide-differentiated U937 cells, *J. Biol. Chem.* 267:17849–17857, 1992; Lam, B. K., Penrose, J. F., Freeman, G. J., and Austen, K. F., Expression cloning of a cDNA for human leukotriene C_4 synthase, an integral membrane protein conjugating reduced glutathione to leukotriene A_4, *Proc. Natl. Acad. Sci. U.S.A.* 91:7663–7667, 1994.

11. Reviewed in: Ketterer, B., Detoxication reactions of glutathione and glutathione transferases, *Xenobiotica* 16:957–973, 1986.

12. Ji, X., Armstrong, R. N., and Gilliland, G. L., Snapshots along the reaction coordinate of an S_NAr reaction catalyzed by glutathione transferase, *Biochemistry* 32:12949–12954, 1993.

13. Ålin, P., Jensson, H., Guthenberg, C., Danielson, U. H., Tahir, M. K., and Mannervik, B., Purification of major basic glutathione transferase isoenzymes from rat liver by use of affinity chromatography and fast protein liquid chromatofocusing, *Anal. Biochem.* 146:313–320, 1985.

14. Mannervik, B., and Jensson, H., Binary combinations of four protein subunits with different catalytic specificities explain the relationship between six basic glutathione *S*-transferases in rat liver cytosol, *J. Biol. Chem.* 257:9909–9912, 1982; Mannervik, B., and Danielson, U. H., Glutathione transferases—structure and catalytic activity, *CRC Crit. Rev. Biochem.* 23:283–337, 1988.

15. Mannervik, B., and Widersten, M., Human glutathione transferases: classification, tissue distribution, structure, and functional properties, in: *Advances in Drug Metabolism in Man* (G. M. Pacifici and G. N. Fracchia, eds.), European Commission, Luxembourg, 1995, pp. 407–459.

16. Mannervik, B., Ålin, P., Guthenberg, C., Jensson, H., Tahir, M. K., Warholm, M., and Jörnvall, H., Identification of three classes of cytosolic glutathione transferase common to several mammalian species: correlation between structural data and enzymatic properties, *Proc. Natl. Acad. Sci. U.S.A.* 82:7202–7206, 1985.

17. Jakoby, W. B., Ketterer, B., and Mannervik, B., Glutathione transferases: nomenclature, *Biochem. Pharmacol.* 33:2539–2540, 1984.

18. Mannervik, B., Awasthi, Y. C., Board, P. G., Hayes, J. D., Di Ilio, C., Ketterer, B., Listowsky, I., Morgenstern, R., Muramatsu, M., Pearson, W. R., Pickett, C. B., Sato, K., Widersten, M., and Wolf, C. R., Nomenclature for human glutathione transferases, *Biochem. J.* 282:305–306, 1992.

19. Tahir, M. K., and Mannervik, B., Simple inhibition studies for distinction between homodimeric and heterodimeric isoenzymes of glutathione transferase, *J. Biol. Chem.* 261:1048–1051, 1986.

20. Dirr, H., Reinemer, P., and Huber, R., X-ray crystal structures of cytosolic glutathione *S*-transferases—Implications for protein architecture, substrate recognition and catalytic function, *Eur. J. Biochem.* 220:645–661, 1994.

21. Sinning, I., Kleywegt, G. J., Cowan, S. W., Reinemer, P., Dirr, H. W., Huber, R., Gilliland, G. L., Armstrong, R. N., Ji, X., Board, P. G., Olin, B., Mannervik, B., and Jones, T. A., Structure determination and refinement of human alpha class glutathione transferase A1-1, and a comparison with the mu and pi class enzymes, *J. Mol. Biol.* 232:192–212, 1993.

22. Fahey, R. C., and Sundquist, A. R., Evolution of glutathione metabolism, *Adv. Enzymol. Relat. Areas Mol. Biol.* 64:1–53, 1991.

23. Lewin, B., *Genes V*, Oxford University Press, New York, 1994, pp. 984–985.

24. Warholm, M., Guthenberg, C., and Mannervik, B., Molecular and catalytic properties of glutathione transferase μ from human liver: an enzyme efficiently conjugating epoxides, *Biochemistry* 22:3610–3617, 1983.

25. Widersten, M., Pearson, W. R., Engström, Å., and Mannervik, B., Heterologous expression of the allelic variant Mu-class glutathione transferase μ and ψ, *Biochem. J.* 276:519–524, 1991.

26. Pearson, W. R., Xu, S., Vorachek, W. R., and Patterson, D., The organisation of human class-Mu glutathione transferase genes *GST M1-GST M5* on chromosome 1p13, in: *Structure and Function of Glutathione Transferases*, K. D. Tew, C. B. Pickett, T. J. Mantle, B. Mannervik, and J. D. Hayes, Eds., CRC Press, Boca Raton, FL, 1993, pp. 279–293.

27. Katoh, T., Inatomi, H., Nagaoka, A., and Sugita, A., Cytochrome P4501A1 gene polymorphism and homozygous deletion of the glutathione S-transferase M1 gene in urothelial cancer patients, *Carcinogenesis* 16:655–657, 1995.

28. Hatayama, I., Satoh, K., and Sato, K., Developmental and hormonal regulation of the major form of hepatic glutathione S-transferase in male mice, *Biochem. Biophys. Res. Commun.* 140:581–588, 1986.

29. Staffas, L., Mankowitz, L., Söderström, M., Blanck, A., Porsch-Hällström, I., Sundberg, C., Mannervik, B., Olin, B., Rydström, J., and DePierre, J. W., Further characterization of hormonal regulation of glutathione transferase in rat liver and adrenal glands. Sex differences and demonstration that growth hormone regulates the hepatic levels, *Biochem. J.* 286:65–72, 1992; Mankowitz, L., Castro, V. M., Mannervik, B., Rydström, J., and DePierre, J. W., Increase in the amount of glutathione transferase 4-4 in the rat adrenal gland after hypophysectomy and down-regulation by subsequent treatment with adrenocorticotropic hormone, *Biochem. J.* 265:147–154, 1990.

30. Dostal, L. A., Guthenberg, C., Mannervik, B., and Bend, J. R., Stereoselectivity and regioselectivity of purified human glutathione transferases π, α–ϵ, and μ with alkene and polycyclic arene oxide substrates, *Drug Metab. Dispos.* 16:420–424, 1988.

31. Robertson, I. G. C., Guthenberg, C., Mannervik, B., and Jernström, B., Differences in stereoselectivity and catalytic efficiency of three human glutathione transferases in the conjugation of glutathione with $7\beta,8\alpha$-dihydroxy-$9\alpha,10\alpha$-oxy-7,8,9,10-tetrahydrobenzo(*a*)pyrene. *Cancer Res.* 46:2220–2224, 1986.

32. Busby, W. F., Jr., and Wogan, G. N., Aflatoxins, in: *Chemical Carcinogens*, 2nd ed. C. E. Searle, Ed., pp. 945–1136, American Chemical Society, Washington, D.C., 1984; Shibamoto, T., and Bjeldanes, L. F., *Introduction to Food Toxicology*, Academic Press, New York, 1993, pp. 103–110.

33. Hayes, J. D., Judah, D. J., McLellan, L. I., and Neal, G. E., Contribution of the glutathione *S*-transferases to the mechanisms of resistance to aflatoxin B_1, *Pharmacol. Ther.* 50:443–472, 1991.

34. Blair, I. A., Boobis, A. R., and Davies, D. S., Paracetamol oxidation: Synthesis and reactivity of *N*-acetyl-*p*-benzoquinoneimine, *Tetrahedron Lett.* 21:4947–4950, 1980.

35. McGirr, L. G., Subrahmanyam, V. V., Moore, G. A., and O'Brien, P. J., Peroxidase-catalyzed 3-glutathion-*S*-yl-*p,p*'-biphenol formation, *Chem. Biol. Interact.* 60:85–99, 1986.

36. Hoffman, K.-J., Streeter, A. J., Axworthy, D. B., and Baillie, T. A., Identification of the major covalent adduct formed in vitro and in vivo between acetaminophen and mouse liver proteins, *Mol. Pharmacol.* 27:566–573, 1985.

37. Savides, M. C., Oehme, F. W., Nash, S. L., and Leipold, H. W., The toxicity and biotransformation of single doses of acetaminophen in dogs and cats, *Toxicol. Appl. Pharmacol.* 74:26–34, 1984.

38. Hazelton, G. A., Hjelle, J. J., and Klaassen, C. D., Effects of cysteine pro-drugs on acetaminophen-induced hepatoxicity, *J. Pharmacol. Exp. Ther.* 237:341–349, 1986.

39. Ware, G. W., *Pesticides: Theory and Application*, W. H. Freeman, San Francisco, 1983, p. 162.

40. Fox, M., and Scott, D., The genetic toxicology of nitrogen and sulfur mustard, *Mutat. Res.* 75:131–168, 1980; Niculescu-Duvăz, I., Baracu, I., and Balaban, A. T., Alkylating agents, in: D. E. V. Wilman, Ed., *The Chemistry of Antitumour Agents*, Chapman and Hall, New York, 1990, pp. 62–130.

41. Montgomery, J. A., and Johnston, T. P., Nitrosoureas, in: *The Chemistry of Antitumour Agents*, D. E. V. Wilman, Ed., Chapman and Hall, New York, 1990, pp. 131–158.

42. Smith, M. T., Evans, C. G., Doane-Setzer, P., Castro, V. M., Tahir, M. K., and Mannervik, B., Denitrosation of 1,3-*bis*(2-chloroethyl)-1-nitrosourea by class Mu glutathione transferases and its role in cellular resistance in rat brain tumor cells, *Cancer Res.* 49:2621–2625, 1989.

43. Abrams, M. J., The chemistry of platinum antitumour agents, in: D. E. V. Wilman, Ed., *The Chemistry of Antitumour Agents*, Chapman and Hall, New York, 1990, pp. 331–341.

44. Suarato, A., Antitumour anthracyclines, in: *The Chemistry of Antitumour Agents*, D. E. V. Wilman, Ed., Chapman and Hall, New York, 1990, pp. 30–62.

45. Myers, C., Gianni, L., Zweier, J., Muindi, J., Sinha, B. K., and Eliot, H., Role of iron in adriamycin biochemistry, *Fed. Proc.* 45:2792–2797, 1986.

46. Dirven, H. A. A. M., van Ommen, B., and van Bladeren, P. J., Glutathione conjugation of alkylating cytostatic drugs with a nitrogen mustard group and the role of glutathione S-transferases, *Chem. Res. Toxicol.* 9:351–360, 1996.

47. Hecht, S. M., The chemistry of activated bleomycin, in: *The Chemistry of Antitumour Agents*, D. E. V. Wilman, Ed., Chapman and Hall, New York, 1990, pp. 395–402.

48. Berhane, K., Widersten, M., Engström, Å., Kozarich, J. W., and Mannervik, B., Detoxication of base propenals and other α,β-unsaturated aldehyde products of radical reactions and lipid peroxidation by human glutathione transferases, *Proc. Natl. Acad. Sci. U.S.A.* 91:1480–1484, 1994.

49. Stenberg, G., Ridderström, M., Engström, Å., Pemble, S. E., and Mannervik, B., Cloning and heterologous expression of cDNA encoding class Alpha rat glutathione transferase 8-8, an enzyme with high catalytic activity towards genotoxic α,β-unsaturated carbonyl compounds, *Biochem. J.* 284:313–319, 1992.

50. Dekant, W., and Vamvakas, S., Glutathione-dependent bioactivation of xenobiotics, *Xenobiotica* 23:873–887, 1993; Monks, T. J., Anders, M. W., Dekant, W., Stevens, J. L., Lau, S. S., and Van Bladeren, P. J., Glutathione conjugate mediated toxicities, *Toxicol. Appl. Pharmacol.* 106:1–19, 1990; Anders, M. W., and Dekant, W., Eds., *Conjugation-Dependent Carcinogenicity and Toxicity of Foreign Compounds, Advances in Pharmacology*, Vol. 27, Academic Press, New York, 1994; Rannug, U., Sundvall, A., and Ramel, C., The mutagenic effect of 1,2-dichloroethane on *Salmonella typhimurium*. I. Activation through conjugation with glutathione in vitro, *Chem.-Biol. Interact.* 20:1–16, 1978.

51. Cmarik, J. L., Humphreys, W. G., Bruner, K. L., Lloyd, R. S., Tibbetts, C., and Guengerich, F. P., Mutation spectrum and sequence alkylation selectivity resulting from modification of bacteriophage M13mp18 DNA with *S*-(2-chloroethyl)glutathione. Evidence for a role of *S*-(2-N7-guanylethyl)glutathione as a mutagenic lesion formed from ethylene dibromide, *J. Biol. Chem.* 267:6672–6679, 1992.

52. McKinney, L. L., Picken, J. C., Jr., Weakley, F. B., Eldridge, A. C., Campbell, R. E., Cowan, J. C., and Biester, H. E., Possible toxic factor of trichloroethylene-extracted soybean oil meal, *J. Am. Chem. Soc.* 81:909–915, 1959.

53. Dekant, W., Vamvakas, S., and Anders, M. W., Bioactivation of hexachlorobutadiene by glutathione conjugation, *Food Chem. Toxicol.* 28:285–293, 1990.

54. Lash, L. H., Nelson, R. M., Van Dyke, R. A., and Anders, M. W., Purification and characterization of human kidney cytosolic cysteine conjugate beta-lyase activity, *Drug Metab. Dispos.* 18:50–54, 1990.

55. Patel, N., Birner, G., Dekant, W., Anders, M. W., Glutathione-dependent biosynthesis and bioactivation of *S*-(1,2-dichlorovinyl)glutathione and *S*-(1,2-dichlorovinyl)-L-cysteine, the glutathione and cysteine *S*-conjugates of dichloroacetylene, in rat tissues and subcellular fractions, *Drug Metab. Dispos.* 22:143–147, 1994.

56. Elam, E. U., Rash, F. H., Dougherty, J. T., Goodlett, V. W., and Brannock, K. C., Di-*t*-butyl-thioketene, *J. Org. Chem.* 33:2738–2741, 1968.

57. Galla, H.-J., Nitric oxide, NO, an intercellular messenger, *Angew. Chem. (Engl.)* 32:378–380, 1993; Stamler, J. S., Singel, D. J., and Loscalzo, J., Biochemistry of nitric oxide and its redox-activated forms, *Science* 258:1898–1902, 1992.

58. Marletta, M. A., Nitric oxide synthase: Structure and mechanism, *J. Biol. Chem.* 268:12231–12234, 1993.

59. Smith, R. P., and Wilcox, D. E., Toxicology of selected nitric oxide-donating xenobiotics, with particular reference to azide, *Crit. Rev. Toxicol.* 24:355–377, 1994.

60. Mathews, W. R., and Kerr, S. W., Biological activity of *S*-nitrosothiols: The role of nitric oxide, *J. Pharmacol. Exp. Ther.* 267:1529–1537, 1993; Josephy, P. D., Rehorek, D., and Janzen, E. G., Electron spin resonance spin trapping of thiyl radicals from the decomposition of thionitrites, *Tetrahedron Lett.* 25:1685–1688, 1984.

61. Lyttle, M. H., Hocker, M. D., Hui, H. C., Caldwell, C. G., Aron, D. T., Engqvist-Goldstein, Å., Flatgaard, J. E., and Bauer, K. E., Isoenzyme-specific glutathione *S*-transferase inhibitors: design and synthesis, *J. Med. Chem.* 37:189–194, 1994.

62. Lyttle, M. H., Satyam, A., Hocker, M. D., Bauer, K. E., Caldwell, C. G., Hui, H. C., Morgan, A. S., Mergia, A., and Kauvar, L. M., Glutathione S-transferase activates novel alkylating agents, *J. Med. Chem.* 37:1501–1507, 1994.

63. Ranganathan, S., Ciaccio, P. J., and Tew, K. D., Principles of drug modulation applied to glutathione *S*-transferases, in: *Structure and Function of Glutathione Transferases*, K. D. Tew, C. B. Pickett, T. J. Mantle, B. Mannervik, and J. D. Hayes, Eds., CRC Press, Boca Raton, FL, 1993, pp. 249–256; Hansson, J., Berhane, K., Castro, V. M., Jungnelius, U., Mannervik, B., and Ringborg, U., Sensitization of human melanoma cells to the cytotoxic effect of melphalan by the glutathione transferase inhibitor ethacrynic acid, *Cancer Res.* 51:94–98, 1991.

64. Cameron, A. D., Sinning, I., L'Hermite, G., Olin, B., Board, P. G., Mannervik, B., and Jones, T. A., Structural analysis of human alpha-class glutathione transferase Al-1 in the apo form and in complex with ethacrynic acid and its glutathione conjugate, *Structure*, 3:717–727, 1995.

12

ARYLAMINE *N*-ACETYLTRANSFERASE

The next phase II enzyme we will discuss is arylamine *N*-acetyltransferase (1). The enzyme was originally characterized on the basis of acetyl coenzyme A-dependent arylamine *N*-acetylation activity, but identical or related enzymes also carry out acetyl coenzyme A-dependent *O*-acetylation of hydroxylamines and acetyl coenzyme A-independent acetyl transfer:

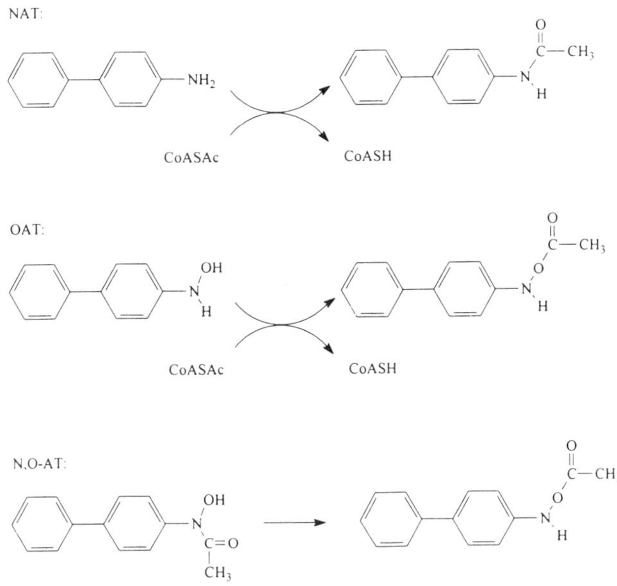

The first of these activities, arylamine *N*-acetyltransferase, is of great pharmacokinetic significance. *N*-Acetylation is a major metabolic route of a wide variety of compounds: natural products, such as caffeine; commercially important synthetic intermediates, such as the carcinogens, benzidine, and β-naphthylamine; the potently mutagenic food pyrolysis product heterocyclic amines; and widely used drugs, including isoniazid, sulfamethazine, and procainamide:

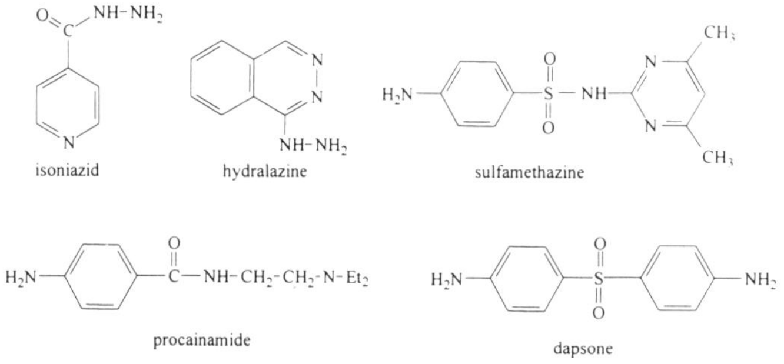

isoniazid   hydralazine   sulfamethazine

procainamide   dapsone

We will return to consideration of many of these compounds in Chapter 20. The hy-droxylamine *O*-acetylation and acetyl transfer reactions also play key roles in aromatic amine activation and are discussed again later.

Individual humans vary greatly in their metabolic capacity to acetylate aromatic amine substrates. This variation in acetylation rates does not follow a simple normal distribution (bell-shaped curve). Instead, the population is divided into "slow" and "fast" acetylators. The molecular basis of this genetic acetylation polymorphism has been elucidated in the last few years. We will return to the molecular biology of *N*-acetyltransferase later in this chapter. First, let's consider the enzymology of the reaction.

ACETYL CoA: ARYLAMINE *N*-ACETYLTRANSFERASE: ASSAY

The conversion of aromatic amines to aromatic amides (see first scheme in this chapter) can be assayed in various ways. For example, the colorimetric reagent dimethyl-aminobenzaldehyde (DMAB) reacts with aromatic amines, but not aromatic amides, to form a yellow Schiff base product; see scheme, p. 190. Thus, the progress of the enzy-matic reaction can be measured by incubating substrate, enzyme source, and acetyl CoA, removing aliquots from the reaction mix at appropriate time intervals and measuring the remaining substrate colorimetrically. Alternatively, high-performance liquid chromatog-raphy (HPLC) can be used to separate and quantitate the substrate and product. With di-amino substrates, such as benzidine (diaminobiphenyl), the latter technique is required, since the reaction occurs in two stages:

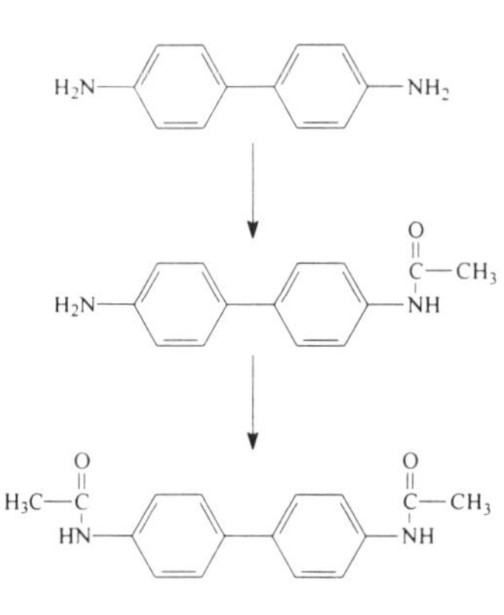

The first metabolite, *N*-acetylbenzidine, also reacts with DMAB, so the colorimetric assay is inappropriate. The mono- and diacetylated products can easily be separated by HPLC.

Acetyl CoA-Dependent *O*-Acetylation of Hydroxylamines

This reaction is also acetyl CoA-dependent; the product is a reactive *N*-acetoxy ester (see further discussion in Chapter 20) which binds spontaneously to nucleic acids in vitro. Therefore, this activity can be assayed by incubating a radiolabeled hydroxylamine substrate (such as [^{3}H]-*N*-OH-aminofluorene), enzyme, acetyl CoA, and calf-thymus DNA. (tRNA can also be used.) After stopping the reaction, the DNA is isolated, and covalent binding of substrate is measured by scintillation counting (2).

Acetyl CoA-Independent Acetyl Transfer

This reaction generates the same reactive intermediate as does acetyl CoA-dependent *O*-acetylation (above) and is assayed similarly. However, the radiolabeled substrate used is [^{3}H]-*N*-OH-acetylaminofluorene, and acetyl CoA is *omitted* from the incubation (3).

ARYLAMINE *N*-ACETYLTRANSFERASES: PURIFICATION

Arylamine *N*-acetyltransferases are cytoplasmic enzymes with relative molecular masses of 33–34 kD. They have been purified from the liver homogenates of pigeons, chickens, hamsters, mice, rats, rabbits, and humans. Purification is hampered by the instability of functional enzyme and by the low abundance of the enzyme proteins, even in tissues where the catalytic activity is high. In humans, *N*-acetyltransferase proteins make up less than 1/20,000 of the total cytoplasmic protein by weight. An NAT enzyme was purified about 1000-fold from human liver cytosol by a series of purification steps, including ammonium sulfate precipitation, anion exchange, hydroxyapatite, gel filtration, and Coenzyme A-Sepharose affinity chromatography. As the guide to purification, an HPLC assay was used, measuring formation of the *N*-acetylated metabolite of sulfamethazine (see structure on page 188). Preparative sodium dodecyl sulfate–polyacrylamide gel electrophoresis (SDS-PAGE) yielded protein sufficient for amino acid sequence determination of selected tryptic peptides (4).

In human liver, two distinct sulfamethazine-acetylating activities (NAT2A and NAT2B) are separable by anion-exchange chromatography. These forms likely arise from the same primary gene product via as-yet-uncharacterized posttranslational modifications. When substrates such as *p*-aminobenzoic acid (PABA) are used, a third, more labile acetyltransferase can be detected (5). This PABA-specific enzyme has been designated NAT1.

ARYLAMINE *N*-ACETYLTRANSFERASES: MECHANISM

The carbonyl C=O bond of an acetate oxy-ester is polarized, such that the carbonyl carbon is electrophilic; in the case of a thioester, the electrophilicity of the carbonyl carbon is much greater. The acetylation reaction is a nucleophilic displacement on the carbonyl carbon, with coenzyme A thiolate anion as the leaving group. An active cysteine thiolate residue of the arylamine *N*-acetyltransferase is involved in catalysis; see scheme B, p. 190. This was first suggested by biochemical studies of the purified rabbit liver enzyme

(6) and supported by site-directed mutagenesis experiments, discussed later, which pinpoint the particular cysteine residue required for catalytic activity. In the biochemical approach, the enzyme was irreversibly inhibited by treatment with either of the electrophilic reagents, iodoacetate or bromoacetanilide (see scheme C):

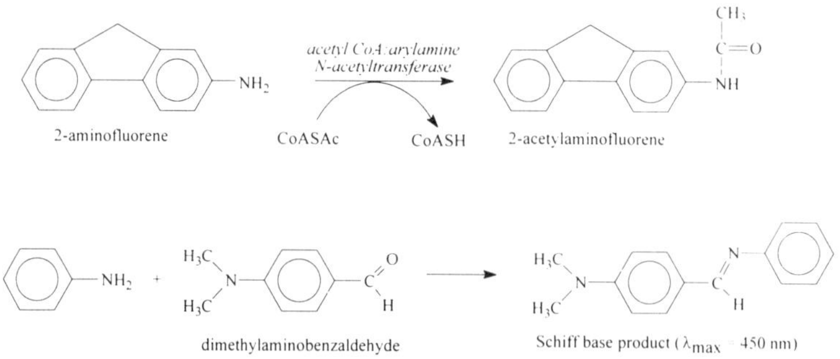

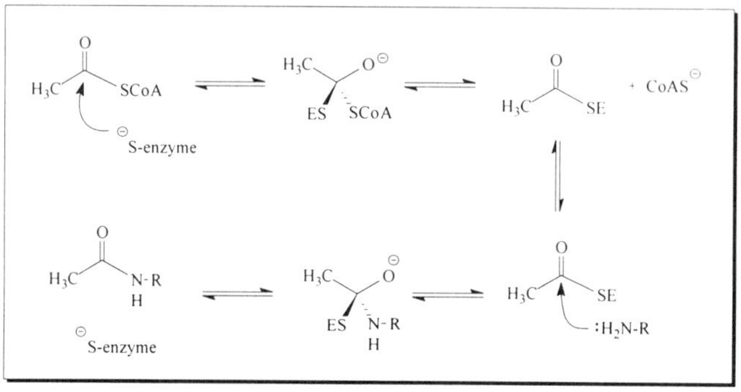

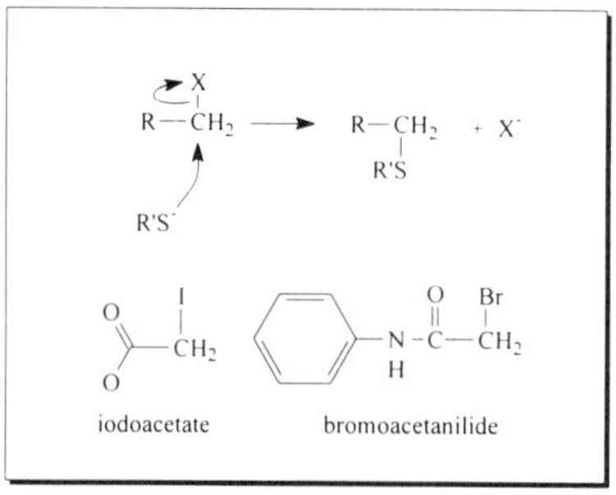

The first of these reagents is often used to modify, selectively, the nucleophilic thiol groups of cysteine residues. Bromoacetanilide was designed as an "affinity alkylator"; that is, an alkylating agent (bromoacyl group) is incorporated into a product analogue (arylamide), which may be expected to bind with high affinity to the enzyme. Indeed, treatment of the enzyme with one-half equivalent of inhibitor resulted in loss of about half of the enzyme activity, consistent with a 1:1 stoichiometric alkylation of the enzyme by the inhibitor, such that *each alkylation event inactivates one molecule of enzyme*. The selective modification of cysteine was proven by amino acid analysis, which showed the loss of one of the five moles of cysteine residues in the protein following treatment with bromoacetanilide.

If an active cysteine residue is involved in catalysis, then the "ping-pong" mechanism shown in the scheme above appears reasonable. First, the enzyme attacks acetyl CoA to form an acyl–enzyme intermediate. Second, the nucleophile (aromatic amine) attacks the acyl–enzyme intermediate, yielding the product amide and the free enzyme. Can the acyl–enzyme intermediate be isolated? Enzyme was incubated with [2-^{3}H]acetyl coenzyme A for 5 min, in the absence of aromatic amine substrate, in the hope that a radiolabeled protein fraction corresponding to the acetyl–enzyme intermediate could be obtained. However, this was unsuccessful; presumably, in the absence of an amine as acceptor, the intermediate is rapidly hydrolyzed to liberate the acyl group as acetate anion. In a second approach, the same incubation was carried out, but the reaction was stopped by addition of 1% SDS solution, quickly denaturing the enzyme. Under these conditions, the acyl–enzyme intermediate could be detected, following separation of the excess radiolabeled CoASAc from the enzyme, by Sephadex G-50 gel filtration chromatography. (This gel separates in the molecular-weight range of 1.5 to 30 kD, so the CoASAc is retained on the column while the enzyme passes through near the void volume.)

ARYLAMINE *N*-ACETYLTRANSFERASE: DISTRIBUTION

The enzyme activity may be very widely distributed throughout the biological world, since it is found in the enterobacterium *Salmonella typhimurium* (7) as well as in humans. The gene was first cloned in that species. On the other hand, there is no detectable NAT enzyme activity in *Escherichia coli. nat⁻* mutants of *S. typhimurium* do not show any obvious growth defects, such as auxotrophies, so the physiological role of the bacterial enzyme remains a mystery. There are no reports of the activity in plants, but this may be "absence of evidence" rather than evidence of absence.

ARYLAMINE *N*-ACETYLTRANSFERASES: HUMAN POLYMORPHISMS

The relevance of experimental studies of hydrazine toxicology suddenly came into focus in the 1950s, when *isoniazid* (isonicotinic hydrazide) was discovered to be a highly effective treatment for tuberculosis ("consumption"). Tuberculosis is a lung infection caused by the bacterium *Mycobacterium tuberculosis*. No medical treatment was available, other than rest and fresh air. The prognosis was very poor. A compelling description of the sense of horror accompanying the diagnosis of tuberculosis was written by the physicist Richard Feynman, whose wife died of the disease in the 1940s (8). The first successful use of isoniazid (9) caused a sensation, similar to the impact of Banting's demonstration of insulin as a treatment for diabetes in 1921.

Very soon after the introduction of isoniazid therapy, clinicians noticed that, occasionally, patients receiving the drug developed peripheral neuropathy, a toxic response characterized by tingling and numbness in the fingers and toes. This problem prompted a careful analysis of the disposition of isoniazid. Histograms of patients' plasma drug concentrations, following a single oral dose of isoniazid, were bimodal; that is, the patient population can be divided phenotypically into *rapid* and *slow* eliminators of the drug. Family studies verified the genetic basis of this polymorphism. The ability to eliminate isoniazid appeared to be a simple Mendelian trait, controlled by the action of two major alleles at a single autosomal gene locus; rapid elimination is genetically dominant. (Later methods allow discrimination among homozygous slow, homozygous rapid, and heterozygous acetylator phenotypes, so the rapid acetylator allele is better described as *codominant* rather than dominant.) Ethnic differences were observed in the proportions of rapid and slow isoniazid eliminators. Caucasian groups in Europe and North America are about equally divided between fast and slow eliminators. Inuit (Eskimo) and Oriental populations have much lower frequencies (as low as 5%) of slow eliminators; North African Arab and sub-Saharan African populations have much higher frequencies (up to 90%).

Isoniazid is eliminated from the body largely as *N*-acetylisoniazid, and the slow excretion phenotype is caused by a reduced rate of isoniazid *N*-acetylation by liver NAT. Moreover, *there is a significant association between the slow acetylator phenotype and the occurrence of neurological side effects*, presumably because "normal" dosing regimens lead to the accumulation of the drug to toxic levels in slow excretors.

(Unfortunately, despite the success of isoniazid therapy, the problem of tuberculosis has become resurgent in the 1990s. This has resulted from several factors. Even in countries where the disease has become rare among the general population, some groups remain at very high risk, due to poverty and inadequate medical care. In 1992, the rate of tuberculosis among status Indians in Canada was more than 40 times higher than among nonaboriginals (10). Second, patients with AIDS are very susceptible to tuberculosis. Also, isoniazid-resistant strains of the disease have emerged.)

During the following decades, many studies documented that this *N*-acetylation polymorphism produces marked interindividual variations in the disposition of aromatic amine and hydrazine drugs and environmental chemicals; some of these compounds are shown on page 188. The clinical and toxicological consequences of this variation have also been studied (11). For example, procainamide therapy for cardiac arrhythmias and hydralazine treatment for hypertension sometimes induce a mimic of systemic *lupus erythematosus*, an autoimmune disease characterized by skin rash, erythema (reddening) on the nose and face, and impaired functioning of the heart and lungs. Many different drugs, especially aromatic amines and hydrazines, can induce lupus. The slow acetylator phenotype is associated with a higher incidence or earlier onset of this adverse drug reaction (12). Drug-induced lupus may be a consequence of oxidative bioactivation of the parent drug, catalyzed by neutrophil myeloperoxidase (see Chapter 6). One proposed mechanism for drug-induced lupus hypothesizes that the activated form of the drug binds to a particular cellular protein, converting it into an altered form, which induces an autoimmune reaction (13). Presumably, the acetylated form of the drug is not a substrate for oxidation by myeloperoxidase.

Several epidemiological studies have suggested that the slow acetylator phenotype is a significant risk factor for the occurrence of bladder cancer, especially in individuals who are occupationally exposed to aromatic amine carcinogens (see Chapter 20). However, the correlation remains controversial (14). The role of *N*-acetyltransferases in pathways of metabolic activation/detoxication of aromatic amine carcinogens are discussed in greater detail in Chapter 20.

In response to the clinical importance of the acetylation polymorphism, numerous methods have been devised in order to determine acetylator phenotype in individuals. These methods involve the administration of low doses of "probe drugs," from whose pharmacokinetic profile, or pattern of urinary metabolite excretion, estimates of *N*-acetyltransferase enzyme activity can be made. Isoniazid, sulfamethazine, procainamide, and dapsone (see structures on page 188) have been used for this purpose. One of the many biotransformation pathways of caffeine depends on the same polymorphic enzyme.

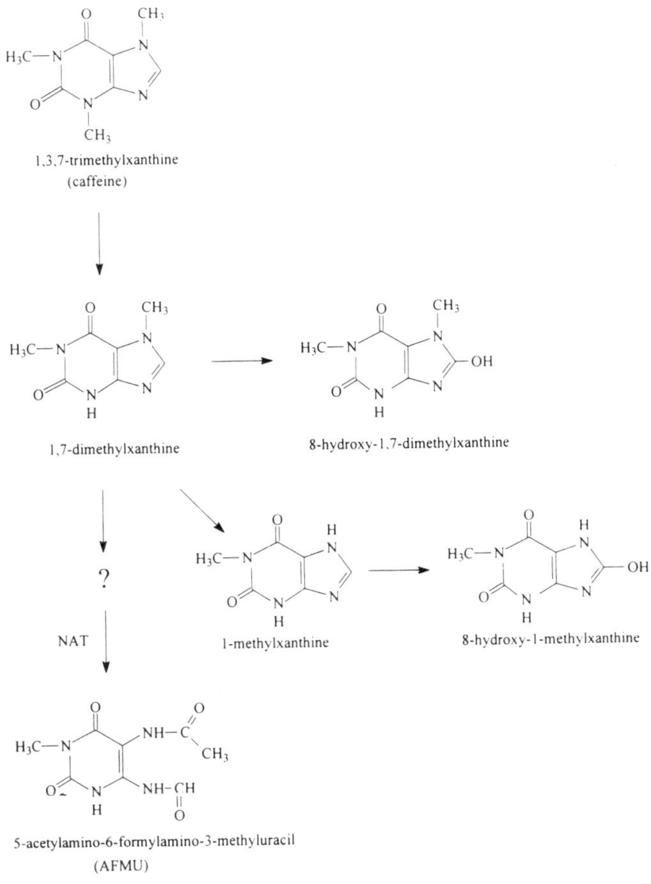

1,3,7-trimethylxanthine
(caffeine)

1,7-dimethylxanthine

8-hydroxy-1,7-dimethylxanthine

?

NAT

1-methylxanthine

8-hydroxy-1-methylxanthine

5-acetylamino-6-formylamino-3-methyluracil
(AFMU)

This has led to a simple test for determining acetylator phenotype, based upon the molar ratio of 5-acetylamino-6-formylamino-3-methyluracil (AFMU) to 1-methylxanthine excreted after administration of a dose of caffeine (15). This test has been widely applied in clinical and epidemiological studies. The use of molecular techniques to determine acetylator *genotype* is discussed below.

SIDEBAR: CAFFEINE

Caffeine (1,3,7-trimethylxanthine) is probably the world's most popular natural-product stimulant, consumed in tea, coffee, and caffeinated soft drinks, as well as in non-prescription pills for combating headache and drowsiness. A cup of tea or coffee can contain 100 mg or more caffeine. Since caffeine contributes little to the flavor and aroma of coffee, but can disturb sleep, there is much demand for caffeine-free coffee. Caffeine can be removed from the green coffee beans by solvent extraction with methylene chloride. Since the solvent is volatile, virtually all traces are removed by the subsequent roasting process. Another decaffeination method ("Swiss water process") uses water extraction followed by activated charcoal filtration. In Germany, supercritical carbon dioxide is used for the extraction. All these methods remove caffeine very effectively, but they also remove many of the volatile and organic-soluble compounds responsible for the flavor of the drink, so decaffeinated coffee tends to be bland-tasting. Caffeine is metabolized by *N*-demethylation [catalyzed by P4501A2 and P4502E1 (see Chapter 14)] and *N*-acetylation.

MOLECULAR GENETICS OF *N*-ACETYLTRANSFERASES

The molecular basis of the drug acetylation polymorphism has been firmly established in the past few years (16). One of the puzzling features of the story had been the observation that several aromatic amines (including PABA)

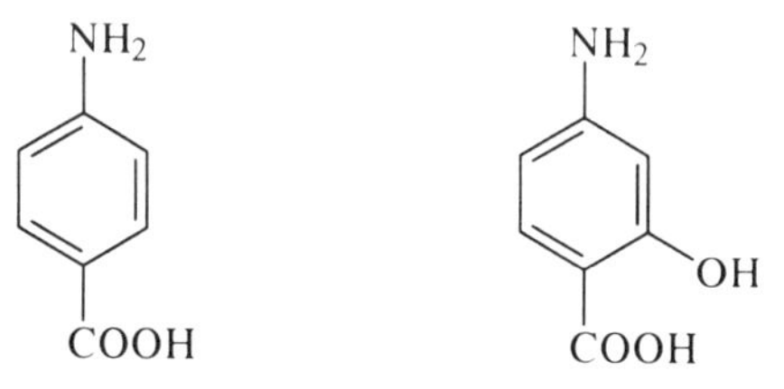

p-aminobenzoic acid

(PABA)

p-aminosalicylic acid

(PABA)

are highly acetylated both in vivo and in vitro, but they display patterns of population variation that are completely unrelated to the acetylation polymorphism affecting compounds such as isoniazid and sulfamethazine. Substrates such as PABA and *p*-aminosalicylic acid are called *monomorphic*, whereas substrates such as isoniazid are called *polymorphic*. *N*-Acetylation polymorphisms are also observed in other mammals, including the rabbit and hamster. Jenne (17) suggested that this phenomenon could be explained by the existence of two distinct acetylating enzymes, one selective for monomorphic substrates and the other selective for polymorphic substrates. An alternative hypothesis is that rapid and slow acetylator individuals possess equal quantities of a single acetylating enzyme, but the enzyme from slow acetylators has an altered or impaired catalytic activity.

Molecular genetic studies have resolved the issue. Cloning, expression, hybridization, and immunoblotting studies in the rabbit (18) demonstrated that there exist two independently regulated genes encoding catalytically distinct *N*-acetyltransferases. The acetylation defect in slow acetylator rabbits is due to deletion of the entire gene encoding one of these enzymes. Using antibody and cDNA probes derived from these animal studies, human *N*-acetyltransferase cDNAs and their corresponding genes were cloned, sequenced, and functionally expressed in heterologous expression systems (19). As is the case in the rabbit, mouse, and hamster, there are two independently regulated *N*-acetyltransferase genes in humans. (A nonfunctional pseudogene also exists.) The genes, mapped on human chromosome 8 (pter-q11), encode the functional *N*-acetyltransferases NAT1 and NAT2. The corresponding proteins share greater than 80% amino acid sequence identity over their entire 290 amino acid lengths, yet display distinct substrate selectivities. Site-directed mutagenesis studies have established that a single conserved cysteine residue at position 68 of the amino acid chain participates directly in the mechanism of acetyl transfer, as described above (20).

As might be expected, one of these enzymes (NAT1) possesses selectivity for the biotransformation of monomorphic substrates, and the other (NAT2) selectively metabolizes polymorphic substrates. NAT2 is the locus of the human acetylation polymorphism, described earlier. At the protein level, the defect in NAT2 function in slow acetylators bears some similarity to that seen in rabbits: the quantity of enzyme protein is drastically reduced (21). However, the genetic basis of the defect differs. The human NAT2 gene is not deleted in any slow acetylator individuals examined to date. Rather, it contains a characteristic pattern of point mutations within the protein coding region; these mutations ultimately result in a reduction in the quantity of NAT2 protein present in human liver. Nine variant alleles, accounting for more than 98% of those present at the NAT2 locus, have now been characterized in human populations (22); eight of these alleles are associated with the slow acetylator phenotype and with markedly reduced content of NAT2 in human liver. Since each of these allelic variants contains at least one point mutation that alters a restriction endonuclease recognition sequence, they can be detected by simple RFLP tests (see Chapter 2) using PCR amplification of the NAT2 gene coding region (23). Several of the mutant NAT2 proteins contain amino acid changes that lead to enzymes which are markedly unstable relative to the wild-type enzyme; this explains the reduced liver NAT2 activity in individuals of the slow acetylator phenotype.

NAT1, as mentioned above, is closely related to NAT2 in structure, but its expression is regulated independently and its substrate specificity is quite different. NAT1 has been described as a "monomorphic enzyme," on the basis of its specificity for so-called monomorphic substrates. However, this is inaccurate. Recent studies have provided evidence that NAT1 activity is also highly variable in human populations, and that part of this variation is genetically based. Use of the NAT1-selective substrate *p*-aminosalicylic acid as a probe drug has revealed that there exist individuals with significantly elevated NAT1 function, as well as those with a marked impairment in this enzyme. Impairment is associated with allelic variation in the NAT1 gene. Thus, independent, genetically based variations in both NAT1 and NAT2 function may affect the disposition of a wide variety of aromatic amines. Some of the carcinogenic arylamines, such as 2-aminofluorene and benzidine, are efficiently metabolized by both NAT1 and NAT2; concurrent and independent variations in these enzymes may play an important role in determining individual predisposition for the occurrence of chemical-induced toxicities from these agents. Further molecular, clinical, and epidemiological analysis will test the roles of these polymorphisms in toxicity and disease.

NOTES

1. Evans, D. A. P., *N*-Acetyltransferase, *Pharmacol. Ther.*, 42:157–239, 1989.
2. Flammang, T. J., and Kadlubar, F. F., Acetyl CoA-dependent, cytosol-catalyzed binding of carcinogenic *N*-hydroxyarylamines to DNA, in: Boobis, A. R., Caldwell, F., de Matteis, F., and

Elcombe, C. R., Ed., *Microsomes and Drug Oxidations*, Taylor and Francis, London, 1985, pp. 190–197.

3. Mattano, S., Land, S., King, C., and Weber, W., Purification of hepatic arylamine *N*-acetyl-transferase from rapid and slow acetylator mice: Identity with arylhydroxamic acid *N,O*-acetyl-transferase, In: C. M. King, L. J. Romano, and D. Schuetzle, Ed., *Carcinogenic and Mutagenic Responses to Aromatic Amines and Nitroarenes*, Elsevier, New York, 1988, pp. 155–159.

4. Grant, D. M., Lottspeich, F., and Meyer U. A., Evidence for two closely related isozymes of arylamine *N*-acetyltransferase in human liver, *FEBS Lett.* 244:203–207, 1989.

5. Grant, D. M., Blum, M., Beer, M., and Meyer, U. A., Monomorphic and polymorphic human arylamine *N*-acetyltransferases: A comparison of liver isozymes and expressed products of two cloned genes, *Mol. Pharmacol.* 39:184–191, 1991.

6. Andres, H. H., Klem, A. J., Schopfer, L. M., Harrison, J. K., and Weber, W. W., On the active site of liver acetyl CoA: Arylamine *N*-acetyltransferase from rapid acetylator rabbits (III/J), *J. Biol. Chem.* 263:7521–7527, 1988.

7. Watanabe, M., Nohmi, T., and Ishidate, M., Jr., New tester strains of *Salmonella typhimurium* highly sensitive to mutagenic nitroarenes, *Biochem. Biophys. Res. Commun.* 147:974–979, 1987.

8. Feynman, R. P., "*What Do You Care What Other People Think?*" Bantam Books, New York, 1989, pp. 34ff.

9. See Weber, W. W., *The Acetylator Genes and Drug Response*, Oxford University Press, New York, 1987.

10. Mitchell, A., Native tuberculosis rate "unbelievable," *Globe and Mail*, Toronto, Nov. 30, 1994.

11. Grant, D. M., Blum, M., and Meyer, U. A., Polymorphisms of *N*-acetyltransferase genes, *Xeno-biotica* 22:1073–1081, 1992.

12. Weber, W. W., and Hein, D. W., *N*-Acetylation pharmacogenetics, *Pharmacol. Rev.* 37:25–79, 1985, §IIIA2.

13. Jiang, X., Khursigara, G., and Rubin, R. L., Transformation of lupus-inducing drugs to cyto-toxic products by activated neutrophils, *Science* 266:810–813, 1994.

14. Hayes, R. B., Bi, W., Rothman, N. Broly, F., Caporaso, N., Feng, P., You, X., Yin, S., Woosley, R. L., and Meyer, U. A., *N*-Acetylation phenotype and genotype and risk of bladder cancer in benzidine-exposed workers, *Carcinogenesis* 14:675–678, 1993.

15. Grant, D. M., Tang, B. K., and Kalow, W., A simple test for acetylator phenotype using caf-feine, *Br. J. Clin. Pharmacol.* 17:459–464, 1984.

16. Meyer, U. A., Blum, M., Grant, D., Heim, M., Broly, F., Hoffman, F., Probst, M., and Garcia-Agundez, J., Acetylation pharmacogenetics, in: *Human Drug Metabolism: From Molecular Bi-ology to Man*, E. H. Jeffery, Ed. CRC Press, Boca Raton, FL, 1993, pp. 117–124.

17. Jenne, J.W., Partial purification and properties of the isoniazid transacetylase in human liver. Its relationship to the acetylation of *p*-aminosalicylic acid, *J. Clin. Invest.* 44:1992–2002, 1965.

18. Blum, M., Grant, D. M., Demierre, A., and Meyer, U. A., *N*-Acetylation pharmacogenetics: A gene deletion causes absence of arylamine *N*-acetyltransferase in liver of slow acetylator rab-bits, *Proc. Natl. Acad. Sci. U.S.A.* 86:9554–9557, 1989.

19. Ohsako, S., and Deguchi, T., Cloning and expression of cDNAs for polymorphic and monomor-phic arylamine *N*-acetyltransferases from human liver, *J. Biol. Chem.* 265:4630–4634, 1990; Blum, M., Grant, D. M, McBride, O. W., Heim, M., and Meyer, U. A., Human arylamine *N*-acetyltransferase genes: Isolation, chromosomal localization and functional expression, *DNA Cell Biol.* 9:193–203, 1990.

20. Dupret, J.-M. and Grant, D.M., Site-directed mutagenesis of recombinant human arylamine *N*-acetyltransferase expressed in *Escherichia coli*: Evidence for direct involvement of Cys68 in the catalytic mechanism of polymorphic human NAT2, *J. Biol. Chem.* 267:7381–7385, 1991; Dupret, J.-M., Goodfellow, G. H., Janezic, S. A., and Grant, D. M., Structure–function studies of human arylamine *N*-acetyltransferases NAT1 and NAT2. Functional analysis of recombinant NAT1/NAT2 chimeras expressed in *Escherichia coli*, *J. Biol. Chem.* 269:26830–26835, 1994.

21. Grant, D. M., Morike, K., Eichelbaum, M., and Meyer, U. A., Acetylation pharmacogenetics: The slow acetylator phenotype is caused by decreased or absent arylamine *N*-acetyltransferase in human liver, *J. Clin. Invest.* 85:968–972, 1990.

22. Grant, D. M., Molecular genetics of the *N*-acetyltransferases, *Pharmacogenetics* 3:45–50, 1993; Hickman, D., Risch, A., Buckle, V., Spurr, N. K., Jeremiah, S. J., McCarthy, A., and Sim, E., Chromosomal localization of human genes for arylamine *N*-acetyltransferase, *Biochem. J.* 297:441–445, 1994.

23. Bell, D. A., Taylor, J. A., Butler, M. A., Stephens, E. A., Wiest, J., Brubaker, L. H., Kadlubar, F. F., and Lucier, G. W., Genotype/phenotype discordance for human arylamine *N*-acetyl-transferase (NAT2) reveals a new slow-acetylator allele common in African-Americans, *Carcinogenesis* 14:1689–1692, 1993.

13

SULFOTRANSFERASE

The next phase II process which we will examine is *sulfate conjugation*. This biotransformation has been known since Victorian times: In 1876, the German chemist Baumann reported the presence of phenyl sulfate in the urine of a person treated with phenol. Although elucidation of the biochemistry of sulfate conjugation has lagged behind that of most other phase II reactions, swift progress is now being made, and the next few years should see the maturation of our understanding of this enzyme family.

SUBSTRATES AND PRODUCTS

As already mentioned (Chapter 9), PAPS is the metabolic donor of sulfate. The general reaction catalyzed by sulfotransferases is

$$R-OH + PAPS \rightarrow R-OSO_3^- + PAP$$

The structure of PAPS is shown on page 129; PAP is 3'-phosphoadenosine-5'-phosphate. The reaction is referred to by some authors as *sulfonation*,* but more commonly as *sulfation*.

Chemical Classes of Sulfate Conjugates

As with glucuronidation, sulfate conjugation provides a route for the biotransformation and elimination of both endogenous and xenobiotic compounds. Several classes of functional groups can be conjugated to sulfate; let's examine the products which result.

If the sulfotransferase acceptor is an alcohol, $R-OH$ (either aliphatic or aromatic), then the product is a sulfate ester, $R-OSO_3^-$ (Figure 13.1). Probably the most familiar representative of this class of compound is sodium dodecyl (or lauryl, C_{12}) sulfate, which is the detergent used in the sodium dodecyl sulfate–polyacrylamide gel electrophoresis (SDS-PAGE) technique (see Chapter 1). The synthesis can be carried out by treating lauryl alcohol with chlorosulfonic acid, $ClSO_3H$, analogous to the use of acetyl chloride for acetylations.

If the sulfate acceptor is a thiol, $R-SH$, then the product is an alkyl thiosulfate, $R-SSO_3^-$, the sulfur analogue of an *O*-sulfate ester (1). This is a very rare case in drug metabolism, but an enzyme-bound thiosulfate is believed to be an intermediate in the formation of sulfite from PAPS in *Escherichia coli* (2).

If the substrate is an amine, $R-NH_2$, then the product is a *sulfamate*, $R-NHSO_3^-$ (by analogy to sulfamic acid, $H_2NSO_3^-$). In the toxicologically important case that the sub-

---

*Do not confuse this reaction with the organic chemist's use of the term *sulfonation* to describe formation of an aryl–sulfur bond: $\phi + H_2SO_4 \rightarrow \phi-SO_3H$.

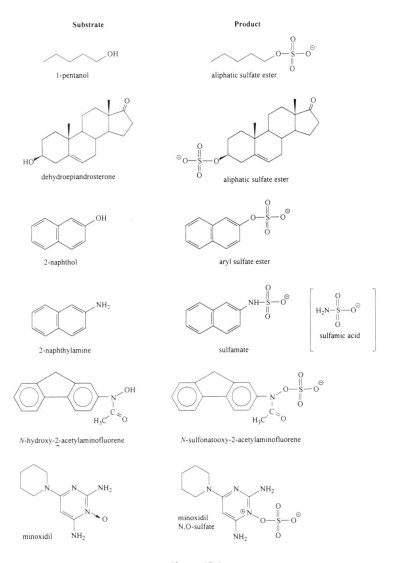

Substrate

Product

1-pentanol

aliphatic sulfate ester

dehydroepiandrosterone

aliphatic sulfate ester

2-naphthol

aryl sulfate ester

2-naphthylamine

sulfamate

sulfamic acid

N-hydroxy-2-acetylaminofluorene

N-sulfonatooxy-2-acetylaminofluorene

minoxidil

minoxidil N,O-sulfate

Figure 13.1.

strate is an aryl hydroxamic acid, $R-N(Ac)OH$, the product is $R-N(Ac)OSO_3^-$, variously called an N-sulfonoxy or N-sulfonatoöxy compound. These compounds are reactive metabolites implicated in aromatic amine carcinogenesis. Heterolytic cleavage of the $N-O$ bond generates a reactive *nitrenium ion* (see p. 361).

SULFOTRANSFERASE: ASSAY

A colorimetric assay for sulfotransferase activity was developed by Fritz Lipmann in the 1950s (3). The assay is based on the observation that the cationic dye methylene blue (see Chapter 8) forms an ion pair with many organic sulfates, and this ion pair can be extracted into organic solvents and quantitated by absorbance. This method is only applicable to the more hydrophobic substrates, such as steroids; the ion pairs formed from sulfates of lower alcohols, for example, are too polar to be extracted in this manner.

The barium salts of inorganic sulfate and PAPS are insoluble, but many substrates give sulfate esters which form soluble barium salts. This observation provides a straightforward assay for sulfotransferase activity, using commercially available [^{35}S]-PAPS. Radioactivity remaining in solution after treatment with Ba^{2+} is determined by scintillation counting. Alternatively (using either [^{35}S]-PAPS or labeled substrate), thin-layer or paper chromatography can be used to separate the sulfated product from the substrates, and activity can be determined by scintillation counting.

Many of the early reports on N-sulfation reactions used 2-naphthylamine as substrate. However, a recent meticulous study (4) using high-performance liquid chromatographic analysis has revealed that commercial lots of 2-naphthylamine contain about 1% 2-naphthol impurity. The contaminating 2-naphthol is a much better substrate than the 2-naphthylamine itself, so earlier assays of "2-naphthylamine sulfotransferase" activity were probably measuring mainly 2-naphthol sulfotransferase activity (O-sulfation). High-performance liquid chromatography purification of the substrate allows genuine 2-naphthylamine sulfotransferase activity to be detected. This case provides an instructive illustration of the importance of using highly purified substrates: Even a small amount of contaminant can mask (or even masquerade as!) the desired activity.

SULFOTRANSFERASES: PURIFICATION

Several sulfotransferases have been obtained in partially pure or homogeneous form (5). Purification methods typically involve ion-exchange and gel filtration chromatography steps. Affinity chromatography has also been used for purification. The agarose-based matrix Affi-Gel Blue (Bio-Rad) incorporates the ligand Cibacron blue, a dye which binds many nucleotide-requiring enzymes; this matrix was used in the purification of rat aryl sulfotransferase IV (6). Hirshey and Falany (7) used ATP-agarose for purification of the minoxidil sulfotransferase; the enzyme was eluted with PAPS-containing buffer. The same group also successfully used adenosine 3',5'-diphosphate-agarose (i.e., a column bearing the PAP product of the sulfotransferase reaction) for purification of a steroid sulfotransferase (8).

ACTIVATION BY SULFATION: MINOXIDIL

In most cases, sulfation is a detoxication pathway leading to readily excreted conjugates. The sulfation of hydroxamic acids is an exception and is considered in more detail in a later chapter (see Chapter 20). Here, we discuss two interesting cases in which sulfation is implicated in the metabolic activation of toxicants to their active/reactive forms.

Minoxidil represents a case of activation, rather than detoxication/inactivation, by a phase II conjugation. The drug was originally introduced as an antihypertensive agent (vasodilator). During clinical trials, it was found to promote facial hair growth in female patients; minoxidil was then shown to be effective at reversing *alopecia* (hair loss). Minoxidil is the first compound shown to have such an effect, despite a long and colorful history of "snake-oil" remedies for baldness! Minoxidil, a pyrimidine N-oxide, is metabolized to an N,O-sulfate ester, and the sulfate appears to be the active form of the drug (9). The sulfate is pharmacologically active in vitro (for example, it induces relaxation of smooth muscle vasculature), although the parent compound is not. Minoxidil sulfate is more soluble in organic solvents than in water, probably because of its zwitterionic character. This unusual lipophilicity of the sulfate may account for its ability to be taken up by cells and exert pharmacological effects (10).

ACTIVATION BY SULFATION: SAFROLE

Safrole is an important constituent of natural flavorings, such as sassafras and cinnamon oils. However, safrole is a rodent hepatocarcinogen when administered at high doses in the diet. Elizabeth and James Miller, of the McArdle Cancer Research Laboratory, University of Wisconsin, investigated the metabolic activation of safrole in the early 1980s (11). The activation pathway they proposed is shown in Figure 13.2C.

Safrole is hydroxylated at the benzylic carbon, in a typical P-450-catalyzed reaction (see Chapter 14); the resulting 1′-hydroxy metabolite is believed to be a substrate for sulfation, as shown in the scheme. Why is the resulting compound a reactive intermediate? To understand this, we need to consider the reactivities of sulfuric acid esters.

Alkyl *di*esters of sulfuric acid, such as dimethyl sulfate (see scheme, part A), are potent alkylating agents, frequently used in organic synthesis. S_N2 reaction with a nucleophile (such as an alcohol or thiol) releases an alkyl sulfate ion; since this ion is the conjugate base of a very strong acid (comparable in strength to sulfuric acid), it is an excellent leaving group. In contrast, with an alkyl *monoester* of sulfuric acid, such as dodecyl sulfate (see scheme, part B), the leaving group would be SO_4^{2-} ion; this ion is the conjugate base of an alkyl bisulfate ion, which is much weaker. Therefore, typical alkyl sulfates are *not* electrophilic alkylating agents.

However, the safrole metabolite (part C) presents a special case. The heterolytic loss of SO_4^{2-} from this sulfate ester should be particularly facile, since it results in a cation which is highly resonance-stabilized since it is both *allylic* and *benzylic* (12). The putative sulfate ester has not been isolated, but the synthetic 1′-acetoxy ester (although not known to be a metabolite of safrole) serves as a model compound for the sulfate ester. 1′-Acetoxysafrole binds to the bases of DNA in vitro to form at least five different adducts.

Mice were injected intraperitoneally with ^{3}H-labeled 1′-hydroxysafrole, and covalent binding to liver DNA, RNA, and protein was observed; the binding was greatly reduced in brachymorphic mice, as expected, given that sulfation is hypothesized to be the final enzymatic step in bioactivation of safrole.

As we will discuss in more detail for other chemical carcinogens, the formation of DNA adducts leads to mutations, following the misincorporation of nucleotides during subsequent rounds of DNA replication. Carcinogenesis may subsequently result from the mutational activation of cellular proto-oncogenes or the inactivation of tumor suppressor genes.

SULFOTRANSFERASE: CLONING AND SEQUENCE ANALYSIS; ISOZYMES

The first successful cloning of a gene encoding a sulfotransferase enzyme was reported in 1989 by Kato and colleagues, in Tokyo (13). Their strategy was to screen a rat liver cDNA expression library with a rabbit antiserum raised against a purified hydroxysteroid sulfotransferase (see below). Since that time, there has been rapid progress in cloning other forms of sulfotransferase, mainly by the use of DNA probes based on partial amino acid sequences of purified proteins or by sequence homology to other forms of the enzyme. The characteristics of more than a dozen sulfotransferase cDNAs are summarized in a recent review (14). Here, we will only mention a few of the results obtained to date, in the rat and human.

At least five isoenzymes are expressed in rat liver, and they are active with aromatic substrates such as *para*-nitrophenol and 2-naphthol. Aryl sulfotransferase IV (AST IV) is the only form which activates the proximate carcinogen, N-OH-2-acetylaminofluorene. The cDNA for AST IV was recently obtained by antibody screening (15); the gene en-

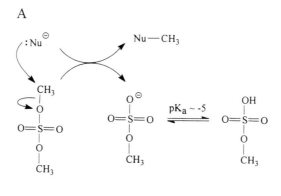

A

B

C

Figure 13.2.

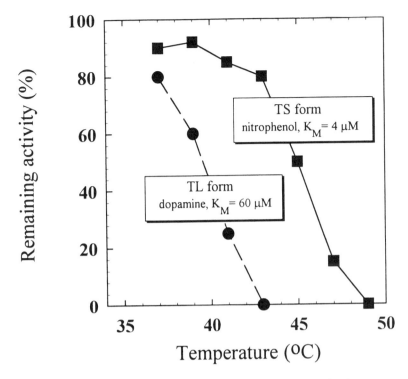

Figure 13.3. Two distinct forms of phenol sulfotransferase occur in human platelets. Homogenates of pooled platelets, obtained from ten subjects, were preincubated at the indicated temperatures for 15 min. Phenol sulfotransferase activity was then assayed with either dopamine or *para*-nitrophenol as substrate, as indicated. [Data from Weinshilboum (29).]

codes a 291-amino-acid protein (33,909 daltons). The same gene was also isolated simultaneously, as the form encoding minoxidil sulfotransferase activity (16).

In human tissues, at least two forms of phenol sulfotransferase and one hydroxysteroid sulfotransferase are found (17). The phenol sulfotransferases can be distinguished by their differential thermal stabilities, as shown in Figure 13.3. The properties of all three enzymes are summarized in Table 13.1.

TL-PST catalyzes sulfation of micromolar levels of dopamine and other naturally occurring monoamines; TS-PST is active with micromolar levels of *para*-nitrophenol. Low levels of these compounds can be used as diagnostic substrates for the enzymes (see Fig. 13.3). For this reason, the two forms are also described as M-PST and P-PST, respec-

Table 13.1. Characteristics of Three Human Sulfotransferases

	Enzyme		
	Thermostable Phenol Sulfotransferase	Thermolabile Phenol Sulfotransferase	Hydroxysteroid Sulfotransferase
Typical substrates	4-Nitrophenol	Dopamine[a]	Dehydroepiandrosterone
Thermal stability	Stable	Labile	Intermediate
Inhibition by DCNP[b]	Sensitive	Resistant	Resistant

[a]Dopamine = 1,2-dihydroxyphenylethylamine.
[b]DCNP = 2,6-dichloro-4-nitrophenol.
Source: Weinshilboum and Otterness (14).

tively, for *m*onoamine and *p*henol sulfotransferases; since dopamine is, in fact, a phenol (catechol) derivative, this nomenclature should probably be avoided. At high substrate concentrations (millimolar), both enzymes metabolize both substrates. TS-PST is the main 2-naphthylamine *N*-sulfotransferase (4). Both genes have been cloned recently (18).

Several regions of high amino acid homology are conserved among all published sulfotransferase sequences, probably including the residues in the PAPS-binding site (14, 15). However, the elucidation of sulfotransferase structure is still at an early stage.

STEROID SULFOTRANSFERASES

As with the glucuronosyltransferases, sulfotransferases also play an important role in the metabolism of endogenous lipophilic compounds. Steroid hormones and bile acids are probably the most important of these endogenous substrates. Steroid sulfation occurs in the liver and in organs which are targets of steroid hormone action, such as adrenal glands, testis, ovary, and uterus. Many milligrams of steroid hormone metabolites are excreted daily by humans, largely in the form of urinary sulfate and glucuronide conjugates. Few details are known about the relationships between individual sulfotransferase isozymes and the sites of sulfation of particular steroids.

Many different sites within the steroid ring system can bear hydroxyl groups, and all of these are probably subject to sulfation. Some of the identified sites are shown in Figure 13.4. Dihydroxy steroids can form disulfates, and mixed sulfate-glucuronide conjugates have also been identified (e.g., pregnanediol 3-sulfate 20-glucuronide).

Some steroid sulfates are transported into cells, via specific carriers, and then subjected to further metabolism, including transformation of the steroid nucleus of the sulfate conjugate (steroid sulfate interconversion). Steroid *sulfatases*, which hydrolyze the sulfates and release the unconjugated steroids, are also known. In summary, then, the complexities of the pathways of steroid sulfate metabolism are most formidable.

Within the cell, steroid sulfates are mainly bound to the protein *ligandin* (see Chapter 11). They are transported in the serum, bound to serum albumin and other proteins, including specific steroid-binding proteins (19). The conjugates also behave as typical phase II conjugates and are excreted in the urine or feces. Some specific examples of steroid sulfation are given here; for more details the reader is referred to the volume by Mulder et al. (20).

The male sex hormone testosterone (see Fig. 13.4) is a substrate for both glucuronidation (see Chapter 9) and sulfation, at the 17β-hydroxyl group. Estrogen (female sex hormone) steroids, such as estradiol (see Fig. 13.4) and estrone, are characterized by an aromatic "A" ring, the absence of C-19, and a phenolic hydroxyl group at the 3-position. Estrogens are synthesized from testosterone in the ovaries, via the action of the cytochrome P-450 *aromatase* enzyme (21). Estrogen sulfotransferases, which catalyze sulfation of the phenolic (3-position) hydroxyl, are found in liver, adrenal gland, uterus, and other tissues; the enzymes are distinct from the phenol sulfotransferases discussed above, and molecular analysis is underway (22). The secondary 17β-hydroxyl group of estradiol, on the other hand, is probably a substrate for sulfation by the testosterone sulfotransferase.

STEROID DRUGS; CONTRACEPTIVES

Many synthetic steroid derivatives are used (or abused) medicinally. Stanozolol (see Fig. 13.4) is an anabolic steroid which has been abused by athletes. It is extensively metabolized by cytochrome P-450-catalyzed hydroxylation. These synthetic steroids are also metabolized to glucuronides (23) and sulfates. The oral contraceptives, such as ethinylestradiol, are sulfated extensively (24, 25). Almost all of the urinary metabolites in humans are glucuronide or sulfate conjugates of these oxidation products (26).

BILE SALT SULFOTRANSFERASES

Quantitatively, the major metabolic fate of cholesterol is conversion to the *bile salts* (or bile acids), such as *deoxycholic acid* (Greek, cholē = bile) and *chenodeoxycholic acid* (see figure). The detailed metabolic pathways for formation of bile salts from cholesterol are discussed by Rawn (27). The liver conjugates bile acids in several ways. The side-chain C-24 carboxylate group of cholic acid can be linked by a peptide bond to the amino groups of either glycine or *taurine* (cysteamine sulfonic acid; see Fig. 13.4). The 3α-hydroxyl group of cholic acid can also be sulfated by a sulfotransferase.

Large amounts of bile salts are secreted by the liver, stored in the gallbladder, and released into the intestines, especially after lipid-rich meals. The bile salts emulsify dietary

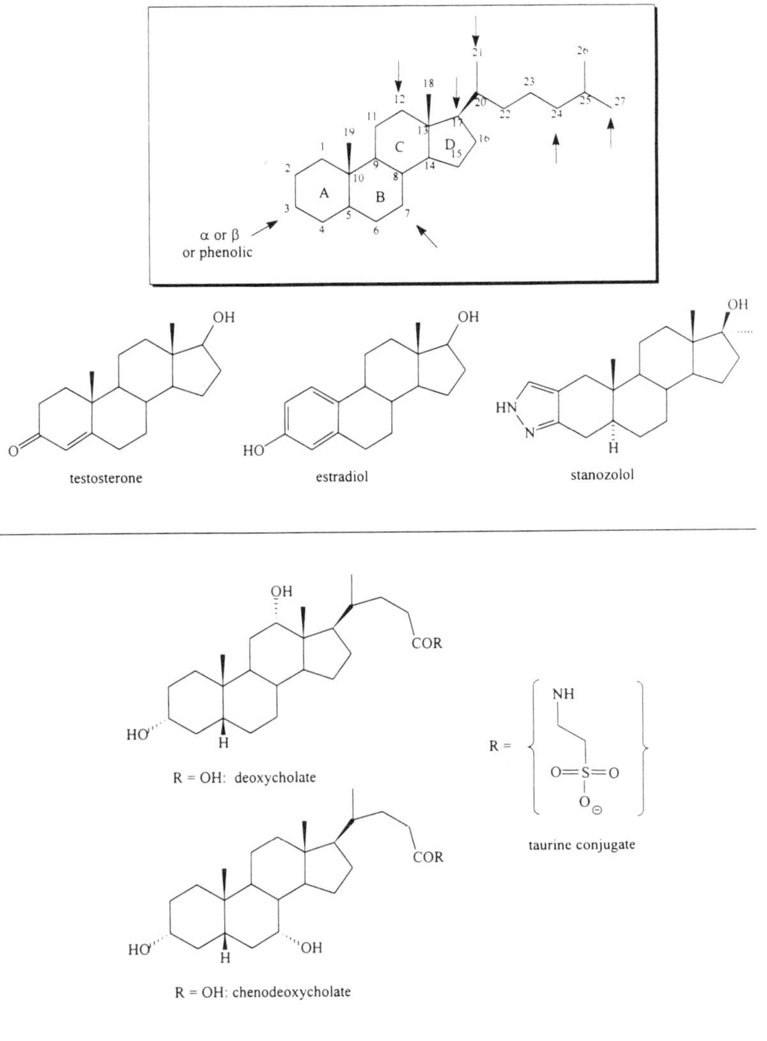

testosterone   estradiol   stanozolol

R = OH: deoxycholate

R = OH: chenodeoxycholate

taurine conjugate

Figure 13.4.

lipids and assist their digestion and absorption. This detergent action of the bile salts is a consequence of their amphipathic structures, which incorporate both hydrophobic and hydrophilic (anionic) moieties.

As much as 50 grams of bile acid is secreted daily by the adult human liver, mainly as glycine and taurine conjugates. Almost all of this material is readsorbed by the intestine, much of it following hydrolysis of the glycine and taurine conjugates by the action of intestinal bacteria. This is another example of the *enterohepatic recirculation* discussed earlier (in the context of glucuronidation). *This efficient reabsorption of bile acids is required to conserve the body pool of these compounds, which totals only a few grams.* Without this "recycling system," the absorption of dietary lipids would require the excretion of a comparable amount of lipid material, in the form of bile acids. In fact, less than 1 gram is excreted in the feces daily.

Under normal circumstances, very little of the bile acid pool is conjugated to sulfate. However, *cholestasis* (impairment of the flow of bile) can result from injury, disease (liver cirrhosis), chemical toxicity, or biliary atresia. This condition leads to accumulation of bile salts (and also bilirubin) in the tissues. Elevated circulating levels of these detergent molecules are acutely toxic. *Under these conditions, bile acid sulfation increases; the sulfates are efficiently cleared by the kidney and excreted in the urine. In effect, sulfation is a "backup" system for the detoxication of bile acids.* Falany and colleagues have shown that a purified human liver steroid sulfotransferase also acts on various bile acids, and they suggest that this enzyme (the dehydroepiandrosterone sulfotransferase listed in Table 13.1) carries out most bile acid sulfation (8).

SULFOTRANSFERASES: DISTRIBUTION AND HUMAN POLYMORPHISM

Sulfotransferase activity has been observed in all mammalian species studied, birds, and reptiles; a bacterial sulfotransferase has been reported, although PAPS is not the sulfate donor (28). In humans, activity is detectable in all tissues. The liver, kidney, and lung are the major sites of xenobiotic sulfation.

There is considerable interindividual variation in sulfation activity, as measured by studies on blood platelets (29). Family studies indicate that this variation is inherited: A genetic polymorphism of the thermostable sulfotransferase exists. There are also substantial racial differences: U.S. blacks have higher levels than U.S. whites (30). Since some sulfotransferase activities can result in bioactivation of carcinogens, these genetic variations may influence susceptibility to environmental carcinogens, but this remains speculative. The development of methods for the genotypic and phenotypic analysis of individual sulfotransferase activities (as is now possible for analysis of *N*-acetyltransferase status, see Chapter 12) should permit rigorous epidemiological tests of this possibility.

NOTES

1. Thiosulfates are also known as *Bunte salts*; see *Angew. Chem. Intl. Ed. (Eng.)* 6:544–553, 1967.
2. Tsang, M. L.-S., and Schiff, J. A., Sulfate-reducing pathway in *Escherichia coli* involving bound intermediates, *J. Bacteriol.* 125:923–933, 1976.
3. Roy, A. B., Sulfotransferases, in: G. J. Mulder, Ed., *Sulfation of Drugs and Related Compounds*, CRC Press, Boca Raton, FL, 1981, pp. 83–130.
4. Hernandez, J. S., Powers, S. P., and Weinshilboum, R. M., Human liver arylamine *N*-sulfotransferase activity: Thermostable phenol sulfotransferase catalyzes the *N*-sulfation of 2-naphthylamine, *Drug Metab. Dispos.* 19:1071–1079, 1991.

5. Sekura, R. D., Duffel, M. W., and Jakoby, W. B., Phenol sulfotransferase, *Methods Enzymol.* 77:197–206, 1981. Falany, C. N., Molecular enzymology of human liver cytosolic sulfotransferases, *Trends Pharmacol. Sci.* 12:255–259, 1991.

6. Mangold, B. L. K., Erickson, J., Lohr, C., McCann, D. J., and Mangold, J. B., Self-catalyzed irreversible inactivation of rat hepatic aryl sulfotransferase IV by N-hydroxy-2-acetylaminofluorene, *Carcinogenesis* 11:1563–1567, 1990.

7. Hirshey, S. J., and Falany, C. N., Purification and characterization of rat-liver minoxidil sulfotransferase, *Biochem. J.* 270:721–728, 1990.

8. Radominska, A., Comer, K. A., Zimniak, P., Falany, J., Iscan, M., and Falany, C. N., Human liver steroid sulphotransferase sulphates bile acids, *Biochem. J.* 272:597–604, 1990.

9. Buhl, A. E., Waldon, D. J., Baker, C. A., and Johnson, G. A., Minoxidil sulfate is the active metabolite that stimulates hair-follicles, *J. Invest. Dermatol.* 95:553–557, 1990.

10. Mulder, G. J., Pharmacological effects of drug conjugates: Is morphine 6-glucuronide an exception? *Trends Pharmacol. Sci.* 13:302–304, 1992.

11. Miller, J. A., and Miller, E. C., The metabolic activation and nucleic acid adducts of naturally-occurring carcinogens: Recent results with ethyl carbamate and the spice flavors safrole and estragole, *Br. J. Cancer* 48:1–15, 1983; Wiseman, R.W., Fennell, T. R., Miller, J. A., and Miller, E. C., Further characterization of the DNA adducts formed by electrophilic esters of the hepatocarcinogens 1′-hydroxysafrole and 1′-hydroxyestragole in vitro and in mouse liver in vivo, including new adducts at C-8 and N-7 of guanine residues, *Cancer Res.* 45:3096–3105, 1985.

12. Streitwieser, A., Jr., and Heathcock, C. H., *Introduction to Organic Chemistry*, 2nd ed., Macmillan, New York, 1981, Sections 20.1.A and 22.5.B.

13. Ogura, K., Kajita, J., Narihata, H., Watabe, T., Ozawa, S., Nagata, K., Yamazoe, Y., and Kato, R., Cloning and sequence analysis of a rat liver cDNA encoding hydroxysteroid sulfotransferase, *Biochem. Biophys. Res. Commun.* 165:168–174, 1989.

14. Weinshilboum, R., and Otterness, D., Sulfotransferase enzymes, In: *Handbook of Experimental Pharmacology*, Vol. 112, *Conjugation–Deconjugation Reactions in Drug Metabolism and Toxicity*, F. C. Kauffman, Ed., Springer, Berlin, 1994, pp. 45–78.

15. Yerokun, T., Etheredge, J. L., Norton, T. R., Carter, H. A., Chung, K. H., Birckbichler, P. J., and Ringer, D. P., Characterization of a complementary DNA for rat liver aryl sulfotransferase IV and use in evaluating the hepatic gene transcript levels of rats at various stages of 2-acetylaminofluorene-induced hepatocarcinogenesis, *Cancer Res.* 52:4779–4786, 1992.

16. Hirshey, S. J., Dooley, T. P., Reardon, I. M., Heinrikson, R. L. and Falany, C. N., Sequence analysis, in vitro translation, and expression of the cDNA for rat liver minoxidil sulfotransferase, *Mol. Pharmacol.* 42:257–264, 1992.

17. Weinshilboum, R. M., Phenol sulfotransferase in humans: Properties, regulation, and function, *Fed. Proc.* 45:2223–2228, 1986.

18. Wilborn, T. W., Comer, K. A., Dooley, T. P., Reardon, I. M., Heinrikson, R. L., and Falany, C. N., Sequence analysis and expression of the cDNA for the phenol-sulfating form of human liver phenol sulfotransferase, *Mol. Pharmacol.* 43:70–77, 1993; Aksoy, I. A., and Weinshilboum, R. M., Human thermolabile phenol sulfotransferase gene (STM): Molecular cloning and structural characterization, *Biochem. Biophys. Res. Commun.* 208:786–795, 1995.

19. Litwack, G., Steroid hormones, Chapter 21 in: *Textbook of Biochemistry with Clinical Correlations*, T. M. Devlin, Ed., Wiley, New York, 1992, pp. 915–916.

20. Mulder, G. J. (Ed.), *Sulfation of Drugs and Related Compounds*, CRC Press, Boca Raton, FL, 1981.

21. Rawn, J. D., *Biochemistry*, Harper and Row, New York, 1983, pp. 810–812; and Okita, R. T., and Masters, B. S. S., Biotransformations: The cytochromes P450, Chapter 23 in: T. M. Devlin, Ed., *Textbook of Biochemistry with Clinical Correlations*, Wiley, New York, 1992, pp. 994–995.

22. Oeda, T., Lee, Y. C., Driscoll, W. J., Chen, H. C., and Strott, C. A., Molecular cloning and expression of a full-length complementary DNA encoding the guinea pig adrenocortical estrogen sulfotransferase, *Mol. Endocrinol.* 6:1216–1226, 1992.

23. Ebner, T., Remmel, R. P., and Burchell, B., Human bilirubin UDP-glucuronyltransferase catalyses the glucuronidation of ethinylestradiol, *Mol. Pharmacol.* 43:649–654, 1993.

24. Reed, M.J., Fotherby, K., and Steele, S. J., Metabolism of ethynylestradiol in man, *J. Endocrinol.* 55:351–361, 1972.

25. See ref. 23.

26. Schänzer, W., Opfermann, G., and Donike, M., Metabolism of stanozolol: Identfication and synthesis of urinary metabolites, *J. Steroid Biochem.* 36:153–174, 1990.

27. Rawn, J. D., *Biochemistry*, Harper and Row, New York, 1983, pp. 812–814.

28. Kim, D. H., Yoon, H. K., Koizumi, M., and Kobashi, K., Sulfation of phenolic antibiotics by sulfotransferase obtained from a human intestinal bacterium, *Chem. Pharm. Bull. (Tokyo)* 40:1056–1057, 1992.

29. Weinshilboum, R. M., Sulfotransferase pharmacogenetics, *Pharmacol. Ther.* 45:93–107, 1990.

30. Kadlubar, F. F., Butler, M. A., Kaderlik, K. R., Chou, H. C., and Lang, N. P., Polymorphisms for aromatic amine metabolism in humans: Relevance for human carcinogenesis, *Environ. Health Perspect.* 98:69–74, 1992.

14

CYTOCHROME P-450

THE CYTOCHROME P-450 SYSTEM

Cytochrome P-450 enzymes play a central role in the metabolism of many xenobiotics, catalyzing both detoxication and bioactivation reactions. P-450 can introduce hydroxyl groups into structures as unreactive as hydrocarbon chains and aromatic rings, initiating the biotransformation of compounds which do not possess functional groups suitable for conjugation.

The capacity of mammalian tissues to oxidize nonpolar xenobiotics, including the hydroxylation of aromatic substrates, was well recognized by the mid-1950s. However, the enzymes responsible for this activity were unknown. The first clue to the nature of these enzymes was obtained in 1955. G. R. Williams and M. Klingenberg, working at the Johnson Foundation, University of Pennsylvania, were studying microsomal heme proteins by optical spectroscopy. Since many ferrous heme proteins form characteristic carbon monoxide complexes, they treated rat liver microsomes with a reducing agent, *sodium dithionite* ($Na_2S_2O_4$), in the presence of CO gas. The resulting ferrous–CO complex was observed by recording an optical *difference spectrum* between CO-bound and CO-free samples. This experiment revealed a strong absorption band at 450 nm, which was unlike any previously known reduced heme–CO complex chromophore. Omura and Sato (Osaka, Japan), who had been working at the Johnson Foundation at the time of the initial observations, first purified the protein responsible for the peculiar 450 nm chromophore in 1962 and confirmed that the absorption was due to a new class of heme proteins (1, 2). They proposed the name *cytochrome P-450*, based on the protein's characteristic absorption maximum. [Note that the ferrous–CO form of the enzyme is not a normal participant in the enzyme's catalytic cycle (see below); it is generated in the laboratory by treatment with dithionite, an artificial reducing agent, and CO. Indeed, CO is a characteristic inhibitor of P-450 catalysis.] Omura and Sato also discovered that P-450 was susceptible to irreversible denaturation, converting the enzyme into an inactive form, with a ferrous–CO complex absorption at 420 nm ("cytochrome P420").

Soon after the identification of P-450, several studies demonstrated that this protein was the hepatic microsomal hydroxylase, an enzyme activity already known from studies of drug biotransformation. A particularly clear piece of evidence was the demonstration that CO inhibition of microsomal hydroxylation could be reversed by photoirradiation (which dissociates the CO complex), with maximal effectiveness occurring at a wavelength of 450 nm. Work at the University of Pennsylvania showed that a cytochrome P-450 enzyme was responsible for sterol C-21 hydroxylation in rat adrenals (3). Final proof of the identity of P-450 and the microsomal hydroxylase came with the reconstitution of hydroxylase activity with purified P-450 (see below). Cytochrome P-450 enzymes catalyze many steps of sterol biosynthesis, the oxidative metabolism of fatty acids, sterols, and other endogenous substrates, as well as the physiological oxidation of the vast majority of drugs and xenobiotics. Cytochrome P-450 enzymes are also responsible for the metabolism of xenobiotics to species responsible for toxic or carcinogenic effects. *Cytochrome P-450 is the key enzyme in the activation and detoxication of a host of substances of toxicological and pharmacological importance.* A distinct hepatic microsomal monoxygenase, a flavoprotein unrelated to P-450, also exists. This enzyme, *flavin-containing monooxygenase* (FMO), plays a more limited catalytic role than P-450, notably in the conversion of tertiary amines to *N*-oxides.*

With the exception of some soluble bacterial proteins, all known cytochrome P-450 enzymes are membrane-bound. Most of the P-450 enzymes involved in the biosynthesis of sterols are found in the membranes of steroidogenic organs, such as the adrenals, testis, ovaries, and placenta; P-450 enzymes involved in the oxidation of drugs and xenobiotics are widely distributed, with high concentrations in the endoplasmic reticulum of the liver, kidney, lung, nasal passages, and gut and significant concentrations in most other tissues. The biosynthetic importance of adrenal cytochrome P-450 and the high concentrations of hepatic cytochrome P-450 enzymes have made these the favored tissues for the investigation of these enzymes in mammals.

The solubilization, purification, and reconstitution of cytochrome P-450 were particularly challenging. The sterol 11β-hydroxylase, a biosynthetic enzyme from adrenal mitochondria, was the first cytochrome P-450 system to be solubilized and separated into its components (4). Purification and reconstitution of active microsomal cytochrome P-450 enzyme was accomplished by A. Y. H. Lu and M. J. Coon, at the University of Michigan, in 1968 (5). This achievement was crucial to the biochemical analysis of P-450 function. Throughout the 1970s and continuing to the present, a very large number of different forms of P-450 were isolated from mammalian liver and other tissues, and their catalytic activities studied in purified, reconstituted systems, following the approach pioneered by Lu and Coon.

Because of the practical difficulties of working with membrane-bound proteins, cytochrome P-450$_{cam}$, a soluble, easily purified bacterial enzyme which hydroxylates camphor,

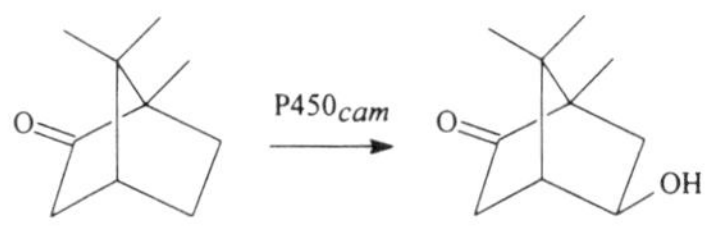

Regiospecific 5-*exo* hydroxylation of camphor by cytochrome P-450$_{cam}$, a bacterial enzyme isolated from *Pseudomonas putida*.

has been a popular system for structural and mechanistic studies. (However, there are several significant functional differences between the soluble bacterial P-450 and membrane-bound microsomal P-450 forms, as discussed later.) P-450$_{cam}$ carries out the first step in the catabolism of camphor by *Pseudomonas putida*, which can grow on this natural product as a sole carbon source.

P-450 ENZYME ASSAYS

P-450 enzymes are monooxygenases: They catalyze reactions in which one oxygen atom of molecular (di)oxygen is inserted into the substrate, and the other atom is reduced to

*For a thorough discussion of FMO, see J. R. Cashman, Structural and catalytic properties of the mammalian flavin-containing monooxygenase, *Chem. Res. Toxicol.* 8:165–181, 1995.

water. Since P-450 monooxygenases catalyze a vast and diverse range of chemical transformations, a wide variety of methods can be used to assay P-450 enzyme activity.

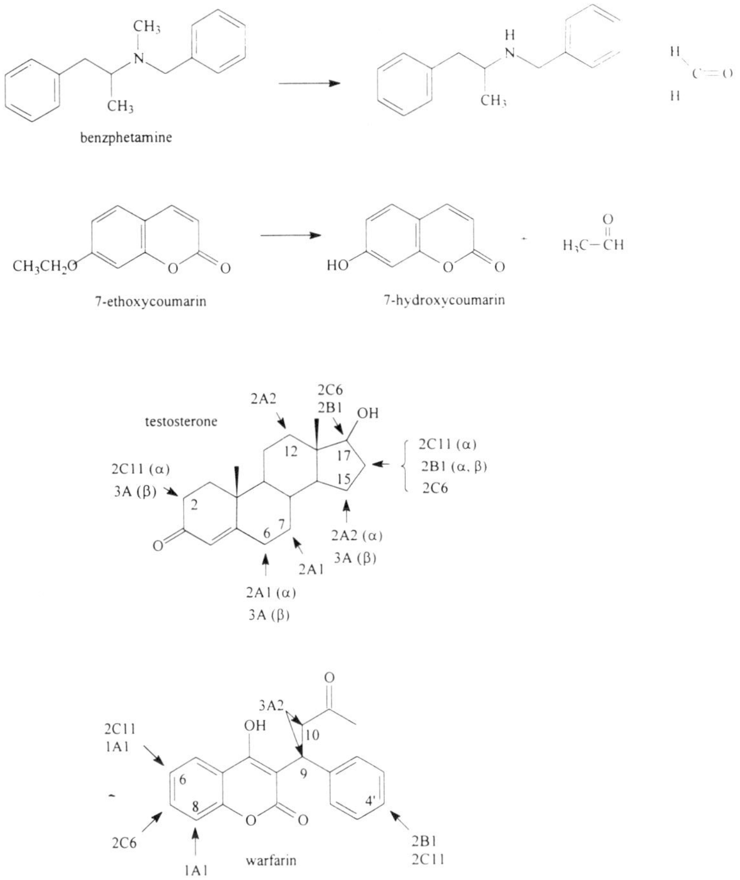

Four of the many assays used to measure the catalytic activities of cytochrome P-450 enzymes. The sites
on testosterone and warfarin hydroxylated by different forms of cytochrome P-450 are indicated. (Warfarin is an anticoagulant used as a rodenticide.) The regiospecificities of these reactions can be used
to identify an enzyme.

The cytochrome P-450-dependent hydroxylation of benzphetamine causes *N*-dealkylation
and release of a methyl group as *formaldehyde* (CH_2O). Formaldehyde formation can be
assayed easily by means of the *Nash assay*:

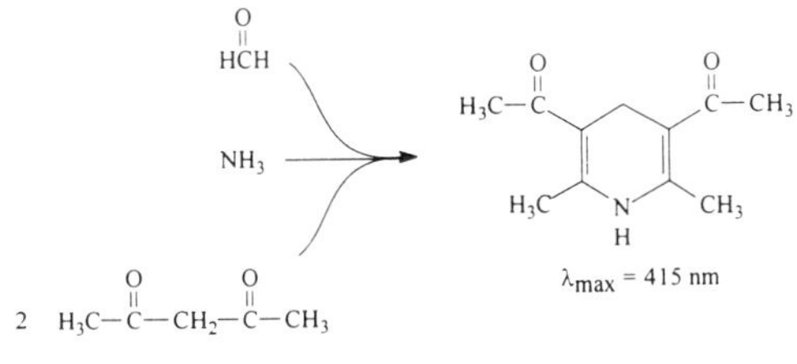

where formaldehyde reacts with ammonia and acetylacetone (2,4-pentanedione) to give a dihydropyridine product with an absorption maximum at 415 nm. This product is readily quantitated by colorimetric methods. Another common assay measures the O-deethylation of 7-ethoxycoumarin to give 7-hydroxycoumarin. The product formed in this reaction is fluorescent, whereas the substrate is not, so that the intensity of the fluorescence maximum provides a simple measure of the amount of product formed. Other widely used P-450 enzyme assays include: aryl hydrocarbon hydroxylase (AHH), the conversion of the polycyclic aromatic hydrocarbon, benzo[a]pyrene, to a mixture of phenolic metabolites; EROD (7-ethoxyresorufin O-deethylase); and biphenyl hydroxylase.

The selection of an appropriate assay method depends on the nature of the information that is sought. If an estimate of the total activity in a sample containing multiple cytochrome P-450 enzymes is desired, the ideal assay would be based on a compound that is a comparable substrate for all the enzymes present. However, no such "universal" substrate (i.e., a substrate for all or most cytochrome P-450 enzymes) exists.

On the other hand, if one desires to determine the activity of a single, specific form of the enzyme (isozyme),* the assay should be based on a compound that is only a substrate for that enzyme. Again, decisively enzyme-specific substrates are only available for a few P-450 forms. One approach to circumventing the lack of enzyme-specific substrates is to use a single substrate that gives several metabolites, each of which is formed with relative selectivity by a subset of cytochrome P-450 enzymes. Quantitation of the "spectrum" of metabolites in the product mixture (separated by, for example, high-pressure liquid chromatography) gives a simultaneous estimate of the activities of several enzymes. Testosterone and warfarin are commonly used for this type of "fingerprinting" assay (see above). Practical considerations of time, expense, and sensitivity will also influence the selection of an appropriate P-450 assay.

In summary, there is no universal assay for P-450 enzyme activity. Especially in crude sources, such as liver microsomes, each assay will reveal different aspects of the constellation of P-450 enzymes present.

THE P-450 GENE FAMILY

The early studies of P-450 enzyme purification (and the results of studies of P-450 induction, discussed later) revealed the existence of multiple forms of P-450, with differing catalytic activities. This raised the following questions: How many P-450 enzymes are actually present in a given tissue; what are the relationships among them; and what role does each play in metabolism? The difficulty of purifying cytochrome P-450 enzymes (particularly, the difficulty of separating very closely related forms) makes these questions hard to answer by "classical" biochemical approaches of enzyme purification. Molecular biological tools have provided the key. cDNAs for cytochrome P-450 enzymes induced in rodents by treatment with agents such as phenobarbital or β-naphthoflavone (see later) were obtained in the 1980s, and cDNAs for new forms of cytochrome P-450 are now isolated routinely. Indeed, the gene sequences of more than 300 cytochrome P-450 enzymes have already been determined, and more are reported monthly (6)!

---

*The multiple forms of cytochrome P-450 have often been described as *isozymes*. However, these forms share a structural and spectroscopic feature, namely, the 450-nm chromophore; they do not necessarily share a particular catalytic activity. Thus it is more accurate to refer to "isoforms" of P450, or simply to "P450 enzymes."

Nomenclature of P-450 Enzymes

Analysis of this wealth of sequence information allowed the development of a rational nomenclature for cytochrome P-450 enzymes. Previous nomenclature systems were based on relative electrophoretic mobility, chromophore λ_{max}, or substrate specificity and differed among laboratories: The same enzyme could be identified by several different names. This haphazard nomenclature has been replaced recently by a systematic, molecular-evolutionary approach. The basis for this system is that the extent of sequence (although not necessarily functional) identity between two enzymes decreases with evolutionary distance from a common ancestor. Thus, two enzymes that differ very little in sequence, such as cytochromes P-450 2B1 and 2B2, are likely to have extensive structural/functional similarity, whereas enzymes with markedly different sequences are least likely to retain such similarity. Enzymes sharing >40% sequence identity are (arbitrarily) assigned to the same *family*; those that share >55% identity are considered as members of the same *subfamily*. Individual enzymes are identified by a family number, subfamily letter, and finally another number, identifying the specific member of the subfamily (Table 14.1). For example, P-450 3A4 is the fourth member of subfamily A of family 3. A more abbreviated form of nomenclature is obtained by replacing cytochrome P-450 with the letters CYP (CYP3A4) (Table 14.2). The latter nomenclature, when italicized, is used to designate the genes for the corresponding proteins. Enzymatic function usually correlates with sequence similarity. For example, all cytochrome P-450 4A enzymes catalyze the ω-hydroxylation of fatty acids [i.e., oxidation at the terminal (or ω) carbon]; the 3A enzymes have related (but not identical) specificities. Family numbers below 100 are reserved for eukaryotic enzymes; those above 100 are used for microbial enzymes.

Although the new system is based on arbitrary cutoff values for sequence identity, it has brought order to a previously chaotic nomenclature. In some instances the trivial (non-

Table 14.1. Selected Forms of Hepatic Cytochrome P-450 Involved in Xenobiotic Metabolism (7–9)

P-450 Family	Enzyme	Rat	Mouse	Rabbit	Typical Substrate or Activity	Typical Inducing Agent
1	1A1	c	P_1	LM_6	EROD, aryl hydrocarbon hydroxylase (AHH)	PAH, TCDD, β-NF (*Ah* receptor)
	1A2	d	P_3	LM_4	2-AAF, IQ, N-hydroxylation	Isosafrole, TCDD
2	2A1	a			Testosterone, 7α-hydroxylase (steroid metabolism)	PB
	2B1	b		LM_2	Hexobarbital, PB	PB also constitutive
	2D6	UT-H			Debrisoquine, sparteine	Noninducible
	2E1	j		LM_{3a}	Dimethylnitrosamine	Ethanol, isoniazid
3	3A4	p			Nifedipine	Steroids, dexamethasone
4	4A1	P-452			ω-Hydroxylase	Peroxisome proliferators

Abbreviations: AAF = 2-acetylaminofluorene; EROD = 7-ethoxyresorufin O-deethylase; PB = phenobarbital; PAH = polycyclic aromatic hydrocarbon; TCDD = 2,3,7,8-tetrachlorodibenzodioxin; β-NF = β-naphthoflavone; IQ = 2-amino-3-methylimidazo[4,5-f]quinoline.
Notes: Family numbers were originally given in Roman numerals (e.g., P-450 III).
Many different notations have been used for the rat liver enzymes (10).

Table 14.2. Selected Substrates of Human Cytochrome P-450 Enzymes (11)

Enzyme	Substrates	Enzyme	Substrates
CYP1A1	Benzo[*a*]pyrene 2-Acetylaminofluorene	CYP2E1	Aniline Aflatoxin *N*-Nitrosodimethylamine
CYP1A2	2-Acetylaminofluorene Ethoxyresorufin Phenacetin Acetaminophen		Acetaminophen Chlorzoxazone Caffeine
	Caffeine Aflatoxin B1	CYP2F1	2-Naphthylamine
		CYP3A4	Aldrin
CYP2A6	Coumarin *N*-Nitrosodiethylamine		Cortisol Cyclosporin A Diltiazem
CYP2B6	7-Ethoxycoumarin		Erythromycin 17β-Estradiol
CYP2C9	Aminopyrene Benzphetamine Hexobarbital Tienilic acid Tolbutamide		Lidocaine Nifedipine Sterigmatocystin Quinidine Taxol Dapsone
CYP2C19	Mephenytoin		Alfentanil Warfarin
CYP2D6	Bufuralol Sparteine Debrisoquine		Lovastatin Ethynylestradiol
	Desipramine Dextromethorphan Propranolol Sparteine	CYP4A	Arachidonic acid

systematic) names continue to be widely used, since they state the function of the enzyme in question. For example, lanosterol-14-demethylase (CYP51) catalyzes lanosterol demethylation during the biosynthesis of cholesterol; aromatase (CYP19A) removes the 19-methyl carbon and aromatizes the A-ring of androstenedione, in the biosynthesis of estradiol; cytochrome P-450$_{cam}$ (CYP101) catalyzes the hydroxylation of camphor.

Cytochrome P-448

Administration of agents such as 3-methylcholanthrene to rodents (see below) leads to the induction of a class of P-450 enzymes which form only a small fraction of the P-450 complement in noninduced animals. By the 1970s, it became clear that these 3-MC-inducible forms represented a distinct class of P-450. First, the enzymes had characteristic reduced-CO absorption peaks around 447–448 nm, rather than 450 nm. Second, *the enzymes catalyze several reactions associated with carcinogen activation*, including the hydroxylation of polycyclic aromatic hydrocarbons and the *N*-oxidation of aromatic amines. Many authors referred to these forms as "cytochrome P-448." The forms involved were later identified as principally 1A1 and 1A2. The modern systematic nomenclature has largely displaced the term cytochrome P-448 from the current literature.

The cytochrome P-450 metabolism of xenobiotics and drugs is primarily catalyzed by enzymes of the CYP1, CYP2, CYP3, and CYP4 families. In humans, the CYP3A family represents up to 60% of the cytochrome P-450 in the liver and is particularly important.

SIDEBAR: NITROSAMINES

Cytochrome P-4502E1 is the most significant enzyme for the activation of *nitrosamines*. Dialkylnitrosamines ($R_1R_2-N-N=O$; nitrosodialkylamines) are synthesized by treating dialkylamines (secondary amines) with nitrous acid, HNO_2. The same synthetic reaction can potentially occur in the stomach: Secondary amines are present in the diet, and nitrous acid can be formed from dietary nitrite at the acid pH of the stomach. In addition to such endogenous synthesis, certain nitrosamines are also found in tobacco, where they are formed by nitrosation of amines related to nicotine.

Many nitrosamines are mutagenic and carcinogenic in animals. Like nitrosoureas (see Chapter 11), nitrosamines are alkylating agents, and cause covalent modification of DNA bases. However, nitrosamines per se are chemically unreactive, and thus they require metabolic activation:

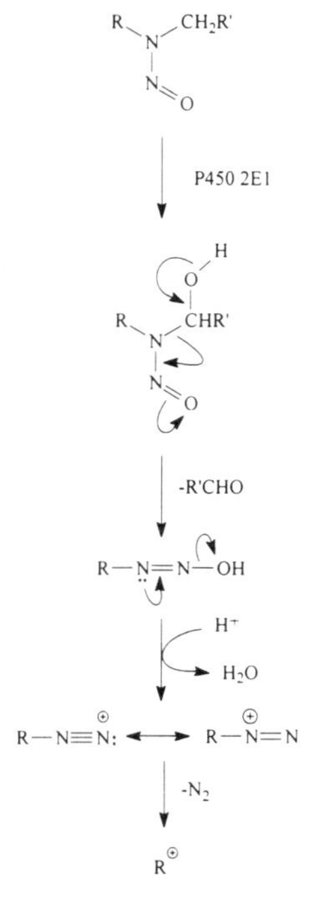

The key step is α-hydroxylation (12), catalyzed principally by P-4502E1. The resulting α-hydroxy metabolites are unstable and cannot be isolated. However, α-acetoxy nitrosamines have been synthesized and these precursors can be converted to the α-hydroxy form by the action of esterases.

α-Hydroxynitrosamines spontaneously decompose to yield reactive electrophiles. The nature of the reactive intermediate remains the subject of debate. One possibility (see scheme above) is the generation of alkyl cations, but the lifetime of such intermediates in solution would be exceedingly short, such that they might not survive diffusion from their site of formation to critical macromolecular targets.

SPECTROSCOPIC PROPERTIES OF CYTOCHROME P-450 ENZYMES

The heme group is a very strong chromophore and its spectroscopic properties are sensitive to the *nature of the ligands* bound to the heme iron, to the iron *oxidation state*, and to the *protein environment* in which the heme is located. The unique feature of the cytochrome P-450 class of enzymes, which led to their discovery and accounts for their name, is the ~450-nm absorption maximum of the reduced (ferrous, Fe^{2+}) carbon monoxide complex of the protein. Among different cytochrome P-450 enzymes, λ_{max} ranges from 447 to 452 nm. The analogous $Fe^{2+}CO$ complex of a spectroscopically typical heme protein is near 420 nm; myoglobin, for example, has $\lambda_{max} = 423$ nm. The position of λ_{max} for the $Fe^{2+}CO$ complex of a hemoprotein is strongly influenced by the identity of the ligand coordinated to the iron on the side opposite to that occupied by CO. This axial ligand, in myoglobin and most other hemoproteins, is a nitrogen atom of a histidine imidazole ring. The unusual P-450 chromophore suggested the presence of an unusual ligand: Earlier evidence from chemical model systems was consistent with a thiolate ligand, and the X-ray crystal structure of P-450$_{cam}$ showed directly that the *cytochrome P-450 axial ligand is the deprotonated sulfur of a cysteine (thiolate)*. Only proteins with a thiolate ligand have reduced CO complexes with λ_{max} near 450 nm (13). The thiolate ligand causes the Soret absorption band to split into the absorbance band at about 450 nm and a second band, of comparable intensity, with a maximum at about 370 nm. A few other proteins, notably thromboxane synthase, prostacyclin synthase, allene oxide synthase, nitric oxide synthase, and chloroperoxidase, also have a thiolate ligand and, therefore, an $Fe^{2+}CO$ complex λ_{max} near 450 nm. From the original work of Omura and Sato, it was already clear that denaturation of cytochrome P-450 caused a shift in λ_{max} from 450 nm to about 420 nm. *The unique spectroscopic signature of P-450 is due to a structural feature—the thiolate ligand—that is required for P-450 monooxygenase enzyme activity.*

P-450 Spin States

The absorption maximum of the "resting" (ferric, Fe^{3+}) state of cytochrome P-450 also depends on the ligation state of the iron. Two such states are known, and they often exist in equilibrium. The *low-spin* state is characterized by $\lambda_{max} = 416$–419 nm, and the *high-spin* state is characterized by $\lambda_{max} = 390$–416 nm (Fig. 14.1). The meaning of low- and high-spin states is readily understood on the basis of an elementary "crystal field" model of the electronic structure of the metal ion (14) and is supported by more sophisticated theoretical analysis. The valence electrons in iron and other transition metals occupy the five *d*-orbitals, so the influence of ligands on the energies of these *d* orbitals underlies the relationship between ligation and spin state. If the iron atom were suspended in free space, all five *d* orbitals (Fig. 14.2) would be degenerate (identical energies). In ferric iron, which has five *d* electrons, each of the orbitals would then be occupied by a single electron; this configuration satisfies Hund's rule and avoids the energy cost of putting two electrons with paired spins into a single orbital. This orbital occupancy, with an unpaired electron spin of 5/2 (1/2 for each unpaired electron), maximizes the number of unpaired electrons and is known as the *high-spin state*. Let us now consider what would happen if we bring negative charges (from ligand atoms) close to the $d_{x^2-y^2}$ and d_{z^2} orbitals, but *not* near to the d_{xy}, d_{xz}, or d_{yz} orbitals. (This "thought" experiment models the formation of an octahedral complex.) Electron repulsion makes placing an electron into the first two orbitals less favorable than for the other three; that is, the energies of the two orbitals vicinal to the negative charges are increased. The *d* orbitals are no longer degenerate, but are split into two groups as shown in Fig. 14.2. If the energy gap (Δ) that sep-

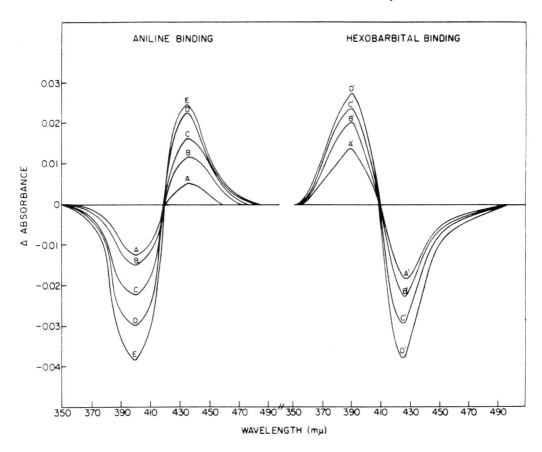

ANILINE BINDING   HEXOBARBITAL BINDING

WAVELENGTH (mμ)

Figure 14.1. Difference spectrum observed when hexobarbital, a "type I" substrate, or aniline, a "type II" substrate, is added to one side of a set of cuvettes containing rat liver microsomes. In a type I spectrum, the decrease in the low-spin species produces a trough at 419 nm while the increase in the absorption of the high-spin species produces the maximum of 390 nm. Approximately the reverse is observed with a type II spectrum. (Adapted with permission from G. J. Mannering, Microsomal enzyme systems which catalyze drug metabolism, in: *Fundamentals of Drug Metabolism and Drug Disposition*, B. La Du, H. G. Mandel, and E. L. Way, Eds., Williams and Wilkins, Baltimore, 1971, pp. 206–222.)

arates the higher from the lower energy orbitals is greater than the spin pairing energy, the five Fe^{3+} d electrons will occupy the lower three orbitals, giving rise to a net unpaired electron spin of 1/2. This state is known as a *low-spin state*.

The iron in a heme group is surrounded by the four nitrogen atoms of the porphyrin, the axial ligand provided by the protein (cysteine in cytochrome P-450), and, possibly, a sixth, distal ligand (e.g., O_2 or CO). The principle that governs the spin state in hemoproteins is similar to that outlined above. If the iron is hexacoordinated, the d_{z^2} orbital points at the proximal and distal ligands, and the $d_{x^2-y^2}$ orbital points toward the porphyrin nitrogen atoms. On the other hand, the d_{xz}, d_{yz}, and d_{xy} orbitals point between the ligands (Fig. 14.2). Two of the d orbitals in the hexacoordinated heme group are therefore at higher energies than the other three, resulting in a low-spin state. Removal of the distal ligand gives a pentacoordinated species in which the split in the energy levels is lower than the electron spin pairing energy, giving rise to a high-spin species, in which one electron occupies each orbital. The decrease in the energy of the $d_{x^2-y^2}$ as well as the d_{z^2} orbital in the pentacoordinate state is not obvious. However, the iron atom (which, in

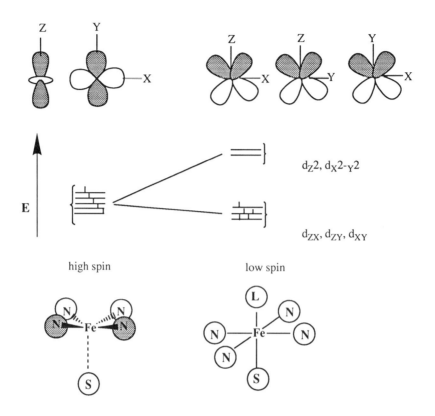

Figure 14.2. Splitting of the iron *d*-orbitals caused by placing the iron in a ligand field of either five or six electron-rich or negatively charged atoms. The shapes of the five *d*-orbitals are shown at the top and the ligand arrangements that give rise to low and high spin states are shown at the bottom.

its hexacoordinate state, lies in the plane of the porphyrin) moves out of the plane, toward the fifth ligand, in the pentacoordinate state. Therefore the $d_{x^2-y^2}$ orbital points less directly at the porphyrin nitrogens, and the d_{z^2} orbital is relieved of the interaction with the distal ligand. *Thus, the spin state indicates whether the iron in a hemoprotein is coordinated to a sixth ligand.*

Difference Spectra of Compounds Which Bind to P-450

Binding of compounds to microsomal cytochromes P-450 is often measured by monitoring the *difference spectrum* between the substrate-free microsomal sample and a second sample to which the compound of interest has been added (15). (This experimental approach suppresses background absorbances and increases the sensitivity and specificity of the measurement.) Measurement of difference spectra provides an experimental probe for studying the interaction between the enzyme and its substrates.

In cytochromes P-450$_{cam}$, P-450$_{terp}$, and P-450BM-3, the only members of the family for which crystal structures are available (see below), the distal ligand in the hexacoordinate resting state is a water molecule. This probably also holds for membrane-bound cytochrome P-450 enzymes. The binding of camphor to cytochrome P-450$_{cam}$ results in displacement of the water ligand, a shift from the hexacoordinate to the pentacoordinate state, and a consequent shift from the low- to the high-spin state. In the absolute optical spectrum, this causes a blue shift of λ_{max}. A typical difference spectrum is shown in Fig. 14.1. The low-spin species (419 nm) has decreased in concentration, while the high-spin species (390 nm) has increased. This type of spectrum, with a maximum at approximately 385–390 and a trough at approximately 420 nm, is known as a *type I difference spectrum*; it indicates the binding of a compound that displaces the distal ligand (H_2O) and causes a low-to-high spin shift. Many compounds induce a type I difference spectrum, including caffeine, DDT, phenobarbital, and chlorpromazine. Some, but not all, are P-450 substrates. In some cytochrome P-450 enzymes, the high-spin form is present as a significant component, even in the absence of added compounds. Apparently, no water molecule is co-ordinated to the iron in these enzymes, although the structural reasons for this are not known.

A distinct type of difference spectrum is observed when certain compounds, particularly those containing nitrogen heterocycles or other nitrogen functions, are added to cytochrome P-450 enzymes. Examples of such compounds are aniline, imidazole, pyridine, and nicotine. This spectrum has a maximum at approximately 425–435 nm and a trough at 390–405 nm, very nearly the inverse of the type I spectrum already described. This *type II difference spectrum* is associated with the binding of compounds which coordinate to the iron *even more strongly than water*. Some compounds resemble water in their coordination to the iron and produce a variant of the type II spectrum, known as a *reverse type I spectrum*. In this spectrum the maximum is at approximately 420 nm and the trough at 388–390 nm. The mixture of P-450 states present in a sample is shifted from the pentacoordinate, high-spin state toward the hexacoordinated, low-spin state by compounds that give either type II or reverse type I spectra. Finally, a few compounds bind without perturbing the ligation state of the heme iron and therefore do not give rise to a difference spectrum at all.

CATALYTIC CYCLE OF CYTOCHROME P-450

The overall stoichiometry of substrate hydroxylation by cytochrome P-450 is represented by the following equation:

$$NAD(P)H + O_2 + SH + H^+ \rightarrow NAD(P)^+ + SOH + H_2O$$

For all mammalian cytochrome P-450, the reducing cofactor is NADPH, but for some bacterial forms, such as P-450$_{cam}$, NADH is used. As will be described below, the reducing equivalents are passed to cytochrome P-450 via an accessory enzyme.

From the stoichiometry alone, we can deduce that several distinct chemical events must occur during the catalytic cycle. The enzyme must bind substrate and oxygen, accept two reducing equivalents and two protons, split the bond between the oxygen atoms, insert the oxygen atom into the substrate, and release the products, water and the oxygenated substrate. In what order do these molecular events occur, and what intermediate states of the enzyme exist? Much effort has been devoted to answering these questions. The tools for studying the reaction cycle include spectroscopy and enzyme kinetics, including isotope substitution methods. Our present understanding of the catalytic cycle is outlined here.

The catalytic cycle of cytochrome P-450 has been most thoroughly defined for the bacterial enzyme cytochrome P-450$_{cam}$ (16), but the essential features seem to apply to mitochondrial and microsomal enzymes as well.

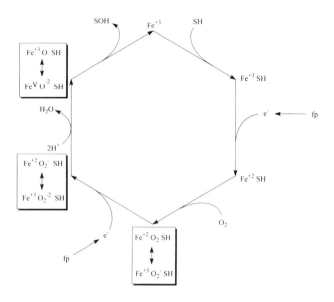

Catalytic cycle of cytochrome P-450 enzymes. Fe represents the iron atom of the prosthetic heme group of P-450; SH represents a substrate; fp represents flavoprotein (P-450-reductase). Formal charges are assigned to the Fe and oxygen atoms to facilitate electron "bookkeeping," but the heme ring, apoprotein (cysteine thiolate), and substrate also participate in the redox chemistry. For further discussion, see also V. Ullrich, Dioxygen activation by heme-sulfur proteins, *J. Molec. Catal.* 7:159–167, 1980; J. H. Dawson and K. S. Eble, Cytochrome P-450: Heme iron coordination structure and mechanisms of action, *Adv. Inorg. Bioinorg. Mech.* 4:1–64, 1986; T. D. Porter and M. J. Coon, Cytochrome P-450: Multiplicity of isoforms, substrates, and catalytic and regulatory mechanisms, *J. Biol. Chem.* 266:13469–13472, 1991; and P. R. Ortiz de Montellano, Ed., *Cytochrome P-450: Structure, Mechanism, and Biochemistry*, 2nd ed., Plenum, New York, 1995.

As already described, the binding of a substrate is usually accompanied by a shift from the low- to the high-spin state. The substrate-bound form is stable, in the absence of reducing equivalents and oxygen, so it is amenable to detailed study. (The crystal structures of complexes of cytochrome P-450$_{cam}$ with various substrates have been solved.) In the case of cytochrome P-450$_{cam}$, this shift in spin state changes the measured redox potential from -300 to -170 mV. *The substrate-bound enzyme is thus much more susceptible to reduction.* Electrons are transferred to cytochrome P-450 by an accessory enzyme: cytochrome P-450 reductase, in the case of hepatic microsomal P-450; adrenodoxin (adrenal mitochondrial P-450); or putidaredoxin (cytochrome P-450$_{cam}$). (These proteins are discussed in more detail in a later section). In at least one case, P-450BM-3, the reductase, and P-450 constitute separate domains of a single protein (see later). Putidaredoxin has a redox potential of -196 mV when bound to cytochrome P-450$_{cam}$. Thus, reduction of cytochrome P-450$_{cam}$ by putidaredoxin becomes thermodynamically accessible once substrate binds to P-450. Consequently, the P-450 enzyme is quiescent, in the absence of substrate, but becomes catalytically activated when a substrate is available. One-electron reduction of the ferric, substrate-bound enzyme to the ferrous form can be studied spectroscopically. The ferrous substrate-bound form of the enzyme rapidly reacts with oxygen to give the ferrous dioxygen-bound complex. Binding of oxygen to the ferrous form of P-450 is formally analogous to the binding of oxygen to hemoglobin or myoglobin, which function as reversible oxygen carriers in the ferrous state (see Chapter 8). However, one must bear in mind that the liganded thiolate anion also contributes to the electronic structure of the iron environment in P-450. The P-450 oxygen-binding step is reversible, but the dioxy form is much less stable in cytochrome P-450 with respect to autooxidation (to generate the ferric enzyme and superoxide ion) than in the case of hemoglobin/myoglobin: P-450 (Fe^{2+}) O_2 SH $\rightleftarrows$ P-450 (Fe^{3+}) $O_2^{\cdot-}$ SH. However, under physiological conditions the second electron transfer usually intervenes before such autoxidation can occur.

The unstable ferrous dioxygen-bound form of the enzyme can be observed by means of cryogenic, stopped-flow, or even conventional spectrophotometry. Addition of a second electron to the dioxygen complex, however, initiates a series of steps that occur too rapidly to be observed directly. Understanding of the sequence of events subsequent to the second electron transfer is based on inferences from chemical model systems and on indirect evidence. This is regrettable, since these later steps of the cycle are the events of greatest mechanistic interest.

Transfer of the second electron produces a complex which is electronically equivalent to that expected from coordination of the hydrogen peroxide dianion with the ferric enzyme:

$$Fe^{1+} O_2 \leftrightarrow Fe^{2+} O_2^{\cdot-} \leftrightarrow Fe^{3+} O_2^{2-}$$

The detailed electron distribution and structure of this complex remain unknown.

The remaining steps of the catalytic cycle are proton uptake, dioxygen cleavage, and substrate hydroxylation. In principle, dioxygen cleavage might occur either before or after substrate hydroxylation. That is to say, the active hydroxylating enzyme intermediate might contain one or two oxygen atoms. The former possibility is almost certainly the major route. Uptake of two protons followed by heterolytic cleavage of the dioxygen bond, with loss of a molecule of water, would give a catalytically active *ferryl* (Fe=O) heme species:

$$Fe^{3+} O_2^{2-} + 2H^+ \rightarrow H_2O + Fe^{3+} O \text{ (or } Fe^V O^{2-})$$

This highly oxidized species may be viewed, formally, as a complex of ferric iron with a neutral oxygen atom ["oxene," in analogy to other six-electron species, carbenes (17) and nitrenes] or as a complex of ferryl iron with a reduced oxygen atom (redox state of water). Undoubtedly, interaction with the cysteine thiolate ligand helps to stabilize this reactive form of the enzyme. This species, still poorly characterized, is often called an "oxenoid" intermediate.

A similar (although probably not identical) species is obtained if the ferric enzyme is allowed to react with hydrogen peroxide, in the absence of NADPH and cytochrome P-450 reductase (18). In some instances, *hydrogen peroxide can replace enzymatically reduced molecular oxygen in the catalytic cycle*; that is, P-450 plus hydrogen peroxide can carry out hydroxylation reactions. This evidence suggests that the intermediate prior to the ferryl species resembles a complex of hydrogen peroxide with ferric cytochrome P-450. In fact, the consumption of oxygen and NADPH by cytochrome P-450 results sometimes in the formation (and release) of hydrogen peroxide, rather than in substrate oxidation. Subtle differences in the structure of the "peroxide" complex that precedes the ferryl species may determine whether it (a) releases hydrogen peroxide or (b) fragments to yield the catalytically active ferryl species.

In the final step of the catalytic process, the oxygen atom of the ferryl species reacts with, and is usually transferred to, the substrate. The substrate presumably remains bound to the enzyme throughout the electron transfer and oxygen activation sequence, and it is released after reaction with the ferryl oxygen. In the case of substrates that are relatively difficult to oxidize, the ferryl oxygen can apparently be reduced to water by additional electrons, provided by the accessory reductase or reductase/iron–sulfur protein pair (see below). To the extent that superoxide, hydrogen peroxide, and water are produced during the catalytic turnover of cytochrome P-450, the reaction is said to be *uncoupled*, and it deviates from the ideal monooxygenase stoichiometry given earlier.

ELECTRON TRANSPORT TO CYTOCHROME P-450

P-450 heme iron accepts electrons one at a time, whereas NADPH and NADH are two-electron donors. Therefore, the electrons provided by the pyridine nucleotides to the heme group must pass through a "transformer," which accepts paired electrons (in the form of hydride anion, H^-) but delivers single electrons to the iron atom. These functions are satisfied by either (a) a flavoprotein plus an iron–sulfur protein or (b) a single protein with two flavin prosthetic groups.

Mitochondrial and Bacterial P-450 Systems

The catalytic turnover of mitochondrial cytochrome P-450 enzymes is supported by the two-component system, as is the turnover of cytochrome P-450$_{cam}$ and most other bacterial enzymes (19). The flavoprotein component found in adrenal cortex mitochondria, known as adrenodoxin reductase, has a single FAD prosthetic group and molecular weight of ~ 54 kD. The companion iron–sulfur protein, *adrenodoxin* (MW ~ 12.5 kD), has an active site with two iron atoms, each coordinated to two cysteinyl sulfurs and bridged by two inorganic sulfur atoms ([2Fe–2S] cluster (20)). Transfer of hydride ion from NADPH to the FAD yields a two-electron reduced form of the reductase, which is reoxidized in two discrete, one-electron transfers to each of two molecules of iron–sulfur protein (Fig. 14.3). The iron–sulfur proteins subsequently transfer the electron to the P-450 heme iron atom. In other words, the iron–sulfur protein shuttles electrons between the flavo- and hemoproteins. This two-protein electron transfer system is particularly important for the biosynthesis of steroid hormones in adrenal mitochondria. The corresponding proteins responsible for supplying electrons to cytochrome P-450$_{cam}$ are known, respectively, as *putidaredoxin reductase* (M_r 48 kD) and *putidaredoxin* (M_r 12.5 kD). Putidaredoxin reductase, like adrenodoxin reductase, has a single FAD prosthetic group, but is reduced by NADH rather than NADPH.

The molar ratio of flavoprotein: iron–sulfur protein:hemoprotein in both adrenal mitochondria and *P. putida* is approximately 1:8:8, so that one flavoprotein reductase provides the electrons for several cytochrome P-450 enzymes.

Microsomal P-450 Systems

Electron transfer from reduced pyridine nucleotides to microsomal cytochrome P-450, including the enzymes involved in mammalian xenobiotic metabolism, is mediated by the enzyme *NADPH-cytochrome P-450 reductase*. P-450 reductase was, in fact, discovered long before P-450 itself. In 1950, Horecker identified a hepatic microsomal enzyme which catalyzed the reduction of cytochrome c (Fe^{3+} to Fe^{2+}) by NADPH. The activity was detected by monitoring the shift in the absorbance spectrum of cytochrome c accompanying reduction. Cytochrome c, of course, is a mitochondrial protein; in these experiments, it was used simply as a convenient protein electron acceptor, readily available in pure form. Horecker named the new enzyme *NADPH-cytochrome c reductase*, reflecting the assay method; its physiological function was, presumably, to reduce some then-unidentified microsomal protein. In the 1960s, following the work of Omura and Sato, it became clear that the physiological substrate is cytochrome P-450, and the enzyme was renamed

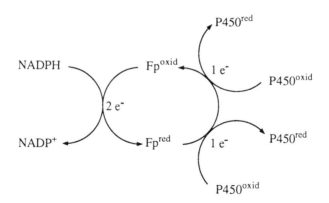

Figure 14.3. The two systems involved in the transfer of electrons from reduced pyridine nucleotides to cytochrome P-450. In one system, a flavoprotein reductase (Fp) transfers electron to an iron-sulfur protein (ISP), which in turn delivers the electrons to the hemoprotein. In the second system, a flavoprotein with two flavin prosthetic groups directly transfers the electrons from NADPH to cytochrome P-450.

NADPH-cytochrome P-450 reductase (or oxidoreductase) (21). Cytochrome c reduction is still used as the standard assay for the reductase.

Lu and Coon, in their original work on reconstitution of P-450 activity from purified microsomal components, demonstrated that the necessary and sufficient constituents required for P-450 enzyme activity are P-450 itself, NADPH-cytochrome P-450 reductase, and phospholipid. (The phospholipid presumably provides a suitable milieu for association of P-450 and reductase, and is not required with soluble forms of P-450.)

The reductase (MW ~78 kD) consists of a large cytosolic domain containing the two flavins and an N-terminal hydrophobic peptide that anchors the protein to the membrane (22, 23). The sequences of NADPH-cytochrome P-450 reductases from many sources, deduced from the sequences of the corresponding genes, are very similar. Reconstitution experiments show that reductase from one species can often reduce cytochrome P-450 from another species. Reductase sequences include (a) two consensus regions associated with flavin binding and (b) a segment indicative of a binding site for a pyridine nucleotide. The sequence evidence agrees with the results of biochemical analysis: The reductase has two flavins, one FMN and one FAD, as prosthetic groups. The protein is reduced by NADPH but not by NADH. Studies of the function of cytochrome P-450 reductase indicate that the pathway of electron flow is from NADPH to reductase-bound FAD, then to bound FMN, and finally to P-450 heme.

Although NADPH-cytochrome P-450 reductase is the only accessory protein absolutely required for reconstitution of P-450 activity in a purified system, the possibility still exists that other microsomal proteins facilitate P-450 activity in vivo. Hepatic microsomes also contain the heme enzyme, cytochrome b5, and the flavoprotein, cytochrome b5 reductase. Microsomal cytochrome b5 is a membrane-bound form of the cytosolic enzyme found in the red blood cell (see Chapter 8). The principal enzymatic activity of the b5/b5 reductase system is desaturation of fatty acids (24). However, the P-450-catalyzed turnover of some substrates can be increased synergistically by electron transfer from cytochrome b5 (25). That is, while NADH alone will not support microsomal P-450 activity, the addition of NADH results in a severalfold increase in product formation, above the maximum rate obtained with excess NADPH. Similar stimulation of product formation is observed, in some instances, when cytochrome b5 is included in a system reconstituted from purified cytochrome P-450 and cytochrome P-450 reductase. (Cytochrome b5 reductase is not required in such reconstitution studies, because cytochrome b5 can be reduced directly by NADPH-cytochrome P-450 reductase.) Kinetic studies show that cytochrome b5 can transfer the second, but not the first, electron required for the catalytic turnover of cytochrome P-450. The synergistic effects of NADH and cytochrome b5 are due, at least in part, to an increase in the coupling of reduced pyridine nucleotide and oxygen consumption to product formation (i.e., to a decrease in the uncoupled reduction of oxygen to give H_2O_2 or water, rather than substrate oxidation). The physiological significance of this "crosstalk" electron flow between the microsomal b5 and P-450 systems remains obscure.

PURIFICATION OF MICROSOMAL P-450

The purification of active P-450 depends on the solubilization of the membrane-bound enzyme. This can be accomplished with nonionic detergents, such as Nonoxynol or octyl glucoside:

Non-ionic detergents for P-450 solubilization

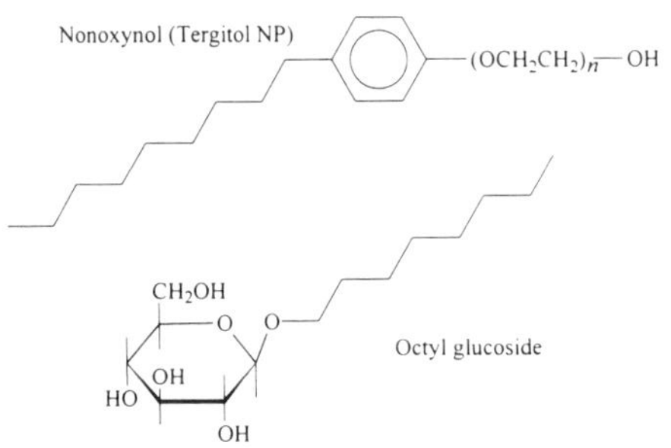

P-450 is stabilized by the presence of 20% glycerol. P-450 protein is purified by column chromatography on media such as hydroxyapatite, n-octylaminosepharose, and DEAE-sepharose. Complete separation of individual forms may be difficult to achieve by column chromatography; isoelectric focusing has been successfully applied to the resolution of phenobarbital-inducible forms (26).

P-450 INHIBITORS

The involvement of P-450 in a microsomal biotransformation can be examined by studying the effects of inhibitors of P-450 activity. CO itself is an inhibitor, since it binds strongly to the ferrous form of P-450, formed during the catalytic cycle. Thus, P-450 reactions are inhibited under an atmosphere of, say, 95% O_2 + 5% CO. CO gas is not applicable in whole animal studies, for obvious reasons, and CO can inhibit many heme proteins other than P-450, so it is not an ideal inhibitor. Several rather nonspecific chemical inhibitors of P-450 activity have been used for many years, notably metyrapone, α-naphthoflavone, and SKF 5252A. In recent years, many researchers have endeavored to develop isoform-selective inhibitors of P-450 activity. Such agents could be used experimentally to test the involvement of particular enzyme forms in bioactivation or detoxication processes, and inhibitor structure–activity relationships could also illuminate our understanding of active-site structure. Since some forms of P-450 (such as CYP 1A1 and CYP1A2) bioactivate carcinogens, isoform-specific inhibitors might also have potential as chemopreventive agents against chemically induced cancer. These developments are discussed in a recent review (27).

CLONING OF P-450 GENES AND THEIR EXPRESSION

The introduction of molecular biological approaches had a particularly profound effect on the study of P-450. Because mammalian P-450 enzymes are membrane-bound and because they are usually present as families of closely related proteins, with levels of expression ranging from very low to very high, their separation and purification presents great difficulties. The cloning of P-450 genes, on the other hand, is relatively straightforward. The well-conserved consensus sequences can be used to design effective DNA probes. For example, degenerate oligonucleotides based on the heme-binding domain were used to PCR-amplify and clone genes encoding P-450 flavonoid hydroxylases, which control flower color in petunias (28). As mentioned earlier, the success of P-450 cloning has brought order to the analysis of P-450 enzymes.

Heterologous expression of individual P-450 forms facilitates the analysis of P-450 structure–function relationships in "clean" cellular systems which do not express endogenous P-450. Also, large amounts of protein may be obtained; this is especially important for P-450 forms which are difficult to obtain from their original sources, such as human forms or forms expressed at low levels. Successful expression of P-450 has been achieved in mammalian, yeast (29), bacterial (30) and insect cells.

P-450 ON THE INTERNET

Computer users familiar with the WorldWideWeb (WWW) service on the InterNet have access to valuable sources of information on P-450 and other proteins. A special Web site for P-450 gene and protein sequence data, known as the "Directory of P-450-Containing

Systems" has been established: The URL access code for this site is http://www.icgeb.tri-este.it/p450/.

P-450 STRUCTURE

Although the gene sequences of more than 300 cytochrome P-450 enzymes are now known, only three X-ray crystal structures[*] have been determined, for P-450$_{cam}$ (31), P-450$_{terp}$ (CYP108) (32), and the heme-containing domain of P-450BM-3 (CYP102) (33). These three P-450 enzymes are soluble bacterial proteins; no membrane-bound mammalian P-450 has yet been crystallized. (Indeed, very few membrane proteins have yielded to the efforts of crystallographers.) Nevertheless, sequence comparisons, supported by a variety of physical, chemical, and biochemical experiments, suggest that the structures of the membrane-bound enzymes are similar to those of the soluble enzymes. The similarities evident among the structures of cytochromes P-450$_{terp}$, P-450BM-3, and P-450$_{cam}$ are consistent with the idea that all P-450s are structurally related (34). Indeed, cytochrome P-450BM-3, like the microsomal P-450 enzymes, can be reduced by cytochrome P-450 reductase, rather than by the flavoprotein/iron–sulfur pairs involved in the reduction of P-450$_{cam}$ and P-450$_{terp}$. P-450BM-3 shares higher sequence similarity with mammalian enzymes of the 4A family (25–30%) than with P-450$_{cam}$ or related bacterial enzymes (15–20%).

Cytochrome P-450$_{cam}$ is roughly a triangular prism, with 12 helical segments encompassing almost half of the amino acid residues (Fig. 14.4). The heme prosthetic group is "sandwiched" between the L helix (on the proximal or thiolate-ligand side) and the I helix (on the distal or substrate-binding side). The proximal helix forms part of the outer surface of the protein; the distal helix extends across the hydrophobic interior of the structure. The heme group is held in place (noncovalently) by hydrophobic contacts with the two helices, hydrogen bonds between the negatively charged propionic acid substituents of the heme and basic residues Arg-299 and His-355, and by the thiolate ligand to the iron, provided by Cys-357. This cysteine residue is located just before the N-terminus of the proximal (L) helix. *The liganded cysteine is absolutely conserved in all cytochrome P-450 enzyme sequences, and many of the residues in its vicinity are also strongly conserved* (see Table 14.3).

The crystal structure of P-450$_{cam}$ with camphor bound in the active site shows that a hydrogen bond exists between the carbonyl group of the substrate and the hydroxyl group of Tyr-96. In addition to this hydrogen bond, camphor makes other contacts, notably with residues Phe-87, Leu-244, Val-247, and Val-295 (9). These interactions position the camphor group approximately 4 Å above the heme plane directly adjacent to the oxygen binding site (Fig. 14.5). Site-specific mutagenesis studies, and the use of camphor analogues from which the carbonyl or methyl groups have been deleted, show that the hydrogen bond and the hydrophobic interactions of the methyl groups with the protein are not essential for catalytic turnover. In the absence of one or more of these interactions, however, the oxidation of camphor no longer exclusively yields 5-*exo*-hydroxy camphor (35, 36). In addition, coupling of oxygen and NADH consumption to substrate oxidation decreases as the interactions that orient and fix the substrate with respect to the oxidizing species are eliminated by substrate modification or site-directed mutagenesis.

---

[*]And now there are four: Cupp-Vickery, J.R., and Poulos, T.L., Strucure of cytochrome P450eryF involved in erythromycin biosynthesis, *Nature Struct. Biol.* 2:144–153, 1995.

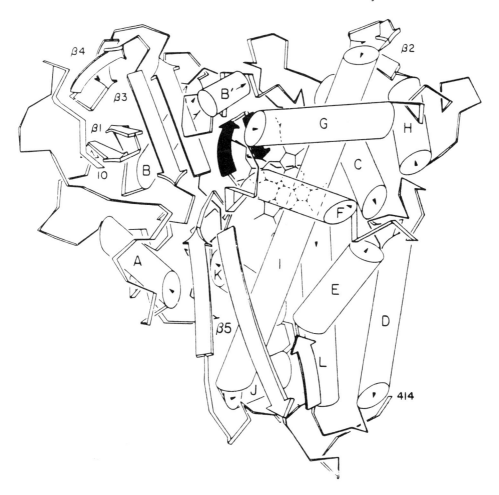

Figure 14.4. Crystal structure of cytochrome P-450$_{cam}$ showing the overall dimensions of the protein and location of the active site in the interior of the protein. (Adapted with permission from T. L. Poulos, B. C. Finzel, and A. J. Howard, High-resolution crystal structure of cytochrome P450$_{cam}$, *J. Mol. Biol.* 195:687–700, 1987.)

Examination of the crystal structure shows that the haem and substrate are buried within the protein. How, then, does the substrate get into the active site? As with many enzymes, entry of the substrate requires conformational changes in the protein structure, opening a channel into the active site. These conformational changes can be thought of as a "breath-

Table 14.3. Amino Acid Sequences in the Conserved Cysteine Region of Cytochrome P-450^a

CYP101	(*P. put.*)	**F**	**G**	H	**G**	S	H	L	**C**^{357}	L	**G**	Q	H	L	**A**	R	R
CYP1A1	(human)	**F**	**G**	M	**G**	K	**R**	K	**C**^{457}	I	**G**	E	T	I	**A**	R	W
CYP1A1	(rat)	**F**	**G**	L	**G**	K	**R**	K	**C**^{461}	I	**G**	E	T	I	G	R	L
CYP1A2	(rat)	**F**	**G**	L	**G**	K	**R**	R	**C**^{456}	I	**G**	E	I	P	**A**	K	W
CYP2C10	(human)	**F**	S	A	**G**	K	**R**	I	**C**^{435}	V	**G**	E	A	L	**A**	G	M
CYP2C12	(rat)	**F**	S	A	**G**	K	**R**	K	**C**^{435}	V	**G**	E	G	L	**A**	S	M
CYP2E1	(rat)	**F**	S	A	**G**	K	**R**	V	**C**^{437}	V	**G**	E	G	L	**A**	R	M
CYP4A1	(rat)	**F**	S	G	**G**	A	**R**	N	**C**^{456}	I	**G**	K	Q	F	**A**	M	S
CYP19A1	(human)	**F**	**G**	F	**G**	P	**R**	G	**C**^{437}	A	**G**	K	Y	I	**A**	M	V

^{a}Conserved residues are shown in **boldface** type. The conserved cysteine in P-450$_{cam}$ is ligated to the heme iron.

ing" motion of the protein, opening and closing the channel. Crystallization of the protein "traps" the structure in one of its conformations and prevents observation of the entry channel, but analysis of the structure suggests that the channel is opened by movement of residues Phe-87, Phe-193, and Ile-395.

Sequence comparisons of cytochrome P-450$_{cam}$ with other cytochrome P-450 enzymes show that a threonine residue analogous to Thr-252 in the I helix of P-450$_{cam}$ is highly conserved, although a few enzymes are known in which it is replaced by Ser or Asn (see Table 14.4). Thr-252 in the P-450$_{cam}$ structure forms a hydrogen bond to the peptide carbonyl of Gly-248 and causes a disruption of the otherwise normal I helix. This "kink" in the I helix, between residues 248 and 252, stabilized by additional hydrogen bond and ionic interactions, forms a cavity close to the heme iron atom; this may be the site in which the distal oxygen is located in the oxygen-bound ferrous enzyme. Site-directed mutation of Thr-252 in P-450$_{cam}$ results in greatly increased uncoupled reduction of molecular oxygen to hydrogen peroxide, although the enzyme retains some catalytic activity. However, in mammalian P-450 enzymes, mutations of the residue believed to correspond to Thr-252 in P-450$_{cam}$ do not always interfere with catalytic activity. In rat CYP1A2, for example, the mutation Thr-319 → Ala suppresses the enzyme's ability to oxidize benzphetamine, but does not alter its ability to oxidize 7-ethoxycoumarin (37). Such experi-

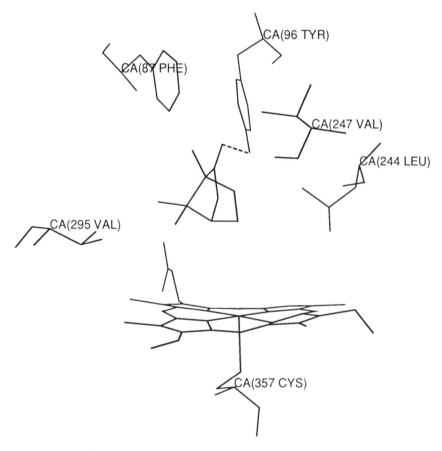

Figure 14.5. Details of the active site of cytochrome P-450$_{cam}$ showing the locations of the bound camphor substrate and several amino acid residues with respect to the heme group.

Table 14.4. Amino Acid Sequences that Correspond to the I Helix of Cytochrome P-450$_{cam}$ in the Vicinity of the Conserved Threonine[a]

CYP101	(*P. put.*)	L	V	G	G	L	D	T^{252}	V	V	N	F	L
CYP1A1	(human)	F	G	A	G	F	D	T^{321}	V	T	T	A	I
CYP1A1	(rat)	F	G	A	G	F	D	T^{325}	I	T	T	A	I
CYP1A2	(rat)	F	G	A	G	F	E	T^{319}	V	T	T	A	I
CYP2C10	(human)	F	G	A	G	T	E	T^{301}	T	S	T	T	L
CYP2C12	(rat)	F	I	G	G	T	E	T^{301}	S	S	L	T	L
CYP2E1	(rat)	F	F	A	G	T	E	T^{303}	T	S	T	T	L
CYP4A1	(rat)	M	F	E	G	H	D	T^{324}	T	A	S	G	V
CYP19A1	(human)	L	I	A	A	P	D	T^{310}	M	S	V	S	L

[a]Conserved residues are shown in **boldface** type.

ments provide indirect evidence which should help to build a model of the active-site environment in mammalian P-450 enzymes.

Cytochrome P-450$_{BM-3}$ is unique among known cytochrome P-450 enzymes: It contains, within a single polypeptide chain, domains that correspond to both "cytochrome P-450" and "cytochrome P-450 reductase." The crystal structure reported in 1993 is that of the hemoprotein domain only; it was obtained by heterologous expression (in *E. coli*) of a gene from which the coding sequence for the flavoprotein domain was deleted. The gross structure of the hemoprotein domain is very similar to that of P-450$_{cam}$, although the individual helices and other structural elements are displaced (as much as 10 Å) from the positions of the corresponding elements in P-450$_{cam}$.

Structures of Mammalian P-450 Enzymes

The solution of the first P-450 structure (P-450$_{cam}$), in 1987, was a breakthrough in the understanding of P-450. However, the mammalian xenobiotic-metabolizing P-450 enzymes are of greater interest to toxicologists and pharmacologists. Since crystallographic evidence is still lacking, we must fall back on indirect approaches to elucidation of their structures: sequence comparison with bacterial P-450 enzymes; site-directed mutagenesis; chemical modification; and so on.

Sequence alignments of membrane-bound cytochrome P-450 enzymes and P-450$_{cam}$ suggest that the main structural features of the membrane-bound enzymes are similar to those of the bacterial protein. The overall structural similarity of P-450BM-3 to P-450$_{cam}$ is reassuring, in this regard, because P-450BM-3 shows higher sequence identity with the mammalian P-450 4A1 family than with P-450$_{cam}$. P-450BM-3 obtains its electrons from a two-flavin protein domain closely resembling the mammalian microsomal cytochrome P-450 reductase, rather than from the iron–sulfur protein plus flavoprotein pair that supports catalytic turnover of the bacterial enzyme. Studies with chemical probes of protein structure provide further experimental evidence that the active sites of mammalian cytochromes P-450 resemble that of P-450$_{cam}$. For example, the I helix, which holds the heme group in place in P-450$_{cam}$, sits above the same pyrrole ring of the heme in the membrane-bound enzymes (38). In general, site-directed mutagenesis studies carried out on the mammalian enzymes, based on sequence alignments with P-450$_{cam}$, cause changes in catalytic activity or substrate-specificity which are consistent with structural homology. On the basis of the sequence alignments and experimental evidence, six regions of the mammalian enzymes are proposed to be involved in determining substrate specificity. These regions are known as *substrate recognitions sites* (SRS). In the case of cytochrome P-450$_{cam}$, the substrate contacts are directly known from the crystal structure and are more limited. Nevertheless, residues in the regions of mammalian enzymes that correspond to the underlined regions of P-450$_{cam}$ are hypothesized to be close to the substrate and to influence its binding. Caution must be used in such extrapolations, of course, because of the ambiguities inherent in sequence alignments. Models of mammalian enzymes based on sequence correlations with the P-450$_{cam}$ structure may give general structural information, but cannot provide the structural precision required for rationalization of substrate specificities.

The membrane topology of microsomal P-450 in the endoplasmic reticulum remains controversial. Amino acid sequences of microsomal P-450 forms always contain a section of about 25 very hydrophobic residues beginning at the amino terminus. This hydrophobic region is recognized by signal recognition particle, which directs insertion of the enzyme into the endoplasmic reticulum membrane, and also functions as a stop-transfer sequence (see Chapter 10). The orientation is *N*-luminal, C-cytoplasmic, as for the UDP-glucuronyltransferases (39). The bulk of the P-450 protein is probably exposed on the cytosolic, rather than the luminal, side of the endoplasmic reticulum (40).

P-450-CATALYZED REACTIONS

The wide variety of metabolites formed by cytochrome P-450-catalyzed reactions is, initially, disconcerting—even bewildering. The student may scarcely believe that such a variety of chemistry can be accounted for by a single class of enzymes. However, many of these metabolites arise by secondary, non-enzyme-catalyzed decompositions of the products formed by the enzymes. Most of the reactions catalyzed by cytochrome P-450 enzymes involve variations on a limited number of chemical possibilities:

> *hydroxylation*: replacement of hydrogen by hydroxyl
> *epoxidation*: addition of oxygen to a carbon–carbon π-bond
> *heteroatom oxidation*: addition of oxygen to an electron lone pair on a nitrogen, sulfur, or other heteroatom

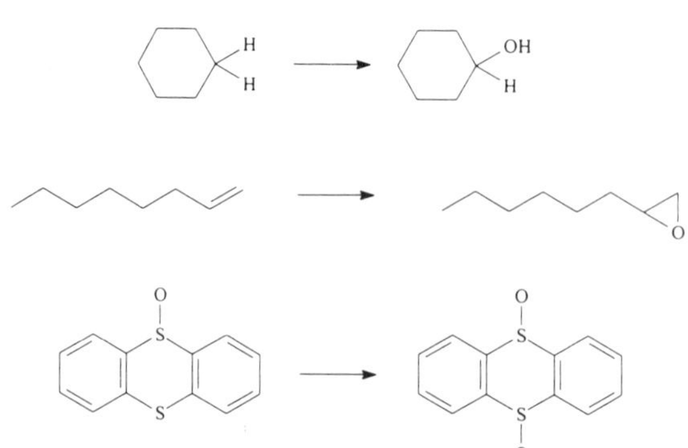

Classes of cytochrome P-450-catalyzed oxidations: hydroxylations, epoxidations, and heteroatom oxidations.

> *reduction*: generally observed only when the supply of molecular oxygen is limited and when an alternate electron acceptor is available (41)

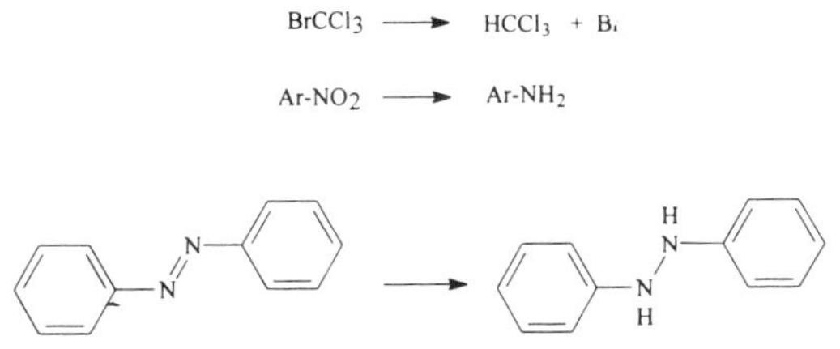

BrCCl$_3$ $\longrightarrow$ HCCl$_3$ + B$_r$

Ar-NO$_2$ $\longrightarrow$ Ar-NH$_2$

Reductions catalyzed by cytochrome P-450.

The main contribution of P-450 is activation of molecular oxygen to a species that is sufficiently reactive to attack relatively inert chemical sites, such as unactivated carbon–hydrogen bonds and aromatic rings.

The reaction of the activated oxygen with the substrate, on the other hand, is apparently not assisted or controlled by the enzyme, other than that *the enzyme juxtaposes the substrate and the reactive oxygen and thus limits the sites on the substrate with which oxygen can react.* The catalytic outcome is thus primarily determined by the nature and relative reactivities of the accessible positions on the substrate.

SIDEBAR: PRIMARY HYDROGEN–DEUTERIUM (OR TRITIUM) KINETIC ISOTOPE EFFECTS

Three isotopes of hydrogen are known: H, D (^{2}H), and T (^{3}H; radioactive). The large mass differences among these isotopes result in substantial chemical isotope effects—much larger than those observed with heavier atoms. These effects can provide valuable information about the mechanisms of reactions involving hydrogen atoms (42). The C$-$H bond is significantly weaker than the C$-$D (or C$-$T) bond, because the quantum-mechanical vibrational zero-point energy of the C$-$D bond is lower, due to the difference in masses. If a C$-$H bond is broken in the transition state of a reaction, then the rate will be faster for a C$-$H than for a C$-$D bond:

The maximum possible kinetic isotope effect (calculated on simple theoretical grounds) is $k_H/k_D = 7$. The effects can be much *lower*, if C$-$H bond breaking is only partially rate-limiting, and much *higher*, if tunneling and other quantum mechanical effects are taken into consideration. In the overall reaction catalyzed by cytochrome P-450, oxygen activation ([e.g., electron transfer from P-450 reductase) is usually the rate-limiting step. Therefore, a small or negligible difference is observed on the *overall rate of product formation* when a hydrogen atom, at the site of the reaction, is replaced by deuterium. However, if the active site is sufficiently flexible to allow the catalytic group of the enzyme to "choose" between equivalent C$-$H and C$-$D bonds *within the same substrate*, substantial *isotopic discrimination* between the two types of bonds can be observed (even in the absence of a significant isotope effect on the overall rate of product formation). This *intramolecular isotope effect* can be calculated from the change in the ratio of hydrogen to deuterium substitution in the substrate and product.

HYDROXYLATION REACTIONS

Carbon hydroxylation is probably the most characteristic P-450 reaction. Even completely unactivated carbon atoms, such as those in saturated fatty acids, can be hydroxylated by P-450, a feat that can hardly be duplicated by the organic chemist. This activity of P-450 is crucial to the biotransformation of a wide range of xenobiotic compounds, such as aliphatic hydrocarbons and polycyclic aromatic hydrocarbons.

Specific substitution of deuterium at one of two equivalent C−H bonds shifts oxidation from the deuterated to the nondeuterated site. This gives rise to large *intramolecular* isotope effects ($k_H/k_D > 7$), in contrast to relatively small isotope effects on the overall rate of the reaction. This result indicates that the reaction outcome is determined by competition between accessible sites (43):

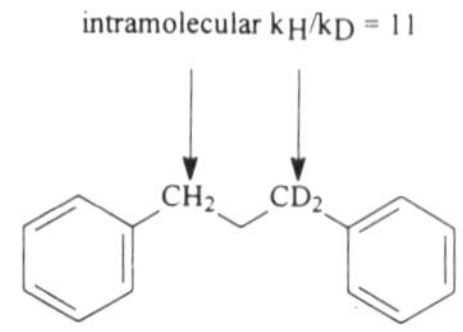

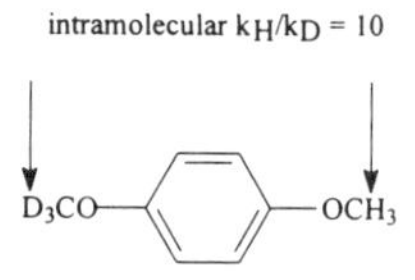

intramolecular k_H/k_D = 11

intramolecular k_H/k_D = 10

Two compounds for which intramolecular isotope effects have been measured by determining the extent of reaction at the deuterated site with respect to the analogous nondeuterated site on the same molecule.

The small kinetic isotope effect on the overall rate of product formation shows that steps other than the oxygen insertion event determine the overall rate of the enzymatic reaction. This is not surprising, in view of the large number of steps in the reaction cycle. The large *intramolecular* isotope effect, on the other hand, indicates that the *energy required to break the C−H bond is a major determinant of the site of the oxygen insertion.*

The intrinsic reactivities of C−H bonds to P-450 hydroxylation decrease in the order tertiary > secondary > primary (44, 45). This observation is consistent with the C−H bond breakage rule just given. Of course, this intrinsic reactivity can be masked by steric effects and by positioning of the substrate in the active site, but it is readily observed when these other factors are minimized. For example, one can examine the proportions of the hydroxylated metabolites formed from small hydrocarbons. Here, the hydroxylation regioselectivity is likely to be controlled primarily by the relative C−H bond energies and by steric effects, rather than by restricted movement within the active site:

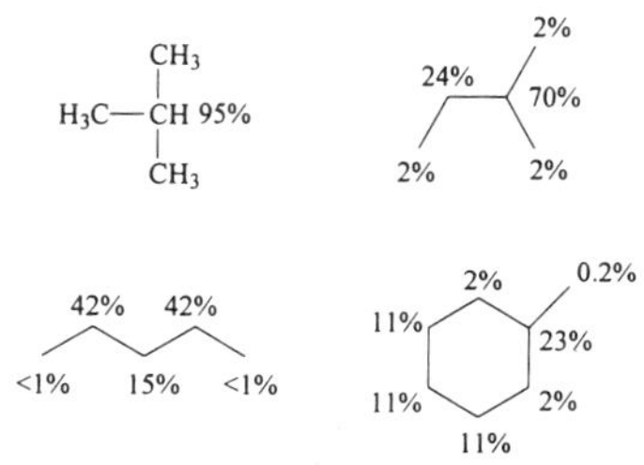

Regiospecificity of the hydroxylation of small hydrocarbons by liver microsomal cytochrome P-450. The proportion of the total hydroxylation reaction occurring at each carbon is indicated.

iso-Butane is hydroxylated primarily at the tertiary carbon, despite the presence of nine primary C−H bonds; methylcyclohexane is hydroxylated to a greater extent at the tertiary carbon than at any individual secondary carbon. Primary carbons are disfavored in all cases.

Hydroxylation mechanisms may be classified as stepwise, postulating discrete activated-carbon intermediates, or concerted, in which the oxygen atom is directly inserted into the C−H bond without intermediates. At first, the observation that regiochemistry and stereochemistry are usually preserved in P-450-catalyzed hydroxylations was taken as evidence for a concerted hydroxylation mechanism. However, the correlation between bond strength and reactivity is consistent with a stepwise "oxygen-rebound" hydroxylation mechanism: hydrogen atom transfer to the reactive oxygen, followed by recombination of the resulting carbon radical with the iron-bound equivalent of a hydroxyl radical:

$$[Fe^V{=}O] + R_3C{-}H \rightarrow [Fe^{IV}{-}OH] + R_3C^{\cdot} \rightarrow [Fe^{III}] + R_3C{-}OH$$

Evidence for this stepwise oxygen insertion mechanism was obtained in a study of the hydroxylation of *exo*-tetradeuterated norbornane, which yields (in part) products in which the deuterium is retained in the *endo* configuration on the hydroxylated carbon (46):

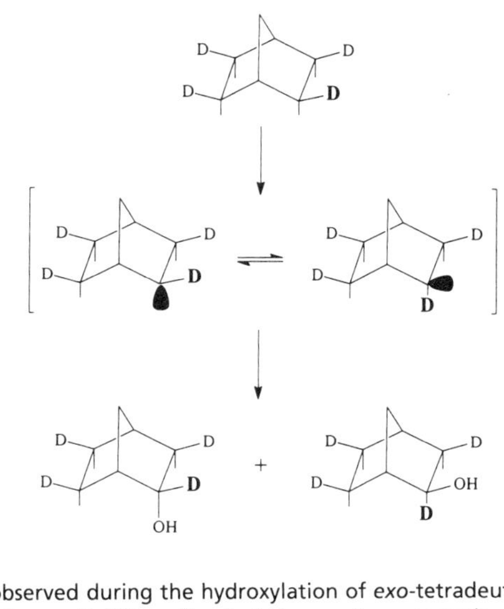

Loss of stereochemistry observed during the hydroxylation of *exo*-tetradeuterated norbornane by rabbit liver microsomal cytochrome P-450 implies that the reaction proceeds, as shown, via an intermediate in which the reaction site can undergo stereochemical inversion.

This inversion of the deuterium stereochemistry during the hydroxylation reaction requires the formation of a discrete intermediate, in which the geometry of the tetrahedral carbon can undergo inversion. Several examples of reactions that occur with loss of stereo- or regiochemistry and which therefore must proceed via an intermediate are now known.

Of course, if the carbon radical intermediate is very short-lived, a stepwise mechanism may be almost indistinguishable from a concerted mechanism. This is thought to describe the P-450 mechanism: The reaction is always stepwise, but the recombination step, in which the carbon radical combines with the ferryl oxygen, is very rapid. The rate of the recombination reaction has been measured by the use of "radical clock" probes. A radical clock is a radical that rearranges to a different radical at a known rate (k_r). If both the initially formed and rearranged radicals are trapped by a common reaction, then the rate of the trapping reaction (kt) can be estimated from the ratio of the rearranged and nonrearranged products and the known rate of the rearrangement. Experiments using this approach indicate that the recombination rate is $\sim 10^{10}$ sec^{-1}.

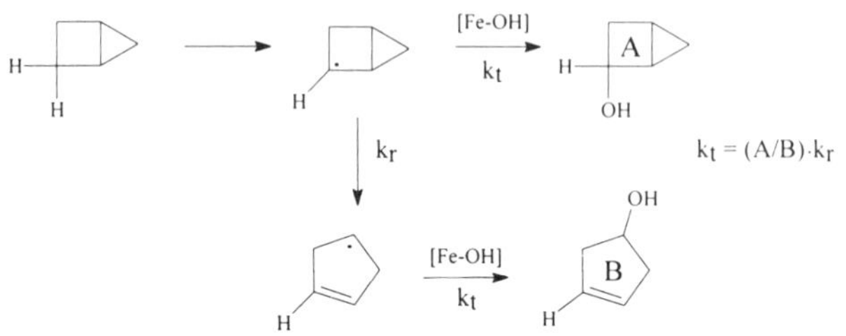

Determination of the approximate rate of the radical recombination step in the hydroxylation of hydrocarbons with the help of a "radical clock" probe. The rate of the recombination step that results in hydroxylation can be calculated, as shown, from the ratio of the rearranged to unrearranged products and the known rate of the rearrangement reaction.

However, Newcomb and colleagues have argued that the recombination rate constants required to explain the radical clock results are, in fact, impossibly high, and they doubt the validity of the oxygen rebound hydroxylation mechanism (47).

Cytochrome P-450 catalyzes the hydroxylation of unactivated hydrocarbon C−H bonds, such as those of octane or cyclohexane. The hydroxylation of hydrocarbon chains usually occurs at a position other than the terminal methyl group, because of the differences in the strengths of primary ($D^0 = \sim 98$ kcal/mol) versus secondary ($D^0 = \sim 95$ kcal/mol) C−H bonds (Table 14.5). *Despite this rule, cytochrome P-450 enzymes of the 4A class preferentially (or exclusively) hydroxylate fatty acid chains at the terminal (ω) position*:

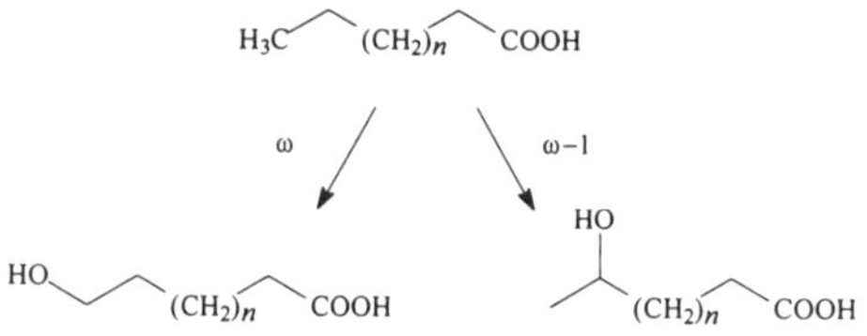

Hydroxylation of lauric acid at the ω- and ω-1 positions. Hydroxylation at positions further down the carbon chain is also possible.

Table 14.5. C−H Bond Dissociation Energies (D⁰) for the Reaction C−H → C· + H· at 25°C (kcal/mol)

Bond	D^0	Bond	D^0
CH_3CH_2-H	98	$CH_2=CH-CH_2-H$	85
$(CH_3)_2CH-H$	95	CH_3O-CH_2-H	93
$(CH_3)_3C-H$	91	$CH_2=CH-H$	110
$PhCH_2-H$	85	C_6H_5-H	110

The mechanistic explanation for ω-specificity is not known; one may hypothesize that the substrate binds in the active site in a manner that limits access of the reactive oxygen species to hydrogens on the terminal methyl group (48). The preferred hydroxylation site on a hydrocarbon chain, in the absence of such control, is the position adjacent ($\omega - 1$) to the terminal methyl group. Presumably, $\omega - 1$ C−H bonds are weaker than those of the ω carbon, but are sterically more accessible than those further down the chain, when the substrate is bound in the active site (see pentane on page 233).

The ω-selectivity of P-450 4A enzymes is a striking illustration of the ability of enzymes to "steer" a reaction into a pathway which, in the uncatalyzed process, is disfavored. Such control is possible because the enzyme itself participates in the transition state of the catalyzed reaction.

Oxygen insertion into C−H bonds stronger than those of a terminal methyl group—for example, vinylic or aromatic C−H bonds—rarely, if ever, occurs. The bond strengths of such C−H bonds ($D^0 = \sim110$ kcal/mol) are so high that hydroxylation does not compete effectively with other possible reactions. *In the case of aromatic rings, hydroxylation can occur by an alternative route, which does not involve oxygen insertion into the C−H bond.* On the other hand, hydroxylation reactions are highly favored when the C−H bond is *weakened* by the presence of an adjacent heteroatom or π-bond. Hydroxylation of a methyl substituent on an aromatic ring is a common process.

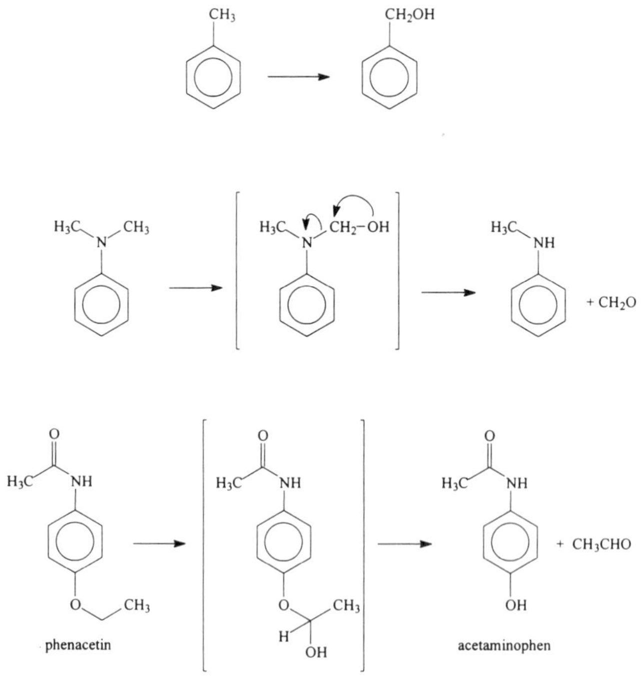

Hydroxylations of benzylic carbons and carbons adjacent to oxygen and nitrogen atoms are generally favored reactions because the corresponding C–H bonds are relatively reactive. Hydroxylation adjacent to a heteroatom produces an alcohol, which usually eliminates the heteroatom to give a carbonyl compound and an alcohol or amine product.

Similarly, hydroxylation of a methyl group attached to an oxygen or nitrogen atom is facile. In the oxygen case, hydroxylation yields a hemiacetal, which usually fragments to give an aldehyde plus an alcohol product. In the nitrogen case, the initial aminal fragments to give an aldehyde plus an amine (see scheme above). *The outcome of hydroxylation adjacent to a nitrogen or oxygen is therefore N- or O-dealkylation.* This is a typical P-450-catalyzed biotransformation. The same sort of fragmentation is observed after hydroxylation adjacent to halogens or other heteroatoms.

Hydroxylation of a carbon bearing more than one halogen atom gives rise to reactive species that can acylate protein residues, perturbing protein structure and function:

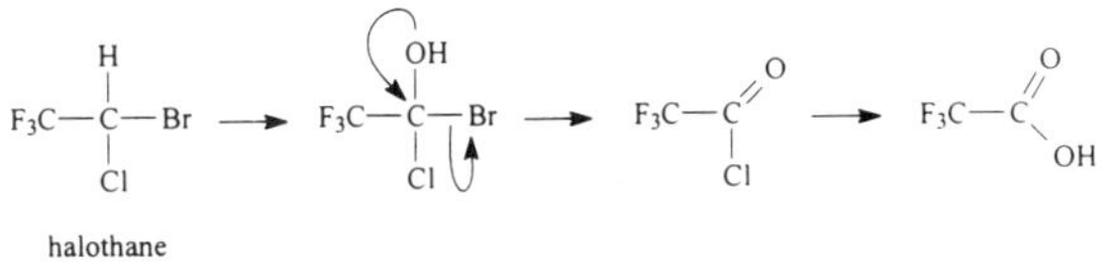

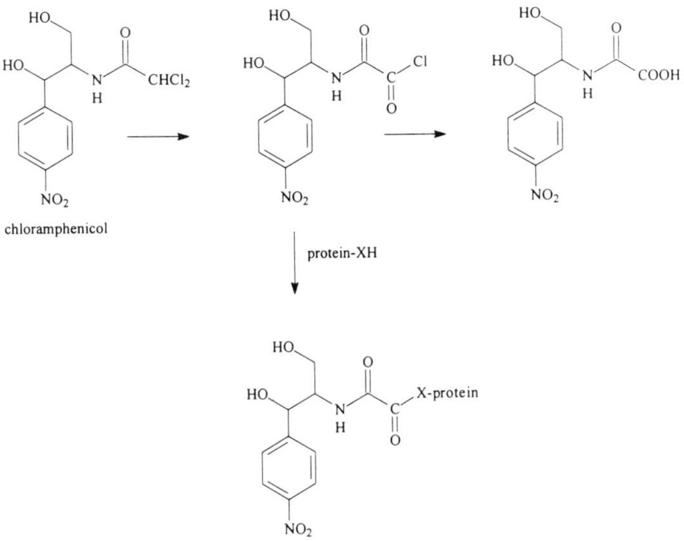

halothane

chloramphenicol

protein-XH

Hydroxylation of substrates with two leaving groups on the carbon that is hydroxylated, a situation often encountered with halogenated compounds, results in the formation of acyl intermediates. The acyl species can react with water to give the corresponding carboxylic acids but can also react with nucleophilic groups on proteins or other macromolecules. Protein acylation is often linked to immunotoxicity. Although not proven, the rare, fatal aplastic anemia associated with chloramphenicol exposure may be due to an immune response triggered by protein acylation.

Halothane (1-bromo-1-chloro-2,2,2,-trifluoroethane) is a widely used inhalation anaesthetic. In rare cases (about one in 100,000 patients), halothane anesthesia causes severe liver damage, which can be fatal (49). Protein acylation by activated halothane may cause direct tissue damage or may give rise to autoimmune sensitivity. Apparently, in sensitive individuals, halothane-acylated liver proteins have become immunogenic, and the liver damage is caused by the "anti-self" immune response.

Cytochrome P-450 can catalyze the hydroxylation of centers other than C−H bonds. The hydroxylation of N−H bonds is a particularly common reaction, although a mechanistic ambiguity exists for these reactions (see below). The oxidations of amines to hydroxylamines and amides to hydroxamic acids are toxicologically important examples:

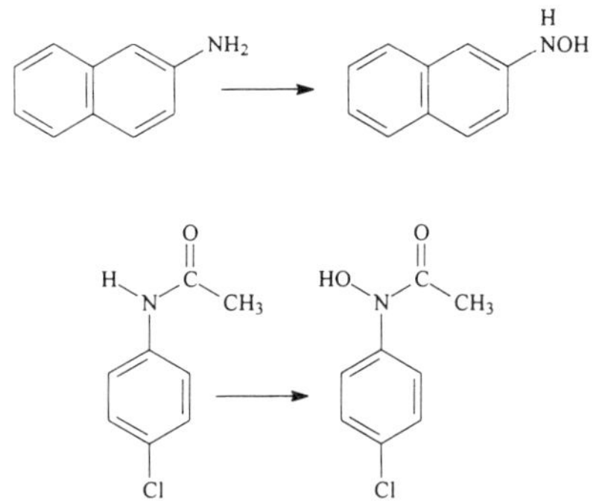

Nitrogen hydroxylation reactions. *N*-Hydroxylation of 2-naphthylamine, followed by sulfate conjugation of the hydroxyl group, is believed to be responsible for the potent carcinogenic properties of the arylamine. Oxidation of *p*-chloroacetanilide, in contrast to the oxidation of acetaminophen (see page 244), gives a stable hydroxylated amide product.

see Chapter 20. The sulfhydryl group can be oxidized to a sulfenic acid (RSH → RSOH); the high electronegativity of oxygen, on the other hand, makes the O−H bond very strong and rules out the hydroxylation of alcohols to peroxides.

EPOXIDATION REACTIONS

Olefins are oxidized by cytochrome P-450 to the corresponding epoxides, with retention of the olefin stereochemistry:

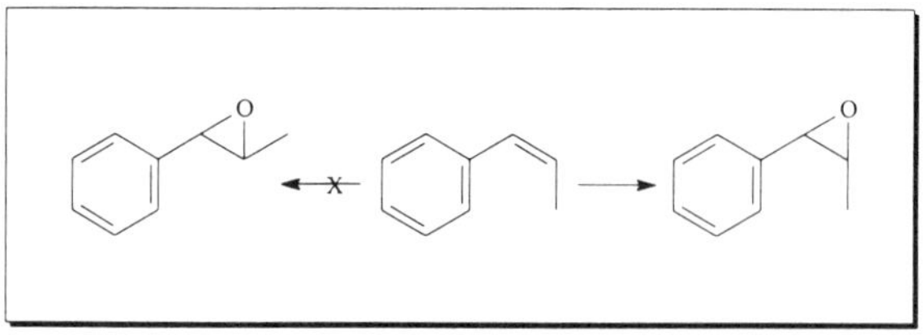

The epoxidation of olefins by cytochrome P-450 proceeds with retention of the olefin stereochemistry. Epoxides are chemically reactive compounds that alkylate proteins (see Chapters 11 and 19).

Therefore, the epoxidation reaction does not proceed via an intermediate that allows free rotation about the carbon–carbon bond. The simplest (not necessarily the correct) explanation for this finding is that the reaction, like nonenzymatic epoxidation by peracids, involves *simultaneous formation of both carbon–oxygen bonds of the epoxide*. The enzymatic reaction, like the peracid reaction, occurs more readily with electron-rich than with electron-poor olefins, consistent with such a mechanism. The occasional formation of carbonyl derivatives as minor reaction products, however, requires either (a) the existence of a second mechanism in addition to a concerted addition or (b) formulation of a more complex mechanism that can account for all the reactions. A concerted mechanism does not explain, for example, the formation of trichloroacetaldehyde from 1,1,2-trichloroethylene, under conditions where it can be shown that the carbonyl products are not formed by rearrangement of the epoxide (50):

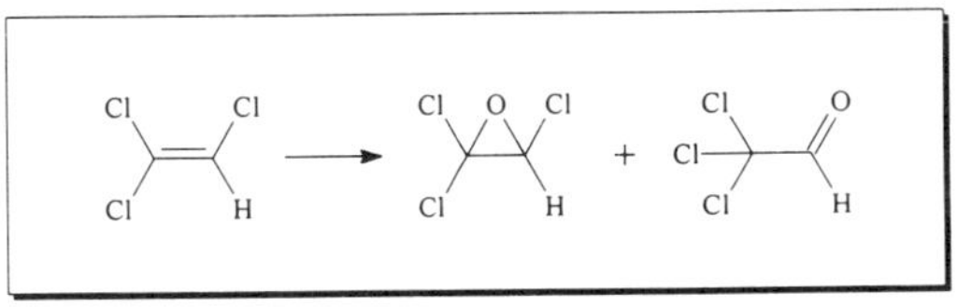

The epoxidation of trichloroethylene produces the corresponding epoxide and trichloroacetaldehyde. The formation of carbonyl products during olefin epoxidation is not common but can modify the toxicological potential of the substrate and provides useful evidence on the mechanism of the reaction.

The 1,2-migration of a hydrogen or halide, required for the formation of such products, indicates that a cationic intermediate is formed in at least the pathway that leads to the rearranged products.

A second, more general phenomenon, not explained by a concerted mechanism, is the inactivation of the enzyme that accompanies the oxidation of terminal olefins, such as ethylene and octene (51). Although each of these olefins is primarily converted to its epoxide, the epoxidation reaction occasionally "goes awry" and results in *alkylation of a pyrrole nitrogen of the enzyme's heme group by the terminal carbon of the olefin*:

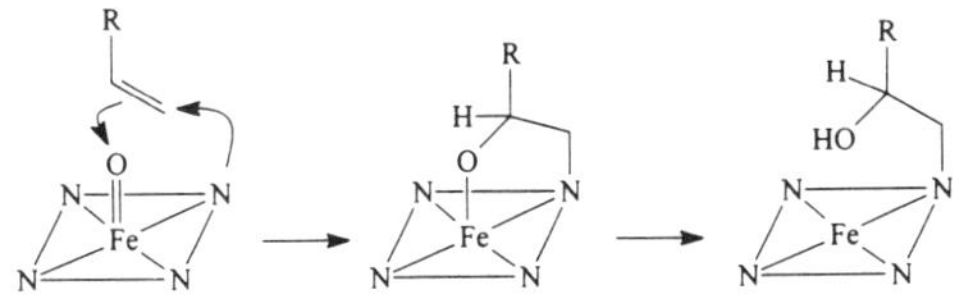

N-Alkylation of the prosthetic haem group of a cytochrome P-450 enzyme during catalytic oxidation of a terminal olefin. This reaction, which inactivates the enzyme, occurs approximately once for every 100 molecules of the olefin converted to the epoxide.

The heme alkylation reaction is triggered by transfer of the activated oxygen to the internal carbon of the double bond.

The N-alkylated prosthetic heme groups obtained with several olefins have been extracted from the protein. Removal of the iron gives an N-alkylated porphyrin, and these have been characterized by nuclear magnetic resonance (NMR) and other techniques. Because the inactivation requires catalytic oxidation of the inhibitor and involves inactivation of the very same enzyme molecule that catalyzes the oxidation, it is known as a *mechanism-based*, or "suicide," inactivation. Although heme alkylation can nominally be explained by reaction of the epoxide with the heme, the involvement of the epoxides in the alkylation process is definitively ruled out by a variety of experiments, including the demonstration that the heme group is not alkylated when the enzyme is incubated with the epoxide metabolites. A compelling mechanism that explains all the available observations has not been established. One possibility is that a key step in the epoxidation reaction is the formation of a charge-transfer complex between the ferryl oxygen and the π-bond (52). This complex then decomposes by one of several pathways that lead to the diverse reaction outcomes. The pathways could include concerted epoxide formation (a) and pathways that proceed via a free radical intermediate (b), a cation intermediate (c), or a metallaoxocyclobutane intermediate in which the iron is simultaneously bound to the oxygen and one of the carbons of the original double bond (d):

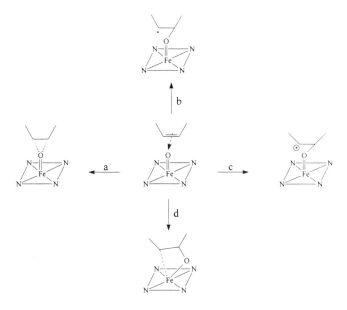

Manifold of possible reaction intermediates in the oxidation of olefins by cytochrome P-450. Formation of a charge transfer complex between the π-bond and the ferryl oxygen could be followed by concerted epoxide formation (a), nonconcerted transfer of the oxygen to the π-bond to give a radical (b) or cationic (c) intermediate, or formation of an intermediate in which both the oxygen and carbon are bound to the iron (d). Some of the intermediates are not mutually exclusive. For example, the radical of path (b) could be oxidized to the cation of path (c) or could collapse to the cyclic product of path (d).

All of these intermediates have been proposed but none has been firmly established, except for the cationic intermediate, which almost certainly is required for the rearrangement reactions that involve migration of an atom to the adjacent carbon (see epoxidation scheme on page 327). The alternative, of course, is that a principal "concerted" mechanism leads to the epoxides whereas minor, alternative mechanisms result in the rearranged products and heme alkylation.

The intermediates in such a scheme could be the same as those shown in the preceding scheme, except that the individual reaction pathways would stem directly from interaction of the olefin with the ferryl oxygen, without the intermediacy of the charge transfer complex that links the intermediates together in the scheme above.

THE OXIDATION OF AROMATIC RINGS

Cytochrome P-450 hydroxylates aromatic substrates. Indeed, the formation of phenolic metabolites incorporating ^{18}O derived from $^{18}O_2$ was the first evidence for monooxygenation reactions in biochemistry, as discussed in an earlier chapter. The hydroxylation of acetanilide by hepatic microsomes was first examined in the 1950s by a group of scientists at the National Institutes of Health, Bethesda, MD (53). These studies first highlighted the pharmacological significance of microsomal drug metabolism and established the existence of a microsomal hydroxylase enzyme several years before the protein cytochrome P-450 was discovered and named by Omura and Sato. Because of the great pharmacological and toxicological significance of aromatic hydroxylation, this biotransformation has been the focus of continuing research in many laboratories.

The NIH group made a surprising discovery during the investigation of acetanilide hydroxylation. When ^{3}H-acetanilide, labeled with tritium at the 4-position, was converted to 4-hydroxyacetanilide (or acetylaminophenol), the tritium was not completely lost to water. Instead, some of the tritium label remained associated with the product! This label could not be at the hydroxylated 4-position, since phenolic hydrogens exchange rapidly with water solvent. Further studies with deuterium labeling proved that *the hydrogen atom at the position of hydroxylation migrated to an adjacent site on the aromatic ring.* This so-called "NIH shift" proved to be a general feature of aromatic hydroxylations catalyzed by P-450. *The NIH shift is discussed further in Chapter 19.*

HETEROATOM OXIDATION

The reactions of molecules bearing nitrogen or sulfur atoms with cytochrome P-450 are dominated by the availability of free electron pairs on the heteroatoms. In general, the more electronegative the atom, the more tightly it holds its electron pairs and the less reactive it is toward oxidation by cytochrome P-450. Nitrogen and sulfur are readily oxidized, but oxygen is not. The simplest reaction of cytochrome P-450 with a heteroatom involves transfer of the electron-deficient ferryl oxygen from the iron to one of the electron pairs of the heteroatom: nitrogen is oxidized to the *N*-oxide ($R_3N \rightarrow O \leftrightarrow R_3N^+ - O^-$) and sulfur to the sulfoxide ($R_2S = O \leftrightarrow R_2S^+ - O^-$). In the case of sulfur, which has two electron pairs, the sulfoxide be further oxidized to the sulfone (R_2SO_2). However, the free electron pair is more difficult to oxidize in the sulfoxide than in the sulfide, because of the partial positive charge on the sulfur. Oxidation of a sulfoxide to a sulfone is therefore more difficult than that of a sulfide to a sulfoxide. Halogen atoms, like oxygen, are highly electronegative and difficult to oxidize, but there is indirect evidence that, in some circumstances, iodide and bromide substituents can be oxidized, resulting in carbon–halogen bond cleavage.

Caution must be used in attributing the formation of *N*-oxides and sulfoxides, either in vivo or in microsomal systems, to the cytochrome P-450 system: These reactions are also catalyzed by the *flavin monooxygenase* enzyme (54) present in many of the same tissues, discussed at the beginning of this chapter. The formation of *N*-oxides, in particular, is often catalyzed by the flavin monooxygenases rather than by cytochrome P-450. The cytochrome P-450-catalyzed reaction normally results in *N*-dealkylation rather than *N*-oxide formation. The flavin monooxygenases, however, do not catalyze the oxidation of $C-H$ or π-bonds.

Dealkylation of alkyl-substituted heteroatoms can occur by hydroxylation of the carbon adjacent to the heteroatom followed by extrusion of the heteroatom to give the carbonyl group. Oxygen and sulfur dealkylation usually follows this reaction pathway. Nitrogen dealkylation, however, could occur by a variant of this mechanism, due to the ease with which an electron can be removed from the nitrogen atom. According to this alternate mechanism, electron transfer to the ferryl oxygen gives a nitrogen radical cation

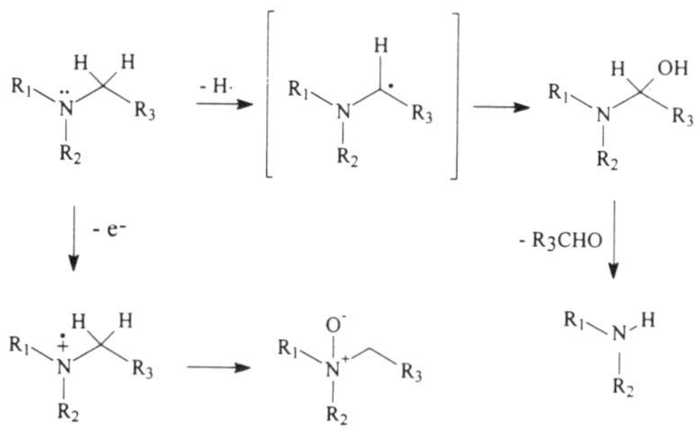

Nitrogen oxidation to the nitrogen radical cation followed by oxygen transfer can produce the *N*-oxide. However, if a hydrogen is present on the carbon adjacent to the nitrogen, proton loss followed by oxygen transfer to the carbon radical is the more commonly observed reaction. The latter reaction is indistinguishable, in terms of reaction outcome, from an *N*-dealkylation reaction initiated by direct hydroxylation of the carbon adjacent to the nitrogen.

The radical cation can, in principle, recombine with the ferryl oxygen to give the *N*-oxide, but this is usually the minor reaction pathway. In the major pathway, the positive charge on the nitrogen acidifies the proton on the carbon attached to it and facilitates its transfer to the ferryl oxygen. Redistribution of the electrons then gives a carbon radical identical to that which would be obtained by conventional hydroxylation of the carbon–hydrogen bond (see scheme above).

Rebound addition of the protonated oxygen to the carbon radical yields the carbinolamine, which fragments to the amine and an aldehyde or ketone. According to this mechanism, the dominance of cytochrome P-450-catalyzed *N*-dealkylation over *N*-oxidation is due to a faster rate of proton transfer to the ferryl oxygen than combination of the nitrogen radical cation with the ferryl oxygen. A similar mechanism can be written for sulfur oxidation, keeping in mind that addition of the oxygen to the sulfur radical cation competes much more effectively with proton transfer than it does in the case of nitrogen. Oxygen dealkylation, however, is achieved by direct hydrogen atom abstraction from the carbon rather than via oxidation of the heteroatom because the high electronegativity of oxygen makes electron removal difficult.

The oxidation of nitrogen atoms bearing at least one hydrogen atom results in formation of either the *N*-dealkylated product, if that reaction is possible, or the *N*-hydroxyl derivative of the substrate (55). *N*-Hydroxylation could occur by a mechanism entirely analogous to that involved in hydrocarbon oxidation—that is, hydrogen abstraction to give a nitrogen radical that combines with the iron-bound hydroxyl radical-equivalent:

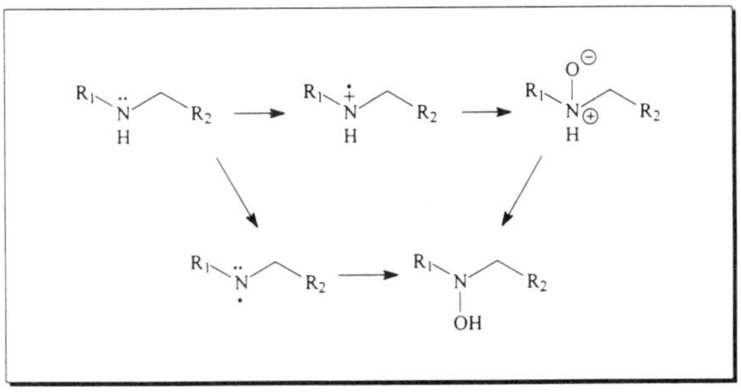

Oxidation of a nitrogen bearing a hydrogen to the *N*-hydroxy product could involve hydrogen abstraction followed by oxygen recombination or could involve formation of the *N*-oxide that tautomerizes to the *N*-hydroxy product.

However, exactly the same product is obtained if the nitrogen is directly converted to the *N*-oxide by addition of the oxygen to the electron pair, because proton tautomerization gives the neutral hydroxylamine. The mechanism is determined by whether hydrogen abstraction or addition of the ferryl oxygen to the nitrogen, possibly preceded by radical cation formation, is favored. At one extreme, it is very likely that hydroxylation of the nitrogen of amides proceeds via a hydrogen abstraction–recombination pathway, because the nitrogen electrons of the amide are highly delocalized and difficult to remove. Conversely, hydroxylamines are probably produced by *N*-oxidation of the amine followed by proton tautomerization. There is little information on cytochrome P-450-catalyzed conversion of sulfhydryl groups to sulfenic acids. This is due, at least in part, to the fact that the sulfenic acids react with the sulfhydryl compound itself, or with glutathione to give disulfides. Nevertheless, similar mechanisms to those invoked for nitrogen can be written for cytochrome P-450-catalyzed sulfhydryl oxidation.

An unusual reaction is observed when a thiocarbonyl group is oxidized by cytochrome P-450:

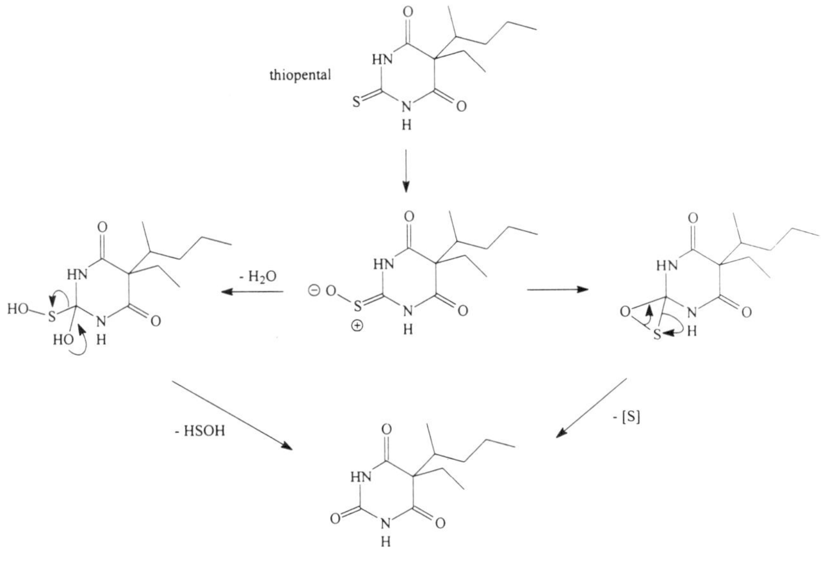

Thiocarbonyl groups are usually oxidized by cytochrome P-450 to carbonyl groups. The reaction involves oxidation of the sulfur followed either by (a) intramolecular rearrangement via a three membered ring with elimination of activated sulfur or (b) addition of water to the activated thiocarbonyl function followed by extrusion of HSOH.

Unlike the oxygen of a carbonyl group, which is too electronegative, the ferryl oxygen can be transferred to one of the electron pairs of a thiocarbonyl sulfur atom. The product is unstable and decomposes, with extrusion of sulfur, to give the oxygen-containing carbonyl group. The decomposition could occur by either of two mechanisms: (i) closure to give a three-member ring that extrudes a sulfur atom or (ii) addition of water to the activated carbon–sulfur double bond followed by elimination of HSOH. In contrast, the *N*-oxide obtained by P-450-catalyzed oxidation of an imine is isolable, although it slowly hydrolyzes to give the carbonyl product.

Acetaminophen (4-hydroxyacetanilide, Tylenol) is a widely used analgesic nonprescription medicine. Although safe at therapeutic doses, acetaminophen overdose is potentially life-threatening; acetaminophen is a frequent cause of accidental poisoning in children and attempted suicide in adults. Acetaminophen metabolism by cytochrome P-450 produces a reactive iminoquinone that is responsible for the hepatotoxic effects of the drug. The oxidation of acetaminophen, which has been the subject of many investigations, illustrates some of the mechanistic complications involved in nitrogen oxidation reactions. The demonstration that the iminoquinone is the reactive species

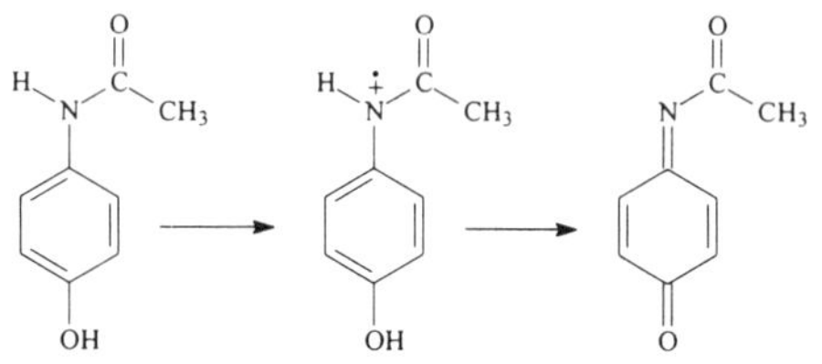

Oxidation of acetaminophen to a reactive iminoquinone that reacts with glutathione, alkylates liver proteins, and causes liver necrosis. Although the reaction was initially thought to involve formation of the *N*-hydroxy derivative, kinetic studies show that the iminoquinone is directly formed in the reaction.

was initially thought to be consistent with *N*-hydroxylation of the amide function, followed by chemical elimination of a molecule of water. Related compounds, such as *p*-chloroacetanilide (see scheme, page 238), give isolable amounts of the *N*-hydroxy derivatives.

Synthesis of the proposed *N*-hydroxy derivative of acetaminophen, however, clearly showed that the water elimination step was too slow to account for the observed rate of formation of the iminoquinone. It is now believed that the *N*-hydroxy intermediate is never formed; one-electron removal from the substrate by cytochrome P-450 gives a radical intermediate; deprotonation and transfer of a second electron to the heme group occurs more rapidly than collapse to give the *N*-hydroxy derivative. Although the detailed sequence of hydrogen and electron transfer steps remains a matter of debate, the evidence strongly suggests that the iminoquinone is formed without the formation of an intermediate other than a transient radical.

INDUCTION OF CYTOCHROME P-450 BY XENOBIOTICS

Exposure to a xenobiotic can markedly enhance the ability to metabolize the same compound and other compounds. The idea that exposure to a small dose of a poison protects against a later, larger dose, goes back to antiquity. The modern experimental analysis of such interactions began with the work of Richardson, Stier, and Borsos-Nachtnebel, in 1952 (56). These researchers discovered that feeding the polycyclic aromatic hydrocarbon 3-methylcholanthrene to rats greatly decreased the carcinogenic activity of a subsequently administered aminoazo dye. This decrease in carcinogenicity was ascribed, two years later, to the fact that 3-methylcholanthrene exposure increased the ability of the rats to metabolize (N-demethylate and reduce) the aminoazo dye (57). The elevation of biotransformation enzyme activities following exposure to xenobiotics is known as *enzyme induction.*

The lipophilic xenobiotics to which animals are exposed present a formidable challenge to the enzyme systems responsible for their metabolism. This is particularly true for the oxidative metabolism mediated by cytochrome P-450. The challenge is met, first of all, by the presence of multiple enzymes with distinct, broad, but overlapping specificities. Second, the metabolic versatility of the detoxication system is greatly enhanced by enzyme induction. Induction is a phenomenon of clinical importance, since induction can cause unexpected drug interactions. The purification and characterization of P-450 enzymes (at least, before the era of gene cloning) was dependent on induction of specific forms. Induction also poses fascinating and fundamental questions about biological regulation.

Structures of some inducers commonly used in experimental studies are shown in the scheme on page 169. Inspection of the figure shows that there is no single chemical theme typifying all of these agents, other than hydrophobicity. Perhaps this is to be expected, since, as discussed below, there are many distinct mechanisms of P-450 induction.

The increased metabolic activities following induction reflect an increase in the amounts of specific forms of cytochrome P-450 present in the tissue (Table 14.6). *The amount of a given P-450 form can be increased by up to two orders of magnitude* by exposure to xenobiotics, although there is usually no more than a two- to three-fold increase in the *total* content of cytochrome P-450 in the tissue. An extraordinary feature of this response is that the forms of cytochrome P-450 that are elevated are often those that are able to bind and oxidize the agent that causes their elevation. Mammals have the ability to respond selectively to many xenobiotics by specifically increasing the production of oxidative enzyme(s) required to metabolize them! Similar, but much less marked, elevations in enzymes such as glucuronyl and glutathione transferases also occur in response to xenobiotics.

The rise in enzyme activities takes hours or days to reach its maximum (Fig. 14.6). The elevation depends on the continued presence of the inducing agent: If the inducing agent is withdrawn, enzyme activities slowly return to baseline, due to normal protein degradation and turnover. The level of induction depends on the concentration of the inducing agent and is saturable. In principle, increases in metabolic enzyme levels could be mediated by several different mechanisms: increasing the rate of transcription of the appropriate gene, stabilizing the RNA derived from it, or stabilizing the protein product against

Table 14.6. Some Drugs That Increase Their Own Metabolism When Administered Chronically (33)

Drug	Species	Drug	Species
Phenylbutazone	Dog, rat	Phenobarbital	Dog, rat
Chlorcyclizine	Dog	Aminopyrine	Rat
Probenecid	Dog	Meprobamate	Man, rat
Tolbutamide	Dog	Glutethimide	Man
Hexobarbital	Dog, rat	Chlorpromazine	Rat
Pentobarbital	Rat, rabbit	Chlordiazepoxide	Rat

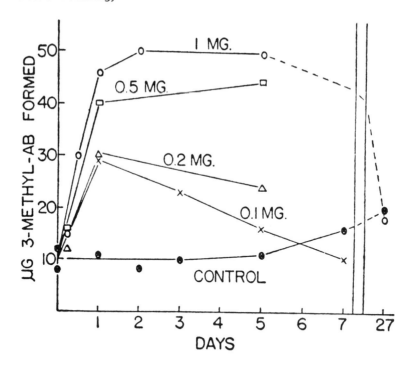

Figure 14.6. Time-dependence of the increase in the cytochrome P-4501A1-catalyzed *N*-demethylation of 3,4′-dimethylaminoazobenzene as a function of time after administration of single increasing doses of the polycyclic aromatic hydrocarbon 3-methylcholanthrene. The enzyme activity increases to a maximum, due to induction of cytochrome P-4501A, and then decays back to control levels. (Copied with permission from A. H. Conney, E. C. Miller, and J. H. Miller, The metabolism of methylated aminoazo dyes. V. Evidence for induction of enzyme synthesis in the rat by 3-methylcholanthrene, *Cancer Res.* 16:450–459, 1956.)

degradation (Table 14.7). All of these mechanisms are involved in P-450 induction; different forms may be induced by different mechanisms.

Two of the prototypical inducers of P-450 are 3-methylcholanthrene (inducer of CYP1 forms) and phenobarbital (58) (CYP2 forms). Besides the distinct pattern of enzymes affected, the actions of these two agents are different in other ways. Notably, phenobarbital causes substantial liver hypertrophy and proliferation of the endoplasmic reticulum, whereas 3-methylcholanthrene does not. The commercial mixture of polychlorinated biphenyls (PCB) known as Aroclor 1254 is often used for P-450 induction, especially when microsomes are prepared for use in genotoxicity assays, such as the Ames test. Aroclor contains PCB isomers which behave as 3-methylcholanthrene-type and phenobarbi-

Table 14.7. Mechanisms of Induction of Cytochrome P-450 Enzymes

Enzyme	Typical Inducers	Mechanism of Induction
CYP1A1	PAH	Transcriptional activation
CYP1A2	PAH	Transcriptional activation mRNA stabilization
CYP2B1, 2B2	Phenobarbital	Transcriptional activation
CYP2E1	Ethanol, acetone	Protein stabilization mRNA stabilization
CYP3A	Dexamethasone, troleandomycin	Transcriptional activation protein stabilization
CYP4A	Clofibrate	Transcriptional activation

Table 14.8. Effect of a Diet Containing Charcoal-Broiled Beef on the Plasma Concentration of Phenacetin in Humans[a]

Diet	Phenacetin Level in Plasma (ng/ml)[b]					
Control (1st)	1328 (1)	925 (2)	313 (3)	149 (4)	66 (5)	17 (7)
Charcoal beef	319 (1)	163 (2)	74 (3)	34 (4)	15 (5)	7 (7)
Control (2nd)	1827 (1)	623 (2)	271 (3)	99 (4)	40 (5)	14 (7)

[a]Subjects were given 900 mg of phenactin orally after each dietary regimen. Each value represents the mean for nine subjects.
[b]Numbers in parentheses indicate the interval after administration, in hours.
Source: Reference 39.

tal-type inducers; therefore, aroclor-induced microsomes contain an array of inducible P-450 enzymes.

CYP2E1, the form implicated in nitrosamine activation (see above), is under unusual control: Its induction is effected mainly by protein stabilization. This form is induced by organic solvents, such as ethanol and acetone, and also by starvation (59) (which probably acts via elevation of circulating levels of ketone bodies, including acetone).

INCREASED GENE TRANSCRIPTION

The mechanisms by which gene transcription is increased are understood best in the case of CYP1A1 induction by agents such as polycyclic aromatic hydrocarbons;* major progress has also been made recently on the mechanism of induction of the CYP4A family of fatty acid ω-hydroxylases (see later). In both cases, protein receptors are responsible for transcriptional activation of the corresponding cytochrome P-450 genes (60, 61). By far the best characterized of the two is the Ah receptor, which mediates induction of the CYP1A1 gene. The Ah receptor plays a central role in the toxicology of halogenated aromatic compounds and is the subject of Chapter 19.

2,3,7,8-Tetrachlorodibenzo-p-dioxin, commonly referred to as TCDD, is a far more potent ligand for the Ah receptor than are the polycyclic aromatic hydrocarbons (36). TCDD is a very powerful inducer of CYP1A1 and the other genes activated by the Ah receptor; this induction appears to be related to the mechanism of TCDD toxicity, although induction of CYP1A1 itself has not been linked to the toxic effects (see Chapter 19).

The effects of xenobiotics on the metabolism of drugs and other xenobiotics in humans are well illustrated by the series of experiments carried out on the effects of eating charcoal-broiled beef on the metabolism of the analgesic, phenacetin (62). Phenacetin is the phenolic ethyl ether derivative of acetaminophen and is metabolized primarily to acetaminophen by cytochrome P-450-catalyzed O-dealkylation. The serum concentration of phenacetin was measured, over time, in volunteers fed controlled diets. The individuals were kept, for several days, on a diet of beef cooked in aluminum foil and were subsequently switched to a diet in which the beef was charcoal-broiled. Phenacetin levels were considerably higher, at all time points, when the volunteers were maintained on the "cooked in foil" diet compared to the "charcoal-broiled" diet (Table 14.8).

Measurements of the acetaminophen metabolite concentrations, in contrast, were found to be higher when the volunteers were on the "broiled-beef" diet. When the volunteers

*Reviewed in M. S. Denison and J. P. Whitlock, Jr., Xenobiotic-inducible transcription of cytochrome P450 genes, *J. Biol. Chem.* 270:18175–18178, 1995.

were put back on the "cooked in foil" diet for several days and phenacetin pharmacoki-netics were subsequently measured, the time dependence of the phenacetin serum con-centration returned to the prebroiled-beef diet status. These results clearly show that a component of the diet associated with broiling the beef increases conversion of phenacetin to acetaminophen, and thereby decreases the half-life of phenacetin and the maximum serum concentration obtainable with a constant dose of the drug in humans. Animal ex-periments have clearly established that these phenomena are caused by induction of cy-tochrome P-450 1A1 by the polycyclic aromatic hydrocarbons produced, in broiling, by carbonization of the animal fat.

The induction of cytochrome P-450 is related to the physical and structural properties (particularly lipophilicity and persistence) of the xenobiotics. Cytochrome P-450 enzymes are induced not only by exposure to drugs and industrial chemicals, but also by factors such as cigarette smoke, ingestion of cruciferous vegetables (e.g., Brussels sprouts, cab-bage), and ethanol. Enzyme induction can decrease drug levels, as shown for the effect of polycyclic aromatic hydrocarbons on phenacetin levels, but can also increase the for-mation of toxic metabolites. The toxicity of acetaminophen, which is triggered by its ox-idation to the iminoquinone, is increased by exposure to agents that elevate the activities of certain cytochrome P-450 enzymes (CYP1A2, CYP2E1) which catalyze this reaction.

The *basal* levels of cytochrome P-450 enzymes are determined by a variety of factors, including gender, age, hormonal and nutritional status, and the presence or absence of dis-ease (63). As the individual cytochrome P-450 enzymes can determine the rate of elimi-nation of a xenobiotic, or of its activation to toxic or carcinogenic products, the suscep-tibility of an individual to the toxic effects of many agents can be influenced by the individual's pattern of cytochrome P-450 enzymes. The role of dietary, environmental, and lifestyle factors in the induction of P-450 enzymes in humans is an area of active in-vestigation.

Clofibrate and related drugs are used in the treatment of hyperlipidemia. These drugs, and other compounds such as the phthalate ester plasticizers, are *peroxisome prolifera-tors*. They induce the production of peroxisomes, organelles responsible for β-oxidation of long-chain fatty acids and other aspects of lipid metabolism (64), in liver cells. Addi-tional hepatic changes induced by peroxisome proliferators include hypertrophy (increased liver size), increased cell proliferation, and tumorigenesis (65). Cytochrome P-450 4A1, the enzyme that catalyzes fatty acid ω-hydroxylation, is induced (both enzyme activity and mRNA levels) by these agents (66).

Genetic factors can give rise to populations that differ widely in the levels of specific cytochrome P-450 enzymes and, consequently, in their ability to metabolize specific xeno-biotics. Large differences in the levels of a few cytochrome P-450 enzymes strongly in-fluence the ability of individuals to oxidize particular drugs, and they should be taken into consideration in the design of appropriate drug regimens. The two best-established ex-amples of cytochrome P-450 genetic polymorphisms are CYP2D6 and 2C19. The levels of cytochrome 2D6 are low in 5–10% of the Caucasian population, who are very slow metabolizers of the antihypertensive drug *debrisoquine* (67). Low levels of cytochrome P-450 2C19, found in 3–5% of Caucasians and 20% of Orientals, are responsible for a group of individuals who metabolize the anticonvulsive drug *mephenytoin* slowly. The low levels of these enzymes have been traced to specific mutations in the genes coding for the proteins, including deletions, insertions, and mutations which prevent the expres-sion of active proteins. Such polymorphisms may be associated with differences in sus-ceptibility to some cancers.

P-450 enzymes catalyze many of the steps of steroid metabolism (68). However, the physiological roles (metabolism of endogenous substances) of the P-450 enzymes associated with drug and carcinogen metabolism remain mysterious. Recently, a transgenic P-4501A2 "knockout" mouse was successfully constructed (69). Remarkably, almost all of these mice die soon after birth, due to failure to the lung surfactant system. The specific metabolic cause of this effect is not yet known, but this surprising discovery indicates that P-450 forms may play important, previously unsuspected roles in mammalian metabolism, in addition to the oxidation of xenobiotics.

NOTES

1. Omura, T., and Sato, R., The carbon monoxide-binding pigment of liver microsomes, *J. Biol. Chem.* 239:2370–2378 and 2379–2385, 1964.
2. Omura, T., Introduction: History of cytochrome P-450, in: *Cytochrome P-450*, 2nd ed., T. Omura, Y. Ishimura, and Y. Fujii-Kuriyama, Eds., VCH, Weinheim, 1993, pp. 1–15.
3. Cooper, O., Discovery of the function of the heme protein P-450: A systematic approach to scientific research, *Life Sci.* 13:1151–1161, 1973.
4. Omura, T., Sanders, E., Estabrook, R. W., Cooper, D. Y., and Rosenthal, O., Isolation from adrenal cortex of a nonheme iron protein and a flavoprotein functional as a reduced triphosphopyridine nucleotide-cytochrome P-450 reductase, *Arch. Biochem. Biophys.* 117:660–673, 1966.
5. Lu, A. Y. H., and Coon, M. J., Role of hemoprotein P450 in fatty acid ω-hydroxylation in a soluble enzyme from liver microsomes, *J. Biol. Chem.* 243:1331–1332, 1968.
6. Nelson, D. R., Kamataki, T., Waxman, D. J., Guengerich, F. P., Estabrook, R. W., Feyereisen, R., Gonzalez, F. J., Coon, M. J., Gunsalus, I. C., Gotoh, O., Okuda, K., and Nebert, D. W., The P450 superfamily: Update on new sequences, gene mapping, accession numbers, early trivial names of enzymes, and nomenclature, *DNA Cell Biol.* 12:1–51, 1993.
7. Murray, M., and Reidy, G. F., Selectivity in the inhibition of mammalian cytochromes P-450 by chemical agents, *Pharmacol. Rev.* 42:85–105, 1990.
8. Ioannides, C., and Parke, D. V., The cytochrome P-450 I gene family of microsomal hemoproteins and their role in the metabolic activation of chemicals, *Drug Metab. Rev.* 22:1–85, 1990.
9. Guengerich, F. P., and Shimada, T., Oxidation of toxic and carcinogenic chemicals by human cytochrome P-450 enzymes, *Chem. Res. Toxicol.* 4:391–407, 1991.
10. See Table 1 in: Ryan, D. E., and Levin, W., Purification and characterization of hepatic microsomal cytochrome P-450, *Pharmacol. Ther.* 45:153–239, 1990, for a comparative listing of designations used by various laboratories.
11. Guengerich, F. P., Human cytochrome P-450 enzymes, *Life Sci.* 50:1471–1478, 1992; Kamataki, T., Metabolism of xenobiotics, in: *Cytochrome P-450*, T. Omura, Y. Ishimura, and Y. Fujii-Kuriyama, Eds., 2nd ed., VCH, Weinheim, pp. 141–158, 1993; Gonzalez, F., Cytochrome P450 in humans, in: J. B. Schenkman and H. Greim, Eds., *Cytochrome P450*, Springer-Verlag, New York, 1993, pp. 239–257.
12. Archer, M. C., and Labuc, G. E., Nitrosamines, in: M. W. Anders, Ed., *Bioactivation of Foreign Compounds*, Academic Press, New York, 1985, Chapter 14, pp. 403–431; Bartsch, H., Shuker, D.E., and Ohshima, H., Human nitrosamine exposure: Recent dosimetry methods and applications, *Prog. Clin. Biol. Res.* 372:197–204, 1991.
13. Dawson, J. H., and Sono, M., Cytochrome P450 and chloroperoxidase: Thiolate-ligated heme enzymes. Spectroscopic determination of their active site structures and mechanistic implications of thiolate ligation, *Chem. Rev.* 87:1255–1276, 1987.
14. Atkins, P. W., *General Chemistry*, Scientific American Books, New York, 1989, pp. 788–795.
15. Schenkman, J. B., Sligar, S. G., and Cinti, D. L., Substrate interaction with cytochrome P450, in: *Hepatic Cytochrome P-450 Monooxygenase System*, J. B. Schenkman, and D. Kupfer, Eds., Pergamon Press, New York, 1982, pp. 587–615.
16. Sligar, S. G., and Murray, R. I., Cytochrome P-450$_{cam}$ and other bacterial P-450 enzymes, in:

Cytochrome P-450: Structure, Mechanism, and Biochemistry, P. R. Ortiz de Montellano, Ed., Plenum Press, New York, 1986, pp. 429–503.

17. Lowry, T. H., and Richardson, K. S., *Mechanism and Theory in Organic Chemistry*, 3rd ed., Harper & Row, New York, 1987.

18. Ortiz de Montellano, P. R., Oxygen activation and transfer, in: *Cytochrome P450: Structure, Mechanism, and Biochemistry*, P. R. Ortiz de Montellano, Ed., Plenum Press, New York, 1986, pp. 217–271.

19. Lambeth, J. D., Seybert, D. W., Lancaster, J. R., Salerno, J. C., and Kamin, H., Steroidogenic electron transport in adrenal cortex mitochondria, *Mol. Cell. Biochem.* 45:13–31, 1982.

20. Stryer, L., *Biochemistry*, 4th ed., W. H. Freeman, New York, 1995, Fig. 21-7.

21. Porter, T. D., and Kasper, C. B., Coding nucleotide sequence of rat NADPH-cytochrome P-450 oxidoreductase and identification of flavin-binding domains, *Proc. Natl. Acad. Sci. U.S.A.* 82:973–977, 1985.

22. Shen, A. L., and Kasper, C. B., Protein and gene structure and regulation of NADPH-cytochrome P450 oxidoreductase, in: *Cytochrome P450*, J. B. Schenkman and H. Greim, Eds., Springer-Verlag, New York, 1993, pp. 35–59.

23. Limited tryptic digestion cuts the peptide bond between the hydrophobic tail and the functional domain at a particularly sensitive site (between Lys-56 and Ile-57) and releases a protein fragment ($\sim$72 kD) that can still be reduced by NADPH and transfer electrons to acceptors such as cytochrome c. The truncated reductase, however, is no longer able to reduce cytochrome P-450.

24. Stryer, L., *Biochemistry*, 4th ed., W. H. Freeman, New York, 1995, pp. 622–623.

25. Bonfils, C., Balny, C., and Maurel, P., Direct evidence for electron transfer from ferrous cytochrome b5 to the oxyferrous intermediate of liver microsomal cytochrome P-450 LM2, *J. Biol. Chem.* 256:9457–9465, 1981.

26. Oertle, M., Filipovic, D., Richter, C., Winterhalter, K. H., and Di Iorio, E. E., Isoelectric focusing of cytochrome P450: Isolation of six phenobarbital-inducible rat liver microsomal isoenzymes, *Arch. Biochem. Biophys.* 291, 24–30, 1991.

27. Halpert, J. R., Guengerich, F. P., Bend, J. R., and Correia, M. A., Selective inhibitors of cytochromes P450, *Toxicol. Appl. Pharmacol.* 125:163–175, 1994.

28. Holton, T. A., Brugliera, F., Lester, D. R., Tanaka, Y., Hyland, C. D., Menting, J. G. T., Lu, C.-Y., Farcy, E., Stevenson, T. W., and Cornish, E. C., Cloning and expression of cytochrome P450 genes controlling flower colour, *Nature* 366:276–279, 1993.

29. Urban, P., Truan, G., Gautier, J.-C., Pompon, D., Xenobiotic metabolism in humanized yeast: Engineered yeast cells producing human NADPH-cytochrome P-450 reductase, cytochrome b5, epoxide hydrolase and P-450s, *Biochem. Soc. Trans.* 21:1028–1034, 1993.

30. Waterman, M. R., Heterologous expression of cytochrome P-450 in *Escherichia coli*, *Biochem. Soc. Trans.* 21:1081–1085, 1993; Gonzalez, F. J., and Korzekwa, K. R., Cytochromes P450 expression systems, *Annu. Rev. Pharmacol. Toxicol.* 35:369–390, 1995.

31. Poulos, T. L., Finzel, B. C., and Howard, A. J., High-resolution crystal structure of cytochrome P450$_{cam}$, *J. Mol. Biol.* 195:687–700, 1987.

32. Boddupalli, S. S., Hasemann, C. A., Ravichandran, K. G., Lu, J.-Y., Goldsmith, E. J., Deisenhofer, J., and Peterson, J. A., Crystallization and preliminary X-ray diffraction analysis of P450$_{terp}$ and the hemoprotein domain of P450BM-3, enzymes belonging to two distinct classes of the cytochrome P450 superfamily, *Proc. Natl. Acad. Sci. U.S.A.* 89:4467–5571, 1992.

33. Ravichandran, K. G., Boddupalli, S. S., Hasemann, C. A., Peterson, J. A., and Deisenhofer, J., Crystal structure of hemoprotein domain of P450BM-3, a prototype for microsomal P450's, *Science* 261:731–736, 1993.

34. Hasemann, C. A., Kurumbail, R. G., Boddupalli, S. S., Peterson, J. A., and Deisenhofer, J., Structure and function of cytochromes P450: A comparative analysis of three crystal structures, *Structure* 3:41–62, 1995.

35. Atkins, W. M., and Sligar, S. G., Molecular recognition in cytochrome P450: Alteration of regioselective alkane hydroxylation via protein engineering, *J. Am. Chem. Soc.* 111:2715–2717, 1989.

36. Atkins, W. M., and Sligar, S. G., The roles of active site hydrogen bonding in cytochrome P-450$_{cam}$ as revealed by site-directed mutagenesis, *J. Biol. Chem.* 263:18842–18849, 1988.

37. Furuya, H., Shimizu, T., Hirano, K., Hatano, M., Fujii-Kuriyama, Y., Raag, R., and Poulos, T. L., Site-directed mutagenesis of rat liver cytochrome P-450d: Catalytic activities toward benzphetamine and 7-ethoxycoumarin, *Biochemistry* 28:6848–6857, 1989.

38. Tuck, S. F., and Ortiz de Montellano, P. R., Topological mapping of the active sites of cytochromes P4502B1 and P4502B2 by in situ rearrangement of their aryl-iron complexes, *Biochemistry* 31:6911–6916, 1992.

39. Murakami, K., Mihara, K., and Omura, T., The transmembrane region of microsomal cytochrome P450 identified as the endoplasmic reticulum retention signal, *J. Biochem. (Tokyo)* 116:164–175, 1994.

40. Black, S. D., Membrane topology of the mammalian P450 cytochromes, *FASEB J.* 6:680–685, 1992.

41. Reviewed by Goeptar, A. R., Scheerens, H., and Vermeulen, N. P. E., Oxygen and xenobiotic reductase activities of cytochrome P450, *Crit. Rev. Toxicol.* 25:25–65, 1995.

42. Pohl, L. R., and Gillette, J. R., Determination of toxic pathways of metabolism by deuterium substitution, *Drug Metab. Rev.* 15:1335–1351, 1985.

43. Hjelmeland, L. M., Aronow, L., and Trudell, J. R., Intramolecular determination of primary kinetic isotope effects in hydroxylations catalyzed by cytochrome P-450, *Biochem. Biophys. Res. Commun.* 76:541–549, 1977.

44. Frommer, U., Ullrich, V., and Staudinger, H., Hydroxylation of aliphatic compounds by liver microsomes. 1. The distribution of isomeric alcohols, *Hoppe-Seyler's Z. Physiol. Chem.* 351:903–912, 1970.

45. White, R. E., McCarthy, M.-B., Egeberg, K. D., and Sligar, S. G., Regioselectivity in the cytochromes P-450: Control by protein constraints and by chemical reactivities, *Arch. Biochem. Biophys.* 228:493–502, 1984.

46. Groves, J. T., McClusky, G. A., White, R. E., and Coon, M. J., Aliphatic hydroxylation by highly purified liver microsomal cytochrome P-450: Evidence for a carbon radical intermediate, *Biochem. Biophys. Res. Commun.* 81:154–160, 1978.

47. Atkinson, J. K., and Ingold, K. U., Cytochrome P450 hydroxylation of hydrocarbons: Variation in the rate of oxygen rebound using cyclopropyl radical clocks including two new ultrafast probes, *Biochemistry* 32:9209–9214, 1993; Atkinson, J. K., Hollenberg, P. F., Ingold, K. U., Johnson, C. C., Le Tadic, M.-H., Newcomb, M., and Putt, D. A., Cytochrome P450-catalyzed hydroxylation of hydrocarbons: Kinetic deuterium isotope effects for the hydroxylation of an ultrafast radical clock, *Biochemistry* 33:10630–10637, 1994; Newcomb, M., Le Tadic, M. H., Putt, D. A., and Hollenberg, P. F., An incredibly fast apparent oxygen rebound rate constant for hydrocarbon hydroxylation by cytochrome P-450 enzymes, *J. Am. Chem. Soc.* 117:3312–3313, 1995.

48. CaJacob, C. A., Chan, W., Shephard, E., and Ortiz de Montellano, P. R., The catalytic site of rat hepatic lauric acid ω-hydroxylase. Protein vs prosthetic heme alkylation in the ω-hydroxylation of acetylenic fatty acids, *J. Biol. Chem.* 263:18640–18649, 1988.

49. Raucy, J. L., Kraner, J. C., and Lasker, J. M., Bioactivation of halogenated hydrocarbons by cytochrome P4502E1, *Crit. Rev. Toxicol.* 23:1–20, 1993; Mehendale, H. M., Roth, R. A., Gandolfi, A. J., Klaunig, J. E., Lemasters, J. J., and Curtis, L. R., Novel mechanisms in chemically induced hepatotoxicity, *FASEB J.* 8:1285–1295, 1994.

50. Miller, R. E., and Guengerich, F. P., Oxidation of trichloroethylene by liver microsomal cytochrome P-450: Evidence for chlorine migration in a transition state not involving trichloroethylene oxide, *Biochemistry* 21:1090–1097, 1982.

51. Ortiz de Montellano, P. R., and Reich, N. O., Inhibition of cytochrome P450 enzymes, in: *Cytochrome P450: Structure, Mechanism, and Biochemistry*, P. R. Ortiz de Montellano, Ed., Plenum Press, New York, pp. 273–214.

52. Ostovic, D., and Bruice, T. C., Mechanism of alkene epoxidation by iron, chromium, and manganese higher valent oxo-metalloporphyrins, *Acc. Chem. Res.* 25:314–320, 1992.

53. Brodie, B. B., Axelrod, J., Cooper, J. R., Gaudette, L., La Du, B. N., Mitoma, C., and Uden-

friend, S., Detoxication of drugs and other foreign compounds by liver microsomes, *Science* 121:603–604, 1955.

54. Lawton, M. P., and Philpot, R. M., Functional characterization of flavin-containing monooxygenase 1B1 expressed in *Saccharomyces cerevisiae* and *Escherichia coli* and analysis of proposed FAD- and membrane-binding domains, *J. Biol. Chem.* 268:5728–5734, 1993.

55. Seto, Y., and Guengerich, F. P., Partitioning between *N*-dealkylation and *N*-oxygenation in the oxidation of *N,N*-dialkylarylamines catalyzed by cytochrome P450 2B1, *J. Biol. Chem.* 268:9986–9997, 1993.

56. Richardson, H. L., Stier, A. R., and Borsos-Nachtnebel, E., Liver tumor inhibition and adrenal histologic responses in rats to which 3′-methyl-4-dimethylaminoazobenzene and 20-methylcholanthrene were simultaneously administered, *Cancer Res.* 12:356–361, 1952.

57. Conney, A. H., Pharmacological implications of microsomal enzyme induction, *Pharmacol. Rev.* 19:317–366, 1967.

58. Waxman, D. J., and Azaroff, L., Phenobarbital induction of cytochrome P-450 gene expression, *Biochem. J.* 281:577–592, 1992.

59. Ueng, T. H., Ueng, Y. F., Chen, T. L., Park, S. S., Iwasaki, M., and Guengerich, F. P., Induction of cytochrome P450-dependent monooxygenases in hamster tissues by fasting, *Toxicol. Appl. Pharmacol.* 119:66–73, 1993.

60. Whitlock, J. P., Genetic and molecular aspects of 2,3,7,8-tetrachlorodibenzo-*p*-dioxin action, *Annu. Rev. Pharmacol. Toxicol.* 30:251–277, 1990.

61. Green, S., Receptor-mediated mechanisms of peroxisome proliferators, *Biochem. Pharmacol.* 43:393–401, 1992.

62. Conney, A.H., Pantuck, E. J., Hsiao, K.-C., Garland, W. A., Anderson, K. E., Alvares, A. P., and Kappas, A., Enhanced phenacetin metabolism in humans fed charcoal-broiled beef, *Clin. Pharmacol. Ther.* 20:633–642, 1976.

63. Anderson, K. E., Pantuck, E. J., Conney, A. H., and Kappas, A., Nutrient regulation of chemical metabolism in humans, *Fed. Proc.* 44:130–133, 1985.

64. Stryer, L., *Biochemistry*, 4th ed., W. H. Freeman, New York, 1995, pp. 931–932.

65. Citron, M., Perplexing peroxisome proliferators, *Env. Health Perspect.* 103:232–235, 1995; Lake, B.G., Mechanisms of hepatocarcinogenicity of peroxisome-proliferating drugs and chemicals, *Annu. Rev. Pharmacol. Toxicol.* 35:483–507, 1995.

66. Bell, D. R., Bars, R. G., Gibson, G. G., and Elcombe, C. R., Localization and differential induction of cytochrome P450IVA and acyl-CoA oxidase in rat liver, *Biochem. J.* 275:247–252, 1991.

67. Smith, C. A. D., Moss, J. E., Gough, A. C., Spurr, N. K., and Wolf, C. R., Molecular genetic analysis of the cytochrome P450-debrisoquine hydroxylase locus and association with cancer susceptibility, *Environ. Health Perspect.* 98:107–112, 1992.

68. Okita, R. T., and Masters, B. S. S., Biotransformations: The cytochromes P450, in: *Textbook of Biochemistry with Clinical Correlations*, T. M. Devlin, Ed., Wiley-Liss, New York, 1992, Section 23.6.

69. Pineau, T., Fernandez-Salguero, P., Lee, S. S. T., McPhail, T., Ward, J. M., and Gonzalez, F. J., Neonatal lethality associated with respiratory distress in mice lacking cytochrome P450 1A2, *Proc. Natl. Acad. Sci. USA* 92:5134–5138, 1995. See also Liang, H.-C.L., Li, H., McKinnon, R.A., Duffy, J.J., Potter, S.S., Puga, A., and Nebert, D.A., *Cyp1a2*(-/-) null mutant mice develop normally but show deficient drug metabolism, *Proc. Natl. Acad. Sci. USA* 93:1671–1676, 1996.

15

THE AH RECEPTOR AND THE TOXICITY OF CHLORINATED AROMATIC COMPOUNDS

The *Ahr* genetic locus* was originally described in the mouse. Some inbred strains of mice (such as C57BL/6) are *responsive* to the polycyclic aromatic hydrocarbon carcinogen 3-methylcholanthrene (3-MC). That is, there is an increase in some P-450 enzyme activities (notably, aryl hydrocarbon hydroxylase, associated with CYP1A1) in microsomes prepared from liver of animals exposed to 3-MC or to the halogenated aromatic compound 2,3,7,8-tetrachlorodibenzo-*p*-dioxin (TCDD). (See page 254.) Other strains, such as DBA/2, are nonresponsive: They show no increase in AHH activity following exposure to 3-MC and are 10- to 100-fold less sensitive to the effects of TCDD. Recognizing the toxicological significance of P-4501A1 activity, many researchers pursued the analysis of this phenomenon.

Cross-breeding experiments showed that inducibility (responsiveness) is an autosomal dominant Mendelian trait, defining a genetic locus originally called the *Ah* locus (and now termed the *Ahr* locus). The *Ah* locus was hypothesized to encode a structural gene for a receptor (binding protein) responsible for regulating the induction process: the AH (aromatic hydrocarbon) receptor (1). The existence of such a TCDD-binding protein was first demonstrated biochemically by Alan Poland and colleagues at the University of Wisconsin, Madison. When ^{3}H-TCDD is incubated with hepatic cytosol and the proteins are separated by sucrose density-gradient ultracentrifugation, the radioactivity associates with a characteristic protein peak. The affinity of binding can be assessed quantitatively by titrating the cytosol with TCDD. (Conforming to pharmacological practice, we refer to TCDD or other activating ligands of the AH receptor as *agonists*.) The observed binding is characterized by high affinity and saturation kinetics, as expected for a receptor interaction. The identity of the biochemically defined AH receptor with the product of the *Ah* genetic locus was established in a straightforward fashion. The AH receptor is readily detected in cytosol prepared from livers of responsive mice; in nonresponsive mice, AH receptor is present in much lower concentrations and has a much reduced affinity for TCDD (2).

TCDD is a potent toxic compound in animals and humans. TCDD is formed as a contaminant in the commercial herbicide 2,4,5-trichlorophenoxyacetic acid (2,4,5-T), a component of the notorious *Agent Orange*. Tens of millions of kilograms of this product were sprayed over Vietnam in the late 1960s as part of the U.S. defoliation campaign during the war.

The toxicity of TCDD (measured as oral LD_{50}) varies considerably among species. In the guinea pig, the LD_{50} is about 1 μg/kg; in the rat and hamster, it is 10- to several thou-

* The newly revised nomenclature follows: *Ahr* refers to the genetic locus; **AH receptor** or **AHR** refers to the protein and cDNA; *Ahr* gene refers to the murine structural gene and promoter; **AHR** refers to the ligand-binding subunit of the AH receptor complex; **AH receptor complex** or **AHR complex** refers to the multimeric protein complex containing the AHR. (Previously, AhR was used for the receptor and *Ah* for the locus.)

sand-fold higher, depending on the sex and strain. In humans, the most notorious incident of TCDD exposure, other than the use of Agent Orange, was the industrial accident in Seveso, Italy, on July 10, 1976. An explosion in a reaction chamber for synthesis of 2,4,5-trichlorophenol released kilogram quantities of TCDD. One of the serious and characteristic consequences of human exposure to TCDD is chloracne, a persistent cystic skin eruption associated with exposure to halogenated aromatic compounds. In animals, toxic effects include loss of body weight ("wasting syndrome") and liver damage. The symptoms of TCDD toxicity are probably mediated via the receptor, but most of the events leading from receptor binding to the manifestations of TCDD toxicity remain obscure.

Progress toward characterization of the AH receptor was long hampered by the difficulty of purification of this protein. The receptor is present in very low concentration, even in the livers of responsive animals. Furthermore, TCDD-binding activity is lost during attempted purification. Poland et al. (3) circumvented this obstacle by developing a method for specifically labeling the receptor, based on the use of a *photoaffinity label*. The TCDD analogue, 2-azido-3-[^{125}I]iodo-7,8-dibromodibenzo-*p*-dioxin, binds noncovalently to the receptor, with high affinity. Irradiation of the agonist–receptor complex with ultraviolet (UV) light activates the azido moiety to a reactive nitrene, which covalently attaches to the adjacent protein:

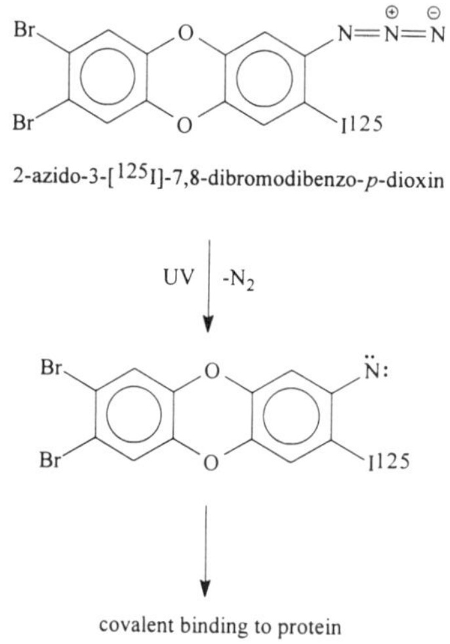

2-azido-3-[^{125}I]-7,8-dibromodibenzo-*p*-dioxin

UV | -N$_2$

covalent binding to protein

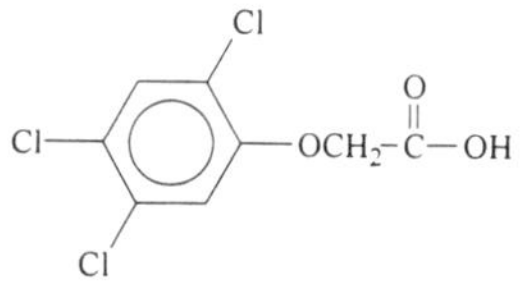

(2,4,5-trichlorophenoxy)acetic acid

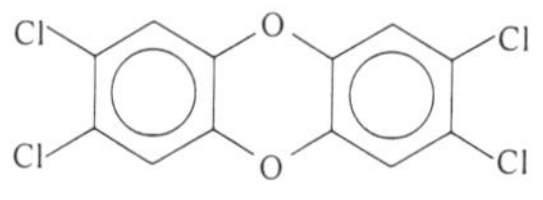

2,3,7,8-tetrachlorodibenzo-*p*-dioxin

The AH receptor was thus radiolabeled and could then be purified to homogeneity by standard techniques, such as ion-exchange chromatography, reversed-phase high-performance liquid chromatography (HPLC), and sodium dodecyl sulfate–polyacrylamide gel electrophoresis (SDS-PAGE). A partial N-terminal amino acid sequence was obtained, and in 1992 the long-anticipated breakthrough was achieved: cloning of cDNAs for the protein (4).

Contrary to prior expectations, the AH receptor does not share any homology with the steroid hormone receptors. Rather, sequence comparisons revealed that it is a member of a family of basic helix–loop–helix proteins, including mammalian ARNT protein (see below), the *Drosophila* neurogenic protein Sim, and the *Drosophila* circadian rhythm protein Per. This group of proteins, all of which have DNA-binding activity, is characterized by a region of homology of approximately 250 amino acids, referred to as the *PAS domain*. In the AhR, the PAS domain plays a role in heterodimer formation and contains the ligand-binding region of the receptor.

A model for AHR action is illustrated in Figure 15.1 (5). Ligands (such as TCDD or 3-MC) bind to the AHR in the cytoplasm. The resulting ligand-receptor complex is converted into a form that is tightly associated with the nucleus, resulting in increased transcription of genes regulated by AHR. The unoccupied AH receptor can be detected in cytosolic fractions prepared from cells and tissues. The molecular mass of mouse cytosolic receptor complex, as determined by hydrodynamic (ultracentrifugation) analysis, is approximately 270 kD. Photoaffinity-labeling and immunoblotting analysis indicate that the molecular mass of the ligand-binding subunit is about 95 kD, very similar to the monomer mass of about 90 kD deduced from the cDNA sequence. Evidence from protein–protein cross-linking and immunoprecipitation experiments indicates that the ligand-binding subunit of cytosolic AH receptor is complexed with the heat shock protein HSP90, and possibly with other proteins. HSP90 appears to associate with the AHR, maintaining it in an active conformation.

Considerable size variability has been observed in AHR from various inbred mouse strains, resulting from the expression of multiple alleles at the Ahr locus. For example, the AH receptor from DBA/2 mice is about 104 kD, whereas the AH receptor from C57BL/6 mice is about 95 kD. Variability among different animal species has also been

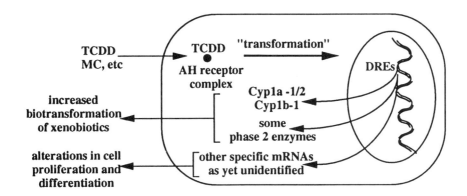

Figure 15.1. General mechanism of AH-receptor-mediated regulation of gene transcription.

reported (6). The human AH receptor is about 110 kD. It is not yet known whether this variation in molecular mass entails variations in AHR function.

After ligand treatment, the AHR is found in the nuclear fraction of cells, rather than the cytosol. Thus, binding of ligand triggers some alteration in receptor function, converting the receptor to a DNA-binding protein. Hydrodynamic characterization has revealed that the AHR complex recovered from the nucleus of mouse hepatoma cells incubated in culture with TCDD has a molecular mass of about 175 kD, quite different from the mass determined for the cytosolic receptor ($\sim$270 kD) or the size of the monomeric ligand-binding subunit ($\sim$95 kD).

Recently, a second protein, the AH receptor nuclear translocator (ARNT), was cloned and identified as a component of the nuclear form of the AH receptor (7). ARNT protein was named for its putative role in the translocation of the AH receptor complex from cytosol to nucleus. ARNT, like AHR, is a member of the PAS family of DNA-binding proteins. Recent evidence indicates that ARNT is a component of the ligand-transformed nuclear AHR complex. The human ARNT-protein-deduced amino acid sequence corresponds to a subunit mass of about 87 kD. Thus, the nuclear form of the AhR appears to be composed of the AHR (which binds ligand) together with ARNT (which does not bind ligand), resulting in a complex of about 175 kD. ARNT is not a component of the ligand-free cytosolic receptor (8).

THE GENOMIC TARGETS OF AHR

Of the multiple effects of exposure to 3-MC-type inducers, mediated by the AHR, the best-characterized response is the induction of cytochrome P4501A1 (CYP1A1) (9). The DNA sites at which transformed AHR acts were identified by molecular manipulation of the regulatory regions upstream from the gene encoding CYP1A1 in mouse cell lines. Selective deletion analysis identified a DNA sequence, containing the core consensus sequence 5'-TNGCGTG-3', in the 5'-flanking region of this gene. The presence of this sequence is necessary and sufficient for AHR-mediated regulation of CYP1A1 mRNA transcription (10).

These specific regions of DNA, which determine the response to 3-MC-type inducers, are known variously as Ah-responsive elements (AhREs), dioxin-responsive elements or dioxin-responsive enhancers (DREs), or xenobiotic response elements (XREs). We will use the first of these designations. This sequence has the properties of an *enhancer* element—that is, a *cis*-acting DNA motif that can influence the expression of a gene when "activated" by protein:DNA complex formation (11). At least 4 AhREs are located about −800 to −1200 bp upstream of the murine *Cyp1a1* gene; each AhRE can confer AHR-mediated responsiveness on gene expression. Recent cross-linking studies have shown that both the AHR and ARNT bind directly to the core consensus sequence (12).

The genes encoding several key enzymes of biotransformation are under direct transcriptional regulation by AHR: CYP1A1, CYP1A2, UDP-glucuronosyltransferase, one form of glutathione *S*-transferase, NAD(P)H:quinone oxidoreductase (NQO$_1$), and aldehyde dehydrogenase. (Several other genes, unrelated to xenobiotic metabolism, are also controlled by AHR.)

Figure 15.2 illustrates a possible sequence of steps resulting from ligand binding to the AHR. Binding of cytosolic AHR with TCDD or other ligand results in dissociation of HSP90 (and, possibly, other proteins). AHR then forms a heterodimer with ARNT, and the AH receptor complex acquires the ability to bind to the AhRE. The AHR complex

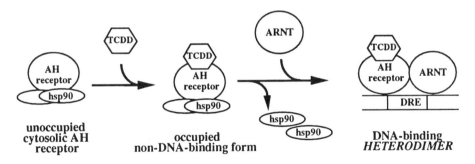

Figure 15.2. TCDD-dependent AH receptor transformation.

activates gene transcription by binding to AhRE sequences as a heterodimer (AHR:ARNT).

Both AHR and ARNT bind directly to the core consensus sequence of the AhRE. The transformation of AH receptor to a DNA-binding complex is not fully understood. Other factors, in addition to those shown in Fig. 15.2, may be involved (both positive and negative effectors). Phosphorylation of the ligand-binding subunit or some other component may be required.

STRUCTURE OF THE AH RECEPTOR PROTEIN

Once the cDNA for murine AHR was isolated, attention turned to mapping the functional domains of the receptor. This was greatly facilitated by the ability to express both AHR and ARNT in an in vitro translation system, consisting of AHR, ARNT, and HSP90, which allowed for the functional expression of these proteins (13). Both TCDD binding to the AHR and ligand-dependent AHR/ARNT recognition of the AhRE-containing DNA were demonstrated. Deletion analysis of the cDNAs encoding murine AHR revealed the localization of several domains within the molecule (Fig. 15.3). The deduced amino acid sequence indicates that the receptor contains a sequence with similarity to the basic region helix–loop–helix motif found in many transcription factors which undergo dimerisation and DNA-binding. Photoaffinity-labeling and peptide mapping techniques indicate that the agonist binds AHR in a region within the PAS domain. A glutamine-rich region in

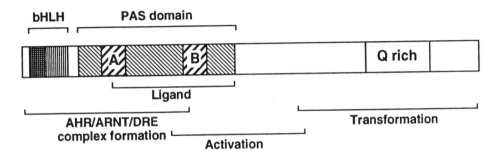

Figure 15.3. Murine AH receptor.

the C-terminal half of the molecule has also been described in several other genes which are developmentally or tissue-specifically regulated. Domain mapping by deletion analysis and functional expression has identified several domains, each serving a different function. The N-terminal region contains residues necessary for AHR:ARNT:AhRE complex formation. There appears to be a repressor region which, if deleted, results in the constitutive binding (i.e., in the absence of agonist) of AHR:ARNT complexes to the AhRE. A region in the C-terminal half of the molecule is important in receptor transformation. Also, the N-terminus of the AHR molecule, which contains the DNA-binding region, ligand-binding region, and PAS domain, appears to be highly conserved across several species. Antibodies raised against this region cross-react with AHR from rat, mouse, guinea pig, hamster, and human AHR.

THE *Ahr* GENE

The murine *Ahr* gene is composed of 11 exons, spanning more than 30 kb. The sequences encoding the helix–loop–helix domain are completely contained within exon 2; the PAS domain is encoded by exons 3 to 9; and the ligand-binding domain is encoded by exons 7 and 8 (4). The promoter is rich in GC nucleotides but contains no TATA or CCAAT boxes, common consensus sequences in eukaryotic promoters (11, pp. 549–552). Sequence analysis has shown the presence of several binding sites for the Sp1 transcription factor (11, p. 562), a potential cAMP response element, AP-1 (11, pp. 553–555) and E-box sites, and two elements which have been demonstrated, in other genes, to confer placental-specific expression.

Using a restriction fragment length polymorphism in exon 7 to examine both responsive and nonresponsive mouse lines, the *Ahr* gene was found to coincide with the phenotypically defined *Ahr* locus (14).

HUMAN AHR

AHR was first identified in rodents. Despite initial reports to the contrary, it is now apparent that the AHR is abundant in many human tissues and cell lines. In general, the mechanism of action of human AHR is very similar to that of rodent tissues (15).

Human receptor binds both TCDD and 3-MC and can be transformed to the AhRE binding state. The core consensus nucleotide sequence recognized by human AHR appears to be the same as that recognized by mouse AHR. There are some distinct differences, however, between human and rodent AHR. The AHR from human tissues, especially placenta, is detected in much higher concentrations if sodium molybdate is present in homogenizing buffers; molybdate ion is not important for the stability of AHR from responsive strains of mice but is crucial for stabilizing AhR in tissues from nonresponsive strains of mice. Secondly, the affinity with which TCDD binds to human AHR is generally lower than the affinity of binding to receptors from rats or responsive mice. The affinity (equilibrium dissociation, K_d) typically ranges from 3 to 15 nM in human samples, compared with a K_d of about 1 nM in cytosols from responsive C57BL/6 mouse liver. In cytosols from livers of nonresponsive mice (strain DBA/2), the K_d is approximately 16 nM. In other words, the affinity with which TCDD binds to human AHR is generally lower than the sensitive, responsive strains of mice but not as low as the nonresponsive strains. However, there is at least a 10-fold variation in the apparent affinity of TCDD for AHR among a series of human placental cytosols from different donors; the biological significance of these differences is unknown (16).

Polymorphisms may exist in the human AHR and might play a role in determining individual response to toxic agents, such as TCDD. The cDNA sequence for the human AHR will be available soon, and molecular pharmacogenetic studies can then be begun (17).

NOTES

1. Poland, A., Glover, E., and Kende, A. S., Stereospecific high affinity binding of 2,3,7,8-tetra-chlorodibenzo-*p*-dioxin by hepatic cytosols. Evidence that the binding species is a receptor for the induction of aryl hydrocarbon hydroxylase, *J. Biol. Chem.* 251:4936–4946, 1976. Poland, A., and Knutson, J. C., 2,3,7,8,-Tetrachlorodibenzo-*p*-dioxin and related halogenated aromatic hydrocarbons: examination of the mechanism of toxicity, *Annu. Rev. Pharmacol. Toxicol.* 22:517–554, 1982.

2. Okey, A. B., Vella, L. M., and Harper, P. A., Detection and characterisation of a 'low affinity' form of the Ah receptor in livers of mice 'non-responsive' to induction of cytochrome P1-450 by 3-methylcholanthrene, *Mol. Pharmacol.* 35:823–830, 1989.

3. Poland, A., Glover, E., Ebetino, F. H., and Kende, A. S., Photoaffinity labeling of the Ah receptor, *J. Biol. Chem.* 261:6352–6365, 1986.

4. Ema, M., Sogawa, K., Watanabe, N., Chujoh, Y., Matsushita, N., Gotoh, O., Funae, Y., and Fujii-Kuriyama, Y., cDNA cloning and structure of mouse putative Ah receptor, *Biochem. Biophys. Res. Commun.* 184:246–253, 1992; Burbach, K. M., Poland, A., and Bradfield, C. A., Cloning of the Ah-receptor cDNA reveals a distinctive ligand-activated transcription factor, *Proc. Natl. Acad. Sci. U.S.A.* 89:8185–8189, 1992; Hankinson, O., Research on the aryl hydrocarbon (dioxin) receptor is primed to take off, *Arch. Biochem. Biophys.* 300:1–5, 1993; Hankinson, O., The aryl hydrocarbon receptor complex, *Annu. Rev. Pharmacol. Toxicol.* 35: 307–340, 1995.

5. Whitlock, J. P., Jr., Mechanistic aspects of dioxin action, *Chem. Res. Toxicol.* 6:754–763, 1993. Okey, A. B., Riddick, D. S., and Harper, P. A., The Ah receptor: mediator of the toxicity of 2,3,7,8-tetrachlorodibenzo-*p*-dioxin (TCDD) and related compounds, *Toxicol. Lett.*, 70:1–22, 1993.

6. Poland, A., and Glover, E., Variation in the molecular mass of the Ah receptor among vertebrate species and strains of rats, *Biochem. Biophys. Res. Commun.* 146:1439–1449, 1987.

7. Hoffman, E. C., Reyes, H., Chu, F.-F., Sander, F., Conley, L. H., Brooks, B. A. and Hankinson, O., Cloning of a factor required for activity of the Ah (dioxin) receptor, *Science* 252:954–958, 1991.

8. Probst, M. R., Reisz-Porszasz, S., Agbunag, R. V., Ong, M. S., and Hankinson, O., Role of the aryl hydrocarbon receptor nuclear translocator protein in aryl hydrocarbon (dioxin) receptor action, *Mol. Pharmacol.* 44:511–518, 1993.

9. Okey, A. B., Enzyme induction in the cytochrome P450 system, in: *Pharmacogenetics of Drug Metabolism*, W. Kalow, Ed., Pergamon Press, New York, 1992, pp. 413–452.

10. Denison, M. S., Fisher, J. M., and Whitlock, J. P., Jr., Inducible, receptor-dependent protein-DNA interactions at a dioxin-responsive transcriptional enhancer, *Proc. Natl. Acad. Sci. U.S.A.* 85:2528–2532, 1988.

11. Lewin, B., *Genes V*, Oxford University Press, Oxford, 1994, pp. 869–873.

12. Elferink, C. J., Gasciewicz, T. A., and Whitlock, J. P., Jr., Protein–DNA interactions at a dioxin responsive enhancer, *J. Biol. Chem.* 265:20708–20712, 1990; Probst, M. R., Reisz-Porszasz, S., Agbunag, R. V., Ong, M. S., and Hankinson, O., Role of the aryl hydrocarbon receptor nuclear translocator protein in aryl hydrocarbon (dioxin) receptor action, *Mol. Pharmacol.* 44:511–518, 1993.

13. Dolwick, K. M., Swanson, H. I, and Bradfield, C. A., In vitro analysis of Ah receptor domains involved in ligand-activated DNA recognition, *Proc. Natl. Acad. Sci. U.S.A.* 90:8566–8570, 1993.

14. Schmidt, J. V., Carver, L. A., and Bradfield, C. A., Molecular characterisation of the murine *Ahr* gene, *J. Biol. Chem.* 268:22203–22209, 1993.

15. Harper, P. A., Prokipcak, R. D., Bush, L. E., Golas, C. L., and Okey, A. B., Detection and characterisation of Ah receptor for 2,3,7,8-tetrachlorodibenzo-*p*-dioxin in the human colon carcinoma cell line LS180, *Arch. Biochem. Biophys.* 290:27–36, 1991; Harper, P. A., Giannone, J. V., Okey, A. B., and Denison, M. S., In vitro transformation of the human Ah receptor and its binding to a dioxin response element, *Mol. Pharmacol.* 42:603–612, 1992.

16. Manchester, D. K., Golas, C. L., Roberts, E. A., and Okey, A. B., Ah receptor in human placentas: stabilisation by molybdate and characterisation of binding of 2,3,7,8-tetrachlorodibenzo-*p*-dioxin, 3-methylcholanthrene, and benzo[*a*]pyrene, *Cancer Res.* 47:4861–4868, 1987.

17. Dolwick, K. M., Schmidt, J. V., Carver, L. A., Swanson, H. I., and Bradfield, C. A., Cloning and expression of the human AH-receptor cDNA, *Molec. Pharmacol.* 44:911–917, 1994.

16

IDENTIFICATION OF DNA ADDUCTS

In this chapter we consider (a) the experimental approaches to identification of the chemical structures of DNA adducts derived from mutagens/carcinogens and (b) the chemical mechanisms of their formation (1). Many chemicals can form covalent adducts to DNA: directly, in some cases, and following metabolic activation, in others. The adducted moiety is a fragment or derivative of the chemical itself: Polycyclic aromatic hydrocarbons form adducts at the exocyclic amino groups of adenine and guanine residues, aromatic amines bind to the C-8 carbon of guanine, and nitrosamines alkylate the exocyclic oxygen atoms of thymine, cytosine, and guanine. The chemical characterization of covalent adducts clarifies the nature of the activated intermediates which reacted with DNA to form them. In the case of xenobiotics which undergo biotransformation, this helps elucidate the mechanisms of metabolic activation.

High-energy radiation also causes characteristic modifications to the DNA structure. Radiation damages may be *direct*, that is, due to the deposition of radiation energy in the DNA molecule itself, or *indirect*, due to the reactions of the energetic products of radiolysis of water (2).* The radiolysis products of water include reducing radicals, such as the solvated electron (e^-_{aq}) and the H· atom, and oxidizing radicals, especially the hydroxyl radical, ·OH. In the presence of molecular oxygen, solvated electrons react rapidly to form superoxide anion: $O_2 + e^-_{aq} \rightarrow O_2^{·-}$ (see Chapter 4; sidebar on radiolysis of water). Thus, as discussed previously, the effects of radiation have much in common with the effects of oxidative stress.

Typically, a single toxic agent, such as a polycyclic aromatic hydrocarbon or a nitrosamine, induces many types of DNA damage. Particular adducts may predominate, but many minor adducts are also formed. For example, alkylating agents react with guanine at several different sites, as in Figure 16.1 (top panel) and also modify other bases (3). In some cases, quantitatively minor adducts may be highly mutagenic (see below) and, hence, biologically significant. The pattern of DNA damages induced by an agent can serve as a distinctive "fingerprint." The recently developed technique of adduct ^{32}P-postlabeling (see page 269) generates a pattern of "spots" corresponding to the positions and intensities of covalent adducts in DNA, separated by two-dimensional planar chromatographic techniques. In principle, if such a pattern is distinctive, then we may be able to work back from an observed spectrum of DNA adducts to deduce the nature of the chemical agent responsible. This raises the prospect of a science of *molecular epidemiology*, in which we detect and identify prior chemical exposures on the basis of persistent DNA (or other macromolecular) adducts (4). For example, placental specimens obtained from smoking mothers showed at least one adduct associated with exposure to a polycyclic aromatic hydrocarbon constituent of cigarette smoke (5).

---

*For a detailed review, see A. P. Breen and J. A. Murphy, Reactions of oxyl radicals with DNA, *Free Radic. Biol. Med.* 18:1033–1077, 1995.

Multiple sites of guanosine alkylation

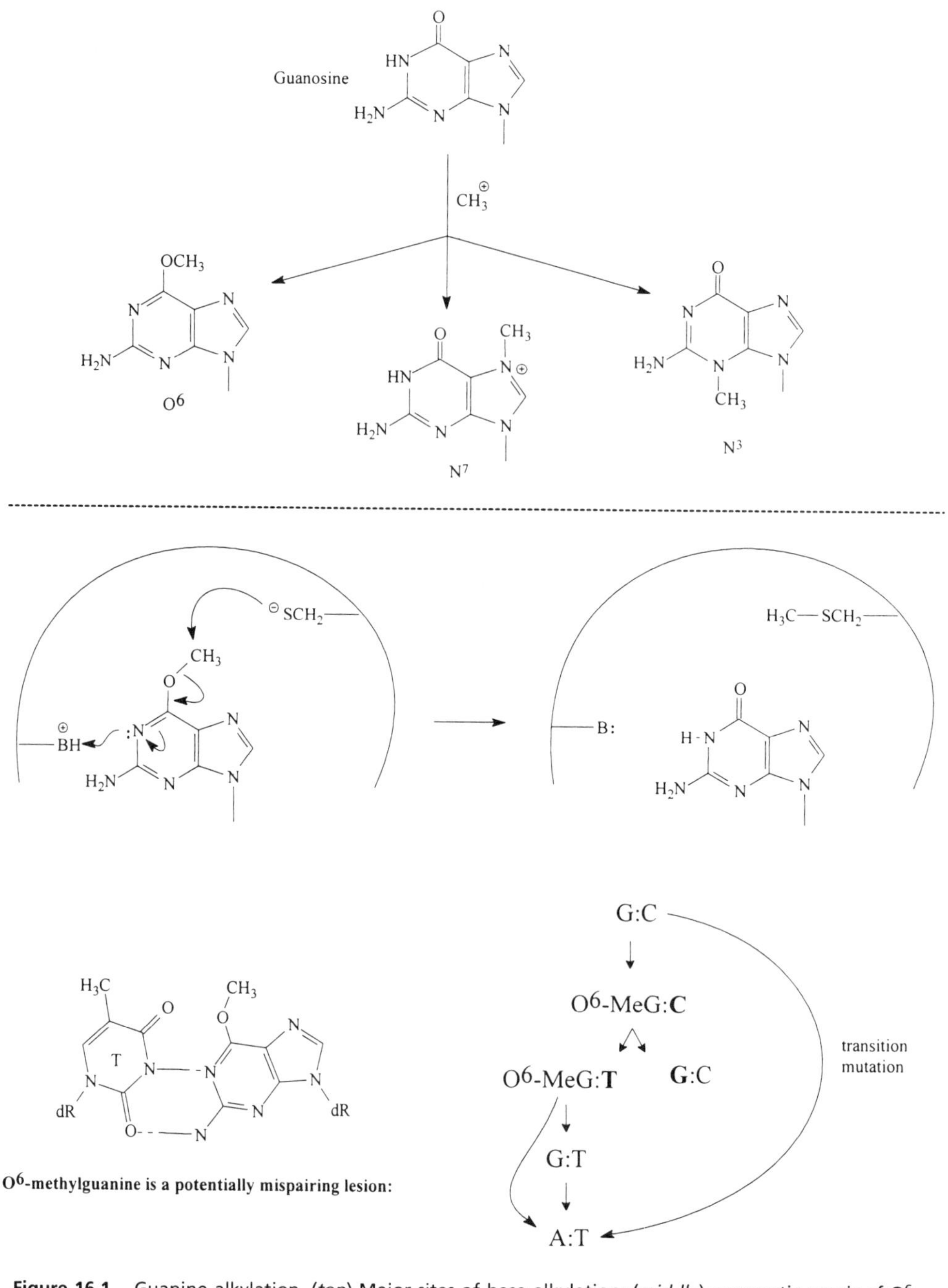

Figure 16.1. Guanine alkylation. (*top*) Major sites of base alkylation; (*middle*) enzymatic repair of O6 methylguanine (see page 287); (*bottom*) O6-methylguanlne-induced mutagenesis (see page 300).

The concentration of DNA in cells is very low when compared to the abundance of protein and RNA. In eukaryotic cells, the DNA is confined to the nucleus; most metabolic activation processes occur in the cytoplasm or endoplasmic reticulum. Therefore, the levels of DNA adducts formed are very low, even following exposure to large doses of a chemical mutagen or carcinogen.

DNA nucleoside or nucleotide adducts are typically large molecules, and structure determination is a challenging problem in organic analysis. The elucidation of the chemical structures of DNA adducts is usually based on spectroscopic identification, especially nuclear magnetic resonance (NMR). NMR analysis, even with very-high-field-strength instruments, is likely to be possible only with the purification of many micrograms of pure material. How can such "large" (by the standards of molecular biology, if not those of organic synthesis) amounts of DNA adducts be obtained? The most productive approach has been to prepare authentic standards of putative DNA adducts by the reaction of synthetic reactive intermediates (or their analogues) with target nucleotides or bases in vitro. Structural analysis is performed on these synthetic standards, and DNA adducts formed in cells or in vivo are identified by co-chromatography, using two or more different systems (stationary and mobile phases).

SYNTHETIC REACTIVE INTERMEDIATES

By definition, reactive intermediates are unstable species (usually electrophiles) and present challenging synthetic targets. The goal of achieving the synthesis of a putative ultimate carcinogenic species is of biological significance, and the quest is all the more exciting if the goal is suspected to be unachievable! In fact, many such intermediates, while highly reactive in a biological milieu, have proven to be isolable when protected from water and other nucleophiles.

The bay-region dihydrodiol epoxide metabolites of benzo[a]pyrene and several other polycyclic aromatic hydrocarbons have been synthesized (see Chapter 19) and are stable in dry organic solvents, such as tetrahydrofuran. They hydrolyze rapidly in water, especially in the presence of acid. N-Acetoxy esters of aromatic amines were first proposed as reactive intermediates formed by enzymatic bioactivation (see Chapter 20). Finally, in the past few years, Gernot Boche and his colleagues (Universität Marburg, Germany) succeeded in preparing several of these compounds by acetylation of the corresponding hydroxylamines with acetyl cyanide. They are isolable at low temperature, but decompose when warmed (6). In one case, N-acetoxysulfamethoxazole, an N-acetoxy ester, proved to be stable even at room temperature (7). In other cases, chemical precursors of the putative reactive metabolites have been prepared, and can be converted to the reactive species themselves, in the presence of the biological target. For example, the α-hydroxy metabolites of nitrosamine have proven to be too reactive for isolation. However, the acetate esters can be prepared, and, either spontaneously or in the presence of esterases, the α-hydroxy metabolites are generated in solution (8). The esters are mutagenic in bacterial assays (see Chapter 17), without metabolic activation by S9 preparation; bacterial esterase activity releases the α-hydroxy compound (9). The diimine oxidation products of aromatic diamines, such as benzidine, can be prepared by chemical or peroxidase-catalyzed oxidation of the parent aromatic amines. At acidic pH (below about pH 5.5), the diimine is protonated, charged, and stable. At higher pH, the diimine becomes deprotonated, neutral, and highly reactive with DNA, with glutathione, or with itself, to form polymers (10).

NUCLEIC ACID TARGETS FOR ADDUCT FORMATION STUDIES

Several kinds of nucleic acid (or constituents) can be used for preparation of adducts in vitro. Generally, the simpler targets allow easier structural characterization, but may be less representative of the interaction with critical biological targets in vivo. So, for example, the monomeric constituents of nucleic acids (bases, nucleosides, or nucleoside 5-monophosphates) are inexpensive, soluble, and homogeneous. However, the monomeric bases are typically less reactive with electrophiles than is DNA itself, because of electronic factors [the electrostatic potential developed by the high negative charge of the sugar–phosphate backbone of DNA (11)]. And, manifestly, the steric effects of DNA structure are missing in electrophile–monomer reactions. These steric interactions are very significant: The bases are shielded in the core of the double helix of B-DNA, and only the edges of the ring systems are exposed in the major and minor grooves. Indeed, the DNA molecule itself is complexed with histone proteins in the eukaryotic chromosomal structure, an effect that cannot be duplicated in an in vitro system containing nucleic acid alone.

POLYMERIC NUCLEIC ACID TARGETS

If we wish to study nucleic acids, rather than their monomeric constituents, several choices are available. Of course, "high molecular weight" DNA can be isolated from animal chromosomal sources, such as calf thymus or salmon sperm, and these materials are commercially available. On the other hand, they are highly heterogeneous in terms of sequence and fragment sizes.

Plasmid or phage DNA is easy to prepare, has defined molecular weight and sequence, and offers the important advantage of providing a biological endpoint. For example, the biological effect of adduct formation in a phage genome preparation can be measured by assaying the remaining plaque-forming capacity of the packaged phage or assaying the subsequent expression of particular genes.

Synthetic homopolymers offer the simplicity of a target containing only a single type of base. A simple and effective approach to analyzing the base specificity of a particular reactive species is to compare its binding in vitro to each of a series of homopolymers, such as poly[G] and poly[A]. Homopolyribonucleotides (RNA) and homopolydeoxyribonucleotides (ssDNA or dsDNA) are both commercially available. RNA homopolymers are prepared by the action of the enzyme *polynucleotide phosphorylase*, an unusual bacterial RNA polymerase, discovered by Marianne Grunberg-Manago and Severo Ochoa in 1955. (Homopolyribonucleotides synthesized in this manner were exploited in the deciphering of the genetic code.) This enzyme assembles nucleoside 5'-diphosphates randomly (i.e., independent of a template) into RNA. Homopolydeoxyribonucleotides are prepared by the action of *terminal deoxynucleotidyl transferase* (12). This enzyme is a unique template-independent DNA polymerase, which adds dNTPS onto the 3' end of a DNA strand; a synthetic oligonucleotide is used as primer. (Synthetic DNA homopolymers prepared in this way are shorter and much more expensive than the corresponding synthetic RNA homopolymers.)

ISOLATION OF DNA ADDUCTS

If a monomer target, such as a DNA base, is reacted with a synthetic electrophile, then adduct purification is a standard organic analytical problem and is approached in the usual way, such as by reversed-phase high-performance liquid chromatography (HPLC) purification. Since bases all absorb in the region of 260 nm, ultraviolet (UV) absorbance may be used to monitor the products.

The isolation of adducts formed with polydeoxyribonucleotide (DNA) targets, in vitro or in vivo, requires isolation of the DNA, followed by hydrolysis into its nucleotide, nucleoside, or base constituents. DNA isolation is usually straightforward in the case of in vitro systems, where the incubation mix is prepared with a large excess of DNA and little or no protein. Isolation of DNA from in vivo systems is a considerably greater challenge. Far more protein than DNA is present; some of the protein (such as histones) is tightly complexed with the DNA. Radiolabeled adduct formation with protein may interfere with measurements of DNA binding.

A typical protocol for isolation of hepatic DNA is as follows (13). Tissue containing adducted DNA is homogenized in buffer, pH 8, containing EDTA (ethylenediaminetetraacetic acid, which chelates metal ions and inhibits DNases) and SDS (sodium dodecyl sulfate); the elevated pH and SDS detergent denature proteins, inhibit enzyme activity, and reduce the positive charge on histone proteins, decreasing their affinity for DNA. Proteinase K (an unusually SDS-resistant enzyme) is added, and the mixture is incubated at 37°C to degrade protein. Two-phase extractions with buffer-saturated CIP (chloroform/*iso*-amyl alcohol/phenol) are used to remove protein from the preparation. Chloroform and phenol are protein denaturants, and *iso*-amyl alcohol reduces foaming at the aqueous–organic interface. These extractions cause much of the protein to denature, precipitate, and collect at the interface. The aqueous layer, containing the DNA, is collected and re-extracted multiple times. Finally, the DNA is precipitated with the addition of two volumes of ethanol and cooling; the DNA is spooled out on a glass rod. To remove residual RNA, the crude DNA is redissolved in buffer and treated with RNase at 37°C, followed by a repeat of the CIP extraction/ethanol precipitation steps. Finally, the DNA is washed with alcohol and acetone and dried. Pure DNA is characterized by a ratio of $A_{260}/A_{280} = 1.8$; lower values indicate residual protein contamination, since protein absorbs more strongly at 280 than at 260 nm.

ENZYMATIC HYDROLYSIS OF DNA

DNA is resistant to base hydrolysis, and concentrated acid hydrolysis causes cleavage of the glycosidic bonds and extensive degradation of the bases and sugars. Mild acid treatment (0.1 M HCl, 70°C) causes hydrolysis of the glycosidic bonds of purine bases, releasing guanine, adenine, and some purine adducts (see below). However, enzymatic hydrolysis methods are the most useful and general tools for adduct analysis (14).

The two distinct modes of nucleic acid hydrolysis yielding 5'-monophosphates or 3'-monophosphates are shown in Figure 16.2. Complete hydrolysis requires the action of both a nonspecific endonuclease, which cuts the polymer into oligonucleotide fragments, and an exonuclease. The most common approach is treatment with pancreatic DNase I and snake venom phosphodiesterase to yield nucleoside 5'-monophosphates. These can then be converted to nucleosides by the action of alkaline phosphatase.

Alternatively, DNA degradation to nucleoside 3'-monophosphates can be carried out with micrococcal nuclease and spleen phosphodiesterase. This approach is used in the Randerath postlabeling method (see below), which requires the presence of the 5'-OH group. In either case, complete hydrolysis is highly desirable to achieve a high yield of nucleotide adducts. Unfortunately, in most cases the presence of covalently bound adducts hinders hydrolysis.

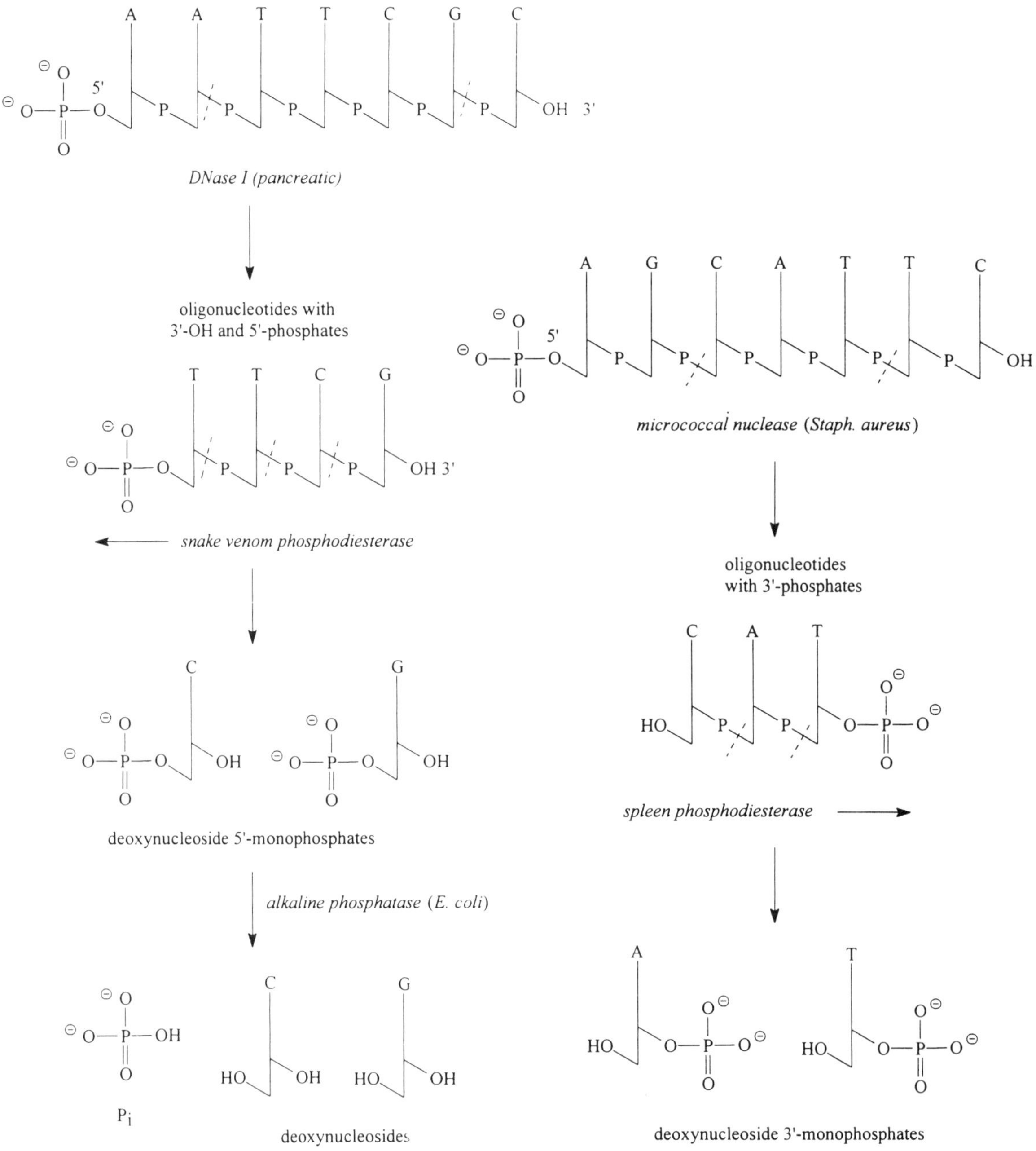

Figure 16.2.

Some adducted DNA residues, notably N^7-alkylated purines, are easily released from DNA as adducted free bases, since alkylation weakens the glycosidic bond between the base and deoxyribose sugar. Analysis of free bases is structurally simpler than the analysis of nucleosides or nucleotides, but there is no general method for cleaving the glycosidic bonds of adducted nucleosides and converting them to adducted bases. Some enzymes are active on particular classes of adducts (15).

SEPARATION OF ADDUCTED NUCLEOSIDES

Let us assume that adducted nucleosides have been successfully prepared by the methods described above. How are they purified from the DNA hydrolyzate and characterized chemically? The purification of the adducted nucleosides is guided by an understanding of their expected chemical characteristics. Even with extensive nucleic acid modification in vitro, nonadducted normal nucleosides will probably outnumber adducts by one million to one, or more. Therefore, one should exploit any substantial chemical differences between the adducts and the normal nucleosides. For example, adducts of polycyclic aromatic hydrocarbons or aromatic amines are much more hydrophobic than nonadducted nucleosides. Preliminary purification on a hydrophobic matrix, such as Sephadex LH-20 (16) or C-18 "Sep-Pak" cartridges (Millipore, Inc.), is often very effective: The normal nucleosides are eluted with water, and the adducts are eluted with methanol. Even adducted nucleotides can be separated this way (17). Another useful technique for separation of hydrophobic adducts is extraction into n-butanol solvent (18). Further purification of adducted nucleosides usually relies on reversed-phase HPLC separation.

Such purification procedures are, of course, greatly facilitated if the mutagen/carcinogen is radioactively labeled; the binding, recovery upon hydrolysis, and purification of the adducts can then be measured by scintillation counting, if the adduct retains the radioactive label. With unlabeled adducts, it may be possible to use fluorescence or UV absorption instead.

Table 16.1. NMR Chemical Shifts of Deoxyribose and Guanine Protons in Deoxyguanosine and Some Covalent Adducts[a]

Proton	Deoxyguanosine	N-(Deoxyguanosin-8-yl)-2-aminofluorene	5-(Deoxyguanosin-N^2-yl)-6-aminochrysene	8-(Benzo-[a]pyren-6-yl)-deoxyguanosine
1'	6.13	6.36	6.33	5.42
2', 2"	2.51, 2.22	2.57, 2.05	2.24; n.r.[b]	2.87, 1.69
3'	4.36	4.45	4.39	3.98
4'	3.83	3.95	3.87	3.10–3.45
5', 5"	3.58, 3.53	3.80, 3.80	3.60, 3.50	
3'-OH	5.11	5.37	n.r.	4.74
5'-OH	4.79	6.02	n.r.	5.58–5.85
C-8	8.38	—	7.77	—
N-1-H	?	10.59	10.81	10.95
2-NH$_2$	?	6.47	8.29	6.69

[a]Structures are shown on page 268. Data were obtained from the following sources:

Deoxyguanosine, N-(deoxyguanosin-8-yl)-2-aminofluorene: Kriek, E., Miller, J. A., Juhl, U., and Miller, E. C., 8-(N-2)-Fluorenylacetamide)guanosine, an arylamidation reaction product of guanosine and the carcinogen N-acetoxy-N-2-fluorenylacetamide in neutral solution, *Biochemistry* 6:177–182, 1967; Evans, F. E., Miller, D. W., and Beland, F. A., Sensitivity of the conformation of deoxyguanosine to binding at the C-8 position by N-acetylated and unacetylated 2-aminofluorene, *Carcinogenesis* 1:955–959, 1980; Beland, F. A., Allaben, W. T., and Evans, F. E., Acyltransferase-mediated binding of N-hydroxyarylamides to nucleic acids, *Cancer Res.* 40:834–840, 1980.

8-(Benzo[a]pyren-6-yl)-deoxyguanosine: Rogan, E. G., Cavalieri, E. L., Tibbels, S. R., Cremonesi, P., Warner, C. D., Nagel, D. L., Tomer, K. B., Cerny, R. L., and Gross, M. L., Synthesis and identification of benzo[a]pyrene-guanine nucleoside adducts formed by electrochemical oxidation and by horseradish peroxidase catalyzed reaction of benzo[a]pyrene with DNA, *J. Am. Chem. Soc.* 110:4023–4029, 1988.

5-(Deoxyguanosin-N^2-yl)-6-aminochrysene: Delclos, K. B., Miller, D. W., Lay, J. O., Jr., Casciano, D. A., Walker, R. P., Fu, P. P., and Kadlubar, F. F., Identification of C8-modified deoxyinosine and N^2- and C8-modified deoxyguanosine as major products of the in vitro reaction of N-hydroxy-6-aminochrysene with DNA and the formation of these adducts in isolated rat hepatocytes treated with 6-nitrochrysene and 6-aminochrysene, *Carcinogenesis* 8:1703–1709, 1987.

[b]n.r., not resolved.

ADDUCT STRUCTURE DETERMINATION

Once purified, the determination of the structure of a nucleoside or base adduct can be approached by the usual techniques of organic analysis. However, the amount of material that can be obtained is often very limited (less than 1 mg). Nuclear magnetic resonance (NMR) is probably the most valuable tool (19). High-field-strength NMR measurements (250–600 MHz) are capable of resolving every proton resonance on an adduct such as the N^2-deoxyguanosine adducts of benzo[a]pyrene dihydrodiol epoxides (20) or the C^8-guanosine adducts of aromatic amines. The resonances corresponding to protons on the adduct moiety can often be assigned by comparison of chemical shifts to those of the parent compound; similarly, the deoxyguanosine moiety resonances (deoxyribose and guanine base) can be compared to the parent nucleoside. Table 16.1 illustrates some typical values obtained for the deoxyribose protons in some typical polycyclic aromatic hydrocarbon and aromatic amine adducts.

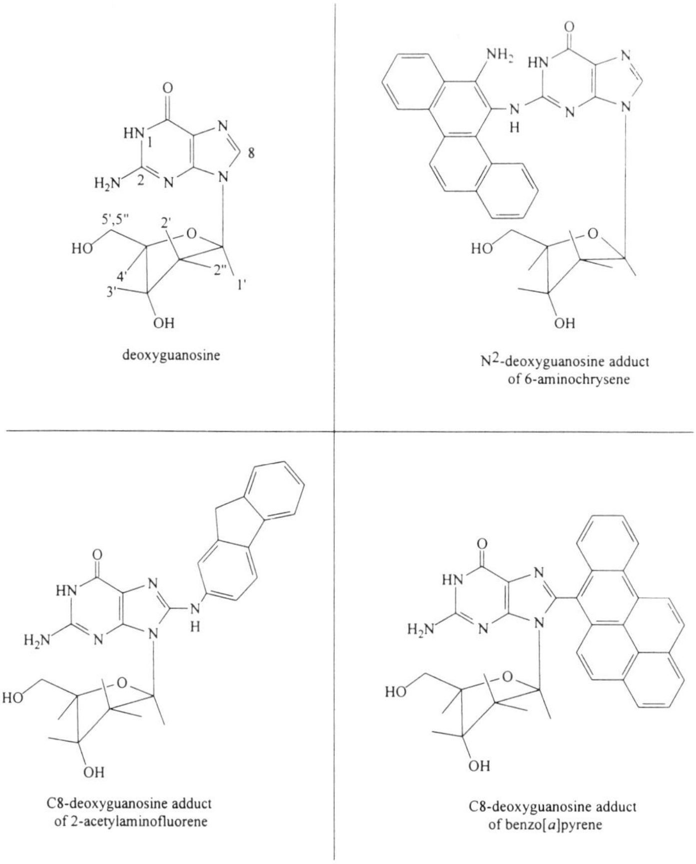

deoxyguanosine

N2-deoxyguanosine adduct
of 6-aminochrysene

C8-deoxyguanosine adduct
of 2-acetylaminofluorene

C8-deoxyguanosine adduct
of benzo[a]pyrene

Small but measurable shifts are observed. NMR assignments can be confirmed by the use of decoupling or two-dimensional COSY techniques (21). ^{13}C-NMR has also been used. As with analysis of glucuronides (Chapter 10), mass spectrometry has become increasingly useful for structure determination of nucleoside adducts, with the development of soft ionization modes, such as fast atom bombardment, thermospray HPLC-MS, and atmospheric pressure chemical ionization.

Once a covalent adduct has been isolated and identified, the adduct can now be used as a standard for the identification, by cochromatography, of adducts formed in vivo or in cells in vitro. The target of interest (such as hepatic DNA in vivo, or the chromosomal DNA of cultured hepatocytes) is exposed to the radiolabeled (^{14}C or ^{3}H) xenobiotic, and DNA adducts are isolated as described above. The quantity of adduct obtained is far too small for direct identification by spectroscopic techniques. Instead, the hydrolyzate is "spiked" by the addition of large amounts of *unlabeled* adduct standards. The spiked hydrolyzate is separated by HPLC, and the eluent is monitored simultaneously for UV absorbance (to detect the unlabeled standards) and radioactivity (to detect the labeled unknown adducts). Coelution in two different chromatographic systems constitutes good evidence of identity (see Fig. 16.3).

POSTLABELING ANALYSIS OF DNA ADDUCTS

The detection of DNA adducts by the direct procedures discussed above is possible when either (i) the adducts are present in sufficiently large amounts for direct spectroscopic detection or (ii) a radiolabeled xenobiotic was used. The first condition will hardly ever be met, except in in vitro systems with purified DNA and synthetic reactive metabolites. The second condition can only be met if a radiolabeled xenobiotic is at hand, and it can be applied in the system of interest. Obviously, this rules out studies on humans; in fact, even

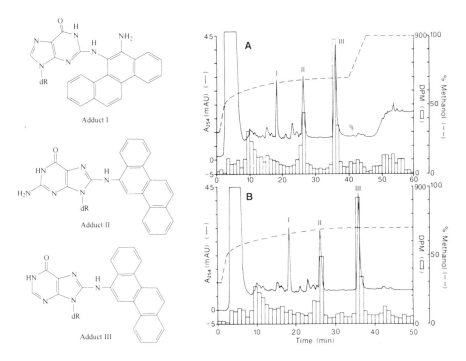

Figure 16.3. Identification of radiolabeled DNA adducts by co-chromatography with synthetic standards. Synthetic standards (unlabeled) of adducts I, II, and III (see structures, left) were mixed with enzymatic hydrolysates of DNA obtained from rat hepatocytes treated (in vitro) with radiolabeled 6-nitrochrysene (A) or radiolabeled 6-aminochrysene (B). Reversed-phase HPLC chromatograms of the samples are shown. (Radioactivity, open bars; UV absorbance, solid line; HPLC gradient profile, dashed line.) Co-chromatography indicates that adducts II and III, but not adduct I, are present in the hepatocyte DNA. From Delclos et al., 1987 (see ref. to Table 16.1, p. 267).

studies on rodents are difficult and expensive, since very large amounts of radiolabeled xenobiotic are required. Furthermore, the technique is fundamentally limited by the relatively low specific activities of ^{14}C and ^3H, determined by their long half-lives.

An entirely new approach to carcinogen–DNA adduct detection was developed in the late 1970s by Kurt Randerath and colleagues, at Baylor College of Medicine in Houston, Texas (22). This approach, known as ^{32}P postlabeling analysis, offers important advantages to previous techniques. Radiolabeled xenobiotics are not required: The label is introduced to the adduct subsequent to DNA hydrolysis. Since ^{32}P is used (half-life = 14 days), extremely high specific activities—and, hence, sensitivities—are achievable.

The postlabeling technique is shown schematically:

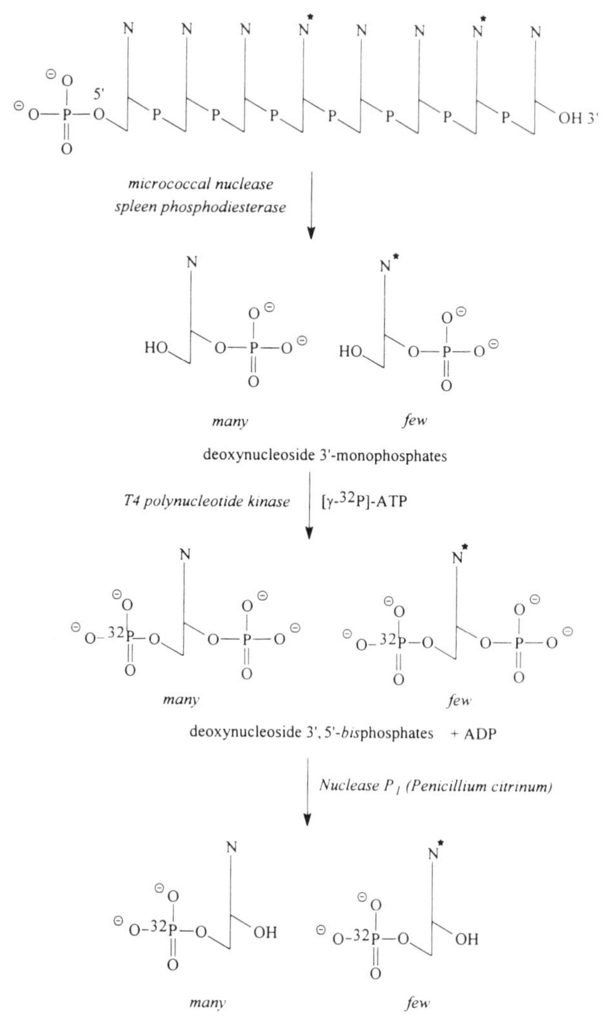

micrococcal nuclease
spleen phosphodiesterase

deoxynucleoside 3'-monophosphates

T4 polynucleotide kinase   [γ-^{32}P]-ATP

deoxynucleoside 3',5'-*bis*phosphates   + ADP

Nuclease P₁ (Penicillium citrinum)

The DNA sample of interest (for example, obtained from the tissue of a carcinogen-treated animal) is purified from other macromolecules and is hydrolyzed with micrococcal endonuclease plus spleen phosphodiesterase, yielding deoxyribonucleoside-3'-monophosphates (dNp's). The hydrolysate dNp mix will consist of a vast excess of "normal" nucleotides (dAp, dGp, dCp, Tp), a considerable amount of methylated nucleotides (5-Me-dCp, 6-Me-dAp), plus a small amount of adducted nucleotides (dN*p). In the next step, the hydrolysate is treated with T4-polynucleotide kinase and [γ-^{32}P]-ATP; this is the method used for end-labeling DNA in standard molecular biology protocols. The dNp's are now phosphorylated to give ^{32}P-deoxyribonucleoside-3',5'-*bis*phosphates (^{32}pdNp's). *If the adducted nucleosides are also phosphorylated by the kinase*, then the mixture will also contain a small quantity of labeled adducts, ^{32}pdN*p's.

The key step in the postlabeling method is separation of the small quantity of radiolabeled adducted nucleotides from the vast excess of "normals." If the chemical properties of the expected adducts are very different from the properties of the normal deoxyribonucleoside-3',5'-*bis*phosphates, this separation may be relatively straightforward. Just as in the case of direct analysis of adducts, discussed earlier, one may take advantage of the hydrophobicity of adducts bearing polycyclic aromatic hydrocarbon moieties, for example, and effect a separation by reversed-phase adsorption chromatography. If the adducts are only slightly different from the normals, as in the case of alkylation damage, separation may still be achievable, using two-dimensional thin-layer chromatography (TLC) separation on polyethylene-imine-cellulose plates.

In some cases, better separation can be achieved following hydrolysis of the deoxyribonucleoside-3',5'-*bis*phosphates to deoxyribonucleoside-5'-phosphates, using nuclease P_1 (see scheme above). Another useful variation is to carry out the labeling step with a limiting concentration of $[\gamma$-^{32}P]-ATP; this exploits the observation that T4-polynucleotide kinase actually labels some adducted nucleotides *preferentially*, relative to normal nucleotides.

Following separation of the normal from the adducted nucleotides, the former are physically removed from the sample (for example, by cutting off a piece of the TLC sheet); otherwise their radioactivity will overwhelm that of the adducts. Finally, the pattern of adduct spots on the plate is determined by autoradiography. The result is a pattern of spots of varying intensities, representing the adducted bases, in the form of deoxyribonucleoside-3',5'-*bis*phosphates.

The sensitivity of the postlabeling technique derives from the very high specific activity of $[\gamma$-^{32}P]-ATP. In favorable cases, as little as one adducted base per mammalian cell can be detected! On the other hand, the amount of material present in such cases is far too small for there to be any possibility of direct chemical identification of the labeled species. In some cases, authentic standards are available for comparison, but in most cases the adducts are identified only as numbered spots. (The TLC mobilities of the adducts may also provides some clues as to their identity.) Nevertheless, the ability to separate and (at least approximately) quantitate the presence of modified bases in DNA from any biological source is a very powerful tool (see Fig. 16.2).

IMMUNOASSAY OF DNA ADDUCTS

Miriam Poirier (National Cancer Institute, Bethesda, MD) has developed the application of immunoassay techniques (see Chapter 1) to the sensitive detection of DNA damage. Carcinogen–nucleoside adducts and carcinogen-modified DNA can elicit an immune response in animals. DNA adducts (small molecule haptens) are conjugated to protein carriers, such as albumin or hemocyanin. (The obvious limitation on the application of immunological methods is that the authentic adduct must be available first, so that the antibody can be raised.) Modified DNA is coupled with methylated proteins to form immunogenic complexes. Both polyclonal and monoclonal antibodies have been prepared successfully. An antiserum raised in rabbits to the adduct guanosin-8-yl-acetylaminofluorene recognizes the DNA adduct-derived nucleosides deoxyguanosin-8-yl-acetylaminofluorene and deoxyguanosin-8-yl-aminofluorene (23), but does not recognize the carcinogen itself, DNA, or several other minor adducts. This antiserum was used in highly

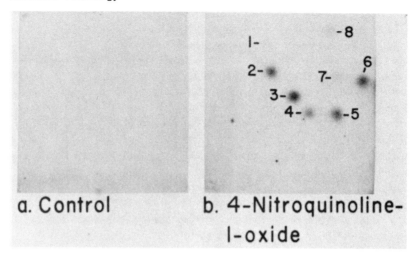

Figure 16.4. ^{32}P-Post-labeling analysis of 4-nitroquinoline-1-oxide DNA adducts formed in DNA of mouse skin. The backs of the mice (two or three mice per group) were shaved, and four doses of the compound (1.2 μmol in 200 μl acetone solvent) were applied at 24-hour intervals. Mice were sacrificed one day after application of the last dose, and skin DNA was extracted, digested to deoxyribonucleoside 3'-monophosphates, labeled, and analyzed by polyethyleneimine-cellulose thin layer chromatography. Normal nucleotides were removed after the second of the four chromatographic development steps. After two further development steps to separate the adducted nucleosides, the plate was visualized by autoradiography. From M. V. Reddy, R. C. Gupta, E. Randerath, and K. Randerath, ^{32}P-Post-labeling test for covalent DNA binding of chemicals in vivo: application to a variety of aromatic carcinogens and methylating agents, *Carcinogenesis* 5:231–243, 1984.

sensitive immunological detection techniques [radioimmunoassay (RIA) or enzyme-linked immunosorbent assay (ELISA) (24)] for these C8 adducts (25).

RIA measures the competition between a radiolabeled standard (Ag*) and the nonlabeled sample (Ag), also called the "inhibitor," which competitively inhibits binding of the standard to the antibody. That is:

in the absence of inhibitor: $Ab + Ag^* \rightarrow AbAg^*$

but, in the presence of inhibitor: $Ab + Ag^* + n[Ag] \rightarrow AbAg$

competes with the formation of AbAg*. The antibody complexes (AbAg and AbAg*) are then separated from the sample, and the bound radioactivity is measured. The amount of Ag present can be calculated from a standard curve prepared with known amounts of inhibitor. In the ELISA approach, the standard (Ag*) is not radiolabeled; instead, it is bound to the surface of a plastic microtiter plate. Ab and Ag are incubated in the plate, and unbound Ab is removed by washing the plate. In the absence of Ag, AbAg* remains attached to the plate. In the presence of Ag, AbAg is formed, and then it is removed during the washing step. The presence of bound Ab can then be quantitated by an enzyme-conjugated second antibody, raised against the constant region of the first Ab (see Chapter 1). [These methods are also discussed by Poirier (26).]

The immunoassay can be used to measure formation of carcinogen–DNA adducts in experimental animals exposed to a known carcinogen; for example, repair of the adducts can be measured as loss of detectable bound adducts following cessation of exposure. Alternatively, the sensitivity of the immunoassay approach can be used to detect carcinogen adducts in human DNA samples. In this case, multiple adducts are likely to be present. For example, smokers are exposed to many similar polycyclic aromatic hydrocarbons, and an antiserum raised against BPDE-modified DNA will cross-react with adducts of some of these compounds. Nevertheless, relative exposure levels can be evaluated, even if the detailed chemical composition of the adduct mixture is unknown (27). Another application of antibodies to DNA adducts is the construction of immunoaffinity columns, with which adducts can be purified from DNA hydrolysates, prior to separation and identification of the adducts by analytical methods, as described earlier in this chapter.

POSITIONS OF ADDUCT FORMATION ON THE DNA BASES

Different reactive species induce different patterns of DNA adduct formation. Earlier in this chapter, we illustrated some of the sites on guanine that are subject to alkylation. In the case of the direct-acting alkylating agent, methylnitrosourea (MNU; ref. 28), guanine N-7 is far the most reactive position, although most of the oxygen and nitrogen atoms, both within the rings and exocyclic, are alkylated to some extent. Dihydrodiol epoxide metabolites of polycyclic aromatic hydrocarbons form adducts mainly at the guanine N-2, a position which is untouched by alkylating agents. Aromatic amines and nitro compounds, activated to nitrenium-ion reactive species, are highly selective for the guanine C-8, a position untouched by dihydrodiol epoxides.

These differing patterns of adduct formation have profound biological consequences. For example, N^7 alkylated purines undergo facile cleavage of the glycosidic bond; this is actually one of the base specific modification reactions of the Maxam–Gilbert DNA sequencing method. The resulting abasic sites are efficiently repaired. On the other hand, guanine O^6-alkylation produces a base (analogous to a rare *enol* tautomeric form of guanine) which is potentially mispairing (see bottom portion of scheme on page 262). As was first pointed out by Loveless in 1969, formation of such a T·O^6-MeG base pair at replication would, if unrepaired, lead to a G·C → A·T transition mutation at the next round of cell division (29). Indeed, such events dominate the mutational spectra of alkylating agents in the *E. coli lacI* gene (30) and account for all of the *ras* oncogene activating mutations observed in lung tumors of mice treated with nitrosamines (31).

What factors account for the different sites of adduct formation by various classes of reactive intermediates? In general, the reactive intermediates are electrophiles (often positively charged) or their precursors: carbonium-ion intermediates derived from the opening of the epoxide ring of a dihydrodiol epoxide; arylnitrenium-ion reactive intermediates from the metabolism of aromatic amines; alkyl cations from alkylating agents, and so on. The target sites on nucleic acids are nucleophilic atoms with lone pairs of electrons (exocyclic keto oxygen and amino nitrogens, as well as ring nitrogens of the bases) or negative charge (phosphate oxygen) (32). Some sites on the bases are particularly susceptible to electrophilic substitution, especially purine N-7.

"Hard" electrophiles (possessing highly localized positive charges), such as carbonium and nitrenium ions, react preferentially with "hard" nucleophilic centers, such as the lone pairs of amino nitrogen and keto oxygen atoms of the bases, rather than with "soft" (polarizable, delocalized negative charge) nucleophilic sites, such as thiol groups in protein and glutathione. These considerations may contribute to determining the relative reactivities of, for example, the guanine O-6 and N-2 sites (33).

The chemistry of adduct formation in DNA cannot be explained simply on the basis of studies of the monomer components of DNA. The reactivities of these sites in native ds-

DNA are often very different from those observed for the bases, nucleosides, or nucleotides. For example, N-1 is a major site of alkylation of guanosine by alkyl iodides in DMSO solution, but is *not* a detectable target in dsDNA. There are probably several reasons for such differences. The electronic environment of the bases is very different in dsDNA: The hyperchromic shift in the UV absorbances of the bases upon DNA denaturation reflects the substantial electronic effect of base stacking in the double helix. Steric factors also play a major role in determining the sites of reactions of electrophiles with dsDNA. Only the "edges" of the bases are potentially exposed to solvent in the major and minor grooves of the double helix (see Chapter 2). Since the major groove is wider and more accessible than is the minor groove, one might expect sites exposed in the major groove to be more susceptible to adduct formation. Indeed, the guanine O-6, N-7, and C-8 positions are prominent reaction sites. The profound differences in reactivities and carcinogenicities of enantiomeric polycyclic aromatic hydrocarbon metabolites (see Chapter 19) presumably reflect their differing interactions with the chiral DNA double helix.

Both polycyclic aromatic hydrocarbons and polycyclic aromatic amines have flat, hydrophobic structures which would seem to be excellent candidates as DNA intercalators. Indeed, the best-known intercalating agent, the fluorescent dye ethidium bromide, is a substituted aromatic amine. It seems plausible that the activated forms of these classes of carcinogens do intercalate between the base pairs of the double helix, and the geometry of this intercalation might well dictate the site of adduct formation. However, the evidence for such mechanisms is indirect at best (34).

GUANINE C-8 MODIFICATIONS

Alkylating agents, which generate cationic reactive species (carbonium ions), do not react at guanine C-8, which appears to be much less nucleophilic than the N-2 or N-7 nitrogens. *However, guanine is the most easily oxidized base in DNA and is especially susceptible to damage by oxidizing species, including free radicals* (35). Methyl radicals, generated in vitro by the peroxidase-catalyzed oxidation of methylhydrazine ($H_3C-NH-NH_2$), alkylates guanine at C-8 (36). Peroxidase-catalyzed or electrochemical oxidation of benzo[*a*]pyrene in the presence of DNA in vitro yields adducts in which the benzo[*a*]pyrene C-6 position is bound to guanine C-8; presumably, the C-6-carbon-centered benzo[*a*]pyrene cation radical is the reactive intermediate in this reaction (37). The structure of this adduct was shown above (see scheme on page 268). However, the toxicological importance of these in vitro radical-derived adducts is not yet clear.

8-HYDROXYGUANOSINE (8-OXOGUANOSINE)

As the most easily oxidized group in DNA, guanine acts as a trap for radiolytically generated oxidant radicals, especially ·OH. In 1984, Kasai and Nishimura (National Cancer Center, Tokyo, Japan) demonstrated the formation of 8-hydroxydeoxyguanosine in DNA, following exposure to chemical systems which generate hydroxyl radical (38). Hydroxyl radical addition to the C-8 position of deoxyguanosine gives a resonance-stabilized neutral radical:

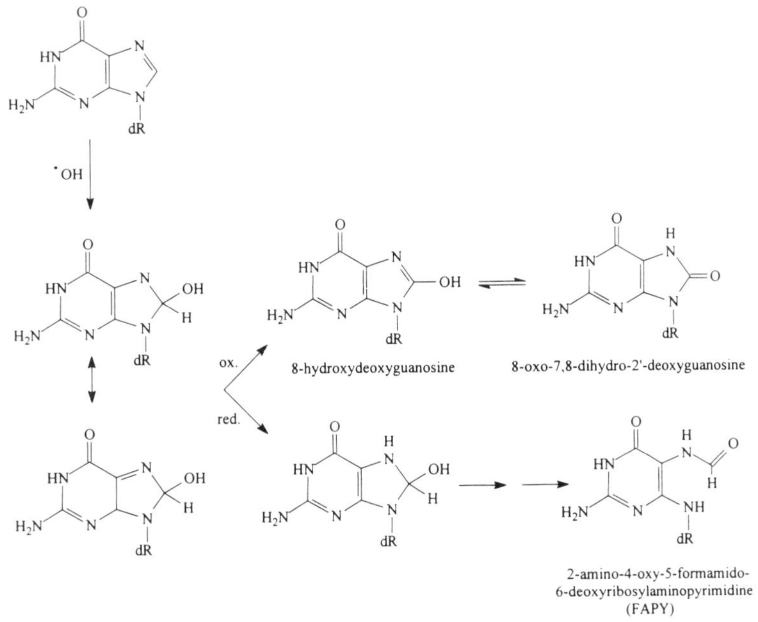

8-hydroxydeoxyguanosine   8-oxo-7,8-dihydro-2'-deoxyguanosine

2-amino-4-oxy-5-formamido-
6-deoxyribosylaminopyrimidine
(FAPY)

(The analogous reaction can also occur with adenosine, but this seems to be much less facile.) The guanine–OH adduct radical can act as either an oxidant or a reductant (34), depending upon subsequent interactions with redox-active species. Oxidation gives 8-hydroxydeoxyguanosine, which tautomerizes to the favored 6,8-diketo form (8-oxodeoxyguanosine). Alternatively, reduction, followed by imidazole ring-opening, gives the formamidopyrimidine product, FAPY. FAPY has also been identified as a product of radiation damage to DNA.

8-Hydroxydeoxyguanosine is also formed by the reaction of *singlet oxygen* with DNA (39). Singlet oxygen is the first electronic exited state of oxygen; the ground state is triplet (see Chapter 3). Singlet oxygen can be produced from some enzymatic processes or following the absorption of light by photosensitizers, such as methylene blue, which transfer excitation energy to oxygen.

The presence of repair enzymes for oxidized guanine products provides important evidence for the biological significance of this type of DNA damage. Several *Escherichia coli* enzymes repair 8-hydroxyguanine damage (40). The *mutT* gene product hydrolyzes 8-hydroxydeoxyguanosine triphosphate (8-OH-dGTP). This modified nucleotide triphosphate would otherwise accumulate in the DNA precursor pool and be incorporated into DNA by DNA polymerase action. 8-Hydroxyguanine is released from DNA by a specific glycosylase (41), the product of the *mutM* gene, which also acts on FAPY sites. The enzyme releases the modified base and also cuts the DNA strand both 5' and 3' to the base, leaving a single nucleotide gap, which is filled by repair synthesis.

8-Hydroxydeoxyguanosine and 8-hydroxyguanine can be detected by HPLC with electrochemical detection; both species are found in human urine and may be useful biomarkers of oxidative damage to cellular DNA. Animal studies have shown that oxidative carcinogens, such as potassium bromate or 2-nitropropane, induce 8-hydroxydeoxyguanosine formation (42). 8-Hydroxydeoxyguanosine is a potentially mispairing modified base, and it induces G:C $\rightarrow$ T:A transversions in several mutation assay systems (43, 44).

GUANINE C-8 ADDUCTS OF AROMATIC AMINES

Adducts at the C-8 carbon atom of deoxyguanosine are very characteristic of N-substituted aromatics, including nitroaraomatics and aromatic amines, although guanine N-2 adducts also occur. A plausible mechanism for this targeting to C-8 has been elucidated recently (45). In this study, the reactive ultimate carcinogen N-acetoxy-2-aminofluorene, precursor to the 2-aminofluorene nitrenium ion (see Chapter 20), was generated by the acetylsalicylic acid-dependent acetylation of N-hydroxy-2-aminofluorene in the presence of guanosine or guanosine derivatives. To prevent formation of the usual C-8 adduct, C^8,N^9-dimethylguanine was used as nucleophilic target. The major adduct proved to be formed by reaction of the aminofluorene nitrogen with the N-7 nitrogen of the base. This suggests that, in the case of deoxyguanosine itself, the initial site of reaction is also at N-7, and the adduct then rearranges to C-8:

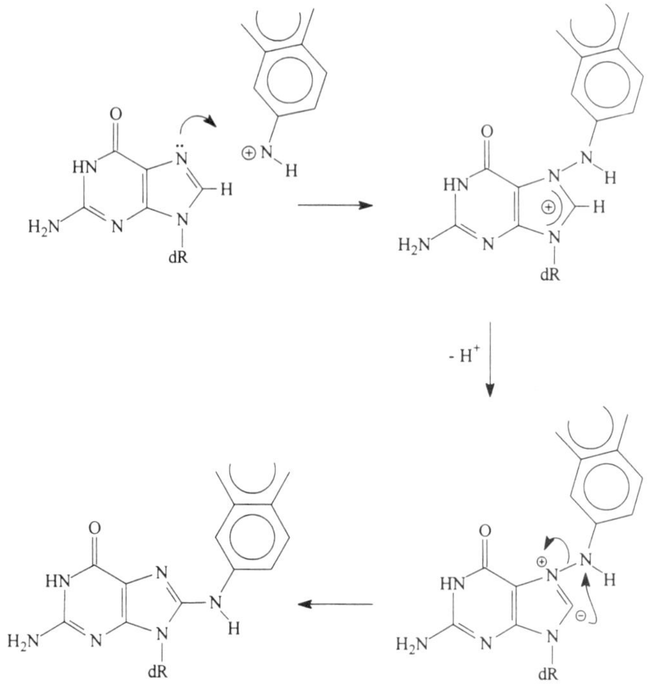

The initial adduct is an imidazolium (purine) cation, resulting from the addition of the nitrenium ion to the N-7 position. The C-8 protons of N^7-alkylated deoxyguanosine adducts are acidic. Loss of the proton at C-8 gives a neutral species with ylide character, which rearranges to form the more stable C-8 adduct, in which the C-8 carbon environment resembles that of the carbon in guanidine. This reaction is an example of the "Stevens rearrangement" of ylides (46).

SEQUENCE CONTEXT

Besides comparing distinct sites *within* a particular base, one can also ask whether particular *base sequences* are susceptible to damage. The observation of mutational "hot spots" (see Chapter 17) is consistent with the idea of nonrandom damage distribution. Striking hot-spot effects are observed in bacteriophage, bacterial, and eukaryotic mutation assays, as well as in the mutational activation of cellular proto-oncogenes (see subsequent chapters). However, such "hot spots" could arise for many reasons other than non-random damage distribution. Differences in the phenotypes of mutations at different sites can lead to large differences in selection efficiency and, hence, recovery of mutants following selection. The most obvious example of this effect is the silent mutation: a DNA sequence alteration that has no effect on the resulting protein sequence, due to the degeneracy of the genetic code. In the case of the *lacI* system, a compilation of the results of numerous investigations of mutational specificity shows that very many different mutations in this gene can be selected phenotypically. Differences in enzymatic repair, or sequence-specific mutational mechanisms such as Streisinger slippage in repeats (see Chapter 17), will also influence the distribution of observed mutations.

Is the distribution of damages induced by DNA-reactive chemicals sequence-dependent? To address this question, one needs to examine initial damage distribution directly, rather than drawing inferences from mutational spectra. The methods for analysis of DNA adduct formation, discussed above, require hydrolysis of the DNA, and thus sequence information is lost. Nevertheless, some experimental systems have been developed for examining damage distribution.

The N-7 position of guanine is, as we have seen, a major site of modification by alkylating agents. N^7-Methylguanine residues undergo facile depurination, and the resulting abasic site can be converted to a single-strand break by piperidine treatment; this reaction is one of the steps used in the Maxam–Gilbert (chemical cleavage) DNA sequencing method. Thus, extent of N^7-methylation at specific sites in a dsDNA fragment following treatment with a methylating agent can be read from a Maxam–Gilbert sequencing gel (47). Some studies based on this methodology have observed substantial effects of the 5' and 3' bases on the N^7-alkylation of guanine residues (48).

N^7-Alkylguanine sites are efficiently repaired, and it would be of greater interest to study the sequence specificity of formation of adducts which play a more important role in mutagenesis, such as O^6-alkylguanine. Unfortunately, no method analogous to the Maxam–Gilbert approach has been devised for detecting these sites in natural DNA sequences. Briscoe and Cotter (49) treated defined synthetic dsDNAs, such as poly(dG-dC)·poly(dG-dC) and poly(dA-dC)·poly(dG-dT), with the alkylating agent N-[^{3}H]-methyl-N-nitrosourea, depurinated the alkylated bases with weak acid, and measured the relative yields of adducts, including N^7-methylguanine and O^6-methylguanine. This approach allows different sequence contexts of guanine residues to be examined. The relative yields of N^7-methylguanine and O^6-methylguanine adducts varied with the sequence context.

ADDUCT EFFECTS ON DNA CONFORMATION

The presence of adducts, especially bulky aromatic carcinogens, can substantially distort the local DNA structure. Many adduct sites, such as guanine O-6 and N-2, are involved in Watson–Crick hydrogen bonding, which would certainly be disrupted. Even if the site of binding (such as guanine C-8) is not involved directly in Watson–Crick base pairing, adduct formation may change the local structure of the double helix (50). Spectroscopic and computer-modeling studies of the interactions of polycyclic aromatic hydrocarbon adducts with DNA indicate that the double-helix structure is substantially altered in the environment of the adduct.

A detailed analysis of the effects of adduct formation on DNA secondary structure would obviously have important implications for understanding how such damaged sites are recognized and repaired. NMR techniques are now being applied to analysis of solution structures of adduct-modified DNA (51, 52; see p. 344). X-ray diffraction analyses of bulky adduct-containing oligonucleotides would also be very informative, but have not yet been achieved. We will return to this topic in the last section of Chapter 19.

NOTES

1. Hemminki, K., and Bartsch, H., Eds., *DNA Adducts of Carcinogenic and Mutagenic Agents: Chemistry, Identification, and Biological Significance*, International Agency for Cancer Research, Lyons, France, 1993; Dipple, A., DNA adducts of chemical carcinogens, *Carcinogenesis* 16:437–441, 1995.

2. von Sonntag, C., *The Chemical Basis of Radiation Biology*, Taylor & Francis, London, 1987.

3. Singer, B., Alkylation, mutagenesis and repair, *Mutat. Res.* 233:289–290, 1990.

4. Schulte, P. A., and Perera, F., Eds., *Molecular Epidemiology, Principles and Practice*, Academic Press, New York, 1993.

5. Everson, R. B., Randerath, E., Santella, R. M., Cefalo, R. C., Avitts, T. A., and Randerath, K., Detection of smoking-related covalent DNA adducts in human placenta, *Science* 231:54–57, 1986.

6. Bosold, F., and Boche, G., The ultimate carcinogen, O-acetyl-N-(2-fluorenyl)hydroxylamine ("N-acetoxy-2-aminofluorene"), and its reaction in vitro to form 2-N-(deoxyguanosin-8-yl)amino]fluorene, *Angew. Chem. Int. Ed.* 29:63–64, 1990.

7. Nakamura, H., Uetrecht, J., Cribb, A. E., Miller, M. A., Zahid, N., Hill, Josephy, P. D., Grant, D. M., and Spielberg, S. P., *In vitro* formation, disposition, and toxicity of N-acetoxysulfamethoxazole, a potential mediator of sulfamethoxazole toxicity, *J. Pharmacol. Expt. Therap.* 274:1099–1104, 1995.

8. Roller, P. P., Shimp, D. R., and Keefer, L. K., Synthesis and solvolysis of methyl(acetoxymethyl)nitrosamine. Solution chemistry of the presumed carcinogenic metabolite of dimethylnitrosamine, *Tetrahedron Lett.* 2065–2068, 1975.

9. Mochizuki, M., Suzuki, E., Anjo, T., Wakabayashi, Y., and Okada, M., Mutagenic and DNA-damaging effects of N-alkyl-N-(α-acetoxy-alkyl)nitrosamines, models for metabolically activated N,N-dialkylnitrosamines, *Gann* 70:663–670, 1979.

10. Josephy, P. D., Activation of aromatic amines by prostaglandin H synthase, *Free Radic. Biol. Med.* 6:533–540, 1989.

11. Pullman, A., and Pullman, B., Electrostatic effect of the macromolecular structure on the biochemical reactivity of the nucleic acids. Significance for chemical carcinogenesis, *Int. J. Quantum Chem: Quantum Biol. Symp.* 7:245–259, 1980.

12. Sambrook, J., Fritsch, E. F., and Maniatis, T., *Molecular Cloning*, 2nd ed., Cold Spring Harbor Laboratory Press, Cold Spring Harbor, New York, 1989, pp. 5.56–5.57.

13. Snell, K., and Mullock, B., Eds., *Biochemical Toxicology: A Practical Approach*, IRL Press, Oxford, UK, 1987, pp. 120–121.

14. Martin, C. N., and Garner, R. C., The identification and assessment of covalent binding in vitro and in vivo, in: *Biochemical Toxicology: A Practical Approach*, K. Snell and B. Mullock, IRL Press, Oxford, UK, 1987, pp. 109–128.

15. Dong, Z., and Jeffrey, A. M., Hydrolysis of carcinogen–DNA adducts by three classes of deoxyribonucleosidase to their corresponding bases, *Carcinogenesis* 12:1125–1128, 1991.

16. Beland, F. A., Allaben, W. T., and Evans, F. E., Acyltransferase-mediated binding of N-hydroxyarylamides to nucleic acids, *Cancer Res.* 40:834–840, 1980.

17. Cheng, S. C., Hilton, B. D., Roman, J. M., and Dipple, A., DNA adducts from carcinogenic and noncarcinogenic enantiomers of benzo[a]pyrene dihydrodiol epoxide, *Chem. Res. Toxicol.* 2:334–340, 1989.

18. Martin, C. N., Beland, F. A., Roth, R. W., and Kadlubar, F. F., Covalent binding of benzidine and N-acetylbenzidine to DNA at the C-8 atom of deoxyguanosine in vivo and in vitro, *Cancer Res.* 42:2678–2686, 1982.

19. Harris, T. M., Stone, M. P., and Harris, C. M., Applications of NMR spectroscopy to studies

of reactive intermediates and their interactions with nucleic acids, *Chem. Res. Toxicol.* 1:79–96, 1988.

20. Sayer, J. M., Chadha, A., Agarwal, S. K., Yeh, H. J. C., Yagi, H., and Jerina, D. M., Covalent nucleoside adducts of benzo[*a*]pyrene 7,8-diol-9,10-epoxides: structural reinvestigation and characterization of a novel adenosine adduct on the ribose moiety, *J. Org. Chem.* 56:20–29, 1991.

21. Koga, N., Inskeep, P. B., Harris, T. M., and Guengerich, F. P., *S*-[2-*N*[7]-guanyl)ethyl)glutathione, the major DNA adduct formed from 1,2-dibromoethane, *Biochemistry* 25:2192–2198, 1986.

22. Randerath, K., Randerath, E., Agrawal, H. P., Gupta, R. C., Schurdak, M. E., and Reddy, M. V., Postlabeling methods for carcinogen–DNA adduct analysis, *Environ. Health Perspect.* 62:57–65, 1985. Phillips, D. H., Castegnaro, M., and Bartsch, H., *Postlabelling Methods for the Detection of DNA Damage*, Oxford University Press, New York, 1993.

23. Poirier, M. C., True, B. A., and Laishes, B. A., Determination of 2-acetylaminofluorene adducts by immunoassay, *Environ. Health Perspect.* 49:93–99, 1982.

24. Holme, D. J., and Peck, H., *Analytical Biochemistry*, 2nd ed., Longman, New York, 1993, pp. 249–260.

25. den Engelse, L., van Benthem, J., and Scherer, E., Immunocytochemical analysis of in vivo DNA modification, *Mutat. Res.* 233:265–287, 1990.

26. Poirier, M. C., Antisera specific for carcinogen–DNA adducts and carcinogen-modified DNA: applications for detection of xenobiotics in biological samples, *Mutat. Res.* 288:31–38, 1993.

27. Perera, F. P., Hemminki, K., Gryzbowska, E., Motykiewicz, G., Michalska, J., Santella, R. M., Young, T.-L., Dickey, C., Brandt-Rauf, P., DeVivo, I., Blaner, W., Tsai, W.-Y., and Chorazy, M., Molecular and genetic damage in humans from environmental pollution in Poland, *Nature* 360:256–258, 1992.

28. Singer, B., and Grunberger, D., *Molecular Biology of Mutagens and Carcinogens*, Plenum Press, New York, 1983.

29. Swann, P. F., Why do O^6-alkylguanine and O^4-alkylthymine miscode? The relationship between the structure of DNA containing O^6-alkylguanine and O^4-alkylthymine and the mutagenic properties of these bases, *Mutat. Res.* 233:81–94, 1990.

30. Horsfall, M. J., Gordon, A. J. E., Burns, P. A., Zielenska, M., Van der Vliet, G. M. E., and Glickman, B. W., Mutational specificity of alkylating agents and the influence of DNA repair, *Environ. Mol. Mutagen.* 15:107–122, 1990.

31. Devereux, T. R., Anderson, M. W., and Belinsky, S. A., Role of *ras* protooncogene activation in the formation of spontaneous and nitrosamine-induced lung tumors in the resistant C3H mouse, *Carcinogenesis* 12:299–303, 1991.

32. Coles, B., Effects of modifying structure on electrophilic reactions with biological nucleophiles, *Drug Metab. Rev.* 15:1307–1334, 1985.

33. Moschel, R. C., Hudgins, W. R., and Dipple, A., Selectivity in nucleoside alkylation and arylation in relation to chemical carcinogenesis, *J. Org. Chem.* 44:3324–3328, 1979.

34. Meehan, T., and Bond, D. M., Hydrolysis of benzo[*a*]pyrene diol epoxide and its covalent binding to DNA proceed through similar rate-determining steps, *Proc. Natl. Acad. Sci. U.S.A.* 81:2635–2639, 1984.

35. Steenken, S., Purine bases, nucleosides, and nucleotides: aqueous solution redox chemistry and transformation reactions of their radical cations and e^- and OH adducts, *Chem. Rev.* 89:503–520, 1989.

36. Augusto, O., Cavalieri, E. L., Rogan, E. G., RamaKrishna, N. V. S., and Kolar, C., Formation of 8-methylguanine as a result of DNA alkylation by methyl radicals generated during horseradish peroxidase-catalyzed oxidation of methylhydrazine, *J. Biol. Chem.* 265:22093–22096, 1990.

37. Rogan, E. G., Cavalieri, E. L., Tibbels, S. R., Cremonesi, P., Warner, C. D., Nagel, D. L., Tomer, K. B., Cerny, R. L., and Gross, M. L., Synthesis and identification of benzo[*a*]pyreneguanine nucleoside adducts formed by electrochemical oxidation and by horseradish peroxidase catalyzed reaction of benzo[*a*]pyrene with DNA, *J. Am. Chem. Soc.* 110:4023–4029, 1988.

38. Kasai, H., and Nishimura, S., Hydroxylation of deoxyguanosine at the C-8 position by ascorbic acid and other reducing agents, *Nucleic Acid Res.* 12:2137–2145, 1984.
39. Devasagayam, T. P. A., Steenken, S., Obendorf, M. S. W., Schulz, W. A., and Sies, H., Formation of 8-hydroxy(deoxy)guanosine and generation of strand breaks at guanine residues in DNA by singlet oxygen, *Biochemistry* 30:6283–6289, 1991.
40. Demple, B., and Harrison, L., Repair of oxidative damage to DNA: enzymology and biology, *Annu. Rev. Biochem.* 63:915–948, 1994.
41. Tchou, J., Kasai, H., Shibutani, S., Chung, M.-H., Laval, J., Grollman, A. P., and Nishimura, S., 8-Oxoguanine (8-hydroxyguanine) DNA glycosylase and its substrate specificity, *Proc. Natl. Acad. Sci. U.S.A.* 88:4690–4694, 1991.
42. Floyd, R. A., The role of 8-hydroxyguanine in carcinogenesis, *Carcinogenesis* 11:1447–1450, 1990.
43. Cheng, K. C., Cahill, D. S., Kasai, H., Nishimura, S., and Loeb, L. A., 8-hydroxyguanine, an abundant form of oxidative DNA damage, causes $G \rightarrow T$ and $A \rightarrow C$ substitutions, *J. Biol. Chem.* 267:166–172, 1992.
44. Grollman, A. P., and Moriya, M., Mutagenesis by 8-oxoguanine: an enemy within, *Trends Genet.* 9:246–249, 1993.
45. Humphreys, W. G., Kadlubar, F. F., and Guengerich, F. P., Mechanism of C^8 alkylation of guanine residues by activated arylamines: evidence for initial adduct formation at the N^7 position, *Proc. Natl. Acad. Sci. U.S.A.* 89:8278–8282, 1992.
46. Lowry, T. H., and Richardson, K. S., *Mechanism and Theory in Organic Chemistry*, 3rd ed., Harper & Row, New York, 1987, p. 541.
47. Wurdeman, R. L., and Gold, B., The effect of DNA sequence, ionic strength, and cationic DNA affinity binders on the methylation of DNA by N-methyl-N-nitrosourea, *Chem. Res. Toxicol.* 1:146–147, 1988.
48. Said, B., and Shank, R. C., Nearest neighbour effects on carcinogen binding to guanine runs in DNA, *Nucl. Acids Res.* 19:1311–1316, 1991.
49. Briscoe, W. T.. and Cotter, L.-E., DNA sequence has an effect on the extent and kinds of alkylation of DNA by a potent carcinogen, *Chem.-Biol. Interact.* 56:321–331, 1985.
50. Santella, R. M., and Grunberger, D., Induction of the base displacement or Z conformation in DNA by N-2-acetylaminofluorene modification, *Environ. Health Perspect.* 49:107–115, 1983.
51. de los Santos, C., Cosman, M., Hingerty, B. E., Ibanez, V., Margulis, L. A., Geacintov, N. E., Broyde, S., and Patel, D. J., Influence of benzo[a]pyrene diol epoxide chirality on solution conformations of DNA covalent adducts: the (−)-*trans-anti*-[BP]G·C adduct structure and comparisons with the (+)-*trans-anti*-[BP]G·C enantiomer, *Biochemistry* 31:5245–5252, 1992.
52. Harvey, R. G., and Geacintov, N. E., Intercalation and binding of carcinogenic hydrocarbon metabolites to nucleic acids, *Acc. Chem. Res.* 21:66–73, 1988.

17

CHEMICAL MUTAGENESIS

DNA AS A TARGET OF CHEMICAL DAMAGE

A major goal of biochemical toxicology has been the characterization of covalently bound DNA adducts formed from carcinogens and mutagens (1). DNA is a critical biological target: DNA damage can lead to mutation—that is, a heritable change in the DNA sequence. Mutation is the raw material for natural selection, the driving force for generation of biological diversity and evolutionary change. But mutation can also have devastating biological consequences: genetic disease and cancer.

A *base-substitution* mutation is the replacement of a given base pair (say, G:C) by another (say, T:A). Twelve base substitution mutations are possible on a single strand: Each of the four bases can be replaced by any of the other three. The requirement of self-complementarity of dsDNA leaves only six distinguishable possibilities. These are classified as follows:

1. *Transversions*. Purine replaced by pyrimidine, or vice versa:

$$G:C \rightarrow T:A; \quad G:C \rightarrow C:G; \quad A:T \rightarrow T:A; \quad A:T \rightarrow C:G$$

2. *Transitions*. Purine replaced by purine, or pyrimidine replaced by pyrimidine:

$$G:C \rightarrow A:T; \quad A:T \rightarrow G:C$$

[An A:T $\rightarrow$ C:G transversion (for example) could arise by the misinsertion, at replication, of a G across from an A (or damaged A) or by the misinsertion of a C across from a T (or damaged T). In most cases we cannot determine which of the two strands of the parental dsDNA molecule was damaged, so the two possibilities are indistinguishable. However, in some mutation assays the target for DNA damage is a single-stranded DNA molecule, such as the bacteriophages ϕX174 and M13. In such assays, we *can* distinguish between the two possibilities, and all 12 base substitutions can be observed.]

Other types of mutations can occur. *Insertions* give daughter DNA molecules with extra base pairs; *deletions* have fewer. If the change in the number of bases is not a multiple of three, then the insertion/deletion event causes a *frameshift* of the triplet reading frame for the genetic code. *Complex* mutations combine more than one event, such as an insertion accompanied by a base substitution.

As we discussed in Chapter 16, different classes of reactive chemicals induce different DNA damages. As we shall see in this chapter, chemical mutagens also cause specific patterns of mutagenesis. To understand how the cause—DNA damage—leads to the effect—mutation—we must first consider the mechanisms of DNA repair and then consider the biochemical processes which convert *unrepaired* DNA damage sites into mutations.

DNA REPAIR

Enzymes continually monitor the integrity of the genome and repair many types of damage, usually with very high efficiency and accuracy. The biochemistry of DNA repair is discussed at length in several books and recent review articles (2–4). Recent progress in our understanding of DNA repair has been swift: the journal *Science* chose "DNA Repair" as the "Molecule of the Year" for 1994, in recognition of the excitement in the field. Here we limit the discussion to an outline of various classes of DNA repair mechanisms and give brief examples of each.

The covalent chemical structure of DNA is remarkably, but not perfectly, stable. The phosphodiester backbone of RNA is readily broken, due to the participation of the ribose $2'$-hydroxyl group in hydrolysis. DNA is more resistant than RNA to hydrolysis, but much more susceptible to cleavage of the glycosidic bond. Many spontaneous chemical processes can act to degrade the DNA structure (5). As we saw earlier (Chapter 16), chemical mutagens cause many additional forms of DNA damage.

DNA repair faithful to the information content of the gene is possible because the DNA molecule is self-complementary; the sequence of the damaged strand can be chemically deduced by the enzymatic repair machinery, which "reads" the complementary strand. The stability of information transmission required for the evolution of complex genomes is only possible on the basis of the principle of self-complementarity (redundant storage of genetic information).

The sine qua non of faithful transmission of genetic information is the fidelity of DNA polymerase, the enzyme which assembles the daughter strands of DNA during replication. There are three DNA polymerases in *Escherichia coli*; the principal replicative enzyme is DNA polymerase III (Pol III). Pol I and Pol II are primarily involved in filling gaps during DNA repair.

Pol III plays a critical role in ensuring that the parent strand is copied faithfully, by selecting the correct complementary dNTP to add to the growing DNA chain. Occasional selection of an incorrect dNTP is inevitable. However, in addition to polymerization activity, Pol III also possesses a $3' \rightarrow 5'$ exonuclease activity, which can remove the last-inserted nucleotide, releasing it as a dNMP. This "proofreading" activity double-checks the action of the polymerase and removes mismatched nucleotides. The combination of faithful polymerization and proofreading reduces the in vitro error rate of Pol III to about 1 misincorporation event per 10^6 nucleotides. (Mutations which inactivate the proofreading activity of Pol III greatly increase spontaneous mutation rates.)

Repair of Chemical Lesions in DNA

Several mechanisms for DNA repair are outlined below. These can be divided into several categories, depending on the manner in which the damaged site is removed. However, like most classification systems, this one is somewhat arbitrary.

Direct Reversal Mechanism.　These mechanisms effect chemical restoration of the damaged site to its intact state. One of the most-studied examples of direct reversal is the activity of the enzyme O^6-methylguanine DNA methyltransferase (6). This "suicide enzyme" (or repair protein) repairs guanine residues bearing alkyl substituents on the O-6 position (see middle panel of scheme on page 262), by transferring the alkyl group *to a cysteine residue in the enzyme active site*. In the process, the guanine residue is returned to its intact state, and the enzyme is irreversibly inactivated: Instead of acting as a catalyst, this unusual "enzyme" is actually a "once-only" reagent. The presence of such an enzyme (in organisms ranging from bacteria to humans) indicates that alkylation has presented a challenge to cells throughout evolutionary history; the cost to the cell of "sacrificing" one molecule of protein per alkylguanosine residue repaired testifies to the biological importance of removal of this lesion (7).

Base Excision Repair.   Most DNA repair systems act by detecting and removing the damage site; excision is followed by repair synthesis, extending the "loose end" by copying the sequence information of the complementary strand. *Base excision repair* systems (8) remove damaged bases by hydrolyzing the glycosidic bond between the base and deoxyribose.

Uracil residues in DNA arise continuously, by the spontaneous (9) or chemically induced deamination of cytosine residues or by the incorporation of dUTP from the nucleotide pool at replication. DNA uracil bases are detected and excised by *uracil DNA N-glycosylase*, an enzyme discovered by Thomas Lindahl in 1974. This discovery answers the riddle posed by the presence of thymine (5-methyluracil), rather than uracil (the corresponding RNA base), in DNA. The G-U base pair resulting from cytosine deamination is a potentially mutagenic mismatch. Were DNA to contain uracil in place of thymine, it would be difficult to discriminate between uracil normally present in an A-U base pair and uracil present in a G-U mismatch, as a result of cytosine deamination. The choice of thymine, instead of uracil, as the base complementary to adenosine in DNA provides an easy "handle," allowing an enzyme to make this discrimination and remove the "unnatural" U residues (10). In the absence of this repair process, spontaneous deamination might lead to an unstoppable mutational drift from G-C toward A-U base pairs and gradually erase the genetic code.

Nevertheless, thymine *can* arise directly in DNA. The modified pyrimidine base 5-methylcytosine is introduced into *E. coli* DNA at the specific sequence $5'$-$CC_T^A GG$-$3'$. This sequence is recognized by the *dcm* (DNA cytosine methylation) gene product, which catalyzes the SAM-dependent 5-methylation of the second cytosine (11). This modification protects chromosomal DNA against degradation by the restriction endonuclease *Eco*RII, which recognizes the same DNA sequence. *Deamination of 5-methylcytosine yields thymine, rather than uracil:*

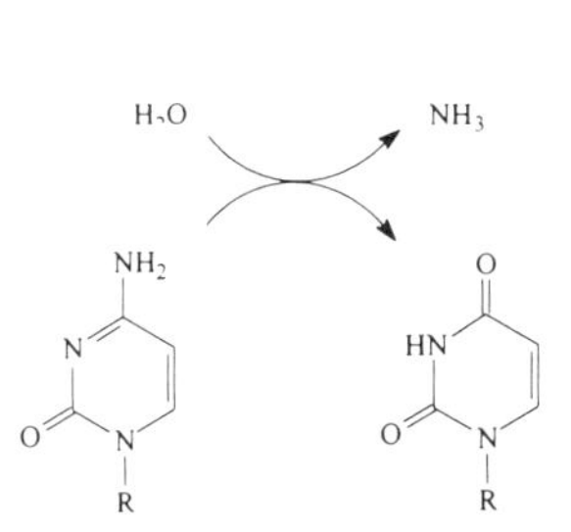

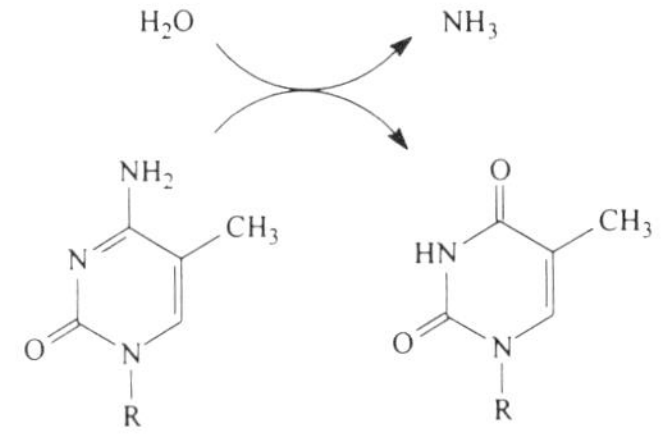

The resulting T residue cannot, of course, be removed by uracil DNA N-glycosylase, and the G-T mismatch represents a possible premutagenic lesion. Indeed, the second C residues in 5'-CCAGG-3' sequences are major hot spots for base-substitution mutations in the *lacI* gene of *E. coli*, and the mutations which occur here are G:C → A:T transitions, as one would predict (12). (The possible role of 5-methylcytosine deamination in mutagenesis in eukaryotes is considered later in this chapter.)

Abasic sites (AP = apurinic/apyrimidinic sites) result from the enzymatic removal of modified DNA bases, including uracil, hypoxanthine (the product of adenine deamination), and oxidized bases, such as 8-hydroxydeoxyguanosine and thymine glycol (13). The repair of AP sites can probably occur by multiple pathways. AP sites can be attacked by endonucleases, which hydrolyze an adjacent phosphodiester bond to create a single-strand break:

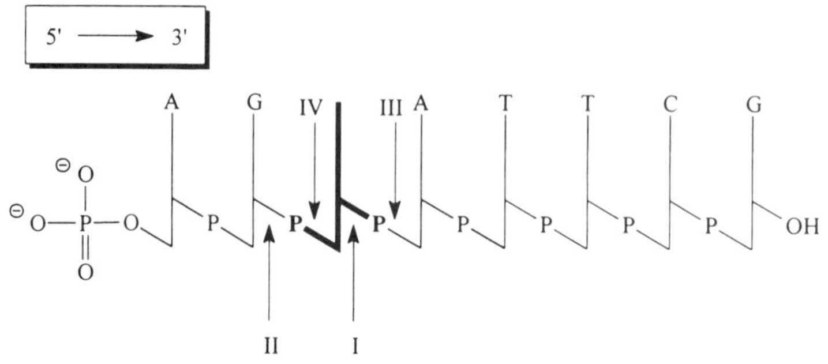

Class I: glycosylase-AP endonucleases, *e.g.*, *M. luteus* endonuclease

Class II: common, *e.g.*, *E. coli* exo III

Class III: *Drosophila* AP endo. I

Class IV: unknown

In principle, any of four distinct modes of cleavage could occur: The phosphodiester bond either 5' or 3' to the AP site could be broken, and either the 5' or 3' side of the bond could be hydrolyzed. These modes are classified as Types I, II, III, and IV, as indicated. Class II AP endonucleases are the most common. Cleavage 5' to the AP site, catalyzed by a Type II enzyme [e.g., *E. coli* endonuclease IV and the human *APE* gene product (14)], leaves (a) the 5' strand bearing a normal 3'-hydroxyl end and (b) the 3' strand bearing a 5' phosphate and an abasic sugar:

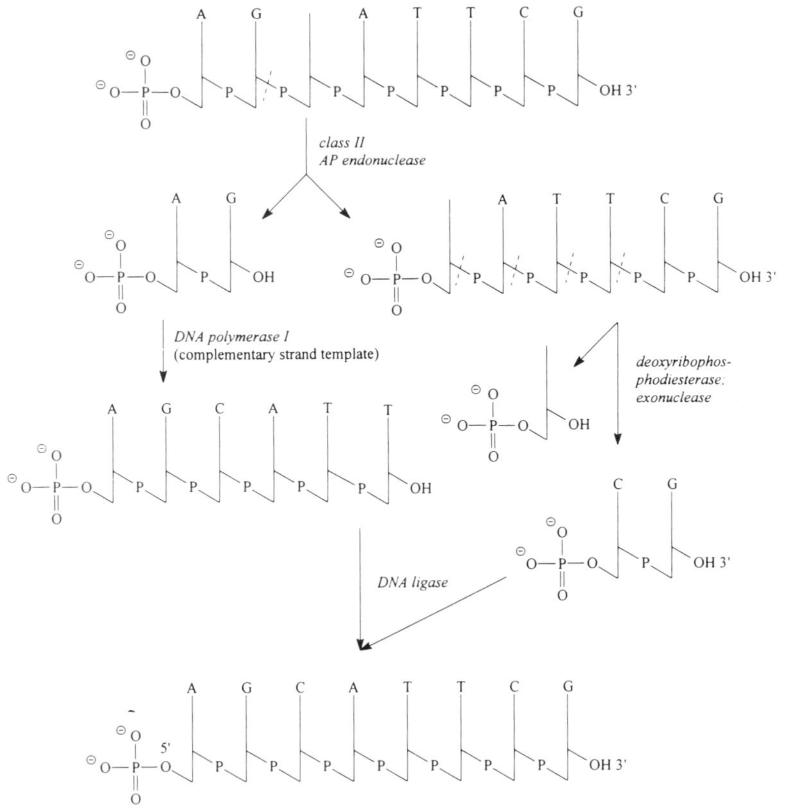

The 3' hydroxyl is a substrate for extension by DNA polymerase; the abasic site on the 3' strand is recognized and removed by deoxyribophosphodiesterase; the strand can then be trimmed by an exonuclease, and the two strands rejoined by DNA ligase. An alternative route for repair of abasic sites is shown below:

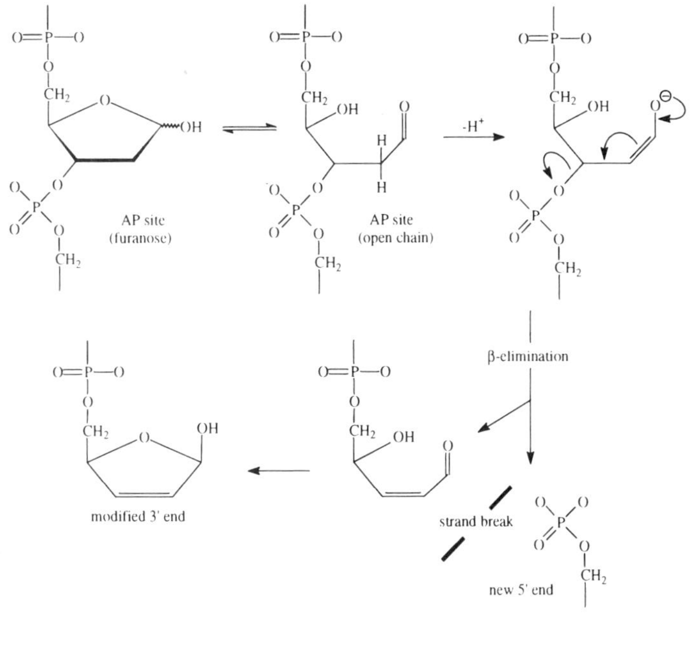

This route begins with incision of the phosphodiester bond 3' to the AP site by an AP lyase; this reaction leaves a normal 5' phosphate on the 3' strand and a damaged sugar (4-hydroxy-2-pentenal) residue blocking the 3' terminus of the 5' strand.* The blocked 3' terminus is processed by enzymatic 3' trimming. Finally, DNA polymerase and ligase complete the repair.

Nucleotide Excision Repair.   Nucleotide excision repair systems remove one or more nucleotide units at the site of damage. The UvrABC complex excision repair system of *E. coli* removes certain damages formed by UV irradiation and many bulky DNA adducts (15). Among the products of UV damage to DNA are thymine–cytosine "6–4" photoproducts (16), believed to be the most important premutagenic lesion induced by UV (17), and *thymine dimers*, in which two adjacent thymines dimerize to form a bridging cyclobutane ring:

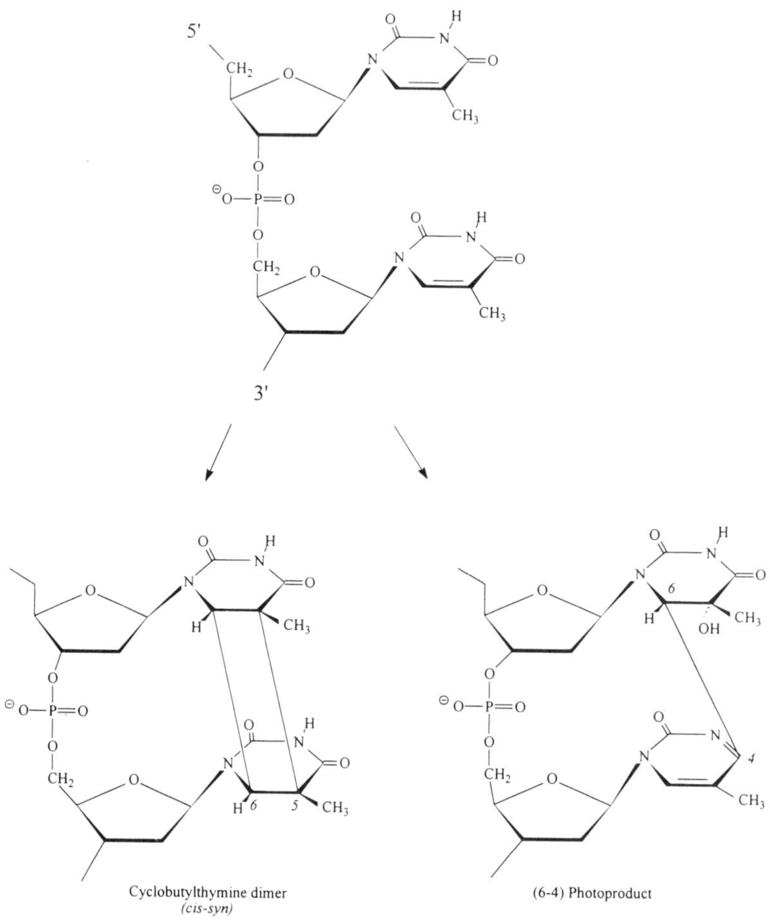

Cyclobutylthymine dimer
(*cis-syn*)

(6-4) Photoproduct

Both forms of damage are repaired by the UvrABC system. In *E. coli* the excision repair process involves the exonuclease activity of the products of the *uvrABC* loci in conjunction with DNA helicase II (*uvrD* gene), DNA polymerase I, and DNA ligase. The UvrA

*Figure based on Povirk, L. F., and Steighner, R. J., Oxidized apurinic/apyrimidinic sites formed in DNA by oxidative mutagens, *Mutat. Res.* 214:13–22, 1989, and Suzuki, T., Ohsumi, S., and Makino, K., Mechanistic studies in depurination and apurinic site chain breakage in oligodeoxyribonucleotides, *Nucl. Acids Res.* 22:4997–5003, 1994.

dimer binds to UvrB protein to form a complex, which recognizes sites of DNA damage and binds to DNA at these sites. Upon interaction of the UvrC protein with the UvrAB–DNA complex, the eighth phosphodiester bond 5′ to the DNA adduct and the fifth phosphodiester bond 3′ to the adduct are hydrolyzed. DNA helicase II and DNA polymerase I displace the UvrABC complex, along with the excised damage-containing oligonucleotide (12 or 13 nucleotides long), and the polymerase fills in the gap. DNA ligase then seals the 3′ end of the newly synthesized oligonucleotide. The enzymology of nucleotide excision repair in eukaryotic cells is discussed in detail elslwhere (2, 4, 8) and is beyond the scope of the present text.

Human Diseases Associated with Defective DNA Excision Repair.

Excision repair is also a critical DNA repair process in human cells. Defects in excision repair systems are responsible for several rare human genetic diseases, including xeroderma pigmentosum (XP), ataxia telangiectasia (AT), Fanconi's anemia, and Bloom's syndrome. These conditions provide one of the clearest pieces of evidence for the link between DNA damage and carcinogenesis (18). Although these recessive diseases are rare in the homozygous state, carriers (heterozygotes) are much more common. AT carriers may show significantly greater radiation sensitivity than noncarriers and comprise a subpopulation at substantially greater risk of radiation carcinogenesis (19). The AT gene has just been cloned (20), and we can expect swift progress in elucidating the molecular basis of the disease.

The clinical symptoms of XP include extreme sensitivity to ultraviolet radiation, leading to severe sunburn and a very high incidence of skin cancer. This sensitivity is also observed in vitro: Cultured cells from XP patients are sensitive to UV (and some chemical mutagens) relative to cells from control individuals. The XP defect can be demonstrated in individual cells by measuring clonogenic survival (colony-forming ability) or unscheduled DNA synthesis (UDS). In the UDS technique, cells are exposed to UV and then dosed with [³H]thymidine. Normal cells will incorporate this labeled base into chromosomal DNA during repair, and the incorporation can be measured by scintillation counting or autoradiography. Such "unscheduled" repair synthesis can readily be distinguished from the much greater incorporation of thymidine during "scheduled" synthesis at mitosis.

The sensitivity of XP cells in vitro has provided a powerful tool for the analysis of the genetics and biochemistry of this disease. Cells from different individuals can be fused into heterokaryon hybrids, by treatment with polyethylene glycol (21). When such hybrids are examined for UDS, it is observed that hybrids from certain pairs of individuals exhibit normal repair, while other pairs are defective. This method allows XP individuals to be classified into distinct *complementation groups*, representing lesions in different genes (different enzymatic steps in repair). At least eight XP complementation groups exist. In some cases the clinical manifestations of the disease correlate with the complementation group classification. Multiple complementation groups of AT have also been identified (22).

Repair-defective mammalian cells can also be isolated experimentally, in vitro. James Cleaver and colleagues isolated several UV-sensitive mutant derivatives of the commonly used CHO (Chinese hamster ovary) mammalian cell line. It is generally much more difficult to isolate *sensitive*, as opposed to resistant, mutants, since "sensitives" cannot be selected for growth. Instead, one must rely on the replica-plating technique and carry out mass screening. Cleaver's group developed semiautomated methods for screening very large numbers of CHO colonies to identify UV-sensitive mutants (23). Much effort has been directed to characterizing the complementation groups, enzymatic defects, and mutant genes in these clones. Some of these ERCC (excision repair cross-complementing) genes complement XP defects in vitro (for review, see refs. 4 and 8).

Transfection of repair-deficient rodent cells with genomic DNA from a normal individual, followed by selection of UV-resistant transfectants, allows the cloning of the normal gene which complements the defect. This approach has led to breakthroughs in the molecular analysis of eukaryotic DNA repair (24). Unexpectedly, it proved more difficult to extend this approach to complementation of human cells, which proved to be difficult to transfect stably. This obstacle has been overcome by the development of Epstein-Barr virus-derived expression shuttle vectors for cloning cDNAs, and genes complementing several FA and XP cell lines have been cloned (25). At least 12 human gene products play a role in nucleotide excision repair (26).

DNA STRAND BREAKS

DNA strand breaks can arise from the action of repair endonucleases, as we have seen above, or by the action of ionizing radiation on DNA. The DNA backbone consists of deoxyribose units linked by phosphodiester bonds; chemical agents which attack either the sugar or the phosphate can lead to strand breakage.

We can make an operational distinction between single strand breaks (SSBs) and double strand breaks (DSBs): SSBs are breaks measured in single-stranded (denatured) DNA, and DSBs are breaks measured in native DNA. What this means in detail is less clear: How close do two breaks, on opposing strands, need to be, so that we have a DSB rather than two SSBs? This may depend on the way in which we measure the break. Intuitively, one would expect a DSB to be much more difficult to repair. A DSB causes a dsDNA molecule to fragment into two separate pieces, whereas an SSB does not.

> Clown: . . . I am resolv'd on two points.
>
> Maria: That if one break, the other will hold; or if both break, your gaskins fall.
>
> *Twelfth Night,* I:5

Even in the case of a DSB, other molecules, such as histone proteins, might hold the broken ends in proximity and allow repair. Nevertheless, DSBs are likely precursors of chromosome breakage or rearrangement events, clastogenic damages associated with some forms of cancer (see Chapter 18). Chromosome breaks can probably lead to cell death at, or following, mitosis. Many researchers have tried to measure SSB and DSB induction, with a range of techniques; unfortunately, they sometimes give conflicting results.

In the case of small "naked" DNA targets, such as defined oligonucleotides or restriction fragments in vitro, or plasmid DNA in bacterial cells, DSBs can be measured directly by electrophoresis. SSBs can also be studied by electrophoresis of plasmid DNA, since the covalently closed circular (ccc) and open circular (nicked) molecules have different mobilities.

The extremely long molecules of chromosomal DNA are so fragile that any standard protocol for DNA purification (as would be used to prepare genomic libraries, for example) will introduce large numbers of strand breaks. Thus, to examine strand breaks in chromosomal DNA, special techniques are needed. Analysis can be carried out either at alkaline pH (pH 12 or greater) or at "neutral" pH (below 10). DNA is the only cellular macromolecule which can resist hydrolysis by strong base. Under alkaline conditions, DNA is denatured into single strands, so SSBs* can be measured. DSBs can, of course, only be measured with the double helix intact.

---

*More accurately, one measures the combination of "true" SSBs and *alkali-labile sites*—that is, damages which are converted into SSBs by alkali treatment. These include abasic sites and many forms of base damage.

For the analysis of eukaryotic chromosomal DNA, the pulsed-field technique extends the applicability of gel electrophoresis methods into the megabase range and can be used for the measurement of strand breakage induced by ionizing radiation (27). Another promising method for electrophoretic analysis of DNA damage is the so-called "comet" assay (28). Individual cells are embedded in agarose and lysed by immersion in a sodium dodecyl sulfate (SDS) solution (alkaline or neutral conditions for SSB or DSB analysis, respectively) to release DNA. Electrophoresis is carried out, and the gel is then soaked in propidium iodide solution, a fluorescent stain for DNA (and RNA). The cells are then examined with a fluorescence microscope system. The electrophoresed DNA gives the appearance of a "comet" streaming away from the cell; increasing DNA damage results in greater electrophoretic mobility and, hence, a longer "comet." This method allows the analysis of individual cells, rather than averaging the response of a large population.

The hydrodynamic mobility of DNA can be measured by ultracentrifugation through sucrose density gradients (29). This allows estimation of relative molecular weight via the Svedberg equation. (Note that the density gradient serves only to minimize convectional mixing of the sample during the centrifuge run.) However, this analysis relies on the assumption that the frictional coefficient, f, remains unchanged following damage induction. This may not be the case if, for example, DNA–protein cross-linking occurs.

Transmission electron microscopy images can be analyzed to determine the contour length of individual DNA molecules, from which molecular weight can be deduced.

In the filter elution method (30), the DNA is deposited on a membrane filter with pore size of about 1 μm. The DNA is then slowly "squeezed" through the filter by pumping an eluting solution. The physical basis of the elution process is complicated and remains poorly understood. Intact cells can be applied to the gradients or filters. Lysis is accomplished by application of detergents, such as SDS, and treatment with nonspecific proteases, such as proteinase K. If an alkaline solution is used, noncovalent protein–DNA or DNA–RNA interactions, which might complicate the analysis, should be completely broken. However, DNA-damaging treatments may induce forms of covalent damage, other than strand breaks, which could also greatly alter the molecular weight and conformation of the DNA molecules. These include covalent crosslinks between separate DNA strands and protein–DNA crosslinks and might not be broken by detergent, enzyme, or alkali treatment.

Many classes of chemical carcinogens, including aromatic amines, polycyclic aromatic hydrocarbons, and alkylating agents, cause SSBs in treated hepatocytes, and there appears to be some correlation between carcinogenic potency and SSB induction. Some of these agents are likely to cause SSBs indirectly, via base damage followed by repair endonuclease action. Other agents [such as radiation (31), oxidants, and the chemotherapeutic drug bleomycin; see Chapter 11) cause strand breaks directly, by attacking the DNA backbone itself.

REPLICATION OF DAMAGED DNA

DNA damage which escapes repair, and persists until the next round of replication, presents a challenge to the replication fidelity of DNA polymerase. Some lesions allow replication to proceed, but with reduced fidelity (*error promoting*). Other lesions strongly inhibit DNA replication (*replication blocking*). Studies of in vitro replication of templates containing abasic sites or pyrimidine dimers reveal that synthesis of the nascent strand stops either at or near the lesion on the template strand. Such a replication block is potentially catastrophic, since DNA replication is required for normal cell division.

How can cells resume DNA synthesis on templates with replication blocks? One way is to reinitiate DNA synthesis farther along the template. This leaves a gap in the daughter strand, which may be filled after replication (postreplication repair). Alternatively, after the initial pause, synthesis may be resumed past the lesion (translesion synthesis). The damaged strand is used as a template, even though the lesion may be noninstructive. In this second method of recovery, a replication blocking lesion is converted to an error promoting lesion. Put simply, it is preferable for the cell to mutate rather than to die. The accumulation of replication blocking lesions in *E. coli* results in the induction of the "SOS" repair system (see Fig. 17.1), which promotes translesion synthesis (32–34).

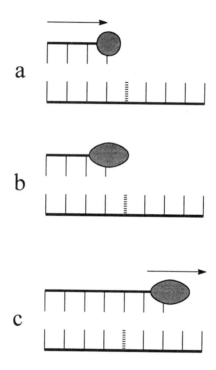

Figure 17.1.   The SOS system in *E. coli*. (*a*) The lower dark line represents the parental DNA strand, with the vertical bars representing bases. Many forms of DNA damage, such as UV-induced base damage (represented by the dashed line), block DNA replication by polymerase (circle on upper, daughter strand) and induce the SOS response. Single-stranded DNA regions are continuously exposed during replication; replication-blocking DNA damage sites lead to the accumulation of such ssDNA regions. The RecA protein binds to these ssDNA regions, and this complex, in turn, activates the LexA protein. LexA is the repressor of the genes in the SOS regulon, including *recA*, *lexA* itself, the *uvrA* and *uvrB* genes, and many others. LexA protein binds to a consensus sequence present in the operators of these genes. *Activation of LexA converts the protein into a protease which degrades other LexA molecules.* Therefore, the activation of LexA (as a protease) *inactivates* LexA (as a repressor of transcription), and transcription of the genes of the SOS response is greatly increased. (*b*) Activation of the SOS response alters the DNA polymerase activity, in a manner which is not understood in detail. This alteration depends on the products of the *umuC* and *umuD* (*UV* mutagenesis) genes, which form part of the SOS regulon. (*c*) The altered polymerase (represented by the oblong) can replicate past the damaged site, although with reduced fidelity. DNA replication, essential for cell replication, can continue, but at the cost of the introduction of mutations.

MISMATCH REPAIR

If DNA polymerase inserts an incorrect base during replication, or if a 5-methylcytosine residue deaminates to form thymine, then a mismatch arises: Normal bases are present, but they are joined in a non-Watson–Crick pair. If, for example, a G-A mismatch persists to the next round of replication, then normal Watson–Crick base pairing will give rise to a G-C base pair on one daughter double strand and generate a T-A base pair on the other: one wild-type molecule and one mutant. The presence of mismatched base pairs in DNA can, in principle, be detected. For example, the mismatch may cause a local distortion of the backbone of the double helix. However, high-resolution X-ray diffraction analysis of a DNA oligonucleotide containing a G-T mismatch revealed little distortion of the helix backbone; instead, a "wobble" non-Watson–Crick H-bonding (35) of the mismatched bases occurred (36). Computer molecular-dynamics simulations indicate that this wobble-pairing is accompanied by changes in the positions of the mismatched bases with respect to the major and minor grooves, along with changes in the orientations of the glycosidic bonds (37). Therefore, mismatches could be recognized by the altered positions of H-bond acceptor and donor groups on the bases.

Suppose that, for example, the presence of a T-C mismatch has been detected. Which of the two strands should be repaired: T-C → G-C or T-C → T-A? *If the mismatch has arisen during replication, then the newly synthesized strand had best be repaired to complement the parent strand.* How can the strands be distinguished? *E. coli* chromosomal DNA contains N^6-methyl adenines in specific sequences. These residues are formed by the action of the *dam* (DNA adenine methylation) gene product. Immediately following replication, *the newly synthesized daughter strand can be recognized by its low level of adenine methylation*, since insufficient time has elapsed for full *dam*-dependent modification to occur. In *E. coli*, at least three proteins are involved in recognition of mismatches: MutS, MutL, and MutH. The MutH endonuclease specifically nicks the newly synthesized strand (38). A portion of the strand is degraded and resynthesized by DNA polymerase III:*

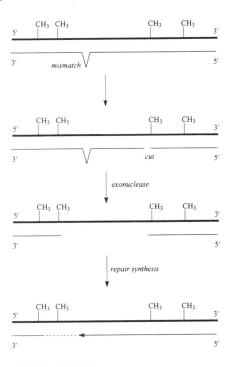

*Figure adapted from *Science* 266:728–730, 1994.

Proteins homologous to the *E. coli* mismatch repair enzymes have been found in yeast and in humans. A gene responsible for the human cancer-prone condition known as *hereditary nonpolyposis colon cancer* (HNPCC) was recently found to be homologous to *E. coli mutS* (39). This finding provides further strong evidence for the role of mutagenesis in cancer development.

5-METHYLCYTOSINE-DEPENDENT MUTAGENESIS IN MAMMALIAN CELLS

Earlier in the chapter we discussed the importance of deamination of 5-methylcytosine as a mutagenic process in *E. coli*. Mammalian cells, of course, do not possess the restriction-modification systems found in bacteria. Nevertheless, a few percent of the C residues in human chromosomes are 5-methylated. The methylation is catalyzed by an enzyme which recognizes CpG sequences (40). Some evidence indicates that this process acts as a regulatory mechanism in cell differentiation, inhibiting expression of hypermethylated genes, but the issue is still controversial (41, 42).

CpG sequences, which are potential sites for methylation, are highly underrepresented in the mammalian genome. The frequencies of the 16 possible dinucleotide sequences can be determined by the method of nearest-neighbor analysis, introduced by Arthur Kornberg in the early 1960s.

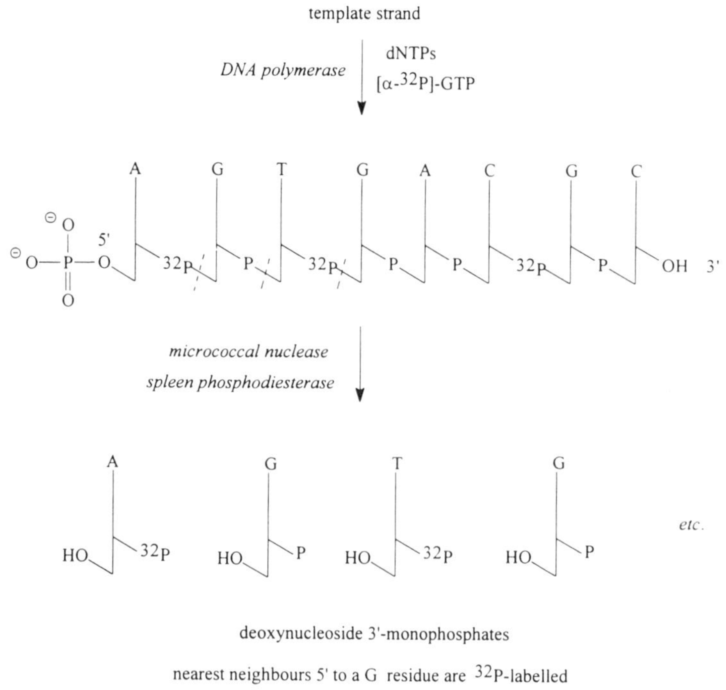

template strand

DNA polymerase | dNTPs
[α-^{32}P]-GTP

microccal nuclease
spleen phosphodiesterase

etc.

deoxynucleoside 3'-monophosphates

nearest neighbours 5' to a G residue are ^{32}P-labelled

First, DNA is synthesized in vitro from the template of interest; in each of four reactions, a different [α-^{32}P]-radiolabeled dNTP is used. After synthesis of the daughter strand, the DNA is digested to deoxynucleoside 3'-monophosphates, using the combined action of the enzymes micrococcal nuclease and spleen phosphodiesterase. (The same enzymatic digestion method is exploited in the Randerath postlabeling method for detection of DNA adducts; see page 270.) The net result is to transfer the labeled phosphate from the originally labeled base to its 5'-upstream nearest-neighbor. By quantitating each of the four labeled nucleotides in each of the four mixes, the frequency of all 16 dinucleotide sequences (5'-XpY-3') can be determined. Since DNA is antiparallel, the frequency 5' CpA 3' equals 5' TpG 3'; 5' GpA 3' equals 5' TpC 3'; and so on. (In fact, Kornberg used this analysis to verify Watson and Crick's prediction that the double helix was antiparallel.) In a random DNA sequence, each dinucleotide XpY would occur at the same frequency (6.25%). *In fact, the CpG sequence is found in vertebrate DNA at only about one-fifth of this frequency (43); this bias results from the highly nonrandom choice of codons for degenerately coded amino acid residues (44).* While there may be many reasons for this bias, one possibility is that CpG sites are relatively unstable due to a tendency to undergo 5-methylcytosine deamination-induced mutations to TpG.

Are 5-methylcytosine residues hotspots for mutagenesis in mammalian cells? To address this question, one must first possess techniques for analysis of the presence of 5-methylcytosines in specific genomic sequences of the cells being studied. Obviously, conventional cloning or PCR, followed by sequencing, does not distinguish between cytosine and 5-methylcytosine. However, some of the ^{me}CpG residues occur within the palindromic sequence CCGG, and these residues can conveniently be detected by restriction analysis. The restriction enzymes *Msp*I and *Hpa*II are *isoschizomers*; that is, they both recognize the same sequence, CCGG. However, the former enzyme cuts at C-methylated sites, while the latter does not (45). Thus, differences in Southern blots of chromosomal DNA cut with either of these restriction enzymes will reveal sites of methylation in CCGG sequences.

A more general approach is direct Maxam–Gilbert (base-specific chemical cleavage) sequencing of genomic DNA; 5-methylcytosine residues are resistant to cleavage by the hydrazine reagent used to cleave at cytosines, and thus they appear as gaps in the sequencing ladder. This method is not limited to CpG residues in specific sequences. However, direct genomic sequencing without prior amplification of the gene (cloning or PCR) is insensitive, and it requires the use of large amounts of DNA and extremely "hot" radiolabelled primers. A recent method, known as *ligation-mediated polymerase chain reaction (PCR)*, greatly facilitates genomic sequencing and methylation analysis. This method combines Maxam–Gilbert genomic sequencing with PCR amplification of the sequencing fragments (46), and it allows sequencing/methylation analysis of microgram quantities of mammalian cell DNA.

Using these techniques, Rideout et al. (47) recently analyzed the methylation patterns of two human genes for which mutations at CpG sites had been characterized: the low-density lipoprotein (LDL) receptor gene and p53. LDL receptor codons 407–408 are AAC GTG; a G → A transition mutation in the first base of codon 408 (val → met) is responsible for one form of *familial hypercholesterolemia*. This mutation is equivalent to a C → T transition in the complementary strand, and it occurs at a potential methylation site. Indeed, the intercodon CpG (wild-type) sequence proved to be methylated in each of several tissues studied, from several individuals. p53 is a tumor suppressor gene (Chapter 18) inactivated in many human tumours. CpG sites known to be targets of mutations which inactivate the p53 gene product in human tumors were also found to be methylated in vivo. The investigators concluded that "a high percentage of mutations in human tumor suppressor genes may be induced by deamination of methylated cytosines to form thymines."

We have already discussed the enzyme uracil DNA *N*-glycosylase, which removes uracil residues from DNA. Josef Jiricny (Friedrich Miescher-Institut, Basel, Switzerland) has discovered an enzyme activity in human (HeLa) cell nuclei, which specifically recognizes G-T mispairs, the mismatch expected to result from deamination of 5-methylcytosine residues (48). A synthetic dsDNA 90-mer substrate was prepared, containing a single G-T mismatch. The mismatch was located at a site cleaved by *Sal*I, in the absence of the mismatch (G-C), so repair could be monitored by restriction digestion and gel elec-trophoresis. Neither the T-containing strand nor a dsDNA containing an A-C mismatch were repaired. This new enzyme activity appears to represent a specific system for the re-pair of mismatches resulting from 5-methylcytosine deamination, and its existence fur-ther supports the hypothesis that such mismatches represent a significant premutagenic lesion in human cells.

MUTATION ASSAYS

Spontaneous mutations are rare events. Even when a cell is treated with high doses of mutagens, selectable mutations in specific target genes are rare. *E. coli* has a genome of about 5×10^6 base pairs, encoding genes for about 4000 proteins (49). If mutations are distributed randomly, then only 1 in 4000 or so will affect the gene of interest, and not all of these will confer a selectable mutant phenotype. The dose of mutagen that can be applied is also limited: If the cell's burden of mutations is too high, the cell will die. Not surprisingly, any mutagen is toxic or growth inhibitory at high concentrations. (Solubil-ity also limits doses achievable in many experiments.) The study of molecular mutagen-esis requires the development of sensitive assays for mutations.

Usually, in genetic analysis of mutagenesis we rely on phenotypic selection to detect the progeny of the mutant organism (e.g., a bacterial strain, yeast strain, or mammalian cell line). That is, we establish selective conditions in which the parent phenotype cannot grow, but the mutant can. One of the major advantages of bacterial mutation assays is that very large numbers of bacterial cells ($>10^8$) can be plated on a single Petri dish. If strong selection for mutant survival can be achieved, very rare events (frequencies of or-der 10^{-8}) can routinely be observed. With mammalian cells in vitro, the number of cells which can be plated per dish is perhaps 100-fold lower; the number of genes is at least 10-fold higher; and the total genomic DNA content is about 100-fold greater, compared to *E. coli*. Each of these factors tends to reduce the sensitivity of mutagenicity assays with mammalian cells, relative to bacteria. Bacteria are haploid organisms, whereas eukaryotic cells are diploid. Thus, many mutations arising in mammalian cells cannot be selected di-rectly, since the second copy of the gene complements the mutation in the first. Het-erozygous cell lines can sometimes be used as targets to circumvent this problem.

FORWARD AND REVERSE MUTATIONS

Forward mutations convert a gene coding for a wild-type (functional) protein product into a mutant form which codes for an altered or nonfunctional product. Some forward muta-tions may confer resistance to a toxic agent, such as an antibiotic, or permit growth on a substrate which does not normally support the organism. For example, wild-type *E. coli* cells are sensitive to the antibiotic rifampicin, which inhibits RNA polymerase activity. Rifampicin-resistant mutants have an altered RNA polymerase, which is less susceptible to inhibition.

Mutation of a biosynthetic gene may give rise to an *auxotrophic* mutant, an organism dependent (for colony growth) upon supply of a particular nutrient (e.g., an amino acid or nucleic acid base). Wild-type *E. coli* grows on minimal medium (salts plus glucose), so auxotrophic mutants can be detected by the replica-plating technique (50).

In contrast to forward mutations, *reversion* mutations restore biological function to a nonfunctional gene. Some auxotrophic mutants will spontaneously revert to prototrophy.

Such an event could occur, for example, by a base-substitution mutation which reverses the original mutation. Note that a reversion mutation does not necessarily restore the original DNA sequence. In the following example, a nonsense mutation (stop codon) reverts by a mutation which restores a sense codon, albeit one coding for a different amino acid. If the original amino acid (in this example, lysine) were not essential for protein function, its replacement by tyrosine might yield an active enzyme.

... CGU AAG GAC CTG ...   wild-type (functional) gene

... arg   lys   asp   leu ...

           ↓

... CGU UAG GAC CTG ...   auxotrophic mutant (nonfunctional) gene

... arg   **stop** asp   leu ...   (stop codon halts translation)

           ↓

... CGU UAC GAC CTG ...   reversion mutation

... arg   tyr   asp   leu ...

Reversion mutants are usually selected by their regained ability to grow on minimal media (*prototrophy*). For example, the various strains of *Salmonella typhimurium* used in the *Ames assay* (51) are auxotrophic for histidine, and revertants are selected by their ability to grow in the absence of this amino acid (see below). Ease of selection is an important advantage of reversion systems for studying mutagenesis, and it compensates for their inherently lower sensitivity: Mutations are more likely to inactivate genes (and, hence, enzymes) than to reactivate them.

In the following sections, we will examine in more detail a forward mutation system (*E. coli lacI*) and a reversion assay (the Ames test in *Salmonella typhimurium*).

THE *lacI* SYSTEM

The *lacI* gene of *E. coli* is often used as a target for the determination of the mutational specificity of forward mutations. In this section, we will discuss the genetic and biochemical basis of this important experimental system (52, 53).

Wild-type *E. coli* can grow on the sugar *lactose* as sole carbon source. The elements of the lactose-utilization system consist of a regulatory gene (*lacI*), control sites (*lacP*, promoter; and *lacO*, operator), and structural genes (*lacZ*, *lacY*, and *lacA*). Together, these units comprise the *lac* operon. The structure of the *lac* operon was elucidated by the elegant studies of Jacques Monod and his co-workers in the 1960s.

The enzymes encoded by the structural genes of the *lac* operon make possible the cell's utilization of lactose, a disaccharide composed of galactose and glucose linked by a β-glycosidic bond. *lacZ* codes for β-galactosidase, an enzyme which cleaves the glycosidic bond in lactose, releasing galactose and glucose. *lacY* codes for galactoside permease, which is required for transport of lactose through the cell membrane. *lacA* encodes an additional enzyme called *transacetylase*, which is not required for lactose metabolism; the biological role of transacetylase is not clear. All three genes are coordinately expressed, since they are transcribed into a single polycistronic mRNA.

lacI codes for the *lac repressor* protein. The *lac* repressor is not an enzyme, but instead a DNA-binding protein. *lac* repressor binds with high affinity to a specific region of DNA, near the beginning of the *lacZ* gene, which is termed the *operator*.

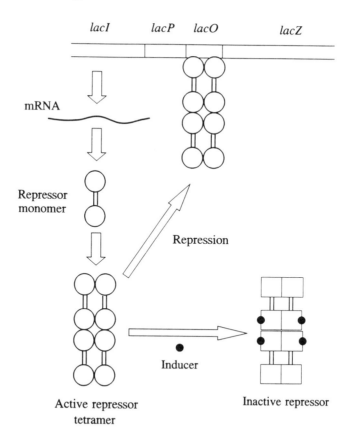

The presence of repressor bound to the operator prevents RNA polymerase from initiating transcription at the nearby *lac* promoter. This negative control prevents the cell from synthesizing the enzymes when they are not required—that is, in the absence of the substrate, lactose. The repressor, operator, and promoter are the control elements of a "genetic switch," which turns on the synthesis of the enzymes in the presence of *inducers*. Lactose itself is an inducer, as are many lactose analogues. How does this genetic switch work?

lac Repressor

The key element of the switch is *lac repressor*, a protein composed of four identical subunits. *lac* repressor is the "transducer" which senses the concentration of lactose in the cell and acts, on the basis of this information, to regulate the transcription of the *lac* operon structural genes. Each repressor subunit consists of two functionally independent domains. The N-terminal (60 amino acids) DNA-binding domain mediates operator binding. The remaining "core" domain (300 amino acids) contains sites for aggregation (formation of repressor tetramers), inducer binding, and transmission of the induction signal from the inducer-binding site to the DNA-binding domain (54). Four repressor monomers associate, through their contacts in the core domains, to form an active repressor tetramer.

The binding of inducer to the repressor is highly cooperative, just as in the case of oxygen binding to hemoglobin: Inducer binding to one monomer facilitates binding to the other monomers. Furthermore, *lac* repressor binding to the operator is also highly cooperative: The operator site has twofold sequence symmetry, and it binds cooperatively to two subunits of the repressor. [In fact, all four subunits bind can bind simultaneously, since there is a second nearby operator site, which is located within the *lacZ* coding sequence (55).] Lactose binds to the C-terminal subunits of the repressor. Inducer binding leads to a change in the conformation of the repressor, including changes in the DNA-binding region. *This conformational change prevents repressor binding to the operator. Consequently, over a narrow range of inducer concentration, the repressor switches from the operator-binding conformation to the nonbinding conformation.* The repressor protein falls off the operator; RNA polymerase can now bind to the promoter sequence and initiate the expression of the genes of the *lac* operon: The lactose-utilization enzymes are produced.

The binding of *lac* repressor to the operator site on the chromosome is mediated by highly specific contacts between the protein's N-terminal domain and the DNA bases of the operator site (56), much as a restriction endonuclease binds to a specific palindromic DNA sequence. Even a single amino acid residue change in the repressor sequence (or a single base pair change in the operator) can greatly weaken the binding of the repressor. Such a mutation will lead to *constitutive* synthesis of the *lac* genes—that is, expression of the genes in the absence of inducer. Since we can select for constitutive mutants (see below), *most mutations occurring in the DNA-binding domain of lacI can be selected phenotypically.* This is one of the main advantages to the use of the *lacI* gene in studies of mutagenesis, since it implies that many different kinds of DNA sequence alterations can be selected phenotypically.

Phenotypic Selection for *lacI⁻* Mutants

Mutants characterized by a defective *lac* repressor are easily selected on the basis of their constitutive expression of one of the *lac* operon gene products. Phenyl-β-D-galactopyranoside (P-gal) is a synthetic analogue of lactose, the natural sugar substrate for β-galactosidase. P-Gal is a substrate, but *not* an inducer of the *lac* operon. Strains which are *lacI⁻ lacZ⁺* synthesize β-galactosidase constitutively, utilize P-gal, and form colonies on minimal medium plates with P-gal as the sole carbon source. (Strains with *lacOᶜ*, a constitutive mutation mapping in the operator region, will also form colonies. In the *lacOᶜ* mutants the operator is altered and does not bind repressor.)

THE AMES MUTAGENICITY ASSAY

The "Ames assay," developed in the 1970s by Bruce N. Ames and co-workers (University of California, Berkeley) is not a single test, but rather encompasses a series of related approaches to the detection of mutagens (57–59). Many components of the Ames test were developed (and are still used) for other mutagenicity assays. However, the assembly of these components into the Ames test system was a highly successful scientific synthesis. The Ames assay remains the most widely used mutagenicity assay.

The Ames assay is a reversion assay: The mutants are prototrophic colonies derived from histidine-auxotrophic mutants (tester strains); only the revertant colonies can grow on minimal agar plates. (A small amount of histidine is incorporated in these plates, to support a few divisions of the auxotrophic cells, sufficient to permit expression of the phenotype in the induced mutants.) After incubation for about 2 days, revertant colonies are counted.

The strains used in the Ames assay are based on several mutants of *Salmonella typhimurium* strain LT-2, which were chosen from among a large collection of histidine-requiring mutants accumulated by Philip Hartman and Ames in the 1960s. Mutants were chosen for high frequencies of chemically induced reversion and low (or at least, tolerable) rates of spontaneous reversion. The subsequent development of the most important tester strains is summarized below:

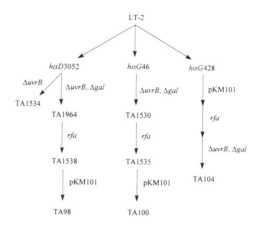

(see refs. 60 and 61 for further discussion). The objective of these additional steps in strain construction was increased sensitivity to induced mutations.

The Δ*uvrB* deletion was introduced by selecting for chlorate resistance, since *chl* is a nearby chromosomal marker; Δ*uvrB* strains lack functional excision repair (see above) and are far more sensitive to many mutagens which form bulky DNA adducts, such as aromatic amines. The LPS coat of the gram-negative bacterial cell serves as a protective barrier against the entry of many mutagens and other foreign compounds. Strain LT-2 is phenotypically "smooth": It possesses a complete LPS coat and, consequently, is serum-resistant and pathogenic in mice. Ames and colleagues introduced either the *gal* (galactose synthesis) mutation, which disrupts the biosynthesis of the O-antigen component of LPS, or the *rfa* ("deep rough") phenotype (selected on the basis of phage C21 resistance). Deep, rough strains retain little more than the lipid A core of the LPS coat and are more sensitive to some mutagens, presumably due to increased uptake of the compounds from the external medium.

Plasmid pKM101, a derivative of a naturally occurring R-factor (antibiotic resistance factor), was constructed by Kristien Mortelmans in the laboratory of Donald MacPhee. pKM101 encodes several genes, including the *mucAB* genes, which enhance UV and chemical mutagenesis; the functions encoded by genes on pKM101 have been analyzed by Graham Walker and colleagues at the Massachusetts Institute of Technology (62). The introduction of the R-factor dramatically increases the mutagenicity of some compounds, such as aflatoxin B1 and benzyl chloride (63).

A relationship between mutagenesis and carcinogenesis had been hypothesized since the early twentieth century. But the inactivity of many chemical carcinogens (such as polycyclic aromatic hydrocarbons and aromatic amines) in bacterial mutation assays appeared to contradict this hypothesis. The missing piece in the puzzle, of course, was metabolic activation. Bacterial assays failed to duplicate the actions of the hepatic mammalian enzymes of biotransformation.

The Ames assay can readily incorporate an activation system—that is, an enzyme preparation capable of metabolic activation of xenobiotics to reactive intermediates—to solve this problem. The most commonly used activation system is mammalian liver homogenate (S9) prepared from rats; often, the animals are pretreated with Aroclor 1254 (polychlorinated biphenyls) or other inducers of P-450 enzymes. $NADP^+$ and glucose-6-phosphate (to support $NADP^+$ reduction via the enzymes of the pentose phosphate pathway) are also added. To carry out the Ames assay with exogenous activation, the test chemical can be incubated with the tester strain bacteria and the activation system, before the mix is plated on the selective (minimal) medium.

Bacterial Enzymatic Activation

The introduction of genetic characteristics enhancing mutagen sensitivity has extended the range of compounds detectable with the Ames assay, as discussed earlier. Another interesting development (see below) is the introduction of genes encoding enzymes of bioactivation into the tester strains themselves. In Chapter 12 we discussed the N-acetyltransferase/O-acetyltransferase enzyme. S. typhimurium possesses this enzyme activity, although E. coli appears not to; this probably explains the high sensitivity of the Ames test to aromatic amine mutagens.

Nitropyrenes

In 1980, Herbert Rosenkranz (then at Case Western Reserve University, Cleveland, Ohio) and colleagues used the Ames test to detect mutagenicity in the carbon black toner used in photocopiers; the active constituents proved to be nitrated polycyclic aromatic hydrocarbons (64). 1,8- and 1,6-Dinitropyrene (DNP) are the most significant members of this class of mutagens, which also proved to be carcinogens (65). Nitrated polycyclic aromatic hydrocarbons were formed during the treatment of carbon black with nitric acid, at one stage in the toner production process. Replacement of this processing step by alternative procedures eliminated the formation of these mutagenic impurities. The detection of these previously unknown mutagens and their speedy elimination from photocopies were important achievements in mutation research and demonstrated the practical value of the Ames test.

Research on the mutagenicity of dinitropyrene led to some interesting discoveries concerning the metabolic capacity of Salmonella to activate mutagens. Following growth of Ames tester strain TA98 on agar plates containing bacteriotoxic levels of 1,8-DNP, a derivative strain was isolated, which proved to be highly resistant to 1,8-DNP mutagenicity. This strain, TA98/1,8-DNP_6, lacks detectable NAT/OAT activity (66). The OAT activates the N-hydroxy metabolites of mutagenic nitro compounds and arylamines, within the bacterial cell, to form reactive N-acetoxy esters (see Chapters 12 and 20).

T. Nohmi and colleagues at the National Institute of Health Sciences, Tokyo, cloned the gene encoding NAT/OAT, by screening on the basis of the gene's enhancement of DNP toxicity. The gene was reintroduced into TA98/1,8-DNP_6 on a multicopy plasmid (pBR322 derivative). The resulting strains are much more sensitive than TA98 to the mutagenicity of aromatic nitro and amino compounds (67). The genes encoding two forms of the human enzyme have also been introduced into tester strains (68). This approach allows the consequences of biotransformation by mammalian hepatic enzymes to be studied in a bacterial mutagenicity assay system.

MUTATION ASSAYS: DNA SEQUENCE ANALYSIS OF MUTANTS

The development of rapid and reliable techniques for the isolation of genes (by cloning or amplification via the polymerase chain reaction) and for DNA sequencing has ushered in a new era in the study of mutagenesis. Whereas mutations were previously studied phenotypically, and genetic analysis was usually limited to mapping, *mutations can now be routinely studied at the DNA sequence level.* This possibility has opened a new window on the study of genetic toxicology. Let's consider some aspects of the study of mutation at the DNA sequence level.

Particular mutagens induce specific mutations in a given biological system (69). For example, the G:C → A:T transition accounts for as many as 98% of the base substitutions induced by alkylating agents, such as N-methyl-N'-nitro-N-nitrosoguanidine (MNNG) and ethyl methane sulfonate (EMS), in the *lacI* gene of *E. coli* (70). This specificity is believed to reflect the mispairing properties of the major premutagenic lesion formed by alkylating agents, O^6-alkylguanine. As shown in the lower panel of the scheme on page 262, an O^6-alkylguanine residue which persists until DNA replication may pair with a thymine, rather than a cytosine. At the next round of DNA replication, the resulting O^6-alkylguanine:thymine mispair (or guanine:thymine mispair, should the alkyl group be removed by DNA methyltransferase) gives rise to a guanine:cytosine pair on one daughter molecule and an adenine:thymine pair on the second daughter molecule, thus fixing a G:C → A:T transition mutation (71).

Other mutagens give rise to very different patterns of mutation. For example, the heterocyclic nitro compound 2-nitro-3,4-dimethylimidazo[4,5-*f*]quinoline (nitro-MeIQ) induced G:C → T:A transversions at three times the rate of G:C → A:T transitions (72). G:C → T:A transversions also dominated the spectrum of mutations induced by (±) *anti*-benzo[*a*]pyrene-7,8-dihydrodiol-9,10-epoxide in the *aprt* gene of Chinese hamster ovary cells (73). Finally, the spectrum of base-substitution mutations induced by ionizing radiation in mammalian cells was not dominated by any single class of event (74).

In addition to specificity in the induction of particular classes of mutational events, mutagens may also be *site-specific.* That is, the positional distribution of mutations within a genetic target is nonuniform. Particularly mutable sites are known as *hot spots.* Hot spots were first observed in the pioneering experiments of Seymour Benzer on fine-structure genetic mapping of *rII* mutants in T4 bacteriophage (75, 76), which demonstrated that the base pair is the smallest unit of genetic mutation and recombination.

Many factors influence the distribution of hot spots within a gene. First, phenotypic selection may induce a bias: Certain codons within the gene correspond to critical amino acid residues, whose alteration causes profound changes in protein structure and function. Other codons correspond to residues which may be substituted without significant effects on the protein's function. Different mutagens can target different hot spots. The local DNA sequence may influence the susceptibility of a particular base to chemical damage, via local secondary structure effects. For similar reasons, lesions in different sites may be repaired with different efficiencies. Local sequences, such as palindromes or runs of repeated bases, may also influence mutational mechanisms, as discussed below.

The histidine operon mutations used in the Ames tester strains were chosen on the basis of their phenotypic behavior—that is, sensitivity to chemically induced reversion. The first clues concerning the nature of the target DNA sequences in the tester strains were obtained by protein sequencing of the histidinol dehydrogenase product of the *hisD* gene but the development of DNA sequencing techniques in the 1970s opened up a new era in the analysis of mutation.

The target sequences for reversion of the *his* mutations in Ames tester strains have been determined (77). Some of the mutations are frameshifts, and some are base substitutions (*hisG428, hisG46*). The *hisD3052* mutation in strain TA98 is a −1 frameshift; the high sensitivity of this strain is due to the presence of a hot spot near the site of the original mutation. This hot spot is a repeated sequence: ... CGCGCGCG ..., which is prone to −2 frameshift events by the Streisinger mechanism (see page 303):

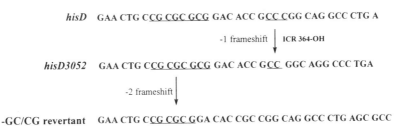

Many other frameshift reversion events are also observed, but this hot spot usually dominates the mutational spectrum. The use of PCR amplification of the target sequences (78) has made the analysis of the mutational spectra of Ames test revertants even simpler.

Jeffrey Miller and colleagues (University of California, Los Angeles) have recently developed an assay system which is an interesting variation on the Ames test approach. They took advantage of the detailed understanding of the structure and sequence of the *lacZ* gene, encoding β-galactosidase, to design a set of tester strains which revert by particular mechanisms. The codon (GAA) for an essential catalytic-site residue in the enzyme, Glu-461, was altered by site-directed mutagenesis. The mutant strains are unable to grow on lactose, since the β-galactosidase product is inactive. Revertants are simply selected by growth on lactose plates.

Six different strains were constructed; each strain can revert to a glutamate codon by one of the six possible base substitution mutations. Thus, a chemical can be tested against this set of six strains to analyze the base substitution-specificity of the mutations which it induces (79).

A set of frameshift-detection strains was also assembled. Whereas the target site in Ames strain TA98 is in a nonessential part of the protein encoded by *hisD*, the frameshift mutations in the Miller strains are near the catalytic site of the *lacZ* gene product and can only restore the *lacZ*⁺ phenotype by an exact reversion to the wild-type sequence. Various frameshift mutations were engineered; each is in a run of repeated single bases or alternating bases, to maximize the likelihood of Streisinger slippage (80).

As with the examination of DNA adduct "fingerprint" patterns, mutational spectra may prove to be diagnostic of particular classes of mutagens and might be used in a molecular epidemiological approach. Examples of chemically induced mutational spectra in the *lacI* gene of *E. coli* are shown in Suzuki, Griffiths, Miller, and Lewontin and in Miller (81).

CONSTRUCTION OF ADDUCTED OLIGONUCLEOTIDES

As discussed in Chapter 16, treatment with a given chemical agent may induce many different types of DNA damage. Since each type of adduct will have different biological effects, it may be difficult to ascribe particular mutational consequences to the processing of particular adducts, even when we study the mutational effects of a single chemical. The development of recombinant DNA technology has provided an approach which circumvents this problem (82). A defined DNA alteration (e.g., an O^6-methylguanine adduct substituted for guanine) can be constructed at a defined position in a piece of DNA, and then test its biological consequences. This approach was pioneered by John Essigman, Massachusetts Institute of Technology, for the study of alkylating agents (83) and has also been applied to damages such as thymine dimers, aminofluorene adducts, and 8-hydroxyguanine.

The synthesis of a defined oligonucleotide containing an adduct can be attempted either by DNA synthesis chemistry (such as the phosphoramidite chemistry used in DNA synthesizers), or by supplying a DNA polymerase with a modified dNTP for in vitro incorporation into a growing strand. *E. coli* Pol I, for example, will readily accept alkylated dNTPs.

The adducted strand can then be used for in vitro mutagenesis assays. A labeled primer is extended by a DNA polymerase, using the adduct-containing strand as template; frequencies of misincorporation opposite the adduct are measured by sequencing the extended primer strand.

The adducted oligonucleotide can also be incorporated into a construct, such as a plasmid, viral genome, or shuttle vector, which can be propagated in cells; mutant progeny are selected phenotypically. This approach allows the study of in vivo mutagenesis by specific adducts.

SPONTANEOUS MUTATIONS

Mutations can arise even in the absence of treatment with chemical mutagens. Spontaneous mutations may be due to several factors. DNA polymerase action involves a finite but small misincorporation frequency; postreplication mismatch repair corrects most, but not all, of these errors. Bases exist in equilibrium between the common keto/imino and rare enol/amino tautomers; the rare tautomers can form mismatched base pairs (such as enol-thymidine with guanosine), which may "fool" DNA polymerase into inserting the incorrect base in the daughter strand. The biological significance of this mechanism has been disputed, however, since there is very little direct evidence concerning the prevalence of rare tautomers in DNA (as opposed to monomeric bases or nucleosides) (84). Natural background radiation is ubiquitous, and endogenous production of reactive oxygen species confronts all aerobic organisms with the challenge of oxidative damage to DNA. Spontaneous chemical lesions also occur in DNA; for example, depurination (hydrolysis of the glycosidic bond between deoxyribose and a purine base) generates an abasic site. Oxidized or missing bases are repairable, but failure of repair will leave a premutagenic lesion at the time of replication.

Any mutation assay will detect spontaneous as well as induced mutations, so studies of mutational specificity of induced mutations should be carried out at sufficiently high doses such that the induced mutations predominate.

MUTATIONAL MECHANISMS

If we wish to understand the molecular mechanisms of mutation, and hence of the generation of genetic diversity, we need to elucidate the detailed chemical/biochemical pathways leading from DNA damage to mutation: *mutational mechanisms*. Many different factors have to be considered here. For example, different types of DNA adducts will be subject to enzymatic recognition and repair with different efficiencies, depending on the ability of enzymatic repair machinery to recognize the presence of the adducted nucleosides and excise them from DNA. Adducts which persist until DNA replication may lead to base misincorporation by DNA polymerase, but the pattern of misincorporation will vary, depending on the structure of the adduct. Adducts or other forms of DNA damage may cause effects other than simple base misincorporation. For example, adducts occurring in runs of repeated bases may promote strand slippage during replication, leading to deletion or insertion mutations. This idea was first proposed by Streisinger et al. in 1966 (85, 86).

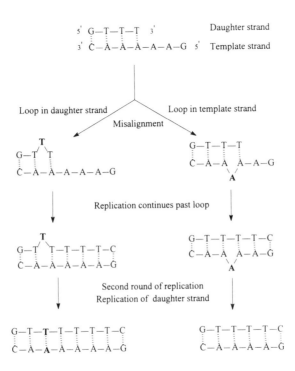

As we discussed earlier, Streisinger slippage explains the hot-spot reversion event in Ames strain *hisD3052*.

The sequence-dependent local secondary structure of DNA may also play a role in mutagenesis. An example of such an effect (87) is shown on the following page:

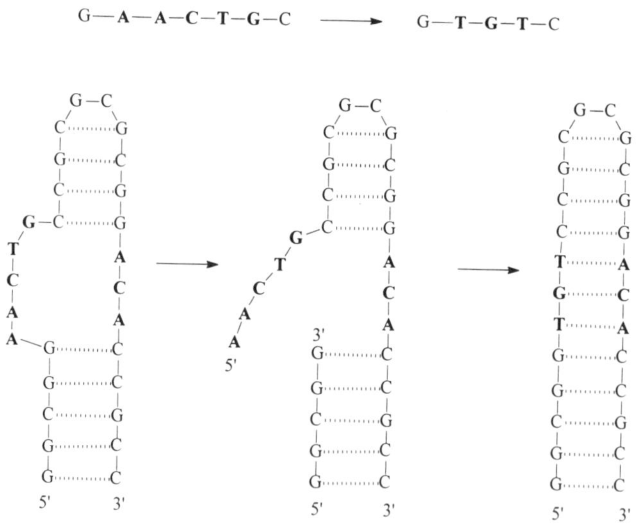

G—A—A—C—T—G—C ⟶ G—T—G—T—C

Here, a complex mutation arose in a study of spontaneous mutations in the *hisD3052* allele. The mutation was a deletion of the five bases AACTG accompanied by the insertion, at the same site, of the three base sequence TGT. The origin of the mutation seems obscure until the local sequence context is examined. A partial palindrome is present, and the mutation converts the sequence into a perfect 26-base-pair palindrome. Apparently, a local "hairpin loop" structure formed during replication; the mismatched five-base sequence (or a longer stretch) was excised and repaired, *using the same strand as template*. Such events may occur spontaneously, or they may be induced by conformational changes resulting from DNA damage.

NOTES

1. Singer, B., and Grunberger, D., *Molecular Biology of Mutagens and Carcinogens*, Plenum Press, New York, 1983.

2. Friedberg, E. C.,Walker, G. C., and Siede, W., *DNA Repair and Mutagenesis*, ASM Press, Washington, DC, 1995; Friedberg, E. C., DNA repair: Looking back and peering forward, *BioEssays* 16:645–649, 1994.

3. Adams, R. L. P., Knowler, J. T., and Leader, D. P., *The Biochemistry of the Nucleic Acids*, 10th ed., Chapman and Hall, London, 1986.

4. Myles, G. M., and Sancar, A., DNA repair, *Chem. Res. Toxicol.* 2:197–226, 1989.

5. Lindahl, T., Instability and decay of the primary structure of DNA, *Nature* 362:709–715, 1993.

6. Demple, B., Self-methylation by suicide DNA repair enzymes, in: *Protein Methylation*, W. K. Paik and S. Kim, Eds., CRC Press, Boca Raton, FL, 1990, pp. 285–304.

7. Pegg, A. E., and Byers, T. L., Repair of DNA containing O^6-alkylguanine, *FASEB J.* 6:2302–2310, 1992; Samson, L., The suicidal DNA repair methyltransferases of microbes, *Mol. Microbiol.* 6:825–831, 1992; Yamada, M., Sedgwick, B., Sofuni, T., and Nohmi, T., Construction and characterization of mutants of *Salmonella typhimurium* deficient in DNA repair of O⁶-methylguanine, *J. Bacteriol.* 177:1511–1519, 1995.

8. Sancar, A., Mechanisms of DNA excision repair, *Science* 266:1954–1956, 1994; Seeberg, E., Eide, L., and Bjørås, M., The base excision repair pathway, *Trends Biochem. Sci.* 20:391–397, 1995.

9. Shapiro, R., and Klein, R. S., The deamination of cytidine and cytosine by acidic buffer solutions. Mutagenic implications, *Biochemistry* 5:2358–2362, 1966.

10. Savva, R., McAuley-Hecht, K., Brown, T., and Pearl, L., The structural basis of specific base-excision repair by uracil-DNA glycosylase, *Nature* 373:487–493, 1995.

11. Marinus, M. G., Methylation of DNA, in: *Escherichia coli and Salmonella typhimurium: Cellular and Molecular Biology*, Vol. 1, F. C. Neidhardt, J. L. Ingraham, K. B. Low, B. Magasanik, M. Schaechter, and H. E. Umbarger, Eds., American Society for Microbiology, Washington, D.C., 1987, pp. 697–702.

12. Glickman, B. W., Mechanisms of mutation in DNA, in: *Genetics of Bacteria*, J. Scaife, D. Leach, and A. Galizzi, Eds., Academic Press, London, 1985, pp. 41–48.

13. Demple, B., and Harrison, L., Repair of oxidative damage to DNA: enzymology and biology, *Annu. Rev. Biochem.* 63:915–948, 1994.

14. Reviewed in Price, A., The repair of ionising radiation-induced damage to DNA, *Semin. Cancer Biol.* 4:61–71, 1993.

15. Lin, J.-j., and Sancar, A., (A)BC excinuclease: the *Escherichia coli* nucleotide excision repair enzyme, *Mol. Microbiol.* 6:2219–2224, 1992.

16. Taylor, J.-S., DNA, sunlight, and skin cancer, *J. Chem. Educ.* 67:835–841, 1990.

17. Livneh, Z., Cohen-Fix, O., Skaliter, R., and Elizur, T., Replication of damaged DNA and the molecular mechanism of ultraviolet light mutagenesis, *Crit. Rev. Biochem. Mol. Biol.* 28:465–513, 1993.

18. Cleaver, J. E., Do we know the cause of XP carcinogenesis? *Carcinogenesis* 11:875–883, 1990.

19. Paterson, M. C., Bech-Hansen, N. T., Smith, P. J., and Mulvihill, J. J., Radiogenic neoplasia, cellular radiosensitivity, and faulty DNA repair, in: *Radiation Carcinogenesis: Epidemiology and Biological Significance*, J. D. Boice, Jr., and J. F. Fraumeni (Eds.), Raven Press, New York, 1984, pp. 319–336.

20. Savitsky, K., Bar-Shira, A., Gilad, S., Rotman, G., Ziv, Y., Vanagaite, L., Tagle, D. A., Smith, S., Uziel, T., Sfez, S., Ashkenazi, M., Pecker, I., Frydman, M., Harnik, R., Patanjali, S. R., Simmons, A., Clines, G. A., Sartiel, A., Gatti, R. A., Chessa, L., Sanal, O., Lavin, M. F., Jaspers, N. G. J., and Shiloh, Y., A single ataxia telangiectasia gene with a product similar to PI-3 kinase, *Science* 268:1749–1753, 1995.

21. Darnell, J., Lodish, H., and Baltimore, D., *Molecular Cell Biology*, 2nd ed., W. H. Freeman, New York, 1990, pp. 170–171, Fig. 5-20.

22. Jaspers, N. G. J., and Bootsma, D., Genetic heterogeneity in ataxia–telangiectasia studied by cell fusion, *Proc. Natl. Acad. Sci. U.S.A.* 79:2641–2644, 1982.

23. Busch, D. B., Cleaver, J. E., and Glaser, D. A., Large-scale isolation of UV-sensitive clones of CHO cells, *Somat. Cell Genet.* 6:407–418, 1980; Busch, D., Greiner, C., Lewis, K., Ford, R., Adair, A., and Thompson, L. H., Summary of complementation groups of UV-sensitive CHO cell mutants isolated by large-scale screening, *Mutagenesis* 4:349–354, 1989.

24. Tanaka, K., Analysis of DNA excision repair genes in XP, in: *Frontiers of Photobiology*, A. Shima, M. Ichihashi, Y. Fujiwara, and H. Takebe, Eds., Excerpta Medica, Amsterdam, 1993, pp. 293–302.

25. Reviewed by Barnes, D. E., Damage-limitation exercises, *Nature* 359:12–13, 1992.

26. Tanaka, K., and Wood, R. W., Xeroderma pigmentosum and nucleotide excision repair of DNA, *Trends Biochem. Sci.* 19:83–86, 1994; Marx, J., DNA repair comes into its own, *Science* 266:728–730, 1994; Hanawalt, P.C., Transcription-coupled repair and human disease, *Science* 266:1957–1958, 1994.

27. Arrand, J. E., and Michael, B. D., Recent advances in the study of ionising radiation damage and repair, *Int. J. Radiat. Biol.* 61:717–720, 1992; Nevaldine, B., Longo, J. A., King, G. A., Vilenchik, M., Sagerman, R. H., and Hahn, P. J., Induction and repair of DNA double-strand breaks, *Radiat. Res.* 133:370–374, 1993.

28. Fairbairn, D. W., Olive, P. L., and O'Neill, K. L., The comet assay: A comprehensive review, *Mutat. Res.* 339:37–59, 1995.

29. von Sonntag, C., *The Chemical Basis of Radiation Biology*, Taylor & Francis, London, 1987, Section 8.2.

30. Hutchinson, F., On the measurement of DNA double-strand breaks by neutral elution, *Radiat. Res.* 120:182–186, 1989.

31. Hutchinson, F., Molecular biology of mutagenesis of mammalian cells by ionizing radiation, *Semin. Cancer Biol.* 4:85–92, 1993.

32. Murli, S., and Walker, G.C., SOS mutagenesis, *Curr. Op. Genet. Devel.* 3:719–725, 1993.

33. Voet, D., and Voet, J. G., *Biochemistry*, 2nd ed., Wiley, New York, 1995, pp. 1051–1052.

34. Woodgate, R., and Sedgwick, S.G., Mutagenesis induced by bacterial UmuDC proteins and their plasmid homologues, *Mol. Microbiol.* 6:2213–2218, 1992.

35. See Voet and Voet, p. 911.

36. Brown, T., Kennard, O., Kneale, G., and Rabinovich, D., High-resolution structure of a DNA helix containing mismatched base pairs, *Nature* 315:604–606, 1985.

37. Shibata, M., Zielinski, T. J., and Rein, R., A molecular dynamics study of the effect of G·T mispairs on the conformation of DNA in solution, *Biopolymers* 31:211–232, 1991.

38. Modrich, P., Mechanisms and biological effects of mismatch repair, *Annu. Rev. Genet.* 25:229–253, 1991.

39. Cleaver, J. E., It was a very good year for DNA repair, *Cell* 76:1–4, 1994; Nicolaides, N. C., Papadopoulos, N., Liu, B., Wei, Y.-F., Carter, K. C., Ruben, S. M., Rosen, C. A., Haseltine, W. A., Fleischmann, R. D., Fraser, C. M., Adams, M. D., Venter, J. C., Dunlop, M. G., Hamilton, S. R., Petersen, G. M., De la Chapelle, A., Vogelstein, B., and Kinzler, K. W., Mutations of two PMS homologues in hereditary nonpolyposis colon cancer, *Nature* 371:75–80, 1994; Modrich, P., Mismatch repair, genetic stability, and cancer, *Science* 266:1959–1960, 1994.

40. Cedar, H., DNA methylation and gene activity, *Cell* 53:3–4, 1988.

41. Li, E., Bestor, T. H., and Jaensich, R., Targeted mutation of the DNA methyltransferase gene results in embryonic lethality, *Cell* 69:915–926, 1992.

42. Jost, J. P., *DNA Methylation: Molecular Biology and Biological Significance*, Basel, Birkhauser Verlag, 1992.

43. Russell, G. J., Walker, P. M. B., Elton, R. A., and Subak-Sharpe, J. H., Doublet frequency analysis of fractionated vertebrate nuclear DNA, *J. Mol. Biol.* 108:1–23, 1976.

44. Lathe, R., Synthetic oligonucleotide probes deduced from amino acid sequence data: theoretical and practical considerations, *J. Mol. Biol.* 183:1–12, 1985.

45. McCelland, M., The effect of sequence specific DNA methylation on restriction endonuclease cleavage, *Nucleic Acids Res.* 9:5859–5866, 1981.

46. Pfeifer, G. P., Steigerwald, S. D., Mueller, P. R., Wold,. B., and Riggs, A. D., Genomic sequencing and methylation analysis by ligation mediated PCR, *Science* 246:810–813, 1989.

47. Rideout III, W. M., Coetzee, G. A., Olumi, A. F., and Jones, P. A., 5-Methylcytosine as an endogenous mutagen in the human LDL receptor and p53 genes, *Science* 249:1288–1290, 1990.

48. Wiebauer, K., and Jiricny, J., In vitro correction of G·T mispairs to G·C pairs in nuclear extracts from human cells, *Nature* 339:234–236, 1989.

49. Neidhardt, F. C., Ingraham, J. L., and Schaechter, M., *Physiology of the Bacterial Cell*, Sinauer, Sunderland, MA, 1990, p. 14.

50. Suzuki, D. T., Griffiths, A. J. F., Miller, J. H., and Lewontin, R. C., *An Introduction to Genetic Analysis*, 4th ed., W. H. Freeman, New York, 1989, pp. 161–162.

51. Suzuki, D. T., Griffiths, A. J. F., Miller, J. H., and Lewontin, R. C., *An Introduction to Genetic Analysis*, 4th ed., W. H. Freeman, New York, 1989, pp. 497–499.

52. Suzuki, D. T., Griffiths, A. J. F., Miller, J. H., and Lewontin, R. C., *An Introduction to Genetic Analysis*, 4th ed., W. H. Freeman, New York, 1989, pp. 445–454.

53. Lewin, B., *Genes V*, Oxford University Press, New York, 1994, Chapter 15.

54. Friedman, A. M., Fischmann, T. O., and Steitz, T. A., Crystal structure of *lac* repressor core tetramer and its implications for DNA looping, *Science* 268:1721–1727, 1995.

55. Reznikoff, W. S., The lactose operon-controlling elements: a complex paradigm, *Mol. Microbiol.* 6:2419–2422, 1992.

56. Lewis, M., Chang, G., Horton, N. C., Kercher, M. A., Pace, H. C., Schumacher, M. A., Brennan, R.G., and Lu, P., Crystal structure of the lactose operon repressor and its complexes with DNA and inducer, *Science* 271:1247–1254, 1996.

57. Ames, B. N., The detection of chemical mutagens with enteric bacteria, in: *Chemical Mutagens, Principles and Methods for Their Detection*, Vol. 1, A. Hollaender, Ed., Plenum, New York, 1971, pp. 267–282; Ames, B. N., Durston, W. E., Yamasaki, E. and Lee, F. D., Carcinogens are mutagens: a simple test system combining liver homogenates for activation and bacteria for detection, *Proc. Natl. Acad. Sci. U.S.A.* 70:2281–2285, 1973.

58. Maron, D. M., and Ames, B. N., Revised methods for the *Salmonella* mutagenicity test, *Mutat. Res.* 113:173–215, 1983.

59. Zeiger, E. The *Salmonella* mutagenicity assay for identification of presumptive carcinogens, in: *Handbook of Carcinogen Testing*, H. A. Milman and E. K. Weisburger, Eds., Noyes Publishing, Park Ridge, NJ, 1985, pp. 83–99.

60. MacPhee, D. G., Development of bacterial mutagenicity tests: a view from afar, *Environ. Mol. Mutagen.* 14(Suppl. 16):35–38, 1989.

61. Busch, D. B., Archer, J., Amos, E. A., Hatcher, J. F., and Bryan, G. T., A protocol for the combined biochemical and serological identification of the Ames mutagen tester strains as *Salmonella typhimurium*, *Environ. Mutagen.* 8:741–751, 1986.

62. Perry, K. L., and Walker, G. C., Identification of plasmid (pKM101)-coded proteins involved in mutagenesis and UV resistance, *Nature* 300:278–281, 1982.

63. McCann, J., Spingarn, N. E., Kobori, J., and Ames, B. N. Detection of carcinogens as mutagens: bacterial tester strains with R factor plasmids, *Proc. Natl. Acad. Sci. U.S.A.* 72:979–983, 1975.

64. Rosenkranz, H. S., McCoy, E. C., Sanders, D. R., Butler, M., Kiriazides, D. K., and Mermelstein, R., Nitropyrenes: isolation, identification, and reduction of mutagenic impurities in carbon black and toners, *Science* 209:1039–1043, 1980.

65. Imaida, K., Tay, L. K., Lee, M.-S., Wang, C. Y., Ito, N., and King, C. M., Tumor induction by nitropyrenes in the female CD rat, in: *Carcinogenic and Mutagenic Responses to Aromatic Amines and Nitroarenes* C. M. King, L. J. Romano, and D. Schuetzle, Eds., Elsevier, New York, 1988, pp. 187–197.

66. Josephy, P. D., New developments in the Ames assay: high-sensitivity detection of mutagenic arylamines, *BioEssays* 11:108–112, 1989.

67. Einistö, P., Watanabe, M., Ishidate, M., Jr., and Nohmi, T., Mutagenicity of 30 chemicals in *Salmonella typhimurium* strains possessing different nitroreductase or *O*-acetyltransferase activities, *Mutat. Res.* 259:95–102, 1991.

68. Grant, D. M., Josephy, P. D., Lord, H. L., and Morrison, L. D., *Salmonella typhimurium* strains expressing human arylamine *N*-acetyltransferases: metabolism and mutagenic activation of aromatic amines, *Cancer Res.* 52:3961–3964, 1992.

69. Miller, J. H., *A Short Course in Bacterial Genetics*, Cold Spring Harbor Laboratory Press, Plainview, NY, 1992, pp. 109–111.

70. Horsfall, M. J., Gordon, A. J. E., Burns, P. A., Zielenska, M., van der Vliet, G. M. E., and Glickman, B. W., Mutational specificity of alkylating agents and the influence of DNA repair, *Environ. Mol. Mutagen.* 15:107–122, 1990.

71. Swann, P. F., Why do O^6-alkylguanine and O^4-alkylthymine miscode? The relationship between the structure of DNA containing O^6-alkylguanine and O^4-alkylthymine and the mutagenic properties of these bases, *Mutat. Res.* 233:81–94, 1990; Vojtechovsky, J., Eaton, M. D., Gaffney, B., Jones, R., and Berman, H. M., Structure of a new crystal form of a DNA dodecamer containing T•(O^6Me)G base pairs, *Biochemistry* 34:16632–16640, 1995.

72. Kosakarn, P., Josephy, P. D., Halliday, J. A., and Glickman, B. W, Mutational specificity of 2-nitro-3,4-dimethylimidazo[4,5-*f*]quinoline in the *lacI* gene of *Escherichia coli*, *Carcinogenesis* 14:511–517, 1993.

73. Mazur, M., and Glickman, B. W., Sequence specificity of mutations induced by benzo[*a*]pyrene-7,8-diol-9,10-epoxide at endogenous *aprt* gene in CHO cells, *Somat. Cell Mol. Genet.* 14:393–400, 1988.

74. Grosovsky, A. J., de Boer, J. G., de Jong, P. J., Drobetsky, E. A., and Glickman, B. W., Base substitutions, frameshifts, and small deletions constitute ionizing radiation-induced point mutations in mammalian cells, *Proc. Natl. Acad. Sci. U.S.A.* 85:185–188, 1988.

75. Benzer, S., On the topography of the genetic fine structure, *Proc. Natl. Acad. Sci. U.S.A.* 47:403–415, 1961.
76. Suzuki, D. T., Griffiths, A. J. F., Miller, J. H., and Lewontin, R. C., *An Introduction to Genetic Analysis*, 4th ed., W. H. Freeman, New York, 1989, pp. 300–309.
77. Hartman, P. E., Ames, B. N., Roth, J. R., Barnes, W. M. and Levin, D. E., Target sequences for mutagenesis in *Salmonella* histidine-requiring mutants. *Environ. Mutagen.* 8:631–641, 1986.
78. Bell, D. A., Levine, J. G., and DeMarini, D. M., DNA sequence analysis of revertants of the *hisD3052* allele of *Salmonella typhimurium* TA98 using the polymerase chain reaction and direct sequencing: application to 1-nitropyrene-induced revertants, *Mutat. Res.* 252:35–44, 1991.
79. Cupples, C., and Miller, J. H., A set of *lacZ* mutations in *Escherichia coli* which allow rapid detection of each of the six base substitutions, *Proc. Natl. Acad. Sci. U.S.A.* 86:5345–5349, 1989.
80. Cupples, C. G., Cabrera, M., Cruz, C., and Miller, J. H., A set of *lacZ* mutations in *Escherichia coli* that allow rapid detection of specific frameshift mutations, *Genetics* 125:275–280, 1990.
81. Suzuki, D. T., Griffiths, A. J. F., Miller, J. H., and Lewontin, R. C., *An Introduction to Genetic Analysis*, 4th ed., W. H. Freeman, New York, 1989, Fig. 17-10; Miller, J. H., *A Short Course in Bacterial Genetics*, Cold Spring Harbor Laboratory Press, Plainview, NY, 1992, Figs. 4-24 and 4-25.
82. Singer, B., and Essigmann, J. M., Site-specific mutagenesis: retrospective and prospective, *Carcinogenesis*, 12:949–955, 1991.
83. Loechler, E. L., Green, C. L., and Essigman, J. M., In vivo mutagenesis by O^6-methylguanine built into a unique site in a viral genome, *Proc. Natl. Acad. Sci. U.S.A.* 81:6271–6275, 1984.
84. Morgan, A. R., Base mismatches and mutagenesis: how important is tautomerism? *Trends Biochem. Sci.* 18:160–163, 1993.
85. Streisinger, G., Okada, Y., Emrich, J., Newton, J., Tsugita, A., Terzaghi, E., and Inouye, M., Frameshift mutations and the genetic code, *Cold Spring Harbor Symp. Quant. Biol.* 31:77–84, 1966.
86. Drake, J. W., Glickman, B. W., and Ripley, L. S., Updating the theory of mutation, *Am. Scient.* 71:621–630, 1983.
87. Wallace, R. E., and Josephy, P. D., Mutational spectrum of benzidine/hydrogen peroxide-induced revertants in the *hisD3052* allele of *Salmonella typhimurium*, *Mutat. Res.* 311:9–20, 1994.

18

CARCINOGENESIS: THE GENETIC TARGETS

Many chemical carcinogens are mutagenic, genotoxic agents (1). What cellular genes are the critical targets in cancer development? Two classes of genes, oncogenes and tumor suppressor genes, have been identified on the basis of their roles in carcinogenesis (2). Generally, *activation* of one allele of an oncogene, or *inactivation* of both alleles of a tumor suppressor gene, contributes to tumor formation. In other words, the activated (mutant) alleles of oncogenes, and the wild-type alleles of tumor suppressor genes are dominant. Oncogene-coded proteins have the normal function of promoting cell growth, while tumor suppressor gene products act as components of growth control mechanisms.

ONCOGENES

The ability of certain viruses to cause tumor formation in animals has been known for many decades (3). These viruses can also *transform* cultured cells; the transformed phenotype is characterized by loss of the normal contact-inhibition of cellular growth in vitro. The properties of transformed cultured cells resemble those of tumor cells. Genetic analysis of one class of tumor viruses, the retroviruses (which carry RNA genomes), revealed that the presence of specific genes (*oncogenes*) was required for tumor induction. Hybridization analysis showed that these viral oncogenes were derived from normal cellular genes; apparently, the viruses captured cellular genes and modified them, thereby producing active oncogenes (4).

In a process independent of viral infection, these cellular genes (*proto-oncogenes*) can be activated by mutation to become active oncogenes, which contribute to malignant transformation. The products of proto-oncogenes normally perform a variety of cellular functions, all leading to cell growth when the appropriate signals are in place. When these signals are overridden, or continually turned on, oncogenesis occurs. Oncoproteins which act as secreted growth factors (*sis*), growth factor receptors (*erbA*), components of signal transduction pathways (*ras*), or transcription factors (*fos* and *jun*) are known (3).

Members of the *ras* family were the first cellular oncogenes to be cloned. Like most oncogenes, *ras* was cloned (5) by a DNA transfection approach. Activated oncogenes are dominant in cell transformation. Normal mouse NIH 3T3 cells were transfected with genomic DNA from a transformed *human* cell line. Foci of transformed cells which grew in the transfected culture were isolated and DNA libraries were prepared from these transformed cell lines. Since human DNA contains characteristic repetitive sequences, the transforming (human) gene could be detected and isolated.

The *ras* proto-oncogenes encode a 21-kD intracellular guanine-nucleotide-binding protein [G-protein (6)]. Point mutations in *ras* have been found in 50% of colon tumors and 90% of pancreatic tumors, as well as in a variety of other tumor types (7). Overexpression of Ras can also contribute to transformation in breast cancer. Ras protein is involved in the transmission of signals from membrane-bound receptor tyrosine kinases to nuclear transcription factors (8). When Ras is in its active state, it is GTP-bound (9). Upon interaction with *GTPase activating protein* (GAP), the intrinsic GTPase activity of Ras hydrolyzes the bound GTP to GDP, leaving Ras in its inactive form. Several activated *ras* mutations correspond to amino acid changes at specific residues involved in GTP hydrolysis. These mutant forms of Ras can still interact with GAP, but lack GTPase activity, and remain in the active, GTP-bound form. When this protein is overexpressed, or present in its activated form, it causes oncogenesis by transmitting a growth-promoting signal continually to its downstream effectors. The identification and characterization of these effectors is the focus of much current research.

A limited number of mutations (those affecting codons 12, 13, and 61) activate *ras* proto-oncogenes (10). In rat mammary carcinomas induced by the alkylating agent MNU (*N*-methyl-*N*-nitrosourea), all the activating mutations detected in tumors from 61 animals were identical: a G:C → A:T transition in the second base of *ras* codon 12 (11).

The study of chronic myelogenous leukemia revealed a pair of oncogenes which, when combined, are involved in the progression of this disease. These cancers often show a characteristic chromosomal rearrangement: A portion of chromosome 9 has become attached to part of chromosome 22 to create the *Philadelphia chromosome* (12). The proto-oncogene *abl* is located at the breakpoint of chromosome 9. When the Philadelphia chromosome is formed, the 3′ end of *abl* becomes fused to the 5′ end of another proto-oncogene, *bcr*, which is located on chromosome 22. The result of this reciprocal translocation is the production of the bcr–abl fusion protein, which has high tyrosine kinase activity (13) and contributes to the development of leukemia.

Another proto-oncogene activated by chromosomal translocation is *myc*. This gene is frequently activated in Burkitt's lymphoma, a B-cell malignancy which is characterized by a translocation between chromosomes 8 and 14. This translocation causes an overproduction of the MYC protein, by juxtaposition of the *myc* gene, on chromosome 8, with immunoglobulin heavy chain genes located on chromosome 14 (14). The MYC protein acts a transcription factor, although the targets of this activity are unknown. Transcriptional activation requires dimerization of MYC with another protein, MAX (15). Mutations in the coding sequence of the myc gene are not required for oncogenesis; overexpression of MYC causes increased transcription and oncogenesis (16).

TUMOR SUPPRESSOR GENES

Whole-cell fusion experiments between tumorigenic and nontumorigenic cell lines can produce hybrids which are nontumorigenic (17, 18). Apparently, a dominant factor from the nontumorigenic cell line can confer its phenotype upon the tumorigenic cell line. This indicates the existence of *tumor suppressor* genes (or anti-oncogenes).

Another piece of evidence for the existence of such genes came from cytogenetic studies. As already mentioned, specific chromosomal abnormalities are associated with particular types of tumors (19). For example, retinoblastoma usually shows chromosomal rearrangements or deletions in a specific region of chromosome 13 (13q14); many colorectal tumors show deletions in chromosome 5 (5q21). Patients who carry one such abnormal chromosome have an elevated risk of developing that cancer. Researchers hypothesized that inactivation of the second copy of the same gene, by a somatic mutational event, would "knock out" the function of the gene product.

Molecular analysis provided additional evidence that the loss of tumor suppressor genes is involved in the progression of some tumors. While normal tissue from an affected individual is often heterozygous for a particular DNA sequence, tumor tissue sometimes shows loss of heterozygosity for the same region (20). This loss of heterozygosity is usually observed in patients who carry one (germ-line) wild-type allele and one mutant allele of a tumor suppressor gene. When the wild-type copy is lost through a deletion, the loss of heterozygosity can be observed in the resulting tumor tissue. These molecular studies complemented the cytogenetic work. In some cases, tumors which usually showed chromosomal abnormalities at specific locations had no such rearrangement. When these same tumors were examined at the molecular level, loss of heterozygosity was observed, even though the chromosomal change was cytogenetically undetectable.

The most frequently used strategy for the cloning of tumour suppressor genes is *positional cloning*. This technique relies upon cytogenetically observed chromosomal abnormalities and loss of heterozygosity in a given tumor type. Once the chromosomal location of a putative tumor suppressor gene has been defined, the laborious task of isolating the gene begins. In many cases, DNA probes from the region of interest were isolated, and a "chromosome walk" was carried out, using these probes as starting point. Along the way, the isolated DNA sequences are checked for the hallmarks of expressed sequences (such as evolutionarily conserved sequences). Once an expressed sequence is found, DNA from many tumors is examined to determine whether this sequence is disrupted. If this is the case, a tumor suppressor gene has probably been identified. Variations of this technique have been successfully used to clone the *Rb* (retinoblastoma), *DCC* (deleted in colorectal cancer), *WT1* (Wilm's tumor), *NF1* (neurofibromatosis type I), and *BRCA1* (breast cancer) tumor suppressor genes.

The protein products of the tumor suppressor genes discovered so far have the common feature of retarding cell growth; the methods by which they perform this function vary. Tumor suppressors that resemble cell adhesion molecules (DCC), control the cell cycle (Rb and p53), or interact with the Ras oncoprotein (rap1) have been identified. One widely studied tumor suppressor gene is the retinoblastoma susceptibility gene, *Rb* (21). The protein product of this gene is involved in the regulation of the cell cycle. While the deletion or mutation of *Rb* is characteristic of retinoblastoma, this gene is also sometimes altered in tumors of the breast and prostate, as well as in osteosarcoma. Most frequently, in retinoblastoma, the *Rb* gene is inactivated by small deletions or duplications (22) which result in a premature stop codon.

A recently cloned tumor suppressor gene, *BRCA1*, is frequently mutated in breast and ovarian cancers (23). Individuals who carry somatic mutations in this gene are predisposed to breast and ovarian cancers, often developing cancer in these organs early in life. The majority of *BRCA1* mutations are nonsense mutations and result in the production of a truncated protein product. Other mutations in *BRCA1* include frameshift and missense mutations; however, the implications of many of these mutations regarding the function of the BRCA1 protein are unclear. Mutations which replace cysteine residues in the zinc-finger domain of the protein (24) are thought to disrupt the putative ability of the BRCA1 protein to bind DNA and act as a transcription factor.

The search for a tumor suppressor gene on chromosome 9p21 (a region known to show frequent abnormalities in malignant melanomas) led to the cloning of the *p16* gene (25). This gene is deleted or mutated in the majority of melanoma cell lines examined and is deleted in many cell lines from other cancers. Mutations in *p16* are associated with familial predisposition to malignant melanoma (26). The sequence of *p16* turned out to be identical to that of a previously described cell cycle regulator which has the ability to block cell division. Thus, it seems that the loss of cell cycle regulation due to deletion or mutation in *p16* is a contributing factor to the development of melanoma (27) and, possibly, other tumors (28).

Another tumor suppressor gene, *p53*, is the most commonly altered gene in human cancers (29). Germline missense mutations in the *p53* gene (in heterozygous individuals) are associated with *Li–Fraumeni syndrome*, a cancer-prone genetic disease (30). Both copies of the gene must be inactivated for tumor formation to occur (see below). In normal individuals, this is a rare event, since two independent *p53* mutations (or "hits") must accumulate in a cell. In the genetic disease, one copy is already knocked out, so the transformation event is just a "one-hit" process.

The many biological roles of p53 protein are now the subject of intense research interest. The cellular functions of p53 protein center on control of the cell cycle (31) and depend on the DNA-binding properties of the protein. The p53 protein binds to DNA sequences containing four repeats of a 5-bp consensus sequence; this reflects the tetrameric structure of the protein (32). As with many other DNA-binding proteins, p53 contains distinct domains involved in DNA binding and oligomerization. The DNA-binding property of p53 is lost in tumorigenic *p53* mutants (33).

p53 protein is thought to enhance the fidelity of the DNA replication process, by acting as a cell cycle "checkpoint" (34). Eukaryotic cells which suffer severe DNA damage undergo a characteristic series of degradative processes, including proteolysis, degradation of chromosomal DNA, and dismantling of the cytoskeleton, culminating in cell disintegration. This process is called *apoptosis* or *programmed cell death* (35). Apoptosis is a normal, "programmed" biological event, occurring during development (e.g., the loss of a tadpole's tail as it matures into a frog) and permitting the turnover of differentiated cells in most mature tissues.* Alternatively, apoptosis can be triggered by DNA damage induced by genotoxic chemicals or radiation. In this latter context, apoptosis can be regarded as a control mechanism or "safety valve" for ridding the organism of severely damaged or excessively mutagenized cells (36). *Functional p53 protein is essential for induction of apoptosis in mutagenized cells.* This role of p53 may explain why loss of p53 function is associated with malignancies. The failure of apoptosis permits transformed cells to escape from the normal regulation of cell proliferation (37).

Targeted gene disruption (38) was used to construct transgenic mice, either homozygous or heterozygous for a mutation which removes much of the *p53* gene coding region, eliminating biosynthesis of the p53 protein (39). Homozygous $p53^\Delta/p53^\Delta$ mice were viable and fertile, but had enormously enhanced susceptibility to cancer. Most animals die within 6 months, from lymphomas, osteosaracomas, teratomas, and other cancers. Heterozygotes (an animal model of the human Li–Fraumeni syndrome) had slightly reduced life spans and increased cancer rates, compared to animals with wild-type p53.

In many tumors involving *p53* mutations, one allele is deleted and the second allele is disrupted by a missense mutation. The type of mutation in *p53* is specific for a particular tumor type and etiology. For example, liver cancers from patients who may have been exposed to aflatoxin have frequent mutations at codon 249, whereas *p53* mutations in colon cancers are found primarily at codons 175, 248, 273, and 282. This suggests that the mutagens responsible for specific tumors may leave their mutational "fingerprints" on the tumor suppressor gene. Since tumor suppressor genes are inactivated by many different mutations, whereas oncogenes are activated only by a few specific mutations, the former are more useful targets for study of the mutational specificity of carcinogens. By analogy to bacterial mutation assays, we may say that tumor suppressor genes correspond to forward mutation assays whereas oncogenes correspond to reversion assays.

---

*Apoptosis should be distinguished from *necrosis* (acute cell death) caused, for example, by mechanical trauma or viral infection. Necrosis is characterized by sudden loss of membrane integrity, release of the cell's contents into the tissue spaces, and consequent inflammation.

NOTES

1. "Nongenotoxic" carcinogens include growth hormones, which promote mitosis and tissue growth; physical carcinogens (e.g., inert materials implanted subcutaneously) which cause inflammation and cell proliferation; and some compounds which induce xenobiotic-metabolizing enzymes.

2. Varmus, J., and Weinberg, R. A., *Genes and the Biology of Cancer*, Scientific American Books, W. H. Freeman, New York, 1993; Weinberg, R. A., The molecular basis of oncogenes and tumor suppressor genes. *Ann. N.Y. Acad. Sci.* 758:331–338, 1995.

3. Watson, J. D., Hopkins, N. H., Roberts, J. W., Steitz, J. A., and Weiner, A. M., *Molecular Biology of the Gene*, Vol. II, 4th ed., Benjamin/Cummings, Menlo Park, CA, 1987, Chapter 26.

4. Sugden, B., How some retroviruses got their oncogenes, *Trends Biochem. Sci.* 18:233–235, 1993.

5. Parada, L. F., Tabin, C. J., Shih, C., and Weinberg, R. A., Human EJ bladder carcinoma oncogene is homologue of Harvey sarcoma virus ras gene, *Nature* 297:474–478, 1982.

6. Linder, M. E., and Gilman, A. G., G proteins, *Sci. Am.* 267(July):56–65, 1992; Stryer, L., *Biochemistry*, 4th ed., W. H. Freeman, New York, 1995, pp. 355–356.

7. McKenzie, S. J., Diagnostic utility of oncogenes and their products in human cancer, *Biochim. Biophys. Acta* 1072:193–214, 1991.

8. Hall, A., Ras-related proteins, *Curr. Opin. Cell Biol.* 5:265–268, 1993.

9. McCormick, F., How receptors turn Ras on, *Nature* 363:15–16, 1993.

10. Diamandis, E.P., Oncogenes and tumor suppressor genes: new biochemical tests, *Crit. Rev. Clin. Lab. Sci.* 29:269–305, 1992.

11. Zarbl, H., Sukumar, S., Arthur, A. V., Martin-Zanca, D., and Barbacid, M., Direct mutagenesis of Ha-*ras*-1 oncogenes by *N*-nitroso-*N*-methylurea during initiation of mammary carcinogenesis in rats, *Nature* 315:382–385, 1985. This result could indicate that MNU induces mutations with extraordinary specificity. However, further analysis of the distribution of mutant cells in MNU-treated mammary tissue was interpreted as indicating that the *ras* mutations were present *before* MNU treatment: Cha, R. S., Thilly, W. G., and Zarbl, H., *N*-Nitroso-*N*-methylurea-induced rat mammary tumors arise from cells with preexisting oncogenic *Hras1* gene mutations, *Proc. Natl. Acad. Sci. U.S.A.* 91:3749–3753, 1994.

12. Groffen, J., Stephenson, J. R., Heisterkamp, N., de Klein, A., Bartram, C. R., and Grosveld, G., Philadelphia chromosome breakpoints are clustered within a limited region, bcr, on chromosome 22, *Cell* 36:93–99, 1984.

13. Konopka, J. B., Watanabe, S. M., and Witte, O. N., An alteration of the human c-abl protein in K562 leukemia cells unmasks associated tyrosine kinase activity, *Cell* 37:1035–1042, 1984.

14. Rabbits, T. H., and Boehm, T., *Adv. Immun.* 50:119–146, 1991.

15. Amati, B., Brooks, M. W., Levy, N., Littlewood, T. D., Evans, G. I., and Land, H., Oncogenic activty of the c-Myc protein requires dimerization with Max, *Cell* 72:233–245, 1993.

16. Penn, L. J. Z., Laufer, E. M., and Land, H., c-Myc: evidence for multiple regulatory functions, *Semin. Cancer Biol.* 1:69–80, 1990.

17. Sager, R., Genetic suppression of tumor formation, *Adv. Cancer Res.* 44:43–68, 1985.

18. Levine, A. J., The tumor suppressor genes, *Annu. Rev. Biochem.* 62:623–651, 1993.

19. Stanbridge, E. J., A genetic basis of tumor suppression, in: *Genetic Analysis of Tumor Suppression*, G. Bock and J. Marsh, Eds., John Wiley & Sons, Chichester, 1989, pp. 149–165.

20. Cavenee, W. K., Hansen, M. F., Scable, H. J., and James, C. D., Loss of genetic information in cancer, in: *Genetic Analysis of Tumor Suppression*, G. Bock and J. Marsh, Eds., John Wiley & Sons, Chichester, 1989, pp. 79–92.

21. Goodrich, D. W., and Lee, W.-H., Molecular characterization of the retinoblastoma susceptibility gene, *Biochim. Biophys. Acta* 1155:43–61, 1993.

22. Dunn, J. M., Zhu, X., Gallie, B. L., and Phillips, R. A., Characterization of mutation in the RB1 gene, in: *Recessive Oncogenes and Tumor Suppression*, W. Cavanee, N. Hastie, and E. Stanbridge, Eds., Cold Spring Harbor Laboratory Press, Cold Spring Harbor, NY, 1989, pp. 93–100.

23. Miki, Y., Swensen, J., Shattuck-Eidens, D., Futreal, P. A., Harshman, K., Tavtigian, S., Liu,

Q., Cochran, C., Bennett, L. M., Ding, W., Bell, R., Rosenthal, J., Hussey, C., Tran, T., Mc-Clure, M., Frye, C., Hattier, T., Phelps, R., Haugen-Strano, A., Katcher, H., Yakumo, K., Gholami, Z., Shaffer, D., Stone, S., Bayer, S., Wray, C., Bogden, R., Dayananth, P., Ward, J., Tonin, P., Narod, S., Bristow, P. K., Norris, F.H., Helvering, L., Morrison, P., Rosteck, P., Lai, M., Barrett, J. C., Lewis, C., Neuhausen, S., Cannon-Albright, L., Goldgar, D., Wiseman, R., Kamb, A., and Skolnick, M. H., A strong candidate for the breast and ovarian cancer susceptibility gene *BRCA1*, *Science* 266:66–71, 1994.

24. Castilla, L. H., Couch, F. J., Erdos, M. R., Hoskins, K. F., Calzone, K., Garber, J. E., Boyd, J., Lubin, M. B., Deshano, M. L., Brody, L. C., Collins, F. S., and Weber, B. L., Mutations in the *BRCA1* gene in families with early-onset breast and ovarian cancer, *Nature Genet.* 8:387–391, 1994.

25. Kamb, A., Gruis, N. A., Weaver-Feldhaus, J., Liu, Q., Harshman, K., Tavtigian, S. V., Stockert, E., Day, R. S., Johnson, B. E., and Skolnick, M. H., A cell cycle regulator potential involved in genesis of many tumour types, *Science* 264:436–440, 1994.

26. Hussussian, C. J., Struewing, J. P., Goldstein, A. M., Higgins, P. A. T., Ally, D. S., Sheahan, M. D., Clark, W. H., Tucker, M. A., and Dracopoli, N. C., Germline p16 mutations in familial melanoma, *Nature Genet.* 8:15–21, 1994.

27. Maestro, R., and Boiocchi, M., Sunlight and melanoma: an answer from MTS1 (p16), *Science* 267:15–16, 1995; Kamb, A., Sunlight and melanoma: an answer from MTS1 (p16). Response, *Science* 267:16, 1995.

28. Marx, J., Link to hereditary melanoma brightens mood for p16 gene, *Science* 265:1364–1365, 1994.

29. Hollstein, M., Sidransky, D., Vogelstein, B., and Harris, C. C., p53 Mutations in human cancers, *Science* 253:49–53, 1991; Greenblatt, M. S., Bennett, W. P., Hollstein, M., and Harris, C. C., Mutations in the p53 tumor suppressor gene: clues to cancer etiology and molecular pathogenesis, *Cancer Res.* 54:4855–4878, 1994.

30. Srivastava, S., Zou, Z., Pirollo, K., Blattner, W., and Chang, E. H., Germ-line transmission of a mutated *p53* gene in a cancer-prone fality with Li–Fraumeni syndrome, *Nature* 348:747–749, 1990; Malkin, D., Germline p53 mutations and heritable cancer, *Annu. Rev. Genet.* 28:443–465, 1994.

31. Prives, C., and Manfreid, J. J., The p53 tumor suppressor protein: meeting review, *Genes Dev.* 7:529–534, 1993.

32. Cho, Y., Gorina, S., Jeffrey, P. D., and Pavletich, N. P., Crystal structure of a p53 tumor suppressor–DNA complex: understanding tumorigenic mutations, *Science* 265:346–355, 1994; Jeffrey, P. D., Gorina, S., and Pavletich, N. P., Crystal structure of the tetramerization domain of the p53 tumor suppressor at 1.7 Angstroms, *Science* 267:1498–1502, 1995.

33. Voet, D., and Voet, J. G., *Biochemistry*, 2nd ed., John Wiley & Sons, New York, 1995, pp. 1188–1189.

34. Cox, L. S., and Lane, D. P., Tumour suppressors, kinases and clamps: How p53 regulates the cell cycle in response to DNA damage, *Bioessays* 17:501–508, 1995; Enoch, T., and Norbury, C., Cellular responses to DNA damage: Cell-cycle checkpoints, apoptosis and the roles of p53 and ATM, *Trends Biochem. Sci.* 20:426–430, 1995.

35. Tomei, L. D., and Cope, F. O., Eds., *Apoptosis: The Molecular Basis of Cell Death*, Cold Spring Harbor Laboratory Press, Cold Spring Harbor, NY, 1991; Tomei, L. D., and Cope, F. O., Eds., *Apoptosis II: The Molecular Basis of Apoptosis in Disease*, Cold Spring Harbor Laboratory Press, Cold Spring Harbor, NY, 1994; Cory, S., Apoptosis: fascinating death factor, *Nature* 367:317–318, 1994; Bortner, C. D., Oldenburg, N. B. E., and Cidlowski, J. A., The role of DNA fragmentation in apoptosis, *Trends Cell Biol.* 5:21–26, 1995.

36. Steller, H., Mechanisms and genes of cellular suicide, *Science* 267:1445–1449, 1995.

37. Thompson, C. B., Apoptosis in the pathogenesis and treatment of disease, *Science* 267:1456–1462, 1995.

38. Capecchi, M. R., Targeted gene replacement, *Sci. Am.*, March 1994, pp. 52–59.

39. Jacks, T., Remington, L., Williams, B. O., Schmitt, E. M., Halachmi, S., Bronson, R. T., and Weinberg, R. A., Tumor spectrum analysis in *p53*-mutant mice, *Curr. Biol.* 4:1–7, 1994.

19

POLYCYCLIC AROMATIC HYDROCARBON CARCINOGENESIS

AN OCCUPATIONAL CARCINOGEN

Coal was the fuel of the industrial revolution; within a few generations in the eighteenth century, coal-burning turned much of the beautiful English countryside black. In the years following the Great Fire of London (1666), coal began to replace wood as the major fuel for residential heating in English urban centers. Coal is no longer commonly used for home heating in the developed world, but coal-fired generating stations supply about half of the electric power production, and 20% of total energy utilization, in North America (1990).

Coal furnace chimneys accumulate combustible soot, and chimney fires posed a serious risk if the narrow flues were not cleaned out during the summer months. The task of crawling up a filthy chimney, often in stifling heat, fell to small children (as young as 5) from poor families, working under conditions of virtual slavery. This abuse was so appalling that it prompted Parliament to enact one of the first bills regulating employment standards, in 1788: The minimum age of employment as a sweep was raised to 8, and the practice of forcing children to go up chimneys which were actually *on fire* was prohibited!

> "This here boy, sir, wot the parish wants to 'prentis," said Mr. Gamfield.
> "Aye, my man," said the gentleman in the white waistcoat, with a condescending smile. "What of him?"
> "If the parish vould like him to learn a light pleasant trade, in a good 'spectable chimbley-sweepin' bisness," said Mr. Gamfield, "I wants a 'prentis, and I'm ready to take him." . . .
> "It's a nasty trade," said Mr. Limbkins, when Gamfield had again stated his wish.
> "Young boys have been smothered in chimneys before now," said another gentleman.
> "That's acause they damped the straw afore they lit it in the chimbley to make 'em come down again," said Gamfield; "that's all smoke, and no blaze; veras smoke ain't o' no use at all in makin' a boy come down, for it only sinds him to sleep, and that's wot he likes. Boys is wery obstinit, and wery lazy, gen'lmen, and there's nothink like a good hot blaze to make 'em come down with a run. It's humane, too, gen'lmen, acause, even if they've stuck in the chimbley, roastin' their feet makes 'em struggle to hextricate theirselves." . . .
> At length . . . Mr. Limbkins said:
> "We have considered your proposition, and we don't approve of it."
>
> Charles Dickens, *Oliver Twist* (1837), Chapter III

In 1775, the eminent surgeon Sir Percivall Pott (1713–1788) observed, in his volume *Chirurgical Works*, that chimney sweeps in London had a very high rate of scrotal cancer. This was the first published description of an occupational cancer. Several aspects of the disease are worth noting, since they were repeated in many subsequent instances of occupational carcinogenesis. First, the disease was hardly ever seen among the general population. Second, the workers suffered repeated exposure to the causative agent (coal soot) at very high levels, extended over years of employment (if they survived the many other life-threatening dangers of the job). Third, the cancer was *site-specific*; since the site affected was a rare one, the connection between the exposure and the disease could be perceived by an insightful clinical observer. Indeed, the link was probably understood by the workers themselves, well before Pott's published findings; sweeps called it the "sooty wart." Despite the gradual improvement in working conditions and general hygiene, the disease was still prevalent among chimney sweeps in Victorian times.

Coal is converted to coke by pyrolysis in the absence of air, supported by the oxygen present in natural coal. Subsequent distillation yields coal gas (CH_4 and other light hydrocarbons), light oil, naphthalene, and other industrial products. The heavy black residue which this process leaves behind is called "coal tar." Millions of tons of this material are produced annually in many industrialized countries. Coal tar can be further processed to yield creosote, asphalt, and pitch, which are used in paving and roofing. Skin cancer and scrotal cancer were reported among workers in coal tar plants and paraffin factories in Germany and England, beginning in the 1880s. (The author reports that industrial roofing practices have changed little in the past century: Shortly after I wrote this section, the roof of the building in which I work was recoated, and a stinking cauldron of black tar bubbled, just outside my window, for 2 weeks!)

Could the association between exposure to coal tar and cancer be demonstrated experimentally? Which particular chemicals in coal tar and soot were the cause of the disease? An animal model was needed to address these questions. Several attempts to induce tumors in animals by treatment with materials such as soot and paraffin were unsuccessful. Finally, in 1915 the physician Yamagiwa and his assistant Ichikawa, in Tokyo, applied coal tar to the inside skin of rabbits' ears and persisted with the treatment protocol, three times a week, for 3 months. Toward the end of this period, the rabbits developed proliferative lesions (papillomas) and, eventually, malignant carcinomas. Soon afterwards, Tsutsui showed that coal tar also caused skin cancer in mice—a much smaller species and easier to maintain in the laboratory. These achievements mark the beginning of the science of experimental chemical carcinogenesis, and they provided a bioassay which could be used to guide the purification of the active constituents of complex mixtures.

The search for the active component of coal tar was undertaken by Kennaway and colleagues, in England (1). Two approaches were attempted simultaneously: synthesizing new polycyclic aromatic hydrocarbons (a relatively unexplored branch of organic chemistry in those days) and fractionating the coal tar. With both approaches, testing for biological activity on mouse skin was a crucial guide to progress. In 1922, Kennaway (2) determined that the active compound had a high boiling point and contained no detectable nitrogen or sulfur. This evidence was consistent with the hypothesis that the active material was a polycyclic aromatic hydrocarbon, such as anthracene. By 1929, Cook and Kennaway had synthesized dozens of new polycyclic aromatic hydrocarbons and had more than 100 mouse skin painting experiments underway! A positive result was finally obtained in 1930 with synthetic dibenz[*a,h*]anthracene:

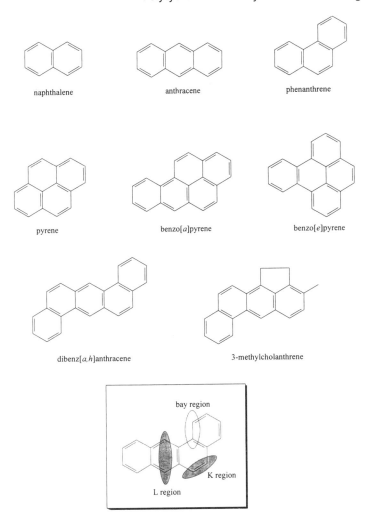

naphthalene   anthracene   phenanthrene

pyrene   benzo[a]pyrene   benzo[e]pyrene

dibenz[a,h]anthracene   3-methylcholanthrene

bay region

K region

L region

For the first time, a single pure chemical had been shown to induce cancer in animals. The demonstration of the carcinogenicity of this polycyclic aromatic hydrocarbon facilitated the isolation of the coal-tar carcinogen. In particular, the observed intense fluorescence of dibenz[a,h]anthracene led the research group to focus their attention on the fluorescent polycyclic components of coal tar.

Two tons of pitch were distilled and extracted with various organic solvents; fractions were tested on mice. By a tedious process of sequential extractions and crystallizations, increasingly active fractions were obtained. After 2 years of these heroic labors, 7 grams of highly active yellow crystals was obtained. By 1933, the active coal-tar carcinogen had been identified as benzo[a]pyrene. The research trail pioneered by Yamagiwa and Ichikawa had culminated in the successful identification of an environmental carcinogen. Later studies have confirmed that benzo[a]pyrene is the most important (although not the only) carcinogenic compound in coal tar and soot.

SIDEBAR: MOLECULAR ORBITAL THEORY OF POLYCYCLIC AROMATIC HYDROCARBONS

Understanding the toxicology of polycyclic aromatic hydrocarbons presents an intriguing challenge: While some compounds are potent carcinogens (e.g., benzo[a]pyrene), close analogues may be inactive (benzo[e]pyrene). Polycyclic aromatic hydrocarbons are particularly amenable to theoretical analysis, because of their structural simplicity. Not surprisingly, then, many attempts have been made to develop a theoretical framework for predicting the biological activity of these compounds. The early efforts in this regard (beginning in the 1950s) were limited to the analysis of the molecular structures of the parent polycyclic aromatic hydrocarbons, because the crucial importance of metabolic activation was not yet understood. More recently, attention has turned to understanding the properties of activated metabolites.

Let's consider some features of the chemistry of the fused-ring polycyclic aromatic hydrocarbons, beginning with the simpler examples such as naphthalene and phenanthrene. In the case of benzene, all bonds are equivalent, by symmetry, and, not surprisingly, have a bond length (1.39 Å) about halfway between that of a $C-C$ single bond and $C=C$ double bond. *This symmetry is broken in fused polycyclic aromatic hydrocarbons.* We can see the effects of asymmetry by simple evaluation of resonance hybrid structures; quantum mechanical analysis bears out these general features. If we consider the five possible resonance hybrid structures of phenanthrene, we see that the 9,10 carbon–carbon bond, isolated from the biphenyl substructure of the remainder of the molecule, bears a double bond in four of the five:

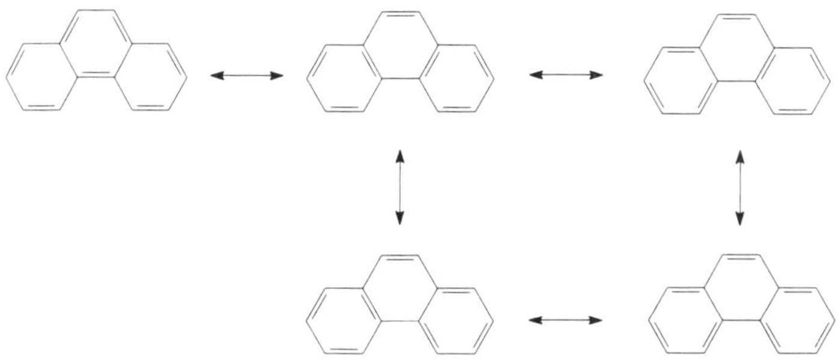

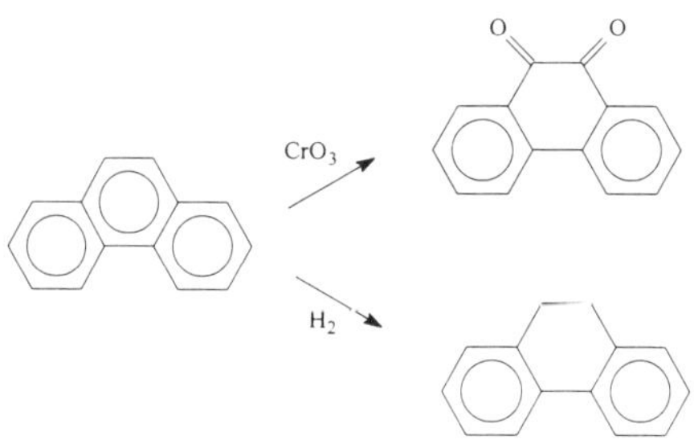

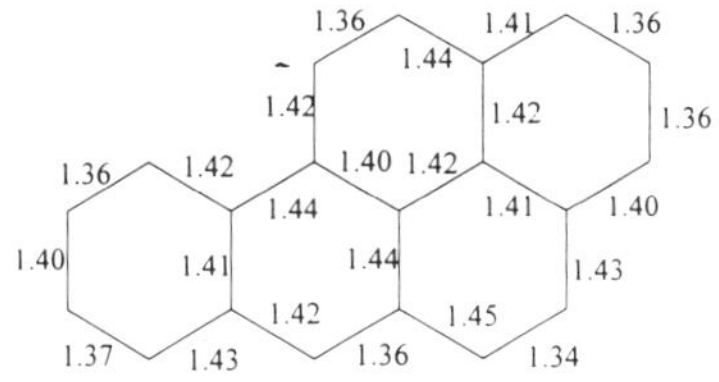

benzo[a]pyrene

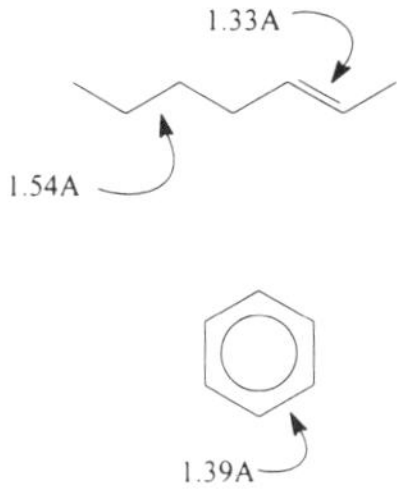

We would expect this bond to be particularly "alkene-like" in its reactivity. The same consideration applies to the 4,5 and 9,10 carbon–carbon bonds of pyrene. This region of high π-electron density is known as the K-region, following the notation introduced by A. and B. Pullman, who pioneered the theoretical study of the chemistry of polycyclic aromatic hydrocarbons in the 1950s.

Crystallography confirms the double-bond character of the K-region: The K-region bond of pyrene, for example, has a bond length of only 1.34 Å, almost the same as that of a typical alkene. The K-region bonds are also particularly reactive. For example, oxidation of phenanthrene with CrO_3 gives red-orange 9,10-phenanthrenequinone, and catalytic hydrogenation of phenanthrene gives 9,10-dihydrophenanthrene; both reactions are entirely regiospecific. Oxidation with hypochlorite or *meta*-chloroperoxybenzoic acid gives the K-region arene oxides (epoxides; see below) (3). The K-region is also a major site of metabolic oxidation.

Two other structural features of polycyclic aromatic hydrocarbons are commonly mentioned in the literature. The so-called "L-region" is the site corresponding to the 9,10-position of anthracene. The "bay region" is the relatively hindered "inner corner" region in phenanthrene and compounds that contain a phenanthrene substructure, such as chrysene and benzo[a]pyrene. We only use the term "bay region" when this structure has a terminal ring on one side:

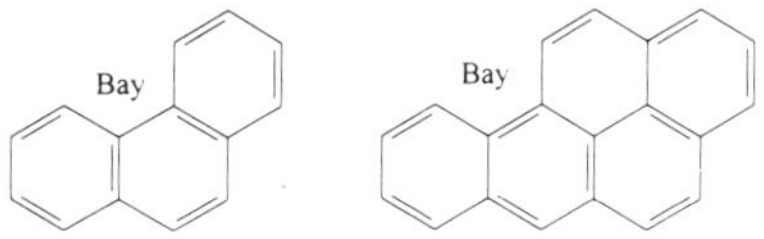

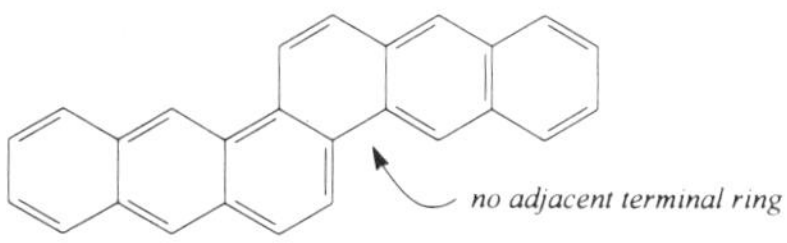

no bay regions in this PAH

As we will see on page 334, metabolic oxidation of the terminal ring is a crucial step in bioactivation of polycyclic aromatic hydrocarbons.

A rigorous theoretical study of the chemistry of polycyclic aromatic hydrocarbons (or any other molecules, for that matter) must be based on quantum mechanical principles. In this section, the elements of the molecular orbital analysis of polycyclic aromatic hydrocarbon structures are presented in a nonmathematical way. We will see that quantum mechanical analysis can readily explain some of the typical features of the chemical behavior of these molecules.

Molecular orbital theory describes the electronic structure of molecules in terms of molecular orbitals constructed from linear combinations of atomic orbitals. As in the simpler case of homonuclear diatomic molecules (4), we can construct a manifold of molecular orbitals for a given molecule; each molecular orbital has a defined energy. In the molecular electronic ground state, electrons fill the molecular orbitals in order, from the lowest energy upwards. Each orbital accommodates two electrons, with opposite spins.

In the case of polycyclic aromatic hydrocarbons, these molecular orbitals are delocalized over the entire conjugated framework. The molecular orbitals at lowest energy have the greatest amount of bonding character. Four of the 14 π molecular orbitals for anthracene are shown below:

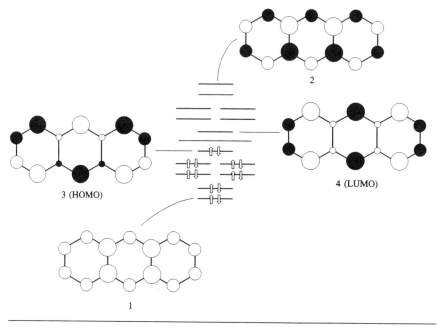

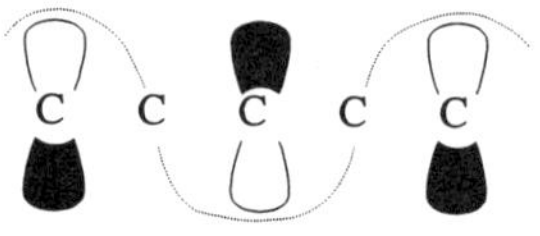

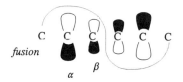

non-bonding MO

typical HOMO

In these sketches, the molecule is viewed from the top. The contribution of each $2p$ atomic orbital to the molecular orbital (MO) is illustrated by the size of the circle (representing the top lobe of the $2p$ orbital). Shaded and unshaded lobes have opposite phases; that is, the shading represents the sign of the atomic orbital's contribution to the molecular orbital wavefunction.

MO1 shows phase agreement (π bonding) between every neighboring pair of carbon atoms. As a result, MO1 is the lowest-energy π molecular orbital. The second molecular orbital illustrated (MO2) shows phase *disagreements* between every pair of neighbors; hence MO2 is at the top of the energy spectrum. In fact, this molecular orbital is just the same as the first, but with each of the phase agreements reversed: MO2 is just as *antibonding* as MO1 is bonding. Hence these two molecular orbitals are referred to as "paired." It can be shown that for π systems containing no odd-numbered rings, *all* the molecular orbitals are paired, at a simple level of quantum mechanical approximation (Hückel theory). Each pair of molecular orbitals straddles the midpoint of the energy spectrum and has the same magnitudes of atomic orbital contributions, but with phases reversed at every other carbon.

The third molecular orbital (MO3) in the preceding scheme shows both phase agreements and disagreements between neighbors. MO3 lies just below the midpoint of the energy spectrum and has a partner (MO4) just *above* the midpoint. It is easily seen that the MO4 can be constructed from MO3 by reversing the phase of every second atomic orbital.

Each carbon atom in the conjugated system uses three of its valence electrons for covalent bonding to its three neighbors (either carbon or hydrogen atoms), through σ bonds. This leaves one electron for contribution to the π system. Anthracene, with 14 conjugated carbons, has 14 π electrons to distribute among the 14 π molecular orbitals. These electrons are placed pairwise, with opposite spins, in the seven lowest-energy molecular orbitals. As a result, any hydrocarbon (without odd-numbered rings) has all π molecular orbitals in the lower half of the energy spectrum filled, and all molecular orbitals above the energy midpoint empty, in its ground electronic state.

Some correlation is observed between those atoms whose atomic orbital coefficients are most prominent contributors to a molecular orbital and that molecular orbital's position in the energy spectrum. Thus the carbon atoms at the ring fusion sites (which are the atoms with the largest number of carbon neighbors) dominate in the lowest-energy molecular orbital and its partner. This arises because these are just the positions from which a π atomic orbital can achieve the most bonding (or antibonding) character, due to the larger number of carbon neighbors. Less-well-connected carbons tend to be dominant in the molecular orbitals nearer the center of the energy spectrum. These characteristics can be seen in the anthracene molecular orbitals (see preceding scheme).

The correlation of molecular orbital energy with atomic orbital dominance is important, because molecular orbital theory uses these two factors in predicting the relative reactivities of different sites in polycyclic aromatic hydrocarbons. A frequently used shortcut in reactivity predictions is to focus only on the highest occupied molecular orbital (HOMO). (Often, the atomic orbitals dominating the HOMO turn out to be the same ones dominating the whole set of molecular orbitals near the energy midpoint.) The partner of this molecular orbital is the lowest unfilled molecular orbital (LUMO). Focusing on these orbitals as a key to understanding chemical reactivity is the basis of the *frontier molecular orbital* approach (5).

An effective way to predict the sites where a molecule is more likely to respond to *electrophilic* attack is to identify the sites that dominate the HOMO. These are atoms having a relatively large amount of π electronic charge density that is not being used very effectively for bonding. (That's why the molecular orbital energies are high.) Conversely, a nucleophilic reaction is likely to occur preferentially at an atom that is prominent in the LUMO. This allows the nucleophile to connect its Lewis-base electron pair charge density to an atom that can accept it. But, for polycyclic aromatic hydrocarbons, the HOMO and LUMO are paired; hence, they are dominated by the same atoms. *Thus, molecular orbital theory predicts that the same sites should be favored for either electrophilic or nucleophilic reactions.*

We can already see that molecular orbital theory will predict the most reactive sites of PAHs to be carbons having two, rather than three, nearest-neighbor carbons. This is because the three-neighbor carbons dominate the π molecular orbitals away from the spectral center (that is, above the LUMO or below the HOMO), leaving the two-neighbor carbons to dominate the π molecular orbitals around the spectral center.

But there are many such two-neighbor carbons. Anthracene has three distinct types (positions 1, 2, and 10). Understanding polycyclic aromatic hydrocarbon metabolism requires knowing the relative reactivities of such sites. Inspection of the HOMO, LUMO pair shown in the preceding scheme leads us to predict a reactivity order of $10 > 1 > 2$, and this agrees with experiment.

In general, polycyclic aromatic hydrocarbons show greater reactivity at carbons that are one bond from a fusion site (α) than at those which are two bonds away (β). There is a simple molecular-orbital-based explanation for this (6). A molecular orbital having its energy right at the midpoint of the spectrum (called a *nonbonding molecular orbital*) is characterized by an atomic orbital pattern where every second carbon π atomic orbital has a zero coefficient. The "wavelength" of the envelope of these atomic orbitals is four carbon–carbon bond lengths. The HOMO in a polycyclic aromatic hydrocarbon lies a bit below the energy midpoint and, hence, has a wavelength slightly longer than this (typically closer to five bond lengths). This gives us a wavelength estimate for a HOMO. We also have a boundary condition, namely, that the *atomic orbital contribution at a fusion site tends to be small* (having been preferentially used up in lowest/highest-energy molecular orbitals). If we draw an envelope wave having wavelength equal to five C–C bonds and place a node at one atom, we find that the resulting wave "dictates" an atomic orbital coefficient that is considerably larger at the carbon one bond from the node than at the carbon two bonds from the node. *This implies that carbons one bond from a fusion site should be more reactive than those two bonds away.* Polycyclic aromatic hydrocarbons sometimes show this pattern very clearly in their HOMO/LUMO pair, as in anthracene. In other cases the connection pattern of the hydrocarbon leads to conflicts that cause this behavior to be spread among several of the higher-energy occupied molecular orbitals. This tends to disguise the cause, but does not alter the general effect: α carbons are more reactive for electrophilic or nucleophilic reactions than are β carbons. In anthracene, carbon atom 10 is α to *two* fusion sites. Such atoms tend to be especially reactive. Atoms of this kind constitute the "L-region," referred to above.

ARENE OXIDES

As early as 1950, Boyland pointed out that epoxides were likely intermediates in the metabolism of polycyclic aromatic hydrocarbons. He noted that *trans*-dihydrodiols were isolable metabolites of naphthalene and phenanthrene. Boyland suggested that *epoxides were the probable precursors to the dihydrodiol metabolites of polycyclic aromatic hydrocarbons.* It had long been understood that the hydrolysis of epoxides proceeds by an S_N2 attack of hydroxide, with resulting stereochemical (Walden) inversion. Thus, for example, the epoxidation and hydrolysis of cyclohexene gives *trans*-cyclohexane-1,2-diol (see lower part of scheme). Polycyclic aromatic hydrocarbon dihydrodiols might arise in the same manner.

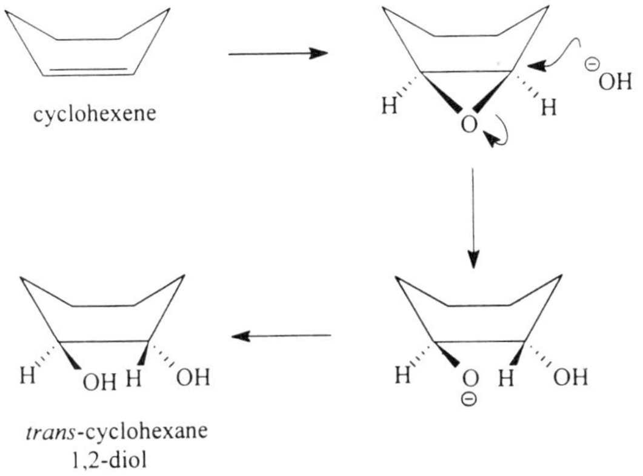

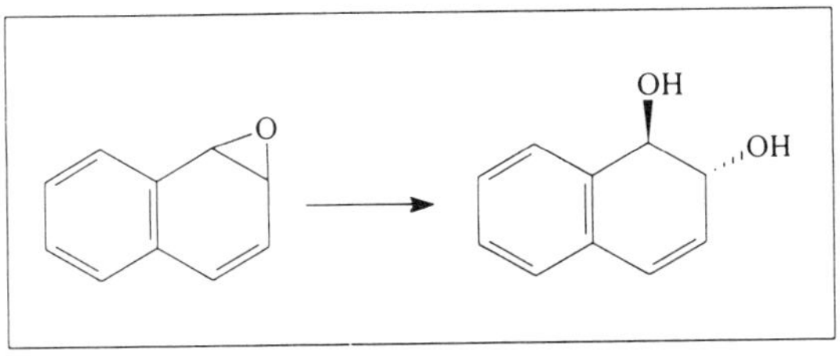

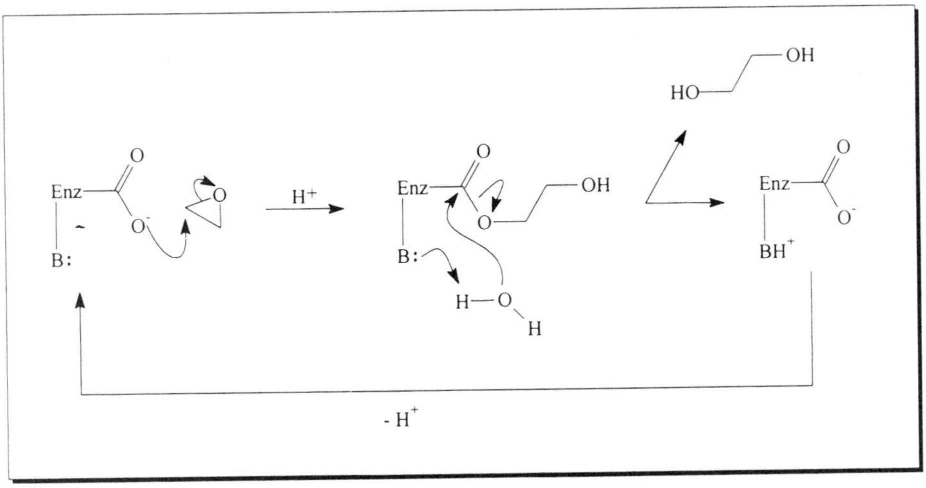

cyclohexene

trans-cyclohexane
1,2-diol

Epoxidation of a polycyclic aromatic hydrocarbon introduces two asymmetric carbon atoms. The three-membered epoxide ring projects either above or below the six-membered ring to which it is attached (7). Thus, two enantiomeric naphthalene 1,2-oxides can be formed.

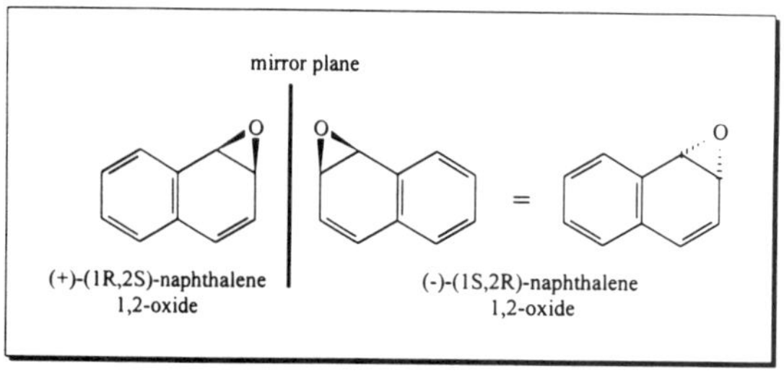

At the time of Boyland's suggestion, arene oxides (the aromatic analogues of olefinic epoxides) were completely unknown. However, with the development of the chemistry of arene oxides, discussed below, Boyland's idea was shown to be correct, and it led to a breakthrough in understanding the toxicity of polycyclic aromatic hydrocarbons. Epoxides are highly reactive because of the strained three-membered ring structure, and the formation of these reactive intermediates suggests an answer to the riddle posed by the potent biological activity of compounds as inherently *unreactive* as hydrocarbons. *Carcinogens are metabolized to reactive intermediates.* This hypothesis was advanced by Elizabeth and James Miller of the McCardle Cancer Research Center, University of Wisconsin.

POLYCYCLIC AROMATIC HYDROCARBONS: METABOLISM AND BIOACTIVATION

In the early 1950s, Elizabeth Miller determined that a metabolite of benzo[*a*]pyrene reacts with the proteins in mouse skin (8). Benzo[*a*]pyrene was painted onto the skin of the animals, and the skin proteins were isolated. Unmetabolized benzo[*a*]pyrene was extracted with organic solvents. The purified protein residue left after extraction was fluorescent, and the fluorescence spectrum resembled that of benzo[*a*]pyrene. Clearly, some reactive metabolite (or metabolites) of the parent hydrocarbon became bound to the protein, and this binding was too strong to be disrupted by exhaustive washings: It was apparently covalent binding.

Miller referred to the then-unknown reactive metabolite as the *ultimate carcinogen*, and he asserted that covalent binding was the key step in bioactivation of polycyclic aromatic hydrocarbon carcinogens. Studies by Miller and Miller on the covalent binding of carcinogenic aminoazo dyes reached similar conclusions, and they suggested that metabolic activation-covalent binding might be a general paradigm for chemical carcinogenesis. Indeed, in the subsequent decades the concept of metabolic activation to reactive intermediates has been verified and extended to several major classes of carcinogens, including aromatic amines and nitrosamines (see Chapter 20).

Since this view has now come to be dogmatic, it is worth remembering that in the 1950s it was novel and controversial. Previous theories of polycyclic aromatic hydrocarbon car-

cinogenesis had been based on quite different concepts, including noncovalent interactions (such as intercalation into DNA) or the actions of hydrocarbons as structural/functional analogues of steroid hormones.

Following the elucidation of the double-helix structure of DNA, the crucial role of nucleic acids as the repository of genetic information was generally appreciated. Cancer had long been suspected to result from chromosomal or genetic changes, so attention soon turned to the nucleic acids as targets for the action of chemical carcinogens.

In 1961, Heidelberger and Davenport demonstrated that ^{14}C-labeled dibenz[*a,h*]anthracene painted onto mouse skin became bound to nucleic acids. DNA was isolated from the skin tissue and freed from contaminating protein and RNA by digestion with proteases and ribonuclease, and covalent binding to DNA was observed. Brookes and Lawley (9) compared the extent of DNA binding by a series of ^{3}H-labeled polycyclic aromatic hydrocarbons, and they reported that the extent of binding correlated with carcinogenic potency. This was consistent with the hypothesis that covalent binding is a prerequisite to chemical carcinogenesis.

SIDEBAR: PAH–DNA BINDING IN VIVO

Although DNA is a biologically important target for covalent binding, it is not present in large amounts in the cell. The composition of liver tissue, for example, is approximately 70% water, 20% protein, 5% lipid, 1% RNA, and only 0.2% DNA, by weight (10). *The fraction of administered dose of a carcinogen which is metabolized to DNA adducts is exceedingly small.* For example, Stowers and Anderson (11) administered ^{3}H-labeled benzo[*a*]pyrene orally to mice, at a dose of 6 mg (about 25 μmol) per mouse. The recovery of DNA adducts in the liver tissue was less than 10 pmol per milligram of DNA. Since 1 gram of liver tissue (wet weight) contains about 2 mg of DNA, this corresponds to about 20 pmol (2×10^{-11} mol) per gram liver, or per mouse. Thus, only about 1 part per million of the administered dose is recovered as hepatic DNA adducts. Similar levels of DNA binding were found in other tissues. Protein specific binding levels were much higher (about 300 pmol per milligram of protein), and total protein mass is about 100 times greater than DNA mass. Clearly, *it is far easier to detect protein binding than DNA binding in vivo*, and the amount of DNA-bound metabolite that can be isolated in vivo is exceedingly small.

Now, the central quest became defined as the search for the ultimate carcinogen. As we will see later, it is now clear that the K-region epoxides, while formed as metabolites, are *not* the key bioactivated forms of polycyclic aromatic hydrocarbons. Instead, the *bay-region dihydrodiol epoxides*, which are chemically a very different class of metabolites, are the most important ultimate carcinogenic metabolites. Before we turn to a discussion of these species, however, the K-region epoxides warrant some further consideration.

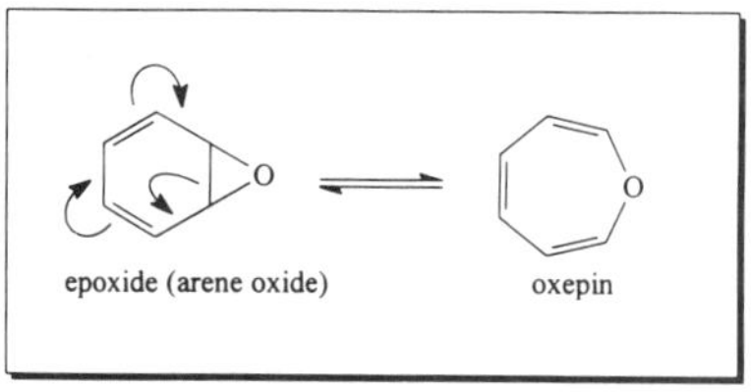

epoxide (arene oxide)   oxepin

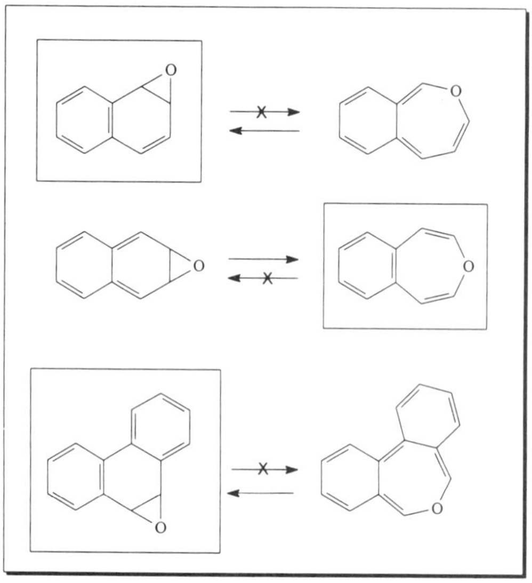

ARENE OXIDE CHEMISTRY: THE NIH SHIFT

The first arene oxide, the K-region 9,10-oxide of phenanthrene, was synthesized by New-man and Blum in 1964. In the following years, a great deal of synthetic and mechanistic progress was made (see ref. 3 for details). Arene oxides can, in principle, rearrange to the isomeric *oxepins* (see preceding scheme), in which the carbon–carbon bond of the epox-ide ring has broken to form a seven-membered ring incorporating the oxygen atom. The equilibrium between the arene oxide and oxepin forms depends on their relative thermo-dynamic stabilities. The colorless benzene oxide rapidly interconverts with the isomeric, conjugated, yellow oxepin valence-bond tautomer. In the case of the naphthalene 1,2- and 2,3-oxides, the forms with aromatic benzene rings predominate—that is, the epoxide form of the former compound and the oxepin form of the latter.

As pointed out above, the epoxide ring can exist in two optically enantiomeric forms ("above" and "below" the plane of the aromatic rings). Reversible equilibration with the oxirane form, of course, results in racemization (loss of optical activity) of an initially pure enantiomer and can be used as a probe of oxepin formation. All K-region epoxides which have been studied exist only in the epoxide form, as would be expected from a consideration of aromaticity (see preceding scheme). Again, this behavior reflects the alkene-like properties of the K-region double bond.

Another important piece of evidence for the metabolic formation of arene oxides was the discovery of the "NIH shift" (12); see also Chapter 14. The first evidence for this shift came from studies on the metabolism of acetanilide by liver microsomes:

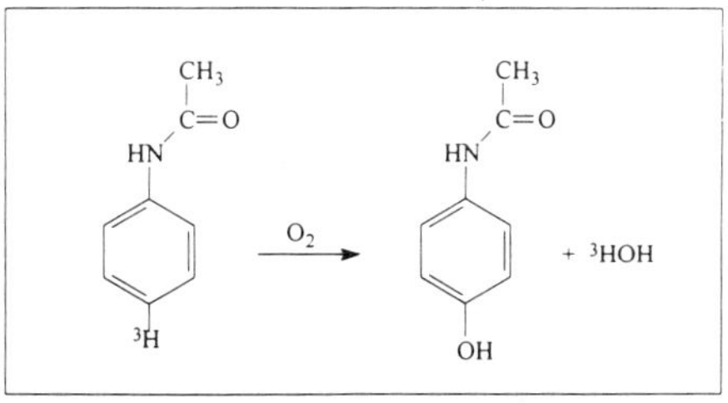

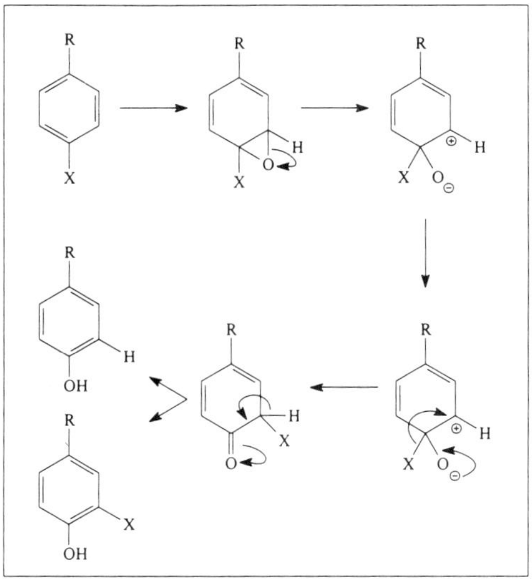

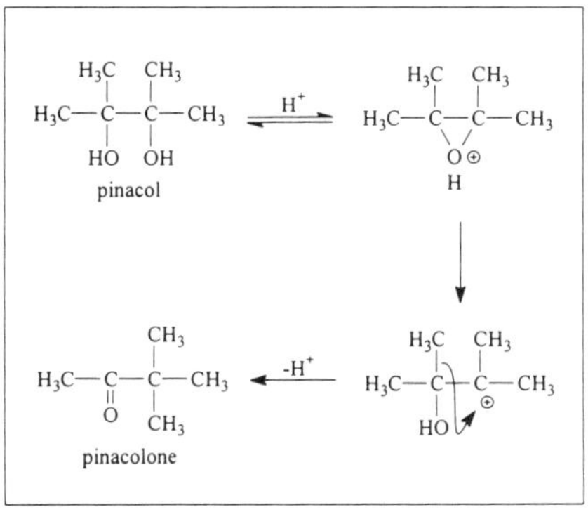

Acetanilide is hydroxylated to *para*-hydroxyacetanilide, in what is now known to be a typical P-450-catalyzed monooxygenase reaction. Udenfriend and colleagues (12) reasoned that a simple enzyme assay for this activity could be devised: They synthesized [4-^{3}H]acetanilide, and they expected that the amount of tritium radioactivity released as tritiated water (HTO) would equal the amount of product *para*-hydroxyacetanilide formed. They were perplexed to discover that the amount of tritium released was variable, and much less than the amount of organic product formed, as measured by a colorimetric assay. Perhaps the radiolabel had been misincorporated into another position on the ring? But the same phenomenon was observed in the enzymatic conversion of [4-^{3}H]phenylalanine into tyrosine. Deuterated [4-^{2}H] substrates were then synthesized; this allowed the position of incorporation, and subsequent fate, of the substituent at the *para* position to be monitored by nuclear magnetic resonance (NMR) spectroscopy. This approach proved that the *para* hydrogen could either be released as water or migrate to the adjacent ring position. This "NIH shift" was subsequently observed for many different aromatic hydroxylation reactions. Not only hydrogen, but also halogen and alkyl substituents, can migrate (13).

What is the mechanism of the NIH shift? The analogous migration of hydrogen, alkyl, or aryl substituents from a β carbon to an adjacent electron-deficient carbon is known as a 1,2-shift and is exemplified by the pinacol rearrangement, discovered by Fittig in 1860 (14). The rearrangement occurs with diols, such as pinacol, and also with epoxides (see preceding scheme). A carbenium ion is formed by the rupture of the epoxide ring, and the migrating substituent moves to this site with its electron pair. In the case of the pinacol rearrangement, the reaction is driven by the favorable formation of the ketone product. By analogy, Jerina and colleagues suggested that the NIH shift proceeded via an arene oxide intermediate, which ruptured to form a carbenium ion. The validity of this model was demonstrated by the direct observation of isotope migration during the isomerization of synthetic arene oxides. For example, [1-^{2}H]-4-methylbenzene 1,2-oxide rearranges to 4-methylphenol and most of the deuterium is retained. *The NIH shift is indirect evidence for the intermediacy of arene oxides in enzymatic aryl hydroxylations.* The first *direct* proof was obtained in 1968, when Jerina and colleagues trapped radiolabeled naphthalene 1,2-oxide as a microsomal metabolite of naphthalene, using unlabeled synthetic oxide as a "trap" for the labile metabolite.

The occurrence of the NIH shift provides a clue to the mechanism of hydroxylation. *The initial products formed in aromatic hydroxylations are epoxides rather than phenols.* However, the epoxides derived from aromatic rings (arene oxides) are much less stable than olefinic epoxides: Cleavage of one of the carbon–oxygen bonds yields a cation which is stabilized by conjugation to the remaining double bonds of the aromatic ring. Formation of this cation initiates the NIH shift rearrangement, which leads to a hydroxylated product. The product is identical to that which would have been formed by direct insertion of oxygen into the C−H bond (15), but a direct mechanism could not account for the NIH shift.

The rearrangement involves shift of a hydride from the carbon retaining the oxygen to the carbocation site, with concomitant formation of the ketone; subsequent proton tautomerization regenerates a fully aromatic ring. The epoxide has two carbon–oxygen bonds, either of which could, in principle, be broken, so the reaction can give rise to two different phenolic products. If cleavage of one of the carbon–oxygen bonds yields a cation that is significantly more stable than that obtained by cleavage of the other, then one product will predominate. For example, if the aromatic ring is substituted with an electron-donating methoxy group, formation of the *para*-hydroxy product is favored; formation of the *meta*-hydroxy product is favored if the substituent is an electron-withdrawing nitro group:

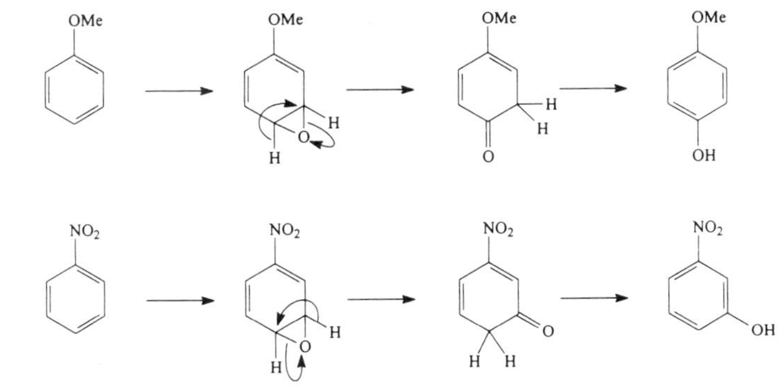

The regiospecificity of the NIH shift expected when the aromatic ring is substituted by an electron-donating methoxy substituent is opposite to that expected when it is substituted by an electron-withdrawing nitro substituent.

The oxidation of aromatic π bonds is subject to mechanistic ambiguities comparable to those that beset the oxidation of simple olefins (Chapter 14). For example, although the epoxides of some aromatic substrates can actually be isolated and shown to undergo the NIH shift, aromatic substrates that have strong electron-donating substituents could possibly proceed to the NIH shift (or other reactions) without actually forming a discrete epoxide intermediate.

This can be envisaged as involving a competition between formation of the second oxygen–carbon bond and electron transfer from the carbon atom to the iron, during the reaction of the aromatic π bond with the ferryl oxygen:

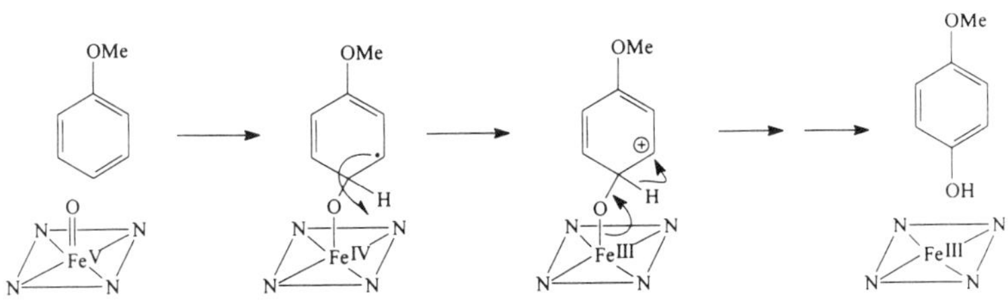

Hydroxylation of aromatic rings with p-electron donor substituents may occur, in some instances, without the actual formation of the epoxide intermediate.

An extreme example of the influence that substituents can have on aromatic ring oxidation is the oxidation of pentafluorophenols to 2,3,5,6-tetrafluoroquinones (16). Recent evidence suggests that oxidation of the polyfluorinated phenol produces a phenoxy radical that combines with the ferryl oxygen at the carbon *para* to the oxygen. The resulting *para*-hydroxylated intermediate eliminates fluoride anion to give the quinone directly:

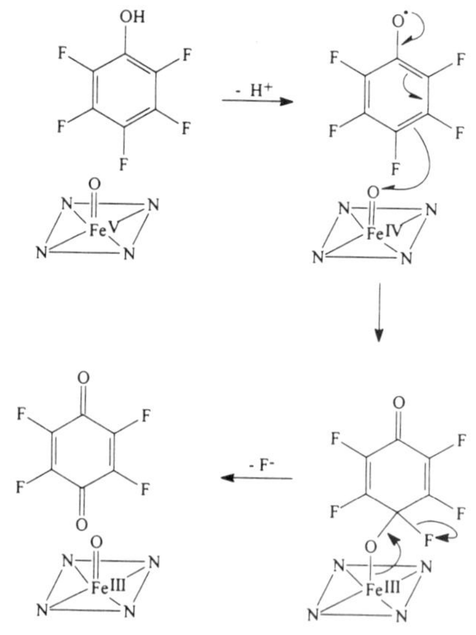

Mechanism for the oxidation of pentafluorophenol that results in fluoride elimination and formation of the tetrafluoro *p*-quinone without formation of an epoxide intermediate.

The reaction with the lowest energy pathway predominates. If substituents sufficiently facilitate electron transfer from the aromatic ring, electron transfer pathways can compete effectively with simple epoxide formation.

METABOLISM OF EPOXIDES

Epoxides metabolites are formed by aromatic hydroxylation, as we have just discussed, and are also common metabolites of olefins, such as the insecticides heptachlor and aldrin, the sedative hexobarbital, and the plastics monomer styrene (17):

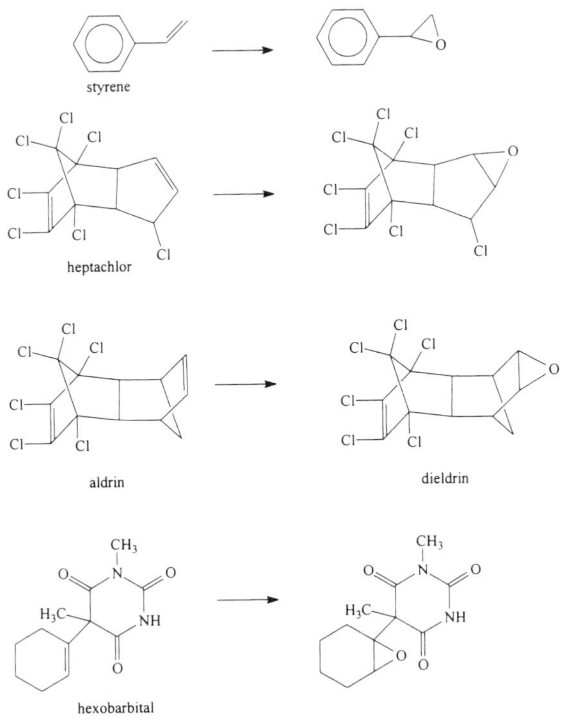

styrene

heptachlor

aldrin   dieldrin

hexobarbital

Before continuing our discussion of polycyclic aromatic hydrocarbon bioactivation, we will consider the metabolism of arene oxides and other epoxides:

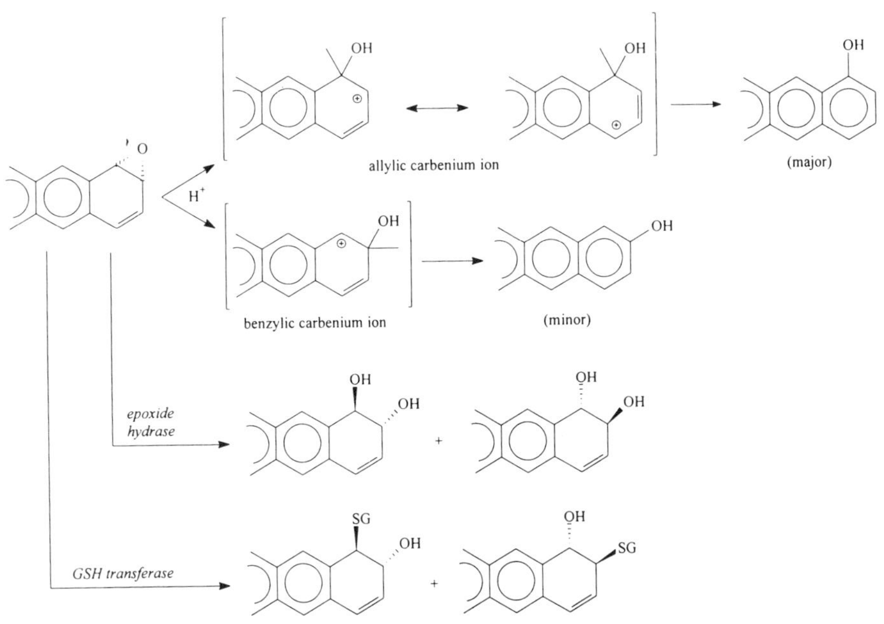

allylic carbenium ion

(major)

benzylic carbenium ion   (minor)

epoxide
hydrase

GSH transferase

The metabolism of an arene oxide metabolite formed at the terminal ring of a polycyclic aromatic hydrocarbon is illustrated. Note that other arene oxides (regioisomers/enantiomers) could also be formed from the parent hydrocarbon, depending on the specificity of the enzyme (cytochrome P-450 form)

EPOXIDE HYDROLASE

Arene oxides and dihydrodiol epoxides are hydrolyzed by a microsomal xenobiotic epoxide hydrolase. (This enzyme has also been called *epoxide hydrase* and *epoxide hydratase*.) The hepatic enzyme can be induced by various agents, including some P-450 inducers, such as phenobarbital. The protein has been purified and the gene has been cloned and sequenced (20). The same enzyme also hydrolyzes many alkene-derived epoxides.

Epoxide hydrolase can be assayed with [³H]styrene oxide as substrate. Following incubation with the enzyme, the substrate is extracted with petroleum ether, and the more polar product, styrene glycol, is extracted with ethyl acetate and quantitated (21). Assays based on chromatographic separation of substrate and product have also been used.

Several forms of epoxide hydrolase have been identified. Cholesterol, a major component of biological membranes, becomes oxidized at the 5,6 double bond during lipid peroxidation. The product, cholesterol 5,6-epoxide, is cytotoxic and may play a role in atherosclerotic processes (22). A steroid-specific epoxide hydrolase metabolizes this compound to cholestane triol. A specific form of the enzyme catalyzes the hydrolysis of leukotriene A₄, an endogenous lipid epoxide derived from arachidonic acid; hydrolysis of leukotriene A₄ yields leukotriene B₄; glutathione conjugation of the epoxide gives rise to leukotrienes C, D, and E (see Chapter 11). A cytosolic epoxide hydrolase also exists (23).

Richard Armstrong, University of Maryland, has proposed a catalytic mechanism for the action of epoxide hydrolase (24). Nucleophilic attack by an active-site carboxylate group on the enzyme generates a transient ester intermediate, which is hydrolyzed to form the diol product and regenerate the enzyme carboxylate (see scheme showing epoxidation and hydrolysis of cyclohexene, page 323).

BAY-REGION DIHYDRODIOL EPOXIDES

As discussed above, the realization that reactive K-region epoxides were metabolic products of polycyclic aromatic hydrocarbons tied in neatly with the observation that these compounds were metabolized to DNA- and protein-binding ultimate carcinogens. Were the K-region epoxides these ultimate reactive species? Indeed, synthetic K-region epoxides were found to cause mutations in bacteria (the Ames assay) and to react with nucleic

---

catalyzing the oxidation. The three major pathways of transformation of the arene oxide are (i) isomerization to phenols, (ii) hydrolysis, catalyzed by epoxide hydrolase, and (iii) glutathione conjugation, catalyzed by glutathione-S-transferase.

Isomerization to phenols proceeds spontaneously by the NIH shift pathway. Here, the acid-catalyzed route is illustrated. The direction of opening of the epoxide ring dictates the phenol isomer formed. The resonance-stabilized allylic intermediate is favored; therefore, for example, naphthalene is metabolized primarily to 1-naphthol, with only a small amount of 2-naphthol formed. Migration (retention) of the substituent originally present at the hydroxylated position (NIH shift) can also occur, but is ignored in this scheme.

Hydrolysis, catalyzed by epoxide hydrolase (see below), generates *trans*-dihydrodiols, since addition of OH⁻ proceeds with inversion of configuration (see scheme showing epoxidation and hydrolysis of cyclohexene, page 323). Both of the enantiomeric *trans*-dihydrodiols can form, depending on the specificity of the enzyme; see ref. 18 for further discussion. Glutathione-S-transferase catalyzes the nucleophilic addition of glutathione to the epoxide, as discussed in Chapter 11. This reaction is analogous to the reaction with water: The products are *trans* glutathione adducts, with the addition of glutathione occurring at either position, under enzymatic control (19).

Note that the terminal ring in the products of arene oxide hydrolysis or glutathione addition is a substituted cyclohexene ring: It is no longer aromatic. Therefore, it is not surprising that the olefinic double bond in this ring is a target for subsequent epoxidation (see text, below).

acids in vitro. However, the role of K-region epoxides had to be reconsidered when they were found to be weak carcinogens in rodents and when the chromatographic characteristics of the epoxide-derived adducts turned out to differ from those of the labeled parent hydrocarbons. Attention then turned to other benzo[*a*]pyrene metabolites (Figure 19.1).

In 1973, Crocker and colleagues (25) studied the microsomal activation of benzo[*a*]pyrene and its 4,5-, 7,8-, and 9,10-dihydrodiol metabolites. Each compound was incubated with DNA and microsomes, and DNA binding was measured. The *trans*-7,8-benzo[*a*]pyrene dihydrodiol was shown to be more than 10 times as potent as benzo[*a*]pyrene or the other dihydrodiols. The dihydrodiol was not directly reactive, but required metabolic activation by the microsomal enzymes. What was the activated metabolite? Since the dihydrodiol metabolites possess an olefinic double bond, epoxidation was an obvious possibility. In 1974, Sims et al. (Chester Beatty Research Institute, Royal Cancer Hospital, London) (26) identified 7,8-benzo[*a*]pyrene dihydrodiol-9,10-epoxide (BPDE) as a potent reactive metabolite of benzo[*a*]pyrene. The key experiments compared the DNA adducts formed from (i) chromosomal DNA prepared from Syrian hamster embryo cells in tissue culture, treated with [³H]- or [¹⁴C]benzo[*a*]pyrene; (ii) purified salmon sperm DNA incubated with synthetic

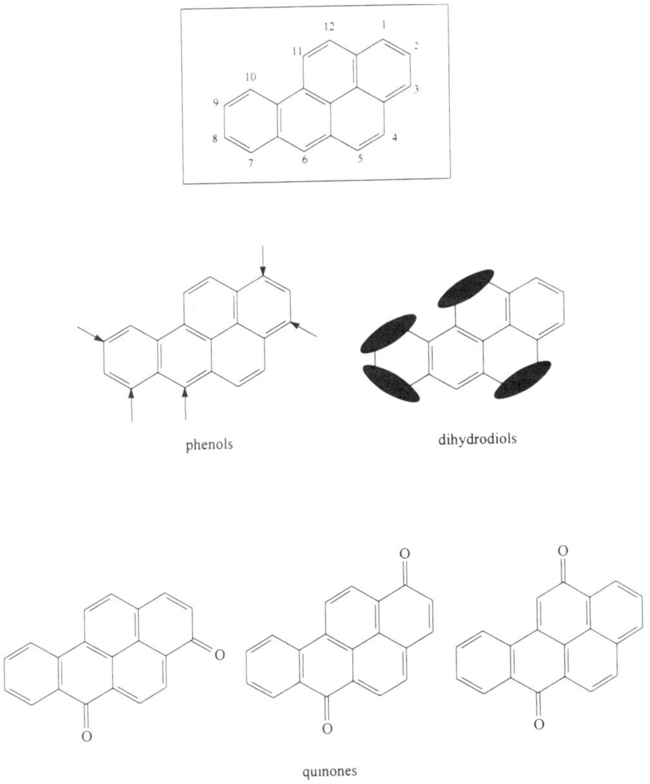

Figure 19.1. Some of the pathways of benzo[a]pyrene metabolism are illustrated. Although epoxidation in the K-region is a major pathway, many other regions of the molecule are also oxidized. *Trans*-dihydrodiols, formed by epoxide hydrase-catalyzed hydrolysis of epoxides, are obtained at the 4,5; 7,8; 9,10; and 11,12 regions. Alternatively, trapping of the epoxide by glutathione yields glutathione adducts (27). Isomerization of the epoxides gives rise to phenolic metabolites at the 1, 3, 6, 7, and 9 positions. Further oxidation of the phenols gives 1,6-, 3,6-, and 6,12-quinones. Metabolites bearing hydroxyl groups (such as dihydrodiols and phenols) are conjugated to form glucuronides and sulfates. Epoxidation of the dihydrodiols, the critical pathway for bioactivation, is discussed separately below.

benzo[a]pyrene-4,5-oxide; (iii) DNA incubated with liver microsomal preparation and [³H]benzo[a]pyrene-7,8-dihydrodiol (isolated from microsomal incubations of [³H]benzo[a]pyrene); and (iv) DNA incubated with [³H]-7,8-benzo[a]pyrene dihydrodiol-9,10-epoxide (prepared by treating the dihydrodiol with *meta*-chloroperoxybenzoic acid). In each case, the DNA was enzymatically hydrolyzed with deoxyribonuclease, phosphodiesterase, and alkaline phosphatase, yielding deoxyribonucleosides. The hydrolysate was then chromatographed on a column of the hydrophobic matrix Sephadex LH20, and adducts were separated by elution with methanol-water gradients. These analyses showed that the adducts formed from cellular metabolism of benzo[a]pyrene coeluted with the BPDE and benzo[a]pyrene dihydrodiol-derived adducts, but were distinct from the K-region epoxide-derived adducts. The critical role of BPDE was soon confirmed when BPDE proved to be highly carcinogenic in rodents, and the DNA adducts formed from benzo[a]pyrene in vivo were also found to coelute with adducts formed from BPDE in vitro (Figure 19.2).

Note that BPDE has never been isolated from a metabolic activation system, due to its reactivity; its presence is usually inferred from a study of the DNA adducts formed.

BPDE Nomenclature

Unfortunately, many different, potentially confusing systems of benzo[a]pyrene-7,8-dihydrodiol-9,10-epoxide (BPDE) nomenclature are in use.

(a) *Chemical designation.* The full name 7,8-dihydroxy-9,10-epoxy-7,8,9,10-tetrahydrobenzo[a]pyrene emphasizes that the terminal ring is completely reduced. This name is cumbersome and is often abbreviated to "7,8-dihydroxy-9,10-epoxybenzo[a]pyrene" or simply to "7,8-diol 9,10-epoxide." This abbreviation is potentially misleading, since the compounds are dihydrodiols, not catechols. The *positions* are sometimes left out also ("BP diol epoxide"), but this can lead to confusion with other regioisomers, such as 9,10-dihydroxy-7,8-epoxybenzo[a]pyrene (not shown).

(b) *Optical isomers.* The four stereoisomers of benzo[a]pyrene-7,8-dihydrodiol-9,10-epoxide form two sets of enantiomers. Enantiomers have identical chemical properties in an optically *in*active environment, but may interact very differently with optically *active* molecules, such as biological macromolecules. Experimentally, enantiomers can be distinguished by *optical polarimetry*: enantiomers have equal and opposite *specific rotatory power*. The enantiomeric forms are designated (+) and (−) on this basis. They also have equal and opposite circular dichroism spectra. Absolute stereochemistry cannot, generally, be deduced from optical measurements alone. For many polycyclic aromatic hydrocarbon metabolites, absolute stereochemistries are not known, and the (+)/(−) system must be used.

(c) *Absolute stereochemistry.* For the compounds shown here, absolute stereochemistries have been established, allowing the use of the systematic (R, S) designations (IUPAC). Absolute stereochemistries were determined by resolution of the racemate (via conversion to separable diastereomeric esters) and use of the exciton chirality circular dichroism method; for details, see ref. 30 and references therein. (In the case of BPDE–purine nucleoside adducts, the optically active purine acts as an "internal standard" and permits construction of rules correlating absolute stereochemistry with the sign of the circular dichroism spectrum; see ref. 31.)

(d) *Synonyms.* The (±) *anti*-BPDE enantiomers are also known as the *trans* dihydrodiol

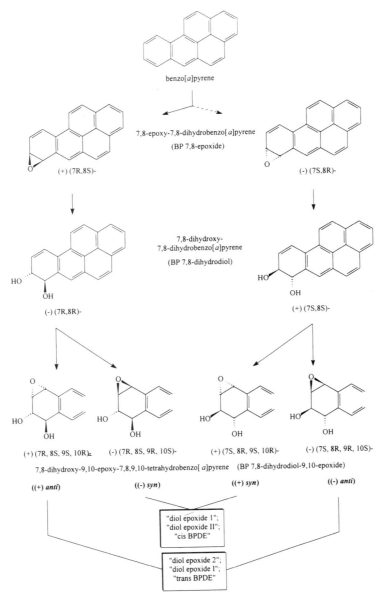

benzo[a]pyrene

7,8-epoxy-7,8-dihydrobenzo[a]pyrene
(BP 7,8-epoxide)

(+) (7R,8S)-

(-) (7S,8R)-

7,8-dihydroxy-
7,8-dihydrobenzo[a]pyrene
(BP 7,8-dihydrodiol)

(-) (7R,8R)-

(+) (7S,8S)-

(+) (7R, 8S, 9S, 10R)-   (-) (7R, 8S, 9R, 10S)-   (+) (7S, 8R, 9S, 10R)-   (-) (7S, 8R, 9R, 10S)-

7,8-dihydroxy-9,10-epoxy-7,8,9,10-tetrahydrobenzo[a]pyrene   (BP 7,8-dihydrodiol-9,10-epoxide)

((+) anti)   ((-) syn)   ((+) syn)   ((-) anti)

"diol epoxide 1";
"diol epoxide II";
"cis BPDE"

"diol epoxide 2";
"diol epoxide I";
"trans BPDE"

Figure 19.2. Metabolism of benzo[a]pyrene to bay region dihydrodiol epoxides. (Other routes of metabolism of benzo[a]pyrene are not shown—see preceding scheme). Cytochrome P-450-catalyzed epoxidation of benzo[a]pyrene is stereospecific. The enantiomeric ratio varies among species and isoforms. Purified rat liver cytochromes P-450 yield the (+) and (−) enantiomers in ratios of between 97:3 and 99:1; among several human liver samples, the ratio was as low as 64:36; see ref. 28. In principle, each enantiomer of the epoxide could be hydrolyzed to both of the dihydrodiols, but the microsomal epoxide hydrolase is regiospecific; water attacks at the 8-position only, so that each of the epoxides gives only a single dihydrodiol, as indicated (29). Cytochrome P-450-catalyzed epoxidation of the dihydrodiols yields the "bay region" benzo[a]pyrene dihydrodiol epoxides (BPDEs). The metabolic conversions show considerable stereospecificity; that is, the ratios of (+) anti to (−) syn, and of (−) anti to (+) syn, are not equal to one. The ratios vary with the enzyme systems studied.

epoxides; both terms refer to the positions of the 7- and 10-position substituents, on *opposite* faces of the ring. The (±) *syn* enantiomers are also known as the *cis* dihydrodiol epoxides (7- and 10-position substituents on the *same* face of the ring). The relationship between the (±) *anti* and the (±) *syn* isomers is diastereomeric. Some authors apply the system used for designation of steroid substituents: α for substituents below the plane of the ring system, and β for substituents above the plane; so, for example, the ((+) *anti*) isomer is named as (+) 7β,8α-dihydroxy-9α,10α-epoxy-7,8,9,10-tetrahydrobenzo[*a*]pyrene.

Two other systems are in use, and, frustratingly, they are mutually contradictory. Following Jerina, the (±) *anti* and the (±) *syn* diastereomers are sometimes called BPDE 2 and BPDE 1, respectively (Arabic numerals). Following Harvey, the (±) *anti* and the (±) *syn* diastereomers are sometimes called BPDE I and BPDE II, respectively (Roman numerals). To minimize this confusion, we will use the *anti/syn* system, but the student will encounter all of these systems in the literature. (Adapted from Dipple, A., Moschel, R. C., and Bigger, C. A. H., Polynuclear aromatic carcinogens, in: *Chemical Carcinogens*, 2nd ed., C. E. Searle, Ed., American Chemical Society, Washington, D.C., 1984, pp. 277–301.)

THE UNUSUAL BIOLOGICAL ACTIVITY OF BAY-REGION DIHYDRODIOL EPOXIDES

Studies of the DNA binding, mutagenicity, and carcinogenicity of polycyclic aromatic hydrocarbon metabolites have repeatedly confirmed the remarkable activity of bay-region dihydrodiol epoxides, compared to any other epoxide metabolites. Bear in mind, as discussed above, that bay region metabolites represent only a small fraction of the total metabolism of the parent hydrocarbon, which occurs at many sites in the molecule (32). What makes the bay region unusual?

To understand this, we need to consider both the chemistry of bay region dihydrodiol epoxides and their metabolic disposition. As mentioned earlier, epoxides can be scavenged enzymatically, by hydrolysis or glutathione conjugation. Epoxides (bay-region or otherwise) are also spontaneously reactive with macromolecules, including DNA. *Bay-region dihydrodiol epoxides are particularly resistant to enzymatic detoxication.* The bay region epoxides are particularly resistant to hydrolysis or conjugation, as can be seen from the data for glutathione transferase, shown in Table 19.1. This resistance is presumably due to

Table 19.1. Glutathione Transferase Activity of Rat Liver Cytosol with Regioisomeric Benzo[a]pyrene Oxides

Substrate	Activity[a]
Benzo[*a*]pyrene-4,5-oxide (K-region)	10
Benzo[*a*]pyrene-7,8-oxide	2.3
Benzo[*a*]pyrene-9,10-oxide (bay region)	0.3
Benzo[*a*]pyrene-11,12-oxide	18

[a]Specific activity: nanomoles per minute per milligram of cytosolic protein.
Hernandez and Bend (19), p. 217.

the steric inaccessibility of the bay region. Bay region dihydrodiol epoxide metabolites of polycyclic aromatic hydrocarbons are, invariably, very poor substrates for epoxide hydrolase.

Studies on the biological activities (carcinogenicity, mutagenicity) of analogues of BPDE have clarified some of the structural features required for activity.

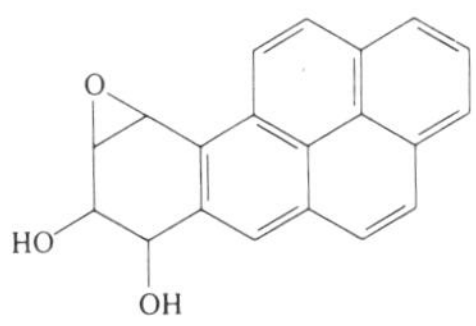

benzo[*a*]pyrene
7,8-dihydrodiol-9,10-epoxide

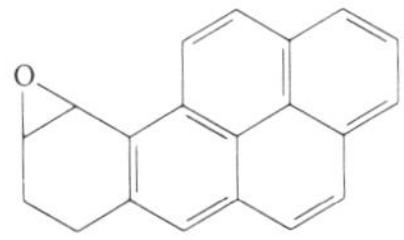

tetrahydrobenzo[*a*]pyrene
9,10-epoxide

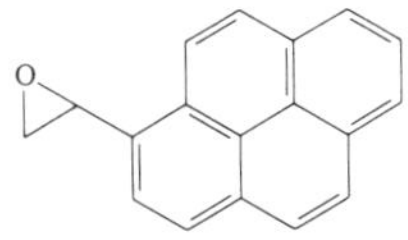

1-oxiranylpyrene

Note that the reduction of the 7,8 double bond (which accompanies conversion to the dihydrodiol functionality) is critical, but the *hydroxyl groups themselves* are not: 7,8-Dihydrobenzo[*a*]pyrene, which is a precursor to a bay region epoxide, is a highly potent carcinogen, but 9,10-dihydrobenzo[*a*]pyrene, precursor to a non-bay-region epoxide, is inactive (33). Indeed, even 1-oxiranylpyrene, in which the 7 and 8 carbon atoms of the terminal ring have "disappeared" altogether, but in which the bay region epoxide is still present, is very active.

In addition to their resistance to enzymatic detoxication, bay region dihydrodiol epoxides yield relatively stable benzylic cation intermediates (34) by the acid-catalyzed opening of the epoxide ring, and the relatively long lifetime of this species may facilitate reaction with DNA.

SIDEBAR: BENZYLIC CATIONS

Based on the earlier discussion of molecular orbital (MO) theory, it is easy to understand why benzylic cations are more effectively stabilized by their attached π-electron systems if they form from bay region dihydrodiol epoxides. In such cations, the benzylic carbon that is produced finds itself bonded to an α site (i.e., on a carbon one bond from a fusion site) in the adjoining unsaturated system. In a non-bay-region epoxide, the analogous process produces a benzylic carbon attached to a β position. (An example is the benzylic carbenium ion shown on page 331.) Since α sites are better able to stabilize attached charged groups, bay region dihydrodiol epoxides produce more stable benzylic cations.

Molecular orbital theory also yields simple rules permitting qualitative predictions of the changes in benzylic cation stability resulting from variations in the parent polycyclic aromatic hydrocarbon, including methylation at various positions, substitution with a heteroatom, or structure change through ring rearrangement (34). In addition, correlation of the Pullman "K-region" reactivity with bay-region carbenium ion stability has been demonstrated. This result explains the correlation of carcinogenicity with K-region activity, first reported in 1954 (35).

The identification of the P-450 forms involved in benzo[a]pyrene bioactivation is being investigated with the help of molecular biological methods. Benzo[a]pyrene metabolism was studied in hepatoma cells expressing human or other animal P-450 forms following infection with recombinant vaccinia viruses (36). Forms 1A1 and 1A2 showed highest activity in conversion of the polycyclic aromatic hydrocarbon to diol and tetrol metabolites. However, the relative importance of each P-450 form in vivo remains to be resolved.

BENZO[a]PYRENE-DERIVED DNA ADDUCTS

Genotoxic carcinogens, such as B[a]P, modify the structure of DNA. DNA adducts (see Chapter 16) lead either to an altered function of a gene product or to disturbance of the normal regulation of the expression of that product. A DNA adduct per se is not a mutation, but rather a premutagenic lesion: The processing of this lesion by polymerases and repair enzymes will either *repair* the lesion (restore the original DNA sequence) or *fix* it as a permanent alteration of the DNA sequence. Once a lesion has been fixed, it comprises a structurally normal DNA molecule containing a heritable alteration in its information content—a mutation (see Chapter 17).

The conversion of a normal cell into a tumor cell is a multistep process; each stage results from the accumulation of an additional genetic lesion affecting a proto-oncogene or a tumor suppressor gene (see Chapter 18). To test the role of a particular reactive carcinogen metabolite, we must examine the link between this metabolite, on the one hand, and, on the other, the specific DNA adducts, genetic lesions, and mutations occurring in target tissues. This link extends our analysis from the molecular level (the reactivities of organic functional groups) to the biological level (the morphological and functional changes in tumor cells and tissues). To bridge this gap, we start at either end and work toward the middle.

The investigation of the reactivity of B[*a*]P metabolites was accomplished by (a) the synthesis and characterization of known or proposed metabolites and (b) the comparison of the stable end products derived from them with the metabolites produced in biological systems. Those stable products include both free metabolites and conjugates, derived from binding to small molecules, such as glutathione, or macromolecules, such as DNA and protein. As in the study of any organic reaction, the identities of the stable end products point to the identity of key reactive intermediates. Such chemical studies have provided unequivocal evidence that bay-region diol epoxides of B[*a*]P (and many other PAH) represent extremely reactive metabolites which alkylate nucleic acids.

As discussed above, following the report (25) that 7,8-dihydroxy-7,8-dihydro-B[*a*]P (BP-7,8-diol) underwent an additional oxygenation step to yield a powerful alkylating agent, several groups achieved the synthesis of *syn*- (or *cis*-) and *anti*- (or *trans*-) BPDE. Intensive study of these diol epoxides revealed that they were highly reactive, formed stable addition products from the attack of water or other nucleophiles, and avidly bound to macromolecules (37). These properties mirrored what was seen when B[*a*]P (or BP-7,8-diol) was activated by microsomal or highly purified cytochrome P-450s.

The hydrolytic and electrophilic behaviours of the two classes of diastereomeric diol epoxides were different: *syn*-BPDE exhibits a half-life of about 40 sec, in aqueous buffer at pH 7.4, whereas *anti*-BPDE has a half-life of about 2 min. This difference apparently results from intramolecular acid catalysis of the opening of the epoxide ring: The 7-hydroxyl proton hydrogen-bonds (and may actually transfer) to the epoxide oxygen. This interaction is geometrically impossible in *anti*-BPDE, and interaction with the 8-hydroxyl proton is not observed. For both diastereomers and, indeed, for all bay-region diol epoxides, the *exceptionally high reactivity results from the stabilization of the benzylic cation resulting from the (acid-catalyzed) opening of the epoxide ring.* Diol epoxides react readily with proteins and nucleic acids.

The characterization of DNA adduct formation by diol epoxides and elucidation of the structures of the adducts were the next steps. Synthetic diol epoxides were reacted with synthetic polynucleotides, which then were hydrolyzed to mononucleosides (see Chapter 16). The adducted mononucleosides were then purified and characterized. While the techniques for the generation, isolation, and structural characterization of these adducts are the same as those used for the study of the products of any reaction, the microscale of product formation and the complexity of the products (adducts) to be characterized made these studies especially challenging. B[*a*]P diol epoxides show a strong preference for reaction with purine residues, particularly guanosine. Adducts are formed by the attack of the exocyclic nitrogen (N-2) of guanosine on the bay-region benzylic carbon (C-10) of the diol epoxide:

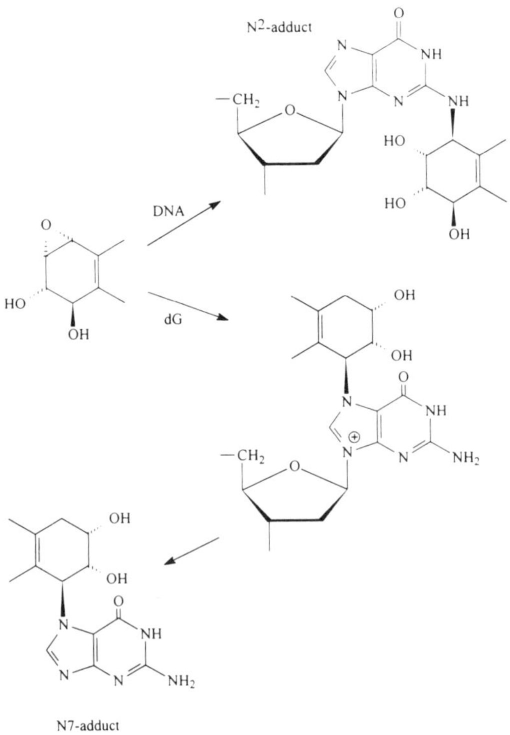

N2-adduct

N7-adduct

This N^2-guanosine adduct is observed with all four B[a]P bay-region diol epoxides.

These synthetic adducts were then used as standards for comparison with adducts isolated from biological systems. Application of B[a]P or its derivatives to cultured cells or to animals was followed by the isolation of DNA, enzymatic hydrolysis to mononucleotides or mononucleosides, and the chromatographic (and, sometimes, spectral) characterization of the adducts. The major adduct observed in these systems is diol epoxide-derived and has been identified as 7R,8S,9R-trihydroxy-10S-(N^2-deoxyguanosyl)-7,8,9,10-tetrahdrobenzo[a]-pyrene [the *trans* adduct formed between the N-2 atom of deoxyguansine and the (+)-enantiomer of *anti*-BPDE (38)]. This adduct, accounting for >90% of total identified adducts, is evidence of profound regio- and stereoselectivity in both the metabolism of B[a]P and the reaction of diol epoxides with DNA, a chiral substrate (39). The attack on N-2 of guanine does not represent substitution at the most nucleophilic site of the purine; indeed, the reaction of deoxyguanosine nucleoside with *anti*-BPDE results in the formation of the N-7 adduct [see scheme above (40)]. The structure of the macromolecule, DNA, steers adduct formation toward the N-2 position.

Although a specific enantiomer of *anti*-BPDE is responsible for the majority of covalent adducts observed, this does not necessarily imply toxicological relevance (41). Other types of DNA damage, not detected in the adduct analyses, might occur in the target cells and be responsible for mutations. This alternative possibility seems unlikely, in view of evidence from a different experimental approach: reverse genetics. Rather than treating intact cells with a B[a]P derivative and then selecting for mutations, DNA constructs were prepared incorporating a few (or a single) diol epoxide-deoxyguanosine adduct (42). These constructs are then transfected into competent cells and processed in those replicating cells; the construct is then isolated from the host cells and sequenced. The types of errors made by polymerases, in their attempts to replicate adducted DNA, can then be established.

A common mutation resulting from the presence of BPDE adducts is the G → T trans-version (43). How might such a mutation arise? The addition of the B[a]P nucleus to N-2 of deoxyguanosine alters the local conformation of the DNA double helix.

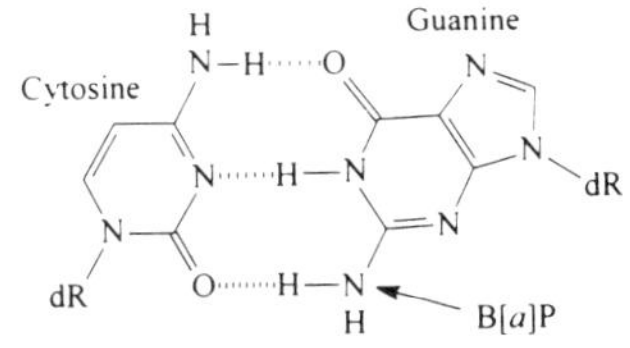

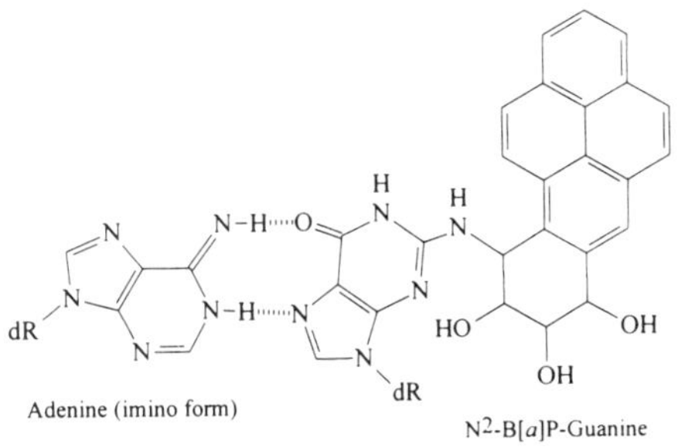

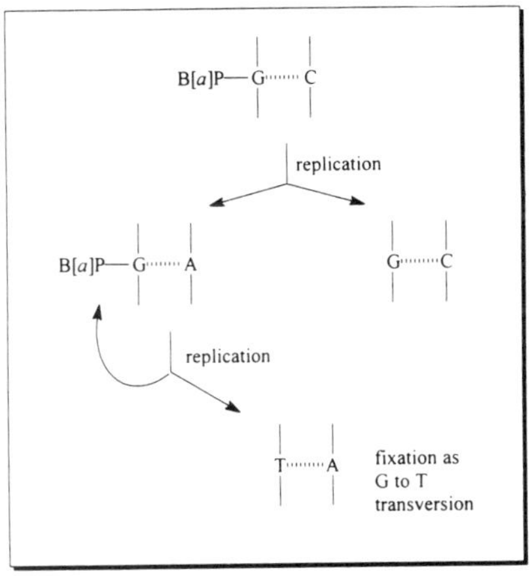

Cytosine — Guanine base pair with B[a]P adduct

Adenine (imino form)   N2-B[a]P-Guanine

B[a]P—G·······C

replication

B[a]P—G·······A   G·······C

replication

T·······A   fixation as G to T transversion

These conformational effects, which are discussed in more detail later, change the effective size and base-pairing character of the purine, which better fits the helix dimensions by pairing to a second purine, deoxyadenosine, in the daughter strand. A second round of replication will result in fixation of the transversion. The distribution of mutational sites resulting from diol epoxide attack demonstrates that these events are also sequence-dependent: The sequence context of a given dG residue strongly influences both its susceptibility to alkylation and the relative efficiencies of fixation versus repair. The mutational spectrum provides us with a framework for understanding how DNA polymerases interact with and "read" the modified structure of adducted DNA; it also gives a "fingerprint" for the types of sequence changes associated with a given carcinogen adduct.

Because of the low yield of transformed cells in a tissue of a carcinogen-treated animal, the process of tumor development is used to select cells which have undergone critical genetic changes relevant to carcinogenesis, such as activating mutations in specific proto-oncogenes. Analysis of B[*a*]P-induced animal tumors, for example, shows that the *ras* oncogene often undergoes an activating mutation. A survey of *ras* mutations resulting from B[*a*]P insult demonstrated that the predominant mutations in both skin and lung tumors are G → T transversions in codon 12 of K-*ras* (44). G → T transversions also predominate *ras* mutations in mouse skin papillomas and carcinomas initiated by B[*a*]P and promoted with phorbol esters (45). Mutations that inactivate tumor suppressor genes also play a role in carcinogenesis. Mouse skin tumors elicited with B[*a*]P show a high incidence of p53 mutations and 71% of those mutations were G → T transversions (46). B[*a*]P- and BPDE-induced mutations, in many systems and target sequences, show this pronounced selectivity for G → T transversions, and evidence from the analysis of key target genes in tumors matches this selectivity. These results are consistent with the postulated role of diol epoxide-derived adducts in B[*a*]P carcinogenesis.

Although a link has been established between the generation of critical B[*a*]P metabolites and mutagenicity, important questions remain regarding the role of these lesions in B[*a*]P carcinogenesis. Stowers and Anderson found that B[*a*]P exposure in mice and rabbits led to N^2-dG adducts as the predominant lesion in the DNA of all tissues examined (11). The levels of DNA binding varied only about fourfold, when comparing the various organs and tissues, and does not correlate with tissue susceptibility to B[*a*]P-induced carcinogenesis. Neither tissue-specific generation of reactive intermediates nor tissue-specific adduct formation can explain the pronounced tissue specificity of B[*a*]P carcinogenesis. Perhaps differences in the packaging of chromatin (related to differential gene expression) render critical genes more susceptible to attack in target cells for tumorigenesis. To extend our understanding of the relationship between DNA adducts, mutations, and cancer to this level will require the ability to determine DNA adduct levels not in whole tissue or cell chromatin, but within specific genes. The techniques to address this target are not yet available.

BIOLOGICAL ACTIVITIES OF BPDE STEREOISOMERS AND DNA ADDUCTS

The mutational spectra of the four BPDE stereoisomers are remarkably different. (+)-*anti*-BPDE is considerably more mutagenic in mammalian cells than (+)-*syn*-BPDE, (−)-*syn*-BPDE, or (−)-*anti*-BPDE stereoisomers; the latter three isomers, however, are more mutagenic to bacterial cells than is (+)-*anti*-BPDE (47). *Mutagenicity of a compound is not a purely chemical property but is also biological; the relative mutagenic potencies of compounds depend on the biological system in which their effects are studied.* All four BPDE stereoisomers are toxic to mammalian cells (48). (+)-*anti*-BPDE is a potent inducer of skin carcinomas in newborn mice, whereas (−)-*anti*-BPDE and both *syn*-BPDE enantiomers are not (49).

(±)-*anti*-BPDE induces mainly G → T transversions in the *E. coli lacI* gene (50), the human c-Ha-*ras1* oncogene (51), and the dihydrofolate reductase gene in Chinese hamster ovary cells (42). (+)-*anti*-BPDE is more mutagenic than (−)-*anti*-BPDE in the *HPRT* locus of Chinese hamster V-79 cells (52). Both (+)- and (−)-*anti*-BPDE induced predominantly base substitution mutations, followed by deletions and frameshifts.

The reaction of BPDE with high-molecular-weight DNA gives rise to a very complex mixture of products. The major products of both (+)- and (−)-*anti*-BPDE reactions with DNA arise from the *trans* addition of the exocyclic amino group of guanine (N^2-dG) to the C10 position of the PAH; in addition, minor products arise from *cis* addition at N^2-dG and from *cis* and *trans* addition at N^7-dG and the exocyclic amino group of adenine

(N^6-dA) (53). However, not all PAH bay region diol epoxides bind to guanines as specifically as does BPDE. For example, benzo[c]phenanthrene diol epoxides bind equally to adenines and guanines (54). The *trans* N^2-dG-BP adducts are the major products formed from the reaction of BPDE and DNA; but nothing is yet known about the biological activities of the minor adducts. These might turn out to be important: The most abundant adduct may not be the most potent.

Deoxyoligonucleotides (i.e., small synthetic DNA molecules) can be modified site-specifically with stereochemically defined *trans* or *cis-anti*-BPDE-N^2-dG lesions (55). These BPDE-modified templates can then be used for in vitro transcription (56) or DNA polymerase-catalyzed primer extension (57). Such studies can shed light on the ways in which adducts interfere with the normal biochemical processing of DNA. (+)-*anti*-BPDE-dG lesions are bypassed by DNA polymerase only with great difficulty, but the normal (deoxycytosine) residue was incorporated opposite the modified G residue in the fully extended primer (57). Primer extension reactions catalyzed DNA polymerase are strongly blocked by each of the stereochemically distinct (+)- and (−)-*trans* and *cis-anti*-[BP]-N^2-dG adducts. When the lesions were bypassed, small amounts of (incorrect) incorporation of A opposite the lesion, as well as one- and two-base deletions, were found in the extended primers. The *trans* and *cis* lesions derived from the (−)-*anti*-BPDE enantiomer had greater miscoding potential than those derived from the (+)-*anti* isomer.

NOMENCLATURE OF BP-DNA COVALENT ADDUCTS

Earlier in this chapter, the (bewildering!) nomenclature of the diastereomeric BP diol epoxides was presented. Unfortunately, further confusion can be engendered by the nomenclature of PAH-DNA adducts. The *trans* and *cis* designations of the BP-N^2-dG adducts refer to the relative orientations of the hydroxyl group at [BP]C9 and the amino group of the nucleic acid base bound to [BP]C10:

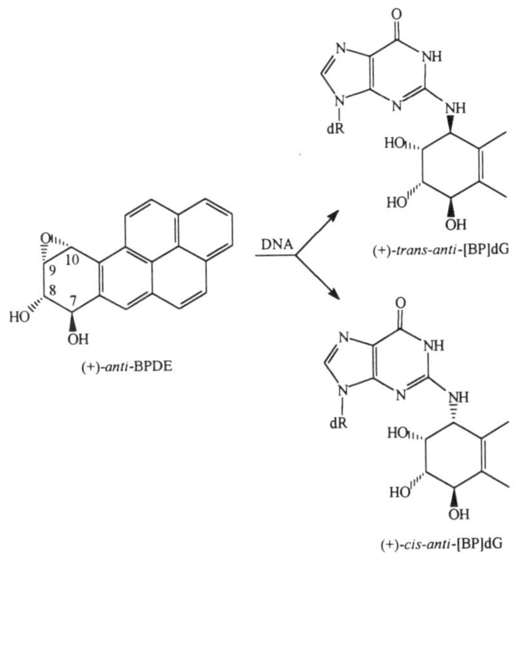

(+)-*anti*-BPDE

(+)-*trans-anti*-[BP]dG

(+)-*cis-anti*-[BP]dG

If these two groups are located on the *same* side of the benzylic ring, then they are *cis* to each other; if on *opposite* sides, then they are *trans* to each other. Reaction of (+)-*anti*-BPDE at N^2-dG results in both (+)-*trans-anti*-[BP]dG and (+)-*cis-anti*-[BP]dG adducts. (The specific adduction site, N^2, is sometimes omitted when only a single site is under discussion. Also, [BP]-N^6-dA adducts are often designated simply as [BP]dA.)

trans and *cis* adducts are diastereomers; they rotate light in opposite directions at long wavelengths (as measured by circular dichroism spectroscopy), so that one of these adducts should be designated (+) and the other (−). However, *the (+) and (−) designations of the parent BPDEs are maintained for designation of the derived adducts.* (The "correct" optical designation of the (+)-*trans-anti*-[BP]dG adduct, based on its circular dichroism spectrum, is actually (−).)

CONFORMATIONS OF PAH-ADDUCTED DNA

Alteration of DNA structure due to the presence of a BP lesion will, presumably, affect the interaction of the nucleic acid with enzymes, such as the replication machinery. The outcome of these interactions may result in mutation. A systematic study of the conformations of DNA duplexes containing site-specific, stereochemically defined PAH adducts and the correlation of structure with biological activity should shed light on the mechanisms of PAH-induced mutations.

Two methods are available for determination of the three-dimensional structures of adducted DNA: X-ray crystallography and nuclear magnetic resonance (NMR) (58). NMR methods are often used in conjunction with "molecular mechanics" computations. Although NMR is a very powerful method for determining solution structures, it is inherently insensitive; in many cases, the most difficult aspect of the structural studies is obtaining sufficient material (5–10 mg). Two types of two-dimensional NMR experiments are used in deducing the structures. "Through-bond" coupling (COrrelation SpectroscopY, COSY) provides information on the pucker conformations of the nucleic acid sugar and the (nonaromatic) benzylic ring of the [BP]dG adduct. "Through-space" connectivities (Nuclear Overhauser Effect SpectroscopY, NOESY) provides information about the distances between protons which are located within 5Å of one another. This information is used to generate a list of proton-proton distance restraints, which are then used to determine the overall structure.

NMR studies of PAH-DNA adducts have provided insights into how the conformation of the modified DNA is influenced by factors such as the stereochemistry of the PAH adduct, whether the modified base is positioned opposite a base or an abasic site, the effect of a bay region methyl group on helix bending, and the location of the binding site (minor versus major groove of the DNA). PAH-DNA structures elucidated to date can be classified into three families, on the basis of adduct location:

1. In the minor groove, without causing significant distortion of the B-DNA duplex [(+) and (−)-*trans-anti*-[BP]dG·dC and (−)-*trans-anti*-[MC]dG·dC duplexes] (38, 59)
2. Intercalated into the helix, by displacing the modified base [(+) and (−)-*cis-anti*-[BP]dG·dC, (+)-*trans*- and (+)-*cis-anti*-[BP]dG·del duplexes] (60)
3. Intercalated into the helix, without disrupting the modified base pair [(+) and (−)-*trans-anti*-[BPh]dA·dT duplexes] (61).

(The shorthand designations are as follows: [BP]dG, benzo[*a*]pyrenyl-N^2-dG adducts; [MC]dG, 5-methylchrysenyl-N^2-dG adducts; [BPh]dA, benzo[*c*]phenanthrenyl-N^6-dA adducts; dC, dT, or "del" indicate whether the modified base was positioned opposite a

C, T, or deletion site, respectively.) Next we will look at some of these structures in more detail.

Monique Cosman and colleagues have determined the conformations of dsDNA oligonucleotides containing each of the four isomeric ((+) and (−), *trans* and *cis*) [BP]dG adducts, in the same 11-mer DNA sequence context:

5′ CCATC<u>G</u>CTACC 3′

3′ GGTAGCGATGG 5′

The modified guanine (underlined) is located in the center of the duplex, positioned opposite a cytosine. Modified duplexes containing a single stereochemically defined [BP]dG lesion were generated by reacting one DNA strand (CCATCGCTACC) with (±)-*anti*-BPDE; the diastereomeric adducts were then separated by HPLC methods. Finally, each purified, modified single strand was annealed to the complementary strand (GGTAGC-GATGG).

Side views (i.e., views perpendicular to the helix axis) of the central 5-bp segments of the four (+)- and (−)-*trans* and *cis-anti*-[BP]dG·dC duplexes are shown in Figure 19.3. First we will consider the *trans* adducts. As discussed earlier, the (+)-*trans* adduct (derived from the binding of the tumourigenic (+)-*anti*-BPDE parent) is the major product found in studies of BPDE-modified DNA, while the (−)-*trans* adduct is obtained from the binding of the nontumorigenic (−)-*anti*-BPDE. In both the (+)- and (−)-*trans-anti*-[BP]dG·dC duplexes (Fig. 19.3A and C), the pyrenyl moiety lies in the minor groove of a minimally perturbed B-DNA helix. In the (+)-*trans* isomer, the long axis of the pyrenyl ring points toward the 5′-end of the modified strand; in the (−)-*trans* isomer, it points in the opposite direction, toward the 3′-end. The stereochemistry of these two adducts differs: the chirality at each of the four benzylic ring carbons is opposite. This change transposes the directionality of the pyrenyl ring with respect to the DNA helix. Perhaps this difference in conformation can help to explain the different biological activities of the enantiomeric parent (+) and (−) diol epoxides.

Unlike the *trans* adducts, which adopt a single conformation in the DNA duplex sequence used in these studies, the two *cis* adducts undergo *conformational exchange* between a major and a minor form. The (+)-*cis-anti*-[BP]dG·dC adduct is also derived from the binding of the tumorigenic (+)-*anti*-BPDE parent; it differs from its (+)-*trans* diastereoisomer by inversion of the chirality at a single benzylic ring carbon ([BP]C10) at the binding site. This results in a dramatic difference in the major conformations of the adducts (Fig. 19.3B). *In the (+)-cis-anti adduct, the pyrenyl ring intercalates between the (intact) flanking dG·dC base pairs by disrupting the hydrogen bonding of the adducted base pair. The modified guanine is displaced into the minor groove, lies perpendicular to the plane of a regular Watson-Crick base pair*, and stacks over the minor groove face of the 5′-side cytosine sugar ring. Its partner cytosine base is displaced into the major groove. Relative to the unmodified (control) 11-mer duplex, large changes in the chemical shifts of the phosphorus resonances are observed in the (proton-decoupled) phosphorus NMR spectrum. This implies that the phosphodiester backbone of the duplex around the lesion site is highly distorted, in order to accommodate the (+)-*cis-anti*-[BP]dG adduct. The relative mutagenic and tumorigenic potencies of the (+)-*trans* and (+)-*cis* adducts are not yet known; although the (+)-*cis* adduct is a minor product, its contribution to the biological activity of (+)-*anti*-BPDE may, nevertheless, be significant.

Finally, consider the (−)-*cis-anti*-[BP]dG·dC duplex, derived from the binding of the nontumorigenic (−)-*anti*-BPDE parent. This adduct differs in stereochemistry from its (−)-*trans* diastereoisomer by inversion of the chirality at the [BP]C10 binding site, and

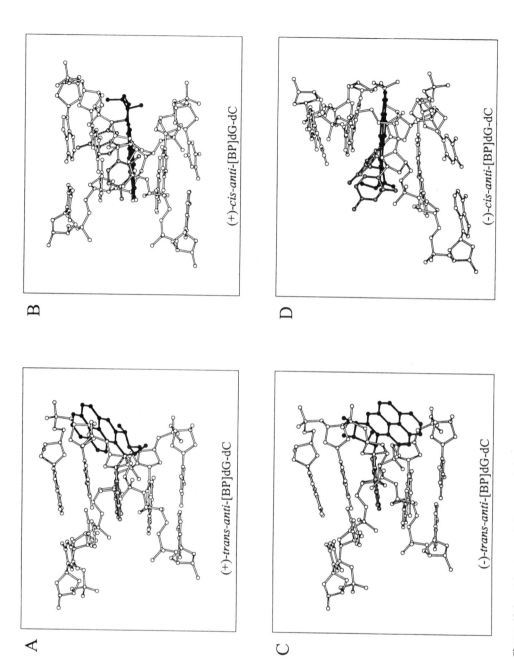

A (+)-*trans-anti*-[BP]dG-dC

B (+)-*cis-anti*-[BP]dG-dC

C (−)-*trans-anti*-[BP]dG-dC

D (−)-*cis-anti*-[BP]dG-dC

Figure 19.3. Side views of the central, five-base-pair segment of 11-mer duplexes containing specific BP-derived adducts. (**A**) (+)-*trans-anti*-[BP]dG-dC; (**B**) (+)-*cis-anti*-[BP]dG-dC; (**C**) (−)-*trans-anti*-[BP]dG-dC; (**D**) (−)-*cis-anti*-[BP]dG-dC. The benzo[a]pyrenyl moiety and the [BP]dG-dC base pair are shown with black and grey bonds, respectively. The figures were prepared using the computer soft-ware Molscript (P. J. Kraulis, *J. Appl. Crystallogr.* 24: 946–950, 1991).

it differs from the (+)-*cis* isomer by a change in chirality at all four benzylic ring carbons. Like the (+)-*cis* isomer, the (−)-*cis* adduct produces a base displacement/intercalation conformation (Fig. 19.3D). However, in this case, both the modified guanine and its partner cytosine are displaced into the major groove and are no longer involved in hydrogen bonding interactions with each other. The modified guanine stacks over the major groove base protons of the 5′-side-cytosine. The "bulging-out" of the modified base pair into the major groove, in the (−)-*cis* isomer, results in a greater distortion of the DNA duplex compared to the previous three adducts.

Let us review the present understanding of PAH-derived DNA adducts. PAH metabolism and the biological activities of the various metabolites are extraordinarily complex. The ultimate carcinogenic metabolites of BP, widely studied as a model PAH, are believed to be the four diastereomeric bay region diol epoxides, (+)-*anti*-BPDE, (+)-*anti*-BPDE, (+)-*syn*-BPDE, and (−)-*syn*-BPDE. Each exhibits different mutagenic and tumorigenic profiles. Each binds to nucleophilic sites on nucleic acids and proteins. The predominant reaction product derived from the binding of BPDE to DNA results from *trans* addition of N^2-dG to the C10 position of BPDE. Minor products result from *cis* addition to N^2-dG and *trans* and *cis* addition to other sites (e.g., N^7-dG and N^6-dA). The solution conformations of several site-specific and stereochemically defined PAH-oligonucleotide adducts have been determined. The stereochemistry of each [BP]dG adduct plays an important role in determining the structural characteristics of the modified duplex. This stereochemically defined distortion of the helix, in turn, may determine the enzymatic processing of the damaged DNA. The analysis of the relationship between the structure of damaged DNA and the toxicological consequences of its formation is a rapidly developing frontier in molecular toxicology.

NOTES

1. Phillips, D. H., Fifty years of benzo[*a*]pyrene, *Nature* 303:468–472, 1983.
2. Waller, R. E., 60 years of chemical carcinogens: Sir Ernest Kennaway in retirement, *J. R. Soc. Med.* 87:96–97, 1994.
3. Boyd, D. R., and Jerina, D. M., Arene oxides-oxepins, Chapter 11 in: A. Hassner, Ed., *Small Ring Heterocycles, Part 3: Oxiranes, Arene Oxides, Oxaziridines, Dioxetanes, Thietanes, Thietes, Thiazetes*, John Wiley & Sons, New York, 1985, pp. 197–282.
4. J. P. Lowe, *Quantum Chemistry*, 2nd ed., Academic Press, New York, 1993, §7-6.
5. J. P. Lowe, *Quantum Chemistry*, 2nd ed., Academic Press, New York, 1993, §14-8.
6. Lowe, J. P., and Silverman, D. B., Simple molecular orbital explanation for "bay-region" carcinogenic reactivity, *J. Am. Chem. Soc.* 103:2582–2585, 1981.
7. Glusker, J. P., X-ray analyses of polycyclic hydrocarbon metabolite structures, Chapter 7 in: *Polycyclic Hydrocarbons and Carcinogenesis*, R. G. Harvey, Ed., American Chemical Society, Washington, D.C., 1985, pp. 125–185.
8. Miller, E. C., Studies on the formation of protein-bound derivatives of 3,4-benzpyrene in epidermal reactions of mouse skin, *Cancer Res.* 11:100–108, 1951.
9. Brookes, P., and Lawley, P. D., Evidence for the binding of polynuclear aromatic hydrocarbons to the nucleic acid of mouse skin: relation between carcinogenic power of hydrocarbons and their binding to deoxyribonucleic acid, *Nature* 202:781–784, 1964.
10. Metzler, D. E., *Biochemistry*, Academic Press, New York, 1977, Table 2-10, p. 118.
11. Stowers, S. J., and Anderson, M. W., Ubiquitous binding of benzo[*a*]pyrene metabolites to DNA and protein in tissues of the mouse and rabbit, *Chem.-Biol. Interact.* 51:151–166, 1984.
12. Guroff, G., Daly, J. W., Jerina, D. M., Renson, J., Witkop, B., and Udenfriend, S., Hydroxylation-induced migration: the NIH shift, *Science* 157:1524–1530, 1967.

13. Daly, J. W., Jerina, D. M., and Witkop, B., Arene oxides and the NIH shift: the metabolism, toxicity, and carcinogenicity of aromatic compounds, *Experientia* 28:1129–1149, 1972.

14. Intramolecular cationic rearrangements, in: *Mechanism and Theory in Organic Chemistry*, 3rd ed., T. H. Lowry and K. S. Richardson, Eds., Harper & Row, New York, 1987.

15. Jerina, D. M., and Daly, J. W., Arene oxides: a new aspect of drug metabolism, *Science* 185:573–582, 1974.

16. Den Besten, C., van Bladeren, P. J., Duizer, E., Vervoort, J., and Rietjens, I. M. C. M., Cytochrome P450-mediated oxidation of pentafluorophenol to tetrafluorobenzoquinone as the primary reaction product, *Chem. Res. Toxicol.* 6:674–680, 1993.

17. Ortiz de Montellano, P. R., Alkenes and alkynes, Chapter 5 in: *Bioactivation of Foreign Compounds*, Vol. 16, M. W. Anders, Ed., Academic Press, New York, 1985, pp. 121–155.

18. van Bladeren, P. J., Sayer, J. M., Ryan, D. E., Thomas, P. E., Levin, W., and Jerina, D. M., Differential stereoselectivity of cytochromes P-450*b* and P-450*c* in the formation of naphthalene and anthracene 1,2-oxides: the role of epoxide hydrolase in determining the enantiomer composition of the 1,2-dihydrodiols formed, *J. Biol. Chem.* 260:10226–10235, 1985.

19. Hernandez, O., and Bend, J. R., Metabolism of epoxides, Chapter 11 in: *Metabolic Basis of Detoxication*, W. B. Jakoby, Ed., Academic Press, New York, 1982.

20. Skoda, R. C., Demierre, A., McBride, O. W., Gonzalez, F. J., and Meyer, U. A., Human microsomal xenobiotic epoxide hydrolase: complementary DNA sequence, complementary DNA-directed expression in COS-1 cells, and chromosomal localization, *J. Biol. Chem.* 263:1549–1554, 1988.

21. Guengerich, F. P., Enzyme assay and purification, Chapter 28 in: *Principles and Methods of Toxicology*, 2nd ed., Hayes, A. W., Ed., Raven Press, New York, 1989, pp. 794–795.

22. Sevanian, A., and Peterson, A. R., The cytotoxic and mutagenic properties of cholesterol oxidation products, *Food Chem. Toxicol.* 24:1103–1110, 1986.

23. Beetham, J. K., Tian, T., and Hammock, B. D., cDNA cloning and expression of a soluble epoxide hydrolase from human liver, *Arch. Biochem. Biophys.* 305:197–201, 1993.

24. Lacourciere, G. M., and Armstrong, R. N., The catalytic mechanism of epoxide hydrolase involves an ester intermediate, *J. Am. Chem. Soc.* 115:10466–10467, 1993.

25. Borgen, A., Darvey, H., Castagnoli, N., Crocker, T. T., Rasmussen, R. E., and Wang, I. Y., Metabolic conversion of benzo[*a*]pyrene by Syrian hamster liver microsomes and binding of metabolites to deoxyribonucleic acid, *J. Med. Chem.* 16:502–506, 1973.

26. Sims, P., Grover, P. L., Swaisland, A., Pal, K., and Hewer, A., Metabolic activation of benzo[*a*]pyrene proceeds by a diol epoxide, *Nature* 252:326–328, 1974; See also: Hulbert, P. B., Carbonium ion as ultimate carcinogen of polycyclic aromatic hydrocarbons, *Nature* 256:146–148, 1975.

27. Hernandez, O., Walker, M., Cox, R. H., Foureman, G. L., Smith, B. R., and Bend, J. R., Regiospecificity and stereospecificity in the enzymatic conjugation of glutathione with (±)-benzo(*a*)pyrene 4,5-oxide, *Biochem. Biophys. Res. Commun.* 96:1494–1502, 1980.

28. Hall, M., Forrester, L. M., Parker, D. K., Grover, P. L., and Wolf, C. R, Relative contribution of various forms of cytochrome P450 to the metabolism of benzo[*a*]pyrene by human liver microsomes, *Carcinogenesis* 10:1815–1821, 1989.

29. Levin, W., Buening, M. K., Wood, A. W., Chang, R. L., Kedzierski, B., Thakker, D. R., Boyd, D. R., Gadaginamath, G. S., Armstrong, R. N., Yagi, H., Karle, J. M., Slaga, T. J., Jerina, D. M., and Conney, A. H., An enantiomeric interaction in the metabolism and tumorigenicity of benzo[*a*]pyrene 7,8-oxide, *J. Biol. Chem.* 255:9067–9074, 1980.

30. Yagi, H., Akagi, H., Thakker, D. R., Mah, H. D., Koreeda, M., and Jerina, D. M., Absolute stereochemistry of the highly mutagenic 7,8-diol-9,10-epoxides derived from the potent carcinogen *trans*-7,8-dihydroxy-7,8-dihydrobenzo[*a*]pyrene, *J. Am. Chem. Soc.* 99:2358–2359, 1977.

31. Sayer, J. M., Chadha, A., Agarwal, S. K., Yeh, H. J. C., Yagi, H., and Jerina, D. M., Covalent nucleoside adducts of benzo[*a*]pyrene 7,8-diol-9,10-epoxides: structural reinvestigation and characterization of a novel adenosine adduct on the ribose moiety, *J. Org. Chem.* 56:20–29, 1991.

32. Conney, A. H., Chang, R. L., Jerina, D. M., and Wei, S. J., Studies on the metabolism of benzo[*a*]pyrene and dose-dependent differences in the mutagenic profile of its ultimate carcinogenic metabolite, *Drug Metab. Rev.* 26:125–163, 1994.

33. Waterfall, J. F., and Sims, P., Epoxy derivatives of aromatic polycyclic hydrocarbons: the preparation and metabolism of epoxides related to benzo[*a*]pyrene and to 7,8- and 9,10-dihydrobenzo[*a*]pyrene, *Biochem. J.* 128:265–277, 1972.

34. Lowe, J. P., and Silverman, D. B., Predicting carcinogenicity of polycyclic aromatic hydrocarbons, *Acc. Chem. Res.* 17:332–338, 1984; Lowe, J. P., and Silverman, D. B., Carcinogenicity of polycyclic aromatic hydrocarbons: a dialogue, *J. Mol. Struct. (Theochem.)* 179:47–81, 1988.

35. Pullman, A., Structure électronique et activité cancérogène des hydrocarbures aromatiques, *Bull. Soc. Chim. France* 595–603, 1954.

36. Gonzalez, F. J., and Gelboin, H. V., Role of human cytochromes P450 in the metabolic activation of chemical carcinogens and toxins, *Drug Metab. Rev.* 26:165–183, 1994; Shou, M., Korzekwa, K. R., Crespi, C. L., Gonzalez, F. J., and Gelboin, H. V., The role of 12 cDNA-expressed human, rodent, and rabbit cytochromes P450 in the metabolism of benzo[*a*]pyrene and benzo[*a*]pyrene *trans*-7,8-dihydrodiol, *Mol. Carcinog.* 10:159–168, 1994.

37. Harvey, R. G., and Geacintov, N. E., Intercalation and binding of carcinogenic hydrocarbon metabolites to nucleic acids, *Acc. Chem. Res.* 21:66–73, 1988; Gräslund, A., and Jernström, B., DNA–carcinogen interaction: covalent DNA adducts of benzo[*a*]pyrene 7,8-dihydrodiol 9,10-epoxides studied by biochemical and biophysical techniques, *Qt. Rev. Biophys.* 22:1–37, 1989; Jernström, B., and Gräslund, A., Covalent binding of benzo[*a*]pyrene 7,8-dihydrodiol 9,10-epoxides to DNA: molecular structures, induced mutations and biological consequences, *Biophys. Chem.* 49:185–199, 1994; Peltonen, K., and Dipple, A., Polycyclic aromatic hydrocarbons: Chemistry of DNA adduct formation, *J. Occup. Environ. Med.* 37:52–58, 1995.

38. Cosman, M., de los Santos, C., Fiala, R., Hingerty, B. E., Singh, S. B., Ibanez, V., Margulis, L. A., Live, D., Geacintov, N. E., Broyde, S., and Patel, D. J., Solution conformation of the major adduct between the carcinogen (+)-*anti*-benzo[*a*]pyrene diol epoxide and DNA, *Proc. Natl. Acad. Sci. U.S.A.* 89:1914–1918, 1992.

39. Koreeda, M., Moore, P. D., Wislocki, P. G., Levin, W., Conney, A. H., Yagi, H., and Jerina, D. M., Binding of benzo[*a*]pyrene 7,8-diol-9,10-epoxides to DNA, RNA, and protein of mouse skin occurs with high stereoselectivity, *Science* 199:778–781, 1978.

40. RamaKrishna, N. V. S., Gao, F., Padmavathi, N. S., Cavalieri, E. L., Rogan, E. G., Cerny, R. L., and Gross, M. L., Model adducts of benzo[*a*]pyrene and nucleosides formed from its radical cation and diol epoxide, *Chem. Res. Toxicol.* 5:293–302, 1992.

41. Bresnick, E., The price of progress or Pandora's purse, *Biochem. Pharmacol.* 32:1331–1336, 1983.

42. Yang, J.-L., Maher, V. M., and McCormick, J. J., Kinds of mutations formed when a shuttle vector containing adducts of (±)-7,8α-dihydroxy-9α,10α-epoxy-7,8,9,10-tetra-hydrobenzo[*a*]pyrene replicates in human cells, *Proc. Natl. Acad. Sci. U.S.A.* 84:3787–3791, 1987.

43. Deletions are also common; Shibutani, S., Margulis, L. A., Geacintov, N. E., and Grollman, A. P., Translesional synthesis on a DNA template containing a single stereoisomer of dG-(+)- or dG-(−)-anti-BPDE (7,8-dihydroxy-anti-9,10-epoxy-7,8,9,10-tetrahydrobenzo[*a*]pyrene), *Biochemistry* 32:7531–7541, 1993.

44. Harris, C. C., Chemical and physical carcinogenesis: Advances and perspectives for the 1990s, *Cancer Res. (Suppl.)* 51:5023s–5044s, 1991.

45. Bailleul, B., Brown, K., Ramsden, M., Akhurst, R. J., Fee, F., and Balmain, A., Chemical induction of oncogene mutations and growth factor activity in mouse skin carcinogenesis, *Env. Health Persp.* 81:23–27, 1989; Colapietro, A. M., Goodell, A. L., and Smart, R. C., Characterization of benzo[*a*]pyrene-initiated mouse skin papillomas for Ha-*ras* mutations and protein kinase C levels, *Carcinogenesis* 14:2289–2295, 1993.

46. Greenblatt, M. S., Bennett, W. P., Hollstein, M., and Harris, C. C., Mutations in the p53 tumor suppressor gene: Clues to cancer etiology and molecular pathogenesis, *Cancer Res.* 54:4855–4878, 1994.

47. Stevens, C. W., Bouck, N., Burgess, J. A., and Fahl, W. E., Benzo[*a*]pyrene diol epoxides: Different mutagenic efficiency in human and bacterial cells, *Mutat. Res.* 152:5–14, 1985.

48. Wood, A. W., Chang, L. R., Levin, W., Yagi, H., Thakker, D. R., Jerina, D., and Conney, A. H., Differences in the mutagenicity of the optical enantiomers of the diastereomeric benzo[*a*]pyrene 7,8-diol-9,10-epoxides, *Biochem. Biophys. Res. Commun.* 77:1389–1396, 1977.

49. Kapitulnik, J., Wislocki, P. G., Levin, W., Yagi, H., Jerina, D. M., and Conney, A. H., Tumorigenicity studies with diol-epoxides of benzo[*a*]pyrene which indicate that ±*trans*-7β,8α-dihydroxy-9α,10α-epoxy-7,8,9,10-tetrahydrobenzo[*a*]pyrene is an ultimate carcinogen in newborn mice, *Cancer Res.* 38:354–358, 1978; Levin, W., Wood, A. W., Yagi, H., Jerina, D. M., and Conney, A. H., ±*trans*-7β,8α-dihydroxy-9α,10α-epoxy-7,8,9,10-tetrahydrobenzo[*a*]pyrene a potent skin carcinogen when applied topically to mice, *Proc. Natl. Acad. Sci. U.S.A.* 73:3867–3871, 1976.

50. Eisenstadt, E., Warren, A. J., Porter, J., Atkins, D., and Miller, J. H., Carcinogenic epoxides of benzo[*a*]pyrene and cyclopenta[*cd*]pyrene induced base substitutions via substitution and specific transversions, *Proc. Natl. Acad. Sci. U.S.A.* 79:1945–1949, 1982; Bernelot-Moens, C., Glickman, B. W., and Gordon, J. E., Induction of specific frameshift and base substitution events by benzo[*a*]pyrene diol epoxide in excision-repair-deficient *Escherichia coli*, *Carcinogenesis*, 11:781–785, 1990.

51. Vousden, K. H., Bos, J. L., Marshall, C. J., and Phillips, D. H., Mutations activating human c-Ha-*ras1* protooncogene (*HRAS1*) induced by chemical carcinogenesis and depurination, *Proc. Natl. Acad. Sci. U.S.A.* 83:1222–1226, 1986.

52. Wei, S-J. C., Chang, R. L., Bhachech, N., Cui, X. X., Merkler, K. A., Wong, C-Q., Henning, E., Yagi, H., Jerina, D. M., and Conney, A. H., Dose-dependent differences in the profile of mutations induced by (+)-7R,8S-dihydroxy-9S,10R-epoxy-7,8,9,10-tetrahydro-benzo[*a*]pyrene in the coding region of the hypoxanthine (guanine) phosphoribosyltransferase gene in Chinese hamster V-79 cells, *Cancer Res.* 53:3294–3301, 1993; Wei, S-J. C., Chang, R. L., Henning, E., Cui, X. X., Merkler, K. A., Wong, C-Q., Yagi, H., Jerina, D. M., and Conney, A. H., Mutagenic selectivity at the HPRT locus in V-79 cells: Comparison of mutations caused by bay-region benzo[*a*]pyrene-7,8-diol-9,10-epoxide enantiomers with high and low carcinogenic activity, *Carcinogenesis* 15:1729–1735, 1994.

53. Weinstein, I. B., Jeffrey, A. M., Jennette, K. W., Blobstein, S. H., Harvey, R. G., Harris, C., Autrup, H., Kasai, H., and Nakanishi, K., Benzo[*a*]pyrene diol epoxides as intermediates in nucleic acid binding *in vitro* and *in vivo*, *Science* 193:592–595, 1976; Jeffrey, A. M., Polycyclic aromatic hydrocarbon-DNA adducts: Formation, detection, and characterization, in: Harvey, R. G., ed., *Polycyclic Hydrocarbons and Carcinogenesis*, American Chemical Society, Washington, 1985, pp. 187–208; Meehan, T., and Straub, K., Double-stranded DNA stereoselectively binds benzo[*a*]pyrene diol epoxides, *Nature* 277:410–412, 1979; Cheng, S. C., Hilton, B. D., Roman, J. M., and Dipple, A., DNA adducts from carcinogenic and noncarcinogenic enantiomers of benzo[*a*]pyrene dihydrodiol epoxide, *Chem. Res. Toxicol.* 2:334–340, 1989.

54. Dipple, A., Pigott, M. A., Agarwal, S. K., Yagi, H., Sayer, J. M., and Jerina, D. M., Optically active benzo[*c*]phenanthrene diol epoxides bind extensively to adenine in DNA, *Nature* 327:535–536, 1987.

55. Cosman, M., Ibanez, V., Geacintov, N. E., and Harvey, R. G., Preparation and isolation of adducts in high yield derived from the binding of two benzo[*a*]pyrene 7,8-dihydroxy-9,10, oxide stereoisomers to the oligonucleotide d(ATATGTATA), *Carcinogenesis* 11:1668–1672, 1990.

56. Choi, D-J., Marino-Alessandri, J. F., Geacintov, N. E., and Scicchitano, D. A., Site-specific benzo[*a*]pyrene diol epoxide-DNA adducts inhibit transcription elongation by bacteriophage T7 RNA polymerase, *Biochemistry* 33:780–787, 1994.

57. Hruszkewicz, A. M., Canella, K. A., Peltonen, K., Lotrappa, L., and Dipple, A., DNA polymerase action on benzo[*a*]pyrene-DNA adducts, *Carcinogenesis* 13:2347–2352, 1992.

58. Wüthrich, K., *NMR of Proteins and Nucleic Acids*, Wiley, New York, 1986; Stassinopoulou, C. I., *NMR of Biological Macromolecules*, Springer, New York, 1994.

59. de los Santos, C., Cosman, M., Hingerty, B. E., Ibanez, V., Margulis, L. A., Geacintov, N. E.,

Broyde, S., and Patel, D. J., Influence of benzo[*a*]pyrene diol epoxide chirality on solution conformations of DNA covalent adducts: The (−)- *trans-anti*-[BP]G·C adduct structure and comparison with the (+)-*trans-anti*-[BP]G·C enantiomer, *Biochemistry* 31:5245–5252, 1992; Cosman, M., Xu, R., Hingerty, B. E., Amin, S., Harvey, R. G., Geacintov, N. E., Broyde, S., and
Patel, D. J., Solution conformation of the (−)-*trans-anti*-5-methylchrysene adduct opposite dC
in a DNA duplex: DNA bending associated with wedging of the methyl group of 5-methylchry-
sene to the 3'-side of the modification site, *Biochemistry* 34:6247–6260, 1995.

60. Cosman, M., de los Santos, C., Fiala, R., Hingerty, B. E., Ibanez, V., Luna, E., Harvey, R.,
Geacintov, N. E., Broyde, S., and Patel, D. J., Solution conformation of the (+)-*cis-anti*-[BP]dG
adduct in a DNA duplex: Intercalation of the covalently attached benzo[*a*]pyrenyl ring into the
helix and displacement of the modified deoxyguanosine, *Biochemistry* 32:4145–4155, 1993;
Cosman, M., Fiala, R., Hingerty, B. E., Amin, S., Geacintov, N. E., Broyde, S., and Patel, D.
J., Solution conformation of (+)-*trans*-[BP]dG adduct opposite a deletion site in a DNA duplex: Intercalation of the covalently attached benzo[*a*]pyrene into the helix with base displacement of the modified deoxyguanosine into the major groove, *Biochemistry* 33:11507–11517,
1994; Cosman, M., Fiala, R., Hingerty, B. E., Amin, S., Geacintov, N. E., Broyde, S., and Patel, D. J., Solution conformation of (+)-*cis*-[BP]dG adduct opposite a deletion site in a DNA
duplex: Intercalation of the covalently attached benzo[*a*]pyrene into the helix with base displacement of the modified deoxyguanosine into the minor groove, *Biochemistry*
33:11518–11527, 1994.

61. Cosman, M., Fiala, R., Hingerty, B. E., Laryea, A., Lee, H., Harvey, R. G., Amin, S., Geacintov, N. E., Broyde, S., and Patel, D., Solution conformation of (+)-*trans*-[BPh]dA adduct opposite dT in a DNA duplex: Intercalation of the covalently attached benzo[*c*]phenanthrene to
the 5'-side of the adduct site without disruption of the modified base pair, *Biochemistry*
32:12488–12497, 1993; Cosman, M., Fiala, R., Hingerty, B. E., Laryea, A., Amin, S., Geacintov, N. E., Broyde, S., and Patel, D., Solution conformation of (−)-*trans-anti*-benzo[*c*]phenan-
threne-dA ([BPh]dA) adduct opposite dT in a DNA duplex: Intercalation of the covalently attached benzo[*c*]phenanthrenyl ring to the 3'-side of the adduct site and comparison with the
(+)-*trans*-[BPh]dA opposite dT stereoisomer, *Biochemistry* 34:1295–1307, 1995.

20

AROMATIC AMINES AND OTHER
N-ARYL COMPOUNDS

In this chapter we look at another important class of chemical carcinogens, the aromatic amines (1). These are compounds of the structural formula Ar-NH$_2$, where R is homoaromatic (phenyl, naphthyl, pyrenyl, etc.) or heteroaromatic (such as imidazolyl). Metabolic processes can interconvert the organic oxidation states of nitrogen, from the most oxidized (nitro, Ar-NO$_2$) to the most reduced (amino, Ar-NH$_2$). These redox processes play a central role in the toxicology of aromatic amines, and so we will also consider these related compounds, such as the environmentally prevalent nitroaromatics.

SYNTHETIC DYES

As mentioned in Chapter 19, the industrial processing and production of chemicals began with the use of coal and coal products for fuel. The organic chemistry required for these purposes was, in the early years of the industrial revolution, limited to pyrolysis and distillation. The industrial application of techniques we would now recognize as *synthetic* began in the latter half of the nineteenth century. In 1856 the 18-year-old Englishman William Henry Perkin, tinkering in his home laboratory, decided to look for a chemical synthesis of the alkaloid drug quinine. Quinine, extracted from the bark of the South American cinchona tree, was the only known effective therapy for malaria (see Chapter 8), and malaria was perhaps the biggest obstacle to the expansion of the British empire. Actually, Perkin was just as likely to fly to the moon as to achieve his synthetic goal, with the primitive knowledge of organic chemistry at that time. He obtained a crude sample of aniline, the simplest aromatic amine, which had been discovered 30 years earlier, and oxidized it with nitric and sulfuric acids. The product was a purple-colored phenazine dye, which he named *mauveine*. (The starting material also contained toluidines, which were essential for formation of this product.) It was certainly not quinine, but he recognized mauveine's commercial potential as a dye. Perkin had the foresight, and the capital, to obtain a patent and embark on the industrial-scale production of this compound, the first important synthetic dye; soon he became a very wealthy young man. The dye was the "hit" of the London Exhibition of 1862, and the 1860s became known as the "mauve decade" because of the wide use of this dye for coloring textiles. Other successful synthetic dyes, such as fuchsin, soon followed. The synthetic chemical boom had begun.

In 1865, August Kekulé conceived of the cyclic structure of benzene during the course of a daydream (brought on when his mind wandered from the task at hand: writing a textbook!). Kekulé thereby laid the keystone of aromatic chemistry. van't Hoff and Le Bel proposed the tetrahedral arrangement of bonds around the asymmetric carbon atom in 1874. These fundamental ideas about molecular structure helped to transform organic chemistry into a systematic science.

In 1860, Griess discovered the diazotization reaction: Treatment of primary aromatic amines with nitrous acid yields unstable diazonium salts. The diazonium group can readily be replaced by hydroxyl, halogen, and other functionalities, so diazonium salts are key synthetic intermediates. Griess' experimental work, and the Kekulé ring structure, stimulated the development of aromatic synthetic chemistry.

BENZIDINE-BASED DYES

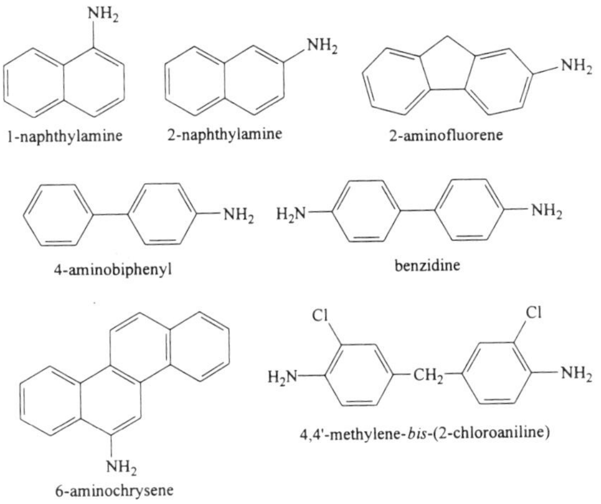

1-naphthylamine   2-naphthylamine   2-aminofluorene

4-aminobiphenyl   benzidine

6-aminochrysene

4,4'-methylene-*bis*-(2-chloroaniline)

The aromatic diamine benzidine was synthesized in 1845 by the acid-catalyzed "benzidine rearrangement" of hydrazobenzene. In 1884 the German chemist Böttiger exploited this reaction to synthesize the first commercially important benzidine-based azo dye:

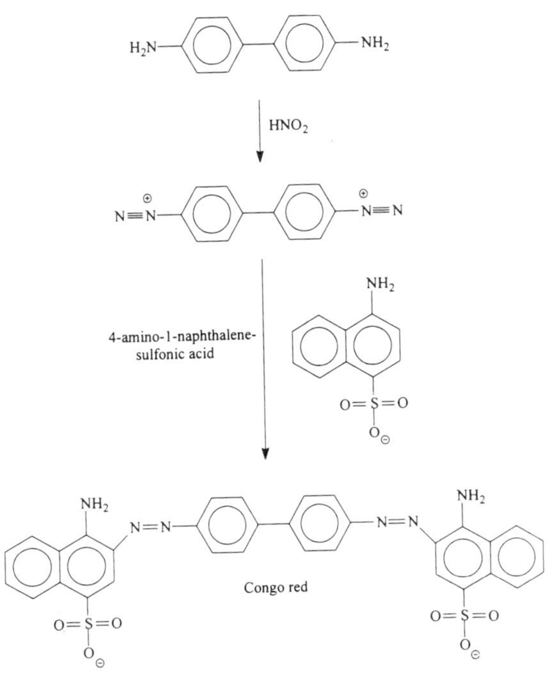

HNO_2

4-amino-1-naphthalene-sulfonic acid

Congo red

Both of the amino groups of benzidine are diazotized, and the reactive electrophilic diazonium groups are trapped by reaction with 4-amino-1-naphthalene sulfonic acid. The extended conjugated systems linked by the azo chromophores make such compounds intensely colored. In honor of the recent German conquests in Africa, Böttiger named the
new dye "Congo Red." By varying the substituents on the benzidine moiety:

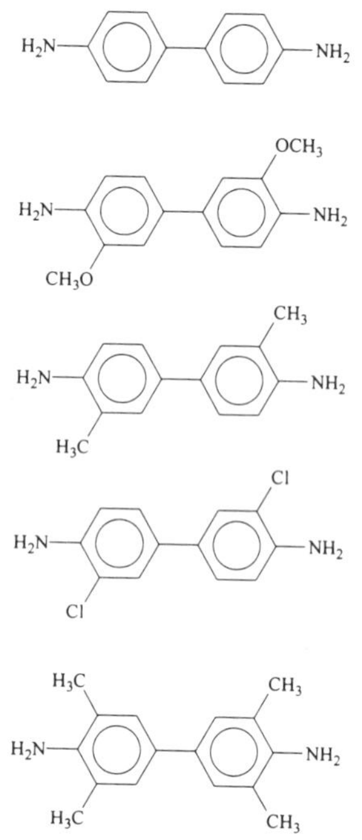

Benzidine congeners (from top to bottom): Benzidine; dianisidine; tolidine; dichlorobenzidine; 3,5,3',5'-
tetramethylbenzidine; see ref. 1.

and choosing various naphthylamine or naphthol coupling components, many useful dyes
in a range of colors can be prepared. The industrial production of benzidine-based dyes
for use on textiles, leather, paper, and other applications grew rapidly, first in Germany
and then in England and the United States, in the latter years of the nineteenth century.

As with polycyclic aromatic hydrocarbons, the first indication of health effects due to
exposure to the substances was a report by a physician. In 1895, L. Rehn described "aniline cancer": bladder cancer among workers involved in the production of fuchsin. (Rehn's
suspicion of aniline as the cause, although reasonable, later proved to be incorrect.) Unfortunately, the "discovery" of aromatic amine-induced bladder cancer had to be made
again and again, because little was done to protect workers from the hazard. Benzidine
was produced in huge cauldrons, and factory workers scoured out the vats by hand after
a batch was prepared. Very large quantities of these compounds were ingested, by breath-
ing the dust, through the skin, or by contamination of hands, clothing, food, and so on.
Within 15 years, Rehn had observed more than 50 cases of bladder cancer among chemical industry workers in the Frankfurt area. However, despite the accumulating evidence,
benzidine production continued in Europe and the United States until the post–World War
II era. The most important improvement (and a relatively easy one to engineer) was "cap-
tive synthesis": Benzidine is produced, diazotized, and coupled to form the dye, in sealed
units.

Later epidemiological studies confirmed the link between occupational exposure to benzidine and bladder cancer incidence (2). For example, a careful follow-up study of workers employed at a benzidine-manufacturing plant which operated in Connecticut, from 1945 to 1965, revealed an incidence of bladder cancer much higher than predicted, based on cancer rates in the general population for that state (8 cases observed, versus 2.3 expected) (3). This plant had operated with relatively high standards of cleanliness and safety. New cases of bladder cancer among dyestuff workers continue to accrue in Europe; these cases probably reflect the late effects of exposures in earlier decades. For example, a recent investigation in the industrial region around Milan, Italy, found a 4.8-fold-elevated risk of bladder cancer among workers in the dyestuff industry (4). The earlier experience in Europe, although less thoroughly documented, was probably worse. The occupational hazard has gradually abated, with improvements in manufacturing practices and workplace hygiene. Benzidine itself is no longer used in dyestuff synthesis, because of its carcinogenicity. Nevertheless, the benzidine congeners, such as dichlorobenzidine, are still widely used in dye manufacture. Some of these congeners are more potent mutagens than benzidine itself (5). Dichlorobenzidine manufacture in a British plant from 1930 to the 1970s appears not to have caused excess bladder cancer incidence, but it is not clear whether this is due to the lower carcinogenicity of dichlorobenzidine or better manufacturing practices and occupational hygiene (6).

Chronic bioassays of two of these benzidine congeners, dimethylbenzidine (tolidine) and dimethoxybenzidine (dianisidine), have been carried out as part of the "Benzidine Dye Initiative" of the National Toxicology Program, U.S.A.; both compounds caused tumors (skin, intestine, liver, etc.) in F344 rats (7). Manufacture of benzidine, although prohibited in North America and Europe, continues in some developing countries. In a recent study, employees of a chemical plant in India, which produces hundreds of kilograms of benzidine daily, were found to excrete urinary benzidine at levels of over 1 μg per ml (8); the long-term consequences of such exposures are all too predictable.

The benzidine dyes, of course, are not aromatic amines, but azo compounds. Hundreds of benzidine congener-based azo dyes are still used in printing inks, textiles, paints and enamels, and other applications. Are these compounds—the articles of commerce—innocuous if ingested by humans? The intestinal contents constitute an almost anaerobic, and highly reducing, microenvironment. Bacteria colonizing the gut can carry out reductions that would not occur in aerobic mammalian tissues. Ingested benzidine-based azo dyes are reduced by the action of azoreductase enzymes found in these bacteria. *The product of azoreduction is the parent benzidine congener.* Animals fed the benzidine dyes Direct Black 38 and Direct Brown 95 excrete benzidine and its metabolites (9). This observation suggests that dye users, not just the persons involved in dye manufacture, may be at risk. Indeed, an increased incidence of bladder cancer has been reported among Japanese kimono painters, who used benzidine-based dyes, and "pointed" brushes with their mouths. Rats treated with oral doses of benzidine-based azo dyes excreted urine containing highly mutagenic metabolites.

NAPHTHYLAMINES

The two isomers of naphthylamine (1- and 2-, also known as α- and β-) have also been used on an industrial scale. Large amounts were produced in the United Kingdom, the United States, and other countries in the first half of the twentieth century. The compounds were used as antioxidants for rubber production, and as chemical intermediates for dye and herbicide production. (One should bear in mind that although the commercial articles were sold as "1-naphthylamine" and "2-naphthylamine," each contained a significant percentage of the other isomer, as well as the corresponding naphthol isomer; many biological studies used impure preparations and should be interpreted cautiously.) Both compounds are also found in that cornucopia of carcinogens, cigarette smoke. Epidemiological studies in the 1950s by Case, in England, implicated 2-naphthylamine as primarily responsible for the large excess rate of bladder cancer in dyestuff workers. Production of 2-naphthylamine in the United States was finally halted in 1972.

AROMATIC AMINE DRUGS

Many aromatic amines are used as drugs, for a variety of therapeutic purposes. Some of these are shown below:

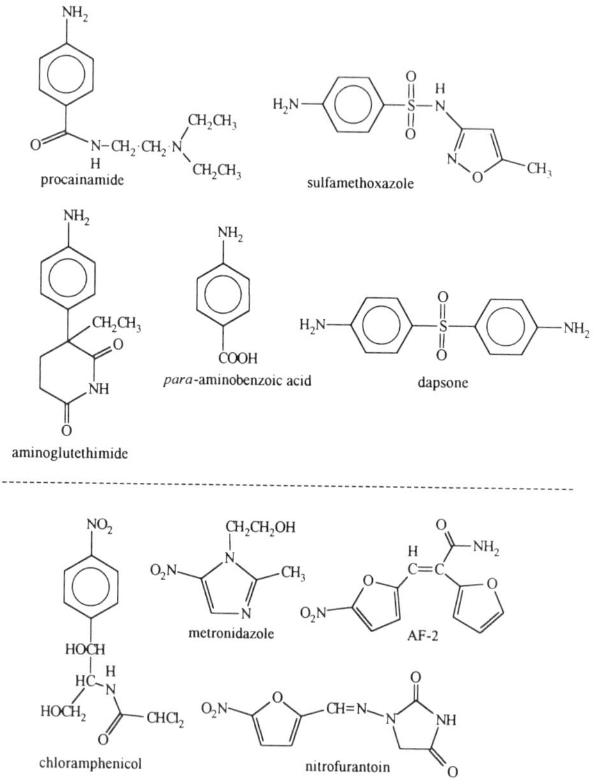

Acetaminophen (para-acetylaminophenol) is a very widely used analgesic, marketed under the brand name Tylenol. The oxidation of acetaminophen by P-450 and its relationship to the drug's overdose hepatotoxicity were discussed in Chapter 19. Phenacetin, the ethyl ether of acetylaminophenol, has been used for the same purpose, and a strong association between heavy phenacetin use and urinary tract cancer has been reported (10). Aromatic amines or nitro compounds used as antibiotics include (a) the antibacterial agents chloramphenicol, the nitrofurans, and the "sulfa" drugs, such as sulfamethazine, and (b) antiprotozoal agents, including metronidazole (antitrichomonal) and dapsone (used to treat leprosy) (see scheme above). Many of these drugs can cause idiosyncratic adverse reactions (11).

FOOD PYROLYSIS PRODUCTS

As we discussed in Chapter 17, the Ames assay is particularly sensitive to the mutagenicity of aromatic amines and nitroaromatics. Several new classes of mutagens have been discovered by testing environmental samples for mutagenicity in the Ames test. In 1976, Takashi Sugimura of the National Cancer Centre, Tokyo, discovered the presence of high mutagenic activity in the charred portion of grilled fish and meat (12). Since grilled foods are popular both in Japan and in the West, this finding raised the possibility that mutagens formed in cooked food play a role in the development of human cancer, and the report stimulated a great deal of research activity. Using mutagenicity as a bioassay, many active compounds were isolated from pyrolyzed foods or from pyrolyzed mixtures of proteins; many active compounds were chemically characterized and synthesized:

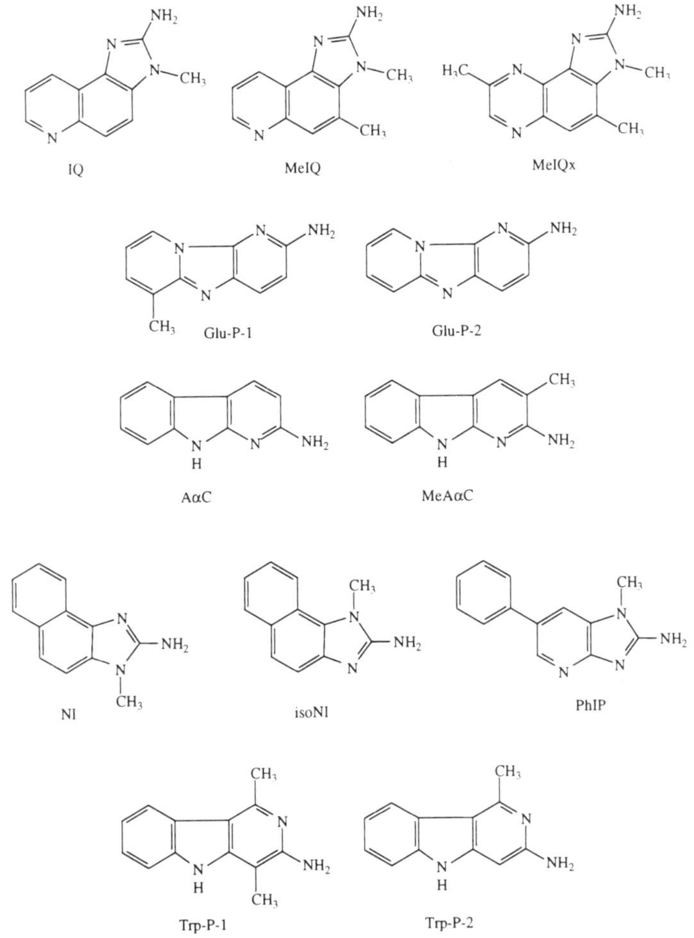

(see Table 20.1 for abbreviations used in this scheme).

Mutagenic pyrolysis products are formed by complex, poorly understood reactions occurring at high temperatures (200–300°C) during grilling; the main precursors are probably amino acids, creatine, and creatinine in the food. These compounds include some of the most potent mutagens known. Many are carcinogenic in rodents (13). The heterocyclic aromatic amine MeIQ is one of the most potent mutagens found in cooked meats (14).

Table 20.1. Food Pyrolysis Product Mutagens*

Abbreviation	Full Name
Glu-P-1	2-Amino-6-methyldipyrido[1,2-*a*:3',2'-*d*]imidazole
Glu-P-2	2-Amino-dipyrido[1,2-*a*:3',2'-*d*]imidazole
IQ	2-Amino-3-methylimidazo[4,5-*f*]quinoline
MeIQ	2-Amino-3,4-dimethylimidazo[4,5-*f*]quinoline
MeIQx	2-Amino-3,8-dimethylimidazo[4,5-*f*]quinoxaline
AαC	2-Amino-α-carboline
MeAαC	2-Amino-3-methyl-α-carboline
NI	2-Amino-3-methylnaphtho[1,2-*d*]imidazole
isoNI	2-Amino-1-methylnaphtho[1,2-*d*]imidazole
PhIP	2-Amino-1-methyl-6-phenylimidazo[4,5-*b*]pyridine
Trp-P-1	3-Amino-1,4-dimethyl-5*H*-pyrido[4,3-*b*]indole
Trp-P-2	3-Amino-1-methyl-5*H*-pyrido[4,3-*b*]indole

*See preceding scheme for structures.

MeIQ causes tumors in the liver and forestomach of mice (15) and in the Zymbal's gland, oral cavity, colon, skin, and mammary gland of rats (16). Although only trace amounts of these mutagens are found in foods, their presence may be cause for concern (17).

OXIDATIVE HAIR DYES

Substituted anilines are components of permanent hair dyes. The chemical basis of permanent hair dyeing is the formation of high-molecular-weight colored products by the hydrogen peroxide-dependent oxidation of aromatic amines and aminophenols. The oxidation occurs within the hair shaft, and the insoluble products remain bound within the hair. The compounds used in hair dyes include phenylenediamines (1,2-, 1,3-, and 1,4-diaminobenzene), 2,4-diaminotoluene (until its use was banned in 1971), anisidine isomers (1,2- and 1,4-aminotoluene), 4-nitro-1,3-diaminobenzene (4-nitro-*ortho*-phenylenediamine), and many others (18). 2,4-Diaminotoluene is still a very important monomer for the production of polyurethane. This plastic was used in the production of the foam covering of the "Meme" implantable breast (mastectomy) prosthesis, and a major public health controversy arose in 1991 when it was discovered that these implants could degrade and release 2,4-diaminotoluene (19).

Some of the components used in hair dyes proved to be mutagens. In 1975, Ames and his colleagues discovered that many hair dye chemicals are mutagenic, and the *oxidation* of hair dye formulations with hydrogen peroxide generates new mutagenic products (20, 21). *o*-Anisidine causes urinary bladder tumors in both mice and rats. *p*-Anisidine is less active, but it increased the incidence of preputial gland tumors in male rats.

NITRO COMPOUNDS

Nitro compounds have been used industrially for a long time, most notably as explosives (such as trinitrotoluene, TNT). Many nitro compounds have antimicrobial activity, as mentioned above. 2-(2-Furyl)-3-(5-nitro-2-furyl)acrylamide, AF-2, was used widely in Japan as a food preservative from 1965 until 1974. Use of AF-2 was banned when it was found to be a rodent carcinogen (22).

Much of the recent interest in nitro compounds stems from discoveries based on the application of the Ames mutagenicity assay. As mentioned earlier (Chapter 17), mutagenicity was detected in carbon black photocopier toners in 1980, and 1,8- and 1,6-dinitropyrene proved to be responsible. Although photocopier toner is now free of dinitropyrenes, they remain important environmental contaminants. 1-Nitropyrene and, in lesser amounts, dinitropyrenes are ubiquitous combustion byproducts, especially from diesel and aircraft jet engines (23). Nitro compounds are activated reductively, and aromatic amines are activated oxidatively; ultimately, the same classes of reactive species can be produced by the two routes.

ENDOGENOUS AROMATIC AMINES

A few endogenous metabolites are also aromatic amines (aniline derivatives). Tryptophan catabolism provides one example: Oxidative opening of the indole ring gives *N*-formylkynurenine, and deformylation gives the substituted aromatic amine, kynurenine. Further metabolism gives 3-hydroxyanthranilic acid:

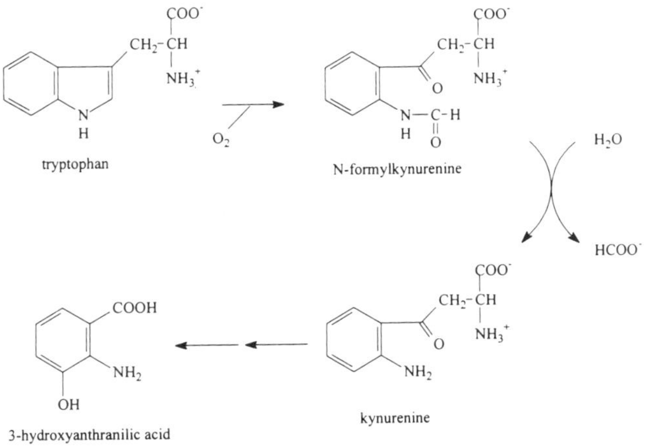

This metabolite is a carcinogen in adult mice and rats, but not in the newborn mouse model (24). *para*-Aminobenzoic acid (see page 356) is a constituent of folic acid, a component of the coenzyme tetrahydrofolate. (Of course, *para*-aminobenzoic acid is also commonly used as an ingredient in sun-tan lotions.) Mammals cannot synthesize folate, but obtain it from dietary sources or via intestinal bacterial synthesis. Sulfonamide antibiotic drugs are *para*-aminobenzoic acid analogues, and they act as competitive inhibitors of bacterial folate synthesis.

2-ACETYLAMINOFLUORENE

In view of the extraordinary diversity of aromatic amine and nitro compound carcinogens, it seems odd that many of the early advances arose from studies on a compound of little environmental significance: 2-acetylaminofluorene. This aromatic amide was synthesized for use as an insecticide, but abandoned when it was found to be a rodent carcinogen (25). 2-Acetylaminofluorene was the first aromatic amine for which detailed studies of oxidative metabolism were carried out, beginning with the work of John Weisburger and James and Elizabeth Miller, in the late 1950s (see below). Since that time, this compound has served as a paradigm for studies of aromatic amine bioactivation.

STRUCTURE–ACTIVITY RELATIONSHIPS

Just as with polycyclic aromatic hydrocarbons, many researchers have tried to establish systematic rules for predicting carcinogenic/ mutagenic potency of aromatic amines. A few structural features stand out. All the potent aromatic amine carcinogens are polycyclic (at least two aromatic rings). None of the aniline derivatives are *potent* carcinogens, although some are apparently positive in high doses (such as phenacetin). Perhaps this is a consequence of the greater lipophilicity of the polycyclic aromatic amines. The most potent compounds (such as the nitropyrenes and the food pyrolysis products, IQ and MeIQ) have three or more aromatic rings in fused structures. Halogenation, which increases lipophilicity, usually increases activity. Extended aromatic conjugation also seems to favor activity. The *para* principle is an empirical rule stating that the most active congeners in extended aromatic structures, such as biphenyl, terphenyl, and fluorene, have one or more amino groups in the *para* positions (e.g., 2-aminofluorene is more potent than 3-aminofluorene; 4,4'-diaminobiphenyl (*para*-benzidine) is more potent than 2,2'-diamino-biphenyl (*ortho*-benzidine).

METABOLIC ACTIVATION

As with the polycyclic aromatic hydrocarbon carcinogens, aromatic amines are generally negative in mutagenicity assays unless an activation system, such as hepatic S9, is supplied. Even before the development of short-term assays, such as the Ames test, it was apparent that aromatic amines per se did not exhibit any of the chemical reactivity expected of mutagens.

John and Elizabeth Weisburger examined the metabolism of 2-acetylaminofluorene by the rat, and they detected several hydroxylated metabolites. Carbon hydroxylation is not a surprising outcome, since we have seen that aromatic and polycyclic aromatic hydrocarbons are commonly metabolized in this way. The key breakthrough in elucidating the metabolic activation of aromatic amines came with the work of James and Elizabeth Miller, around 1960.

The Millers observed that, following prolonged (months) administration of 2-acetylaminofluorene to rats, a new metabolite was observed in the urine. This metabolite was identified as N-hydroxy-2-acetylaminofluorene; its isolation was the first demonstration of metabolic N-hydroxylation (26). We now know that this is a characteristic activity of cytochrome P-450; form CYP1A2 is primarily responsible for aromatic amine N-hydroxylation (see Table 14.2).

N-Hydroxy-2-acetylaminofluorene is an *arylhydroxamic* acid. The presence of the electron-withdrawing hydroxy function renders the nitrogen atom more reactive and electrophilic than the rather inert amide parent. When synthetic N-hydroxy-2-acetylaminofluorene was administered to rats in the diet, it was found to be a more potent carcinogen than 2-acetylaminofluorene (27). Furthermore, N-hydroxy-2-acetylaminofluorene, administered intraperitoneally, induced tumors *at the injection site*, with high frequency; the parent compound, 2-acetylaminofluorene, never caused peritoneal tumors: " ... peritoneal sarcomas were found in 18 of the 22 rats which were injected with N-hydroxy-AAF and which survived for at least 3 months, whereas none were found in the rats similarly treated with AAF. ... The tumors invaded the diaphragm, liver, spleen, mesentery, and body wall...." This striking result suggested that the metabolite did not require further hepatic activation, but was active locally. *The N-hydroxylation of 2-acetylaminofluorene was the first metabolic activation pathway to be elucidated.*

As in the case of polycyclic aromatic hydrocarbon activation, discussed in Chapter 19, multiple enzymatic steps are probably required to convert aromatic amines into directly reactive metabolites. In other words, *N*-hydroxy-2-acetylaminofluorene, like benzo[*a*]pyrene dihydrodiol, is a proximate carcinogen and requires further activation to generate the ultimate reactive species. Subsequent studies of aromatic amine activation have focused on the enzymology of *N*-oxidation and the subsequent metabolism of *N*-hydroxylated metabolites of amines and amides. Some of these pathways are shown for the case of 2-acetylaminofluorene:

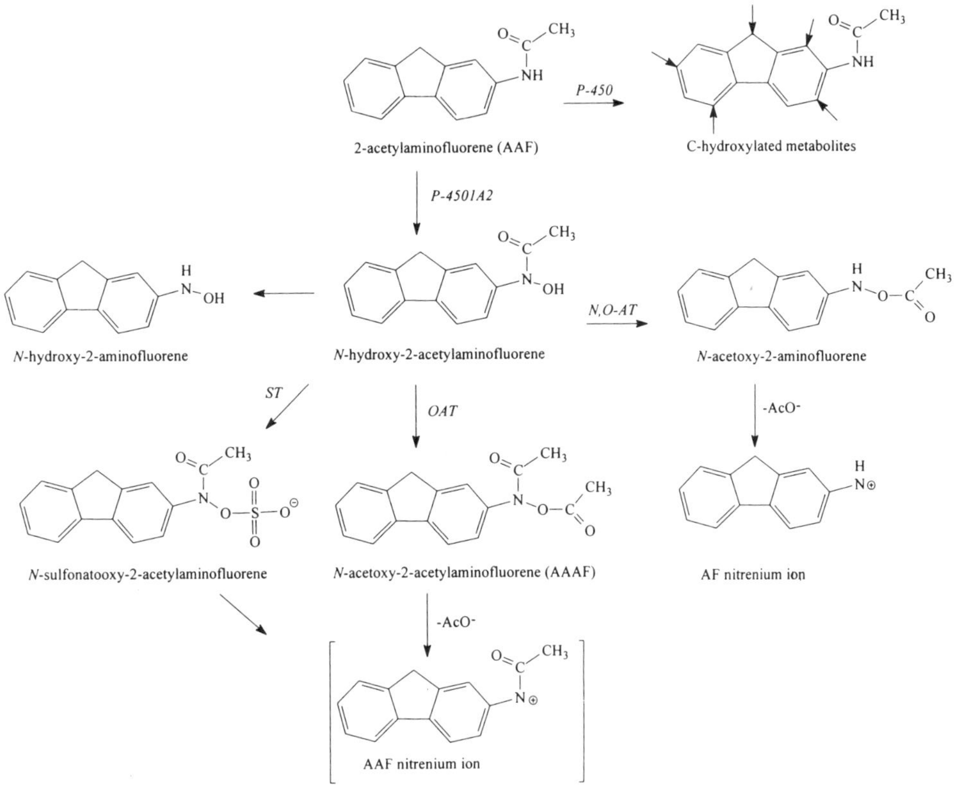

The identification of the DNA adducts derived from administered aromatic amines or amides is discussed in Chapter 16. The most common adducts (in hepatocytes in vitro, or liver tissue in vivo, for example) are formed at the C-8 position of guanine and are (at least, formally) the products of addition of a species of the form $R\overset{+}{N}H$ to the nucleic acid base. $R\overset{+}{N}H$ is a *nitrenium ion*, a six-electron cation analogous to a carbenium ion or oxonium ion. Like those species, it is a reactive, short-lived electrophile. Although nitrenium ions have not been isolated in biological systems, both their metabolic precursors, and adducts consistent with their formation have been identified.

In the case of 2-acetylaminofluorene, both acetylated and nonacetylated (i.e., 2-aminofluorene-derived) DNA adducts have been identified. This suggests that both acetylated and nonacetylated reactive species are formed ($R\overset{+}{N}Ac$ and $R\overset{+}{N}H$). The metabolic routes which could lead from 2-acetylaminofluorene or N-hydroxy-2-acetylaminofluorene to such reactive species can be understood on the basis of the biotransformation reactions discussed in earlier chapters. The key point is that good leaving groups can be introduced into the substrate by conjugation reactions; the product will then be activated as an electrophile and can release a nitrenium ion (or equivalent).

One route is the conjugation of N-hydroxy-2-acetylaminofluorene. O-Acetylation or O-sulfation will produce acetoxy or sulfonooxy esters. Heterolytic loss of acetate anion or sulfate anion, respectively, will generate $R\overset{+}{N}Ac$. Another route is transfer of the acetyl moiety from the N to the O atom of N-hydroxy-2-acetylaminofluorene (N,O-acetyltransfer), yielding the highly reactive N-acetoxyaminofluorene; loss of acetate anion yields $R\overset{+}{N}A$. Alternatively, deacetylation of N-hydroxy-2-acetylaminofluorene gives the arylhydroxylamine, N-hydroxy-2-aminofluorene. Arylhydroxylamines are directly reactive with nucleophiles. They are also substrates for O-acetylation, giving the same N-acetoxy ester that is formed by N,O-acetyltransfer. The enhanced mutagenicity of aromatic amines and arylhydroxylamines in bacterial tester strains with elevated NAT/OAT activity, discussed in Chapter 17, indicates that this activating step is critical.

NOTES

1. Garner, R. C., Martin, C. N., and Clayson, D. B., Carcinogenic aromatic amines and related compounds, in: *Chemical Carcinogens*, 2nd ed., C. E. Searle, Ed., American Chemical Society, Washington, D.C., 1984, pp. 175–276.
2. Parkes, H. G., and Evans, A. E. J., Epidemiology of aromatic amine cancers, in: *Chemical Carcinogens*, 2nd ed., C. E. Searle, Ed., American Chemical Society, Washington, D.C., 1984, pp. 277–301; Cartwright, R. A., Historical and modern epidemiological studies on populations exposed to N-substituted aryl compounds, *Environ. Health Perspect.* 49:13–19, 1983.
3. Meigs, J. W., Marrett, L. D., Ulrich, F. U., and Flannery, J. T., Bladder tumor incidence among workers exposed to benzidine: a thirty-year follow-up, *J. Natl. Cancer Inst.* 76:1–8, 1986.
4. LaVecchia, C., Negri, E., D'Avanzo, B., and Franceschi, S., Occupation and the risk of bladder cancer, *Int. J. Epidemiol.* 19:264–268, 1990.
5. Savard, S., and Josephy, P. D., Synthesis and mutagenicity of 3,3'-dihalogenated benzidines, *Carcinogenesis* 7:1239–1241, 1986.
6. MacIntyre, I., Experience of tumors in a British plant handling 3,3'-dichlorobenzidine, *J. Occup. Med.* 17:23–26, 1975.
7. Morgan, D. L., Dunnick, J. K., Goehl, T., Jokinen, M. P., Matthews, H. B., Zeiger, E., and Mennear, J. H., Summary of the National Toxicology Program benzidine dye initiative, *Environ. Health Perspect.* 102(Suppl. 2):63–78, 1994.
8. Dewan, A., Jani, J. P., Shah, K. S., and Kashyap, S. K., Urinary excretion of benzidine in relation to acetylator status of occupationally exposed subjects, *Human Toxicol.* 5:95–97, 1986.
9. Nony, C. R., Bowman, M. C., Cairns, T., Lowry, L. K., and Tolos, W. P., Metabolism studies of an azo dye and pigment in the hamster based on analysis of the urine for potentially carcinogenic aromatic amine metabolites, *J. Toxicol.* 4:132–140, 1980.
10. See: Hinson, J. A., Reactive metabolites of phenacetin and acetaminophen: a review, *Environ. Health Perspect.* 49:71–79, 1983.
11. Uetrecht, J. P., Mechanism of drug-induced lupus, *Chem. Res. Toxicol.* 1:133–143, 1988.
12. Review: Sugimura, T., Studies on environmental chemical carcinogenesis in Japan, *Science* 233:312–318, 1986.
13. Ohgaki, H., Takayama, S. and Sugimura, T., Carcinogenicity of heterocyclic amines in cooked food, *Mutat. Res.* 259:399–410, 1991.
14. Overvik, E., and Gustafsson, J., Cooked-food mutagens: current knowledge of formation and

biological significance, *Mutagenesis* 5:437–446, 1990; Felton, J. S., and Knize, M. G., Occurrence, identification, and bacterial mutagenicity of heterocyclic amines in cooked food, *Mutat. Res.* 259:205–217, 1991.

15. Ohgaki, H., Hasegawa, H., Suenaga, M., Kato, T., Sato, S., Takayama, S. and Sugimura, T., Induction of hepatocellular carcinoma and highly metastatic squamous cell carcinoma in the forestomach of mice by feeding 2-amino-3,4-dimethylimidazo[4,5-*f*]quinoline, *Carcinogenesis* 7:1889–1893, 1986.

16. Kato, T., Migita, H., Ohgaki, H., Sato, S., Takayama, S., and Sugimura, T., Induction of tumors in the Zymbal gland, oral cavity, colon, skin and mammary gland of F344 rats by a mutagenic compound, 2-amino-3,4-dimethylimidazo[4,5-*f*]quinoline, *Carcinogenesis* 10:601–603, 1989.

17. Layton, D. W., Bogen, K. T., Knize, M. G., Hatch, F. T., Johnson, V. M., and Felton, J. S., Cancer risk of heterocyclic amines in cooked foods: an analysis and implications for research, *Carcinogenesis* 16:39–52, 1995.

18. Marzulli, F. N., Green, S., and Maibach, H.I., Hair dye toxicity—a review, *J. Environ. Pathol. Toxicol.* 1:509–530, 1978.

19. "Ottawa bans Meme breast implant," *Globe and Mail*, Toronto, April 18, 1991.

20. Ames, B. N., Kammen, H. O., and Yamasaki, E., Hair dyes are mutagenic: identification of a variety of mutagenic ingredients, *Proc. Natl. Acad. Sci. U.S.A.* 72:2433–2437, 1975.

21. Watanabe, T., Hirayama, T., and Fukui, S., Mutagenicity of commercial hair dyes and detection of 2,7-diaminophenazine, *Mutat. Res.* 244:303–308, 1990.

22. McCalla, D. R., Nitrofurans, in: *Antibiotics VII: Mechanism of Action of Antibacterial Agents*, F. E. Hahn, Ed., Springer-Verlag, Berlin, 1979, pp. 175–213.

23. Guerin, M. R., and Buchanan, M. V., Environmental exposure to *N*-aryl compounds, in: *Carcinogenic and Mutagenic Responses to Aromatic Amines and Nitroarenes*, King, C. M., Romano, L. J. and Schuetzle, D., Eds., Elsevier, New York, pp. 271–276, 1988.

24. Fujii, K., Evaluation of the newborn mouse model for chemical carcinogenesis, *Carcinogenesis* 12:1409–1415, 1991.

25. Wilson, R. H., DeEds, F., and Cox, A. J., The toxicity and carcinogenic activity of 2-acetaminofluorene, *Cancer Res.* 1:595–608, 1941.

26. Cramer, J. W., Miller, J. A., and Miller, E. C., *N*-Hydroxylation: a new metabolic reaction observed in the rat with the carcinogen 2-acetylaminofluorene, *J. Biol. Chem.* 235:885–888, 1960.

27. Miller, E. C., Miller, J. A., and Hartmann, H. A., *N*-Hydroxy-2-acetylaminofluorene: a metabolite of 2-acetylaminofluorene with increased carcinogenic activity in the rat, *Cancer Res.* 21:815–831, 1961.

Index

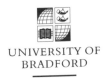

UNIVERSITY OF
BRADFORD

LIBRARY

This book should be returned not later than the last date stamped below.
The loan may be extended on request provided there is no waiting list.

FINES ARE CHARGED ON OVERDUE BOOKS

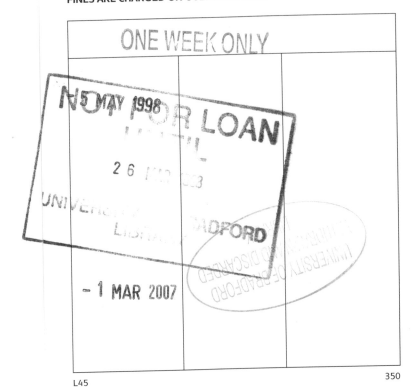